EVIDENCE-BASED PRACTICE IN ACTION

Also from Sona Dimidjian

Behavioral Activation for Depression:
A Clinician's Guide
Christopher R. Martell, Sona Dimidjian, and Ruth Herman-Dunn

Behavioral Activation with Adolescents:
A Clinician's Guide
*Elizabeth McCauley, Kelly A. Schloredt, Gretchen R. Gudmundsen,
Christopher R. Martell, and Sona Dimidjian*

Expecting Mindfully: Nourish Your Emotional Well-Being
and Prevent Depression during Pregnancy and Postpartum
Sona Dimidjian and Sherryl H. Goodman

EVIDENCE-BASED PRACTICE IN ACTION

Bridging Clinical Science and Intervention

edited by
SONA DIMIDJIAN

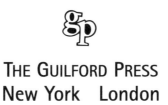

THE GUILFORD PRESS
New York   London

Copyright © 2019 The Guilford Press
A Division of Guilford Publications, Inc.
370 Seventh Avenue, Suite 1200, New York, NY 10001
www.guilford.com

Paperback edition 2021

Printed in the United States of America

This book is printed on acid-free paper.

Last digit is print number: 9 8 7 6 5 4 3 2

The authors have checked with sources believed to be reliable in their efforts to provide
information that is complete and generally in accord with the standards of practice that
are accepted at the time of publication. However, in view of the possibility of human error
or changes in behavioral, mental health, or medical sciences, neither the authors, nor the
editors and publisher, nor any other party who has been involved in the preparation
or publication of this work warrants that the information contained herein is in every
respect accurate or complete, and they are not responsible for any errors or omissions
or the results obtained from the use of such information. Readers are encouraged to
confirm the information contained in this book with other sources.

Library of Congress Cataloging-in-Publication Data

Names: Dimidjian, Sona, editor.
Title: Evidence-based practice in action : bridging clinical science and
   intervention / edited by Sona Dimidjian.
Description: New York : The Guilford Press, [2019] | Includes bibliographical
   references and index.
Identifiers: LCCN 2019000880 | ISBN 9781462539765 (hardback : alk. paper) |
   ISBN 9781462547708 (paperback)
Subjects: | MESH: Mental Health | Evidence-Based Practice |
   Psychotherapy—methods
Classification: LCC RC454 | NLM WM 101 | DDC 616.89—dc23
LC record available at *https://lccn.loc.gov/2019000880*

About the Editor

Sona Dimidjian, PhD, a clinical psychologist, is Director of the Renée Crown Wellness Institute and Professor in the Department of Psychology and Neuroscience at the University of Colorado Boulder. She is a widely recognized expert on women's mental health; the clinical application of contemplative practices, such as mindfulness meditation; and cognitive and behavioral approaches. She has developed successful prevention and treatment programs to promote mental health and wellness in health care, education, and community settings. Dr. Dimidjian is a recipient of multiple awards and the author of widely cited scholarly papers. She is coauthor of the self-help resource *Expecting Mindfully* as well as *Behavioral Activation for Depression* and *Behavioral Activation with Adolescents* (for mental health professionals).

Contributors

Susan E. Abbey, MD, Centre for Mental Health, University Health Network, and Department of Psychiatry, University of Toronto, Toronto, Ontario, Canada

Yoni K. Ashar, PhD, Department of Psychology and Neuroscience, University of Colorado Boulder, Boulder, Colorado

Manuel Barrera, Jr., PhD, Department of Psychology, Arizona State University, Tempe, Arizona

Arielle Baskin-Sommers, PhD, Department of Psychology, Yale University, New Haven, Connecticut

James Bennett-Levy, PhD, University Centre for Rural Health (North Coast), The University of Sydney, Sydney, Australia

Shadi Beshai, PhD, Department of Psychology, University of Regina, Regina, Saskatchewan, Canada

Jennifer N. Carty, PhD, Department of Psychiatry, Michigan State University, East Lansing, Michigan

Felipe González Castro, PhD, MSW, Center for Health Promotion and Disease Prevention, College of Nursing and Health Innovation, Arizona State University, Tempe, Arizona

Richard Trent Codd III, EdS, LPC, BCBA, Cognitive-Behavioral Therapy Center of Western North Carolina, Asheville, North Carolina

Zachary D. Cohen, PhD, Department of Psychiatry, University of California, Los Angeles, Los Angeles, California

Evan Collins, MD, Centre for Mental Health, University Health Network, and Department of Psychiatry, University of Toronto, Toronto, Ontario, Canada

Meghan M. Colosimo, MS, Department of Psychology, Drexel University, Philadelphia, Pennsylvania

Ioana A. Cristea, PhD, Department of Clinical Psychology and Psychotherapy, Babes-Bolyai University, Cluj-Napoca, Romania

Pim Cuijpers, PhD, Department of Clinical, Neuro, and Developmental Psychology, Amsterdam Public Health Research Institute, VU University Amsterdam, Amsterdam, The Netherlands

Catherine D'Avanzato, PhD, Department of Psychiatry and Human Behavior, Alpert Medical School of Brown University and Rhode Island Hospital, Providence, Rhode Island

Robert J. DeRubeis, PhD, Department of Psychology, University of Pennsylvania, Philadelphia, Pennsylvania

Sona Dimidjian, PhD, Department of Psychology and Neuroscience, University of Colorado Boulder, Boulder, Colorado

Jonathan Downar, MD, PhD, Centre for Mental Health, University Health Network; Institute of Medical Science; and Department of Psychiatry, University of Toronto, Toronto, Ontario, Canada

Norman Farb, PhD, Department of Psychology, University of Toronto Mississauga, Mississauga, Ontario, Canada

Rodney K. Goodyear, PhD, Department of Counseling and Human Services and Center for Advanced Professional Education, University of Redlands, Redlands, California

Beverly Haarhoff, PhD, School of Psychology, Massey University, Auckland, New Zealand

Syed Usman Hamdani, PhD, Human Development Research Foundation, Islamabad, Pakistan; Institute of Psychology, Health and Society, University of Liverpool, Liverpool, United Kingdom

Steven D. Hollon, PhD, Department of Psychology, Vanderbilt University, Nashville, Tennessee

Sam Hubley, PhD, Department of Family Medicine, University of Colorado Anschutz Medical Center, Aurora, Colorado

Emily Kemp, BS, Department of Psychology, Louisiana State University, Baton Rouge, Louisiana

Rob Kidney, DClinPsych, College of Life and Environmental Sciences, University of Exeter, Exeter, United Kingdom

Helena Chmura Kraemer, PhD, Department of Psychiatry and Behavioral Sciences, Stanford University, Stanford, California

Jessica Kraus, PhD, Department of Psychology, The New School, New York, New York

Willem Kuyken, PhD, Department of Psychiatry, University of Oxford, Oxford, United Kingdom

Robert D. Latzman, PhD, Department of Psychology, Georgia State University, Atlanta, Georgia

Robert W. Levenson, PhD, Department of Psychology, University of California, Berkeley, Berkeley, California

James W. Lichtenberg, PhD, ABPP, Department of Educational Psychology, University of Kansas, Lawrence, Kansas

Scott O. Lilienfeld, PhD, Department of Psychology, Emory University, Atlanta, Georgia

Marsha M. Linehan, PhD, ABPP, Department of Psychology, University of Washington, Seattle, Washington

Steven Jay Lynn, PhD, ABPP, Department of Psychology, Binghamton University, The State University of New York, Binghamton, New York

Sara Hoffman Marchese, MS, Department of Preventive Medicine, Northwestern University, Chicago, Illinois

Christopher R. Martell, PhD, ABPP, Psychological Services Center, University of Massachusetts Amherst, Amherst, Massachusetts

J. Christopher Muran, PhD, Gordon F. Derner Institute of Advanced Psychological Studies, Adelphi University, Garden City, New York

Rachel K. Narr, MA, Department of Psychology, University of Virginia, Charlottesville, Virginia

Arthur M. Nezu, PhD, Department of Psychology, Drexel University, Philadelphia, Pennsylvania

Christine M. Nezu, PhD, Department of Psychology, Drexel University, Philadelphia, Pennsylvania

Lisa S. Onken, PhD, National Institute on Aging, National Institutes of Health, Bethesda, Maryland

Vyjeyanthi S. Periyakoil, MD, Primary Care and Population Health, Department of Medicine, Stanford University School of Medicine, Stanford, California

Jacqueline B. Persons, PhD, Oakland Cognitive Behavior Therapy Center, Oakland, California; Department of Psychology, University of California, Berkeley, Berkeley, California

Atif Rahman, PhD, Institute of Psychology, Health and Society, University of Liverpool, Liverpool, United Kingdom

Lorie A. Ritschel, PhD, Department of Psychiatry, School of Medicine, University of North Carolina at Chapel Hill, Chapel Hill, North Carolina

Jeremy D. Safran, PhD (deceased), Department of Psychology, The New School, New York, New York

Zindel V. Segal, PhD, Department of Psychological Clinical Science, University of Toronto Scarborough, Toronto, Ontario, Canada

Roz Shafran, ClinPsychol, PhD, UCL Great Ormond Street Institute of Child Health, University College London, London, United Kingdom

Bonnie Spring, PhD, Department of Preventive Medicine, Northwestern University, Chicago, Illinois

Jeremy Steglitz, PhD, private practice, Washington, DC

Donna M. Sudak, MD, Department of Psychiatry, Drexel University College of Medicine, Philadelphia, Pennsylvania

Charles R. Swenson, MD, Department of Psychiatry, University of Massachusetts Medical School, Worcester, Massachusetts

Lisa S. Talbot, PhD, Peninsula Behavioral Health, Palo Alto, California; Department of Psychiatry and Behavioral Science, Stanford University School of Medicine, Stanford, California

Bethany A. Teachman, PhD, Department of Psychology, University of Virginia, Charlottesville, Virginia

Terence J. G. Tracey, PhD, Department of Counseling and Counseling Psychology, Arizona State University, Tempe, Arizona; Departments of Educational and Counselling Psychology and Special Education, University of British Columbia, Vancouver, British Columbia, Canada

Madhukar H. Trivedi, MD, Center for Depression Research and Clinical Care, Department of Psychiatry, University of Texas Southwestern Medical Center, Dallas, Texas

Joseph M. Trombello, PhD, Center for Depression Research and Clinical Care, Department of Psychiatry, University of Texas Southwestern Medical Center, Dallas, Texas

Anna Van Meter, PhD, Feinstein Institute for Medical Research, Glen Oaks, New York

Bruce E. Wampold, PhD, ABPP, Department of Counseling Psychology, University of Wisconsin–Madison, Madison, Wisconsin; Modum Bad Psychiatric Center, Vikersund, Norway

Chelsey R. Wilks, PhD, Department of Psychology, University of Washington, Seattle, Washington

Tim Williams, PhD, School of Psychology and Clinical Language Sciences, University of Reading, Reading, United Kingdom

Eric A. Youngstrom, PhD, Department of Psychology, University of North Carolina at Chapel Hill, Chapel Hill, North Carolina

Mark Zimmerman, MD, Department of Psychiatry and Human Behavior, Alpert Medical School of Brown University and Rhode Island Hospital, Providence, Rhode Island

Eva Zysk, PhD, Department of Psychology, University of British Columbia, Vancouver, British Columbia, Canada

Preface

When I was in my mid-20s, after having completed an undergraduate degree in psychology and a master's degree in social work, I got a job working in a mental health agency that provided outpatient and home-based services to clients in small towns and rural settings. I had worked previously as an intern in a psychiatric research institute with depressed teens and their families, but this was my first job in the "real world."

My coworker and I were assigned to contact a woman in her late 50s who recently had been laid off from a job she had held for many years, with little prospect for employment and mounting bills. We first met with her in her home. She was soft spoken but warm as she welcomed us into her living room. Photographs of her children and ex-husband lined the walls, though the empty rooms echoed with their absence. She had little contact with her adult sons, who were busy in their own lives and had stopped coming home long ago.

I was enthusiastic about my new job—and worried about this client. I was the newest staff person in the clinic, but even with little experience under my belt, I questioned whether she was experiencing any benefit from the treatment that was being provided. I spoke to the director of the agency about my concerns, asking if my client needed something more or different than what she was receiving from the agency. He told me, essentially, that their program had worked for years, with many clients, and he didn't see the need for change in this specific case or in general. The authority of his position took precedence over my questions. Her treatment program remained the same, and she died by suicide a few days later.

That experience fueled within me three enduring commitments. First, I was driven to use the tools of science. It was clear to me the ways in which personal opinion and status could perpetuate practices of questionable quality. Second, I was committed to discovering not only interventions that would be effective for women like her, struggling with severe depression, but also prevention approaches that could help people build skills for wellness early in life that would provide enduring benefit. Third, I pledged to ensure that even the most remote settings had access to good data to guide clinical practice. I applied to clinical psychology doctoral programs and immersed myself in the study of treatments for depression for the next 9 years at the University of Washington, with an amazing group of mentors who over time became also colleagues and friends. When I accepted my first faculty position at the University of Colorado Boulder, I was confident that I was well prepared to share this knowledge with students and mentor them in contributing to the science and practice of psychological interventions. Not surprisingly, I still had a lot to learn, perhaps most importantly from my students and clients. This book is the result of that learning, and the credit for the knowledge and skills that are contained in these pages goes to an incredible group of people with whom I have been fortunate to work over many years.

I would like to acknowledge my current and former students, who are my best teachers, including Sam Hubley, Rosi Kaiser, Blair Kleiber, Kyle Davis, Jennifer Felder, Yoni Ashar, Christina Metcalf, Rachel Vanderkruik, Elizabeth Lemon, Anne Fritzson, and Caitlin McKimmy, and all the other students I have had the privilege of teaching, supervising, and mentoring. My research team today at the University of Colorado Boulder gives me great hope for the future of science and practice in health care and education, and I share particular thanks with Julia Zigarelli, Leah Teeters, Michelle Shedro, Marta Genovez, and Joey Levy. I also want to thank my colleagues at the University of Colorado Boulder, Tina Pittman Wagers and Joanna Arch, who are true partners in thinking about how to bridge psychological science and practice in the clinic and classroom. I am also grateful to Jennifer Sayrs, who is a dear friend and ally on the many paths we have traveled together since graduate school and postdoctoral training.

I also owe a debt of gratitude and respect to the incredible clinical practitioners and researchers from whom I have been honored to learn through their teaching, supervision, mentoring, and collaboration, starting with my graduate advisor, Neil S. Jacobson, and broadening after his death to include Marsha Linehan, Steve Hollon, Bob Kohlenberg, Steve McCutcheon, Elizabeth McCauley, Zindel Segal, and Sherryl Goodman. Their generosity, guidance, and friendship enriched my learning and work and infuses each and every good idea that is part of this volume (I take full responsibility for bad ones!). My collaborators in the health services area, including Arne Beck, Greg Simon, and Vikram Patel, also have helped to anchor my focus in the pragmatic realities of health care systems and the need for practice-relevant research.

Finally, I want to acknowledge my daughter, Serena, who is a powerful embodiment of and advocate for the values that inform this book. Just the other day, she said to me, "My friends are starting to roll their eyes at me when they tell me things because my reply is always something like, 'Well, what's the evidence for that?'" I am so amazed by who she is in the world and the ways in which she and her generation are standing up for the value of science and critical thinking. It is my hope that this book is a small part of ensuring accessible, effective mental health resources that are worthy of her generation and those that follow.

Contents

PART III. ILLUSTRATIONS OF EVIDENCE-BASED PRACTICE IN ACTION

PART IV. TRAINING, SUPERVISION, AND CONSULTATION
TO PROMOTE EVIDENCE-BASED PRACTICE

Introduction

Context, Intention, and Compassion

SONA DIMIDJIAN

The role of science in public life has been challenged in unprecedented ways in recent years. For people who care about the quality of and access to mental health care, this context only amplifies the urgency of addressing the gap that has long existed between clinical research and practice. This edited volume is for those of us—students, trainees, supervisors, practitioners, and researchers—who are drawn to action. As the media and other public spaces reckon with the role of scientific evidence in policy and personal decision making, we have an opportunity to renew a commitment to bridging research and practice as a collective field and as individuals. This book aims to articulate precisely how we can do that, with more specificity and focus than we have done in the past.

When I joined the faculty at the University of Colorado Boulder, I started teaching a course titled "Adult Psychotherapy." It had been a core part of the curriculum for some time, and I was excited to infuse it with my prior learning and ongoing research. It was an exciting time to begin teaching such a course. The framework of evidence-based medicine was explicitly being recognized as valuable and relevant in behavioral and mental health practice. The American Psychological Association specifically adopted this model in 2006, first proposed in medicine about 10 years before. High-quality studies on the efficacy of psychotherapy had amassed

into an impressive evidence base for specific disorders, allowing the students in my class to consider data on the efficacy of specific approaches, and how they worked and for whom. Detailed treatment manuals also provided guides to learning core principles and practical skills. I loved teaching that class! And graduate students often described it as among their most valuable courses in their training. However, over time I began to realize that the students needed more than what I was giving them.

Students in my class struggled to propose treatment approaches based on scientific information about various interventions for specific clients. They struggled to learn *how* to enact these approaches. Students had a plethora of questions that were not addressed by the readings that we discussed in class. They asked for examples of how to do the work of integrating science and practice. Reflecting on their requests, I carefully considered the course reading list. Each year, I included core clinical handbooks and treatment manuals in the field as well as a stack of empirical and review articles. Multiple books were available to help people learn empirically supported treatments, and some great collections provided chapters illustrating a range of specific treatments in action with the clients for whom such treatments had been developed. My colleagues and I had coauthored one such chapter in which we described how to do behavioral activation with a depressed adult (Dimidjian, Martell, Herman-Dunn, & Hubley, 2014). These were indispensable resources, but I had to admit that the students' requests were valid. I realized that the literature available to help students take treatment principles into action was quite limited. The course presented what evidence-based practice was but lacked examples of how to do it.

This lack of modeling was problematic for the class assignments and discussions, but, more importantly, it persisted as the students progressed in their applied clinical training after the course ended. I often had the experience of students returning to me to consult about clients they were seeing under someone else's supervision. They would describe the challenge or uncertainty, and I would ask questions like "What have you found in the literature related to that problem?" or "On what basis are you using a given treatment approach or strategy?" A flash of recognition would pass over students' faces and they would leave my office, returning when a literature review was in hand. Even then, though, it was not clear how to synthesize an increasingly voluminous literature in ways that would guide clinical practice, nor was it clear how to address myriad complexities in client characteristics, context, and training. Similarly, the gap between evidence and practice was problematic in the other direction as well. There were few examples of how to leverage work in the therapy room to inform next steps in research.

I kept thinking, people need more examples of how to do the integration of science and practice. I ordered a shipment of books over one holiday break to see if I could find a comprehensive text that would both explain the framework of evidence-based practice and how to put it into action, a guide for people as they went between the classroom or the lab and the clinic. Not finding one, I started drafting a "wish list" of chapters, which, over time, turned into the table of contents for this book.

Intentions

This book is intended to be part of broader efforts today to bridge science and practice. Ignoring the gap that exists between what we know and what we do is neither effective nor ethical. The realities that became evident in my class exist broadly. We have a robust evidence base that addresses the efficacy and effectiveness of mental health interventions, but we lack a guide for how to research and synthesize the knowledge contained within and across those studies. We have libraries of treatment manuals for specific problems and populations, but we lack a guide for how to integrate and apply that information when facing the complexity of the specific individuals or families seeking help. Similarly, we lack a guide for how to think about applying research findings to people whose experiences and needs have not been foregrounded in past research. We have structures for supervision and training, but we lack a guide for how to use evidence to inform that work. We have conferences and commentaries that champion the importance of using evidence to guide practice, but we often ignore the critical question of how.

Addressing these gaps is critical today. Mental health problems are prevalent among adults and young people (Kessler & Wang, 2008), and the majority of people do not access the care they need (Wang et al., 2005). Moreover, our treatments require improvement to be more effective, precise, and robust. Progress in these areas requires a closer bridge between research and practice. We need contexts where clinicians identify the problems of practice in mental health settings that help set research agendas for clinical scientists. Such partnerships have existed for decades in other areas, such as education, where methods for data sharing, analysis, and interpretation were refined and formalized. For example, the Consortium on Chicago School Research at the University of Chicago, where I attended college, has a near-30-year history of a research–practice partnership with Chicago Public Schools (Roderick, Easton, & Sebring, 2009). This partnership has led to a robust evidence base of actionable knowledge and transformational reform of school policy and practice precisely because researchers are investigating questions of relevance to practitioners and studying outcomes that matter. These methods have not penetrated the field of psychology, medicine, social work, nursing, and the other disciplines that support and guide mental health care.

This book is designed for clinical students, practitioners, educators, and researchers. For the clinical audiences, it provides the conceptual and applied scaffolding necessary to do evidence-based practice in mental health settings. For research audiences, it brings to life the complexity of mental health practice that illuminates multiple questions that demand empirical study. It is intended for fields that are dedicated to promoting and protecting mental health, including psychology, psychiatry, social work, and other disciplines. In four sections, the book addresses what is evidence-based practice, and, perhaps even more importantly, provides clear guidance and examples of how to do it.

Parts I and II provide a foundation of information necessary to engage in evidence-based practice. Part I covers the historical and contemporary contexts relevant to evidence-based practice in mental health settings and current controversies regarding the use of evidence-based practice in mental health. Part II addresses foundational knowledge of the core components of evidence-based practice. Recommendations for evidence-based practice often assume that students and practicing clinicians have the knowledge base required to understand and apply clinically the research literature. This, however, often is not the case. Part conceptual and part methodological, this section provides this requisite knowledge with a succinct and practical emphasis. Specific chapters address research design and methods, systematic reviews and meta-analysis and clinical guidelines, personalizing treatment based on client characteristics, the importance of culture and context, clinical expertise, and assessment.

Part III presents an innovative format in which experts were invited to demonstrate evidence-based practice "in action" through rich, realistic case illustrations. Each author was asked to select a case representative of his or her practice setting, with a premium placed on demonstrating the complex and multifaceted nature of evidence-based practice in action. This section is designed to provide readers across multiple clinical settings an opportunity to learn by example. In planning this section of the book, I consulted with leaders in the field who have dedicated their lives to bridging science and practice—people like like Jacqueline Persons and Steven Hollon. Their feedback was instrumental in underscoring the importance of complexity and diversity in conveying the often-messy work of bridging science and practice. Hence, in this section, you will find examples of both triumphs and tribulations in doing evidence-based practice. Authors were asked to bring the process of their work "to life" and to make explicit the knowledge and skills that are often implicit in typical case presentations.

Thus, for example, authors present not only a summary of the evidence base relevant to treating the target disorder, but a form of "thinking aloud" about how they made sense of this literature and applied the treatment to the particular client, presentation, and clinical setting, giving an opportunity for students and clinicians to learn by example.

Part III also provides examples of working with common clinical problems as well as the comorbidities and complexities that are present in many people's lives. The chapters seek to cover the major mental health problems with which clients typically present for help, as well as common settings in which intervention is delivered and challenges that clinicians often face. We cover anxiety disorders, mood disorders, obsessive–compulsive disorder, borderline personality disorder, substance use disorders, and other critical problem areas. We explore questions that often arise in working with clients for whom life is complicated and with whom the course of intervention involves unexpected twists and turns. We cover a range of settings in which clinicians work and study, including outpatient, inpatient, partial hospitalization, and primary care. We explore the many challenges that arise in the context of doing evidence-based practice, including the doubts and questions that can arise within the clinician and how the evidence base can be utilized as a guide. Knowing that in the future some of the treatments covered here will be displaced by even more effective treatments, readers of this book are also invited to bear in mind the evidence-based framework in order to integrate new scientific findings into their work decade after decade.

A final section serves to focus on key components of training, supervision, and consultation to promote the integration of science and practice in the context of lifelong learning. The role of self-reflection, consultation, and supervision is highlighted in a clinician's learning process.

How can this book be used most effectively? If you are a clinician in private practice or working in an outpatient or inpatient setting, you may have had your fill of evidence-based "this and that." The hope is that this book will be different. The first two sections may help to make explicit what you know implicitly or may help to round out your knowledge of the components of evidence-based practice. The third section invites you to meet friends and allies who, like you, have moments of feeling stuck with this question of "How?" in their clinical practice. The authors of the chapters have been asked to write with authenticity and openness about where they struggle and how they engage scientific evidence to find a clearer path through complexity and uncertainty in the service of their clients. They have shared their experiences and reflections with the hope that it will enrich your practice, support you in being more effective in serving your clients, and make it easier for you to bring the value of evidence into your work and life. Additionally, if you provide supervision or engage in consultation, the final section will speak to you with actionable frameworks and engaging recommendations to make these learning experiences rich and rewarding.

If you are a teacher contemplating how to use this book in your class, the book is organized for ease of course planning and active student engagement. This material can be adapted for both graduate-level and residency training and upper-level undergraduate students who are interested in mental health practice or research. You are encouraged to use Parts I–III as a foundation for your course. The chapters in Part I provide engaging material for learning the historical context of evidence-based practice. Students can be invited to debate with one another, articulating different sides of the controversies about the use of evidence in clinical practice. The chapters in Part II can be assigned independently or in tandem with specific research studies, using the chapters as a guide for making sense of both the content and the context of specific types of research. Also, as an integrated assignment for the first two sections, students can be invited to evaluate the pros and cons of different frameworks and ways of configuring the relationship among the different components of evidence-based practice. They also can be invited to be creative in proposing new models for bridging science and practice for the future. For example, students can be invited to work with one another to visually represent new models. We have created a "gallery walk" of such representations in classes, inviting students to critically evaluate different options for how to integrate components such as the evidence, client characteristics, context, clinical expertise, and so forth. In Part III, it can be helpful for students to work alone, or in pairs or small groups, to present to the class, using the case in the chapter as a centerpiece, building around it with their own evaluation

of relevant studies and exploration of relevant treatment manuals. The complexity of the cases in this section invites students to engage critical thinking and reflection, enlivening class discussions. As the instructor, you can think of these chapters as doors into understanding specific clinical contexts, complexities and comorbidities, and scientific fields. The range of cases and contexts included in this section also allows you flexibility in designing a course or permits you to engage student choice in pursuing topics that are of greatest relevance and interest to them. Finally, students can be invited to read the chapters in the final section and propose an integrated set of guidelines and recommendations for their own training and supervision, making these chapters immediately relevant and actionable.

Finally, if you are a student, it is with a great sense of excitement that these chapters are offered to you. You were the root source of the inspiration for creating this book, and your work will have the most impact on the field for years to come. Through learning the history, thinking critically about controversies, and developing applied skills in finding, synthesizing, and interpreting evidence, you will be prepared for clinical practice with skills that apply across patient populations, problems, and settings. Through immersing yourself in the case examples, you will have guides for finding your way through clinical challenges and being prepared for a wide range of situations. These chapters can help you build skill and confidence. Through reading the recommendations for supervision and consultation, you will be armed with knowledge for asking what you need to promote your learning now and for years to come. In so doing, you will be poised to lead a new generation of clinical practice and inform more actionable, relevant research.

Compassion

Evidence-based practice is, at its core, a practice of compassion for oneself as a clinician and for one's clients. For oneself, evidence-based practice acknowledges the reality of clinical practice as filled with questions and challenges to which clear solutions are not always apparent. Instead of ignoring or oversimplifying this reality in a way that leaves the student or clinician alone, the approach in this book provides a guide to thinking and acting that gives permission and encouragement to not always have all the answers. In fact, it disrupts the commonly held beliefs about being an "expert" to make explicit the ways in which being an expert means being always a learner. Compassion for oneself as a clinician means to embrace always learning.

For one's clients, evidence-based practice means providing the best clinical care and advancing the best research possible. It guides us to bring the best of what we know to being of service, but it also invites humility, recognizing that our field continues to have more questions than answers. The chapters in this volume embrace what William James wrote so many years ago: "The best mark of health that a science can show is this unfinished-seeming front." A dedication to science holds the true interests of our clients at its core.

By bringing together the expertise of people who deeply care about the integration of clinical science and practice and communicating such knowledge in an accessible and practical manner, I believe we have an opportunity to influence the nature of mental health care delivered today and into the future through the training of clinicians and the inspiration of new science that will address increasingly complex and relevant questions.

References

American Psychological Association. (2006). Evidence-based practice in psychology. *American Psychologist, 61*(4), 271–285.

Dimidjian, S., Martell, C. R., Herman-Dunn, R., & Hubley, S. (2014). Behavioral activation for depression. In D. H. Barlow (Ed.), *Clinical handbook of psychological disorders: A step-by-step treatment manual* (5th ed., pp. 353–393). New York: Guilford Press.

Kessler, R. C., & Wang, P. S. (2008). The descriptive epidemiology of commonly occurring mental disorders in the United States. *Annual Review of Public Health, 29*, 115–129.

Roderick, M., Easton, J., & Sebring, P. B. (2009). *The Consortium on Chicago School Research: A new model for the role of research in supporting urban school reform.* Chicago: Consortium on Chicago School Research, University of Chicago Urban Education Institute.

Wang, P. S., Lane, M., Olfson, M., Pincus, H. A., Wells, K. B., & Kessler, R. C. (2005). Twelve-month use of mental health services in the United States: Results from the National Comorbidity Survey Replication. *Archives of General Psychiatry, 62*(6), 629–640.

PART I

CONTEXT AND KEY CONCEPTS

CHAPTER 1

History and Process of Evidence-Based Practice in Mental Health

BONNIE SPRING

SARA HOFFMAN MARCHESE

JEREMY STEGLITZ

The evidence-based practice (EBP) movement has always been about implementing optimal health care practices. Until the start of the 19th century, however, there were very few health interventions that could be considered legitimate (McKeown & Lowe, 1966). Only then did the outcomes of antiseptic surgery, vaccination, and public sanitation start to demonstrate that some practices produced clear health benefit, whereas others did not. Having an ability to identify best practices challenges all health disciplines to implement these within their scope of care. Because the Institute of Medicine (IOM) has declared EBP a core competence for all health professionals and has endorsed its implementation by integrated interprofessional teams (Greiner & Knebel, 2003; IOM, 2012, 2015), a transdisciplinary approach to EBP offers a shared mental model for care teams.

EBP is both a conceptual model and a process involving the "conscientious, explicit, and judicious use of current best evidence in making decisions" about care (Sackett, Rosenberg, Gray, Haynes, & Richardson, 1996, p. 71). This chapter characterizes early milestones in the EBP movement and compares how models of EBP evolved in the several health professions that address behavioral, psychosocial, and mental health interventions.

The History of EBP

Three main factors shaped the emergence of EBP: the Flexner Report, the influence of Archibald Cochrane, and the work of the McMaster University group, as outlined elsewhere (Spring, 2007; Spring et al., 2005; Spring & Neville, 2010; Spring, Ferguson, Russell, Sularz, & Roehrig, 2013).

The Flexner Report

For much of the 19th century, no effective professional regulation of medical education or practice existed in the United States. Attentive, well-meaning doctors were in good supply, due largely to a proliferation of freestanding, for-profit medical schools (Beck, 2004; Duffy, 2011). Rather than requiring college training, these schools' main entry criterion was an ability to pay the fees. Tuition was kept low because faculty members taught only lecture courses and divided the students' tuition revenues among themselves. By the turn of the century, the problem of a substandard medical workforce was recognized, and licensing laws were strengthened to correct the problem. The Carnegie Foundation for the Advancement of Teaching in collaboration with the American

Medical Association (AMA), commissioned educator Abraham Flexner to evaluate the quality of education in U.S. and Canadian medical schools. After visiting 155 medical schools in 18 months, Flexner (1910) filed a blistering report. His conclusion that financial motives had caused gross overproduction of underqualified physicians sounded a death knell to for-profit medical schools unaffiliated with an academic institution.

The Report's mandate that medical schools provide future physicians with high-quality, hands-on laboratory and clinical training was well warranted. However, the exponentially higher cost of providing sound science training to a smaller pool of qualified students who, in turn, contributed shrinking tuition revenue, made survival financially untenable for most freestanding schools. By 1935, the ensuing attrition due to both principles and economics led to the closure of one-third of existing U.S. medical schools (Duffy, 2011). The analogous proliferation of for-profit psychology professional schools today prompts many to call for a similar tear-down of all but university-based graduate psychology training programs that prioritize scientific research (Baker, McFall, & Shoham, 2008).

Archibald Cochrane

Scottish physician and epidemiologist Archibald Cochrane (1909–1988) was a founding figure in the EBP movement whose skepticism about therapies began with his own personal experiences. While still in school, he sought psychoanalytic treatment for a sexual dysfunction from one of Sigmund Freud's students, Theodor Reik. The treatment proved ineffective, although an incidental benefit was that Cochrane became fluent in German, which served him well during the years he later spent in German prisoner of war (POW) camps (Stavrou, Challoumas, & Dimitrakakis, 2014). He described his experiences in the pithy, engaging book *Effectiveness and Efficiency: Random Reflections on Health Service,* an evaluation of the National Health Service (NHS). Cochrane's time in POW camps convinced him that medical treatments are superfluous to the outcome of much disease. As senior medical officer, Cochrane was responsible for the well-being of 20,000 POWs who subsisted on 600 kcal/day. All had diarrhea and were subject to epidemics of typhoid, diphtheria, infections, and jaundice

that swept through the camp. Given that the sole medical remedies available were some aspirin, antacid and skin antiseptic, Cochrane expected hundreds of POWs to die on his watch. Only four did die, however, three of whom were shot by German guards (Cochrane, 1972). The POW experience taught Cochrane that the impact of medical therapeutics often pales in comparison with the recuperative power of the human body and, we might speculate, a therapeutic alliance. Conversely, his later experiences with urban poverty in London taught him that socioeconomic disadvantage can significantly compromise human health.

While studying medicine in London during the 1930s, Cochrane was appalled by the differences he saw between the health care of the rich and the poor. Under a self-designed banner proclaiming that "all effective treatment must be free," he picketed in favor of forming Britain's National Health Service (Cochrane, 1972). But how could one reconcile an inevitably limited supply of health care resources against an unlimited desire for cures? Cochrane (1972) attributed the voracious desire for treatment to a "very widespread belief that for every symptom or group of symptoms there was a bottle of medicine, a pill, an operation, or some other therapy which would at least help. The doctor on his side was hardly to blame for aiding and abetting in the production of this myth. He very earnestly wanted to help" (p. 8). Two problems remained. First, the physician had little knowledge of which of a number of accessible drugs and devices was effective. Second, demand for treatment would always outstrip available resources. Hence, Cochrane argued the need for care decisions to be based on *cost-effectiveness,* or the efficiency with which the health care system used its human and financial assets. He frankly acknowledged his belief "that cure is rare while the need for care is widespread, and that the pursuit of cure at all costs may restrict the supply of care" (p. 7).

Cochrane's own successful experiences conducting randomized clinical trials (RCTs) in the POW camp [stet] subsequently convinced him that RCTs offer the most unbiased way of determining whether a treatment works. He continued to advocate for an organized, continually updated, valid summary of RCTs to be made available to help clinicians make optimal care decisions for their patients. That dream was ultimately realized in 1993 by the formation of the Cochrane Collaboration (*www.cochrane.*

org), a worldwide network of more than 28,000 scientists who have published 6,616 online systematic reviews of health interventions evaluated by RCTs (Cochrane Collaboration, 2004). In addition to systematic evidence reviews, the Trials tab of the Cochrane library links to the Cochrane Central Register of Controlled Trials (CENTRAL), a repository of reports on RCTs and quasi-RCTs. Overall, Cochrane's work laid EBP's foundation by highlighting the value of the RCT and prompting the creation of a centralized resource to make synthesized expert reviews of trials accessible for practicing clinicians and policymakers.

The McMaster University Group

A third major influence on the EBP movement was the clinical epidemiology group led by David Sackett at McMaster University in Canada. Sackett published his first relevant paper in 1969. The problem the McMaster group tackled was the rarity with which clinicians used best research evidence about the effectiveness of treatments when making clinical decisions about patient care. Instead, clinicians' treatment decisions more often were guided by habits acquired during training, advice from colleagues, personal experiences, or worries about liability (Guyatt et al., 1986; Isaacs & Fitzgerald, 1999; Spring et al., 2005). As a corrective, the McMaster group endorsed practicing "scientific medicine," grounded in the *research knowledge base*. That name raised hackles, however, as it appeared to devalue the clinician's and the patient's contributions to clinical decisions. As a compromise, Gordon Guyatt coined the phrase *evidence-based medicine,* which was introduced in 1992 as a new paradigm for practicing clinical medicine (Evidence-Based Medicine Working Group, 1992).

Three-Circles Models of EBP

Whereas "scientific medicine" prioritized only research evidence, the McMaster Group proposed a more complex model of evidence-based medicine that incorporated three data streams, all of which were to be integrated in clinical decision making. The original three-circles model (Haynes, Sackett, Gray, Cook, & Guyatt, 1996; Sackett et al., 1996) displayed clinical expertise, research evidence, and patient preferences as pillars of a three-legged stool, coequal but

with expertise as the topmost circle. Placing clinical expertise on top was a pragmatic strategy to earn clinician buy-in by ceding that, in some contexts, clinical judgment may override research evidence (G. Guyatt, personal communication, June 8, 2005). Although it was subsequently revised, the initial three-circles model remains the best known and served as template for the American Psychological Association's 2006 conceptualization of EBP.

The McMaster Group's revised three-circles model (Haynes, Devereaux, & Guyatt, 2002) corrected an important limitation of the initial version by proposing clinical decision making as a way to cope with discrepancies between the research evidence and either patient preferences or clinical opinion. In the updated model, a "clinical state and circumstances" circle replaced the one that had originally contained clinical expertise. Now, clinical expertise was depicted as an interior circle or decision-making process to actively tie together and resolve contradictions among patients' state and circumstances, their preferences, and the evidence base. Retaining clinical expertise as the central integrating circle expressed respect for the practitioner's pivotal role. Notably, *clinical expertise* was defined more explicitly not as intuition, but rather as skill in performing an EBP process that requires eliciting, appropriately appraising, and ultimately integrating the three potentially disparate sources of data (Haynes et al., 2002).

The Emergence of EBP across the Health Professions

It is ironic that psychology is among the last health professions to adopt the EBP framework because clinical psychologists first contemplated a version of EBP before the movement took root in medicine. In fact, clinical psychologists actually proposed an approach to EBP a year before the McMaster group published its influential initial papers on EBM (Haynes et al., 1996). In 1995, the American Psychological Association's Society of Clinical Psychology (Division 12) released the first report of its Task Force on Promotion and Dissemination of Psychological Procedures, chaired by Dianne Chambless (Chambless et al., 1996). The aim of the Division 12 Task Force was to establish standards of evidence that could be applied to select which psychological treatments warranted inclusion in psychology training programs.

The field of social work also had earlier models for the integration of research and practice (e.g., Gambrill, 1999), but when evidence-based social work practice emerged in the 1990s, it was considered a paradigm shift made feasible by increased practice research and dissemination. Like EBP in medicine and psychology, EBP in social work comprises a three-circles model. However, the model incorporates political, economic, and organizational contextual factors that affect the social worker's roles in management and policy in addition to practice. EBP in social work has flourished since 1999, with organizations such as the international Campbell Collaboration, the U.S. Substance Abuse and Mental Health Services Administration (SAMHSA), and the U.K. Social Care Institute for Excellence (SCIE) providing infrastructure support to curate and disseminate practices supported by research.

Public health resembles social work in emphasizing social determinants of health, but it differs by broadening its unit of analysis and concern from the patient to the population. Hence, EBP in public health was first defined in 1997 as the "use of epidemiological insight while studying and applying research, clinical, and public health experience and findings in clinical practice, health programs, and health policies" (Jenicek, 1997, p. 190). As the entity charged with fostering health in all policies of nations affiliated with the United Nations, the World Health Organization directs and coordinates the translation and implementation of evidence internationally. Consistent with an emphasis on communities and populations, the three-circles model in EBP public health uses surveillance data to contextualize application of the research evidence base, while engaging communities in decision making about policy implementation (Kohatsu, Robinson, & Torner, 2004).

Like psychology's early advocacy of empirically supported treatments, nursing also had an EBP predecessor in its research utilization movement of the 1970s (Titler et al., 2001). Ultimately, the EBP model for nursing garnered greater appeal partly because its three-circles model went beyond sole emphasis on research to also consider patient preferences and nurse expertise when making clinical decisions (Weaver, Warren, Delaney, & International Medical Informatics Association Nursing Informatics Special Interest Group and Evidence-Based Practice Working Group, 2005). Inclusion of EBP competencies as a required component of nursing education (American Association of Colleges of Nursing, 2008; American Nurses Credentialing Center, 2007) helped drive nursing into the EBP movement, as did a similar requirement for hospitals seeking to earn prestigious Magnet accreditation.

Ironically, 100 years after the Flexner Report, some opinion leaders express concerns that, in medical education, the privileging of research over clinical practice, teaching, and service may have gone too far (Cooke, Irby, Sullivan, & Ludmerer, 2006; Duffy, 2011). Flexner's ideas were strongly influenced by the German university system of the late 19th century (Billroth, 1924), a context that also shaped the origins of U.S. graduate training in psychology. Widely recognized as the best educational institutions in the world in that era, German universities placed heavy emphasis on rational analysis, collection of data, and the advancement of scientific knowledge using methods drawn from the natural sciences. Like Flexner, who sought graduate training in Berlin, numerous Americans flocked to study at German universities. One popular mentor was German physician-physiologist Wilhelm Wundt, who taught the first course in scientific psychology, founded the first academic journal devoted to psychological research, and applied experimental methods to study the physiological connection between brain and mind. Upon returning to the United States, a number of Wundt's students instantiated their training by founding psychology departments at Harvard, the University of Pennsylvania, Cornell, and Clark University (Johnson & Henley, 1990). Similarly, Flexner infused his observations of German science-based medical education into the physician training curricula at Harvard, Johns Hopkins, the University of Pennsylvania, and the University of Michigan.

The shared zeitgeist of these new U.S. training programs was their grounding in science as the prime raison d'être for all health disciplines. The chief responsibility of all future health professionals, whether aspiring to teach or to do research, or clinical practice, was held to be the generation of new research data to advance scientific understanding. By 1925, however, Flexner had begun to worry that an overfocus on research was driving out the practical and humanitarian aspects of medical education, a concern that has continued over time (Cooke et al., 2006; Duffy, 2011). One long-standing question has been whether the hyperrational, value-neutral orientation of science sufficiently encourages professionals to see knowledge as in the service of patients, rather than the converse. In 2010, the U.S. Congress took steps to address this concern by authorizing formation of the Patient-Centered Outcomes Research Institute (PCORI), which currently is a significant funder of comparative effectiveness research that addresses the questions most relevant to patients. The program implements its commitment to generating patient-centered evidence by engaging investigators with patients, caregivers, clinicians, and other health care stakeholders throughout the research process.

Also, between 2004 and the present, the IOM, the Association of American Medical Colleges (AAMC), the accrediting bodies for U.S. and Canadian medical schools, and the Josiah Macy Jr. Foundation prompted changes that broadened medical school entry and curricular requirements to lay groundwork for more person-centered care. In particular, 2015 witnessed rollout of a new behavioral and social science subtest of the Medical College Admission Test (MCAT). This change ensures that future physicians enter medical training with foundational knowledge of psychological and social sciences, paralleling what is required for biology, chemistry, and mathematics prerequisites. The goal is to ensure that physicians are mindful that context, culture, and social stratification affect human well-being at least as powerfully as do biological determinants (IOM Committee on Behavioral and Social Sciences in Medical School Curricula, 2004; Kaplan, Satterfield, & Kington, 2012). In the same vein, fostering active exchange and even adversarial collaboration (Kahneman & Klein, 2009) among the different health professions on the integrated health care team has the potential to reinforce the progression toward more patient-centered, equitable health practice. This is because several health professions represented on the care team—particularly social work, public health, and nursing—have strong value traditions in public service, patient collaboration, and equity, balancing other priorities that may drive health care. These roots are reflected by the history of social work, which originated as a vocation in the 1800s out of philanthropic efforts to help impoverished workers who flooded cities because of the Industrial Revolution (Okpych & Yu, 2014). A moral imperative to serve the poor, the infirm, and the outcast also was a cornerstone in the origins of nursing and public health, and indeed, beneficence remains a shared ethic for all health professions.

The Transdisciplinary Model of Evidence-Based Behavioral Practice

Following medicine (Sackett et al., 1996), nursing (Craig & Smyth, 2002), social work (Gibbs, 2003), public health (Brownson, Baker, Leet, Gillespie, & True, 2003), and psychology (American Psychological Association Presidential Task Force on Evidence-Based Practice, 2006; Chambless & Ollendick, 2001) all embraced EBP. Each discipline retained research evidence as one of the three circles but otherwise introduced improvements that adapted the model to its own context (Satterfield et al., 2009). Evidence-based nursing emphasized the need to integrate patient experiences and preferences into clinical decision making. To operationalize and understand patient experience, EBP in nursing gives increased emphasis to research data deriving from qualitative, patient satisfaction, and quality improvement studies (Newhouse, Dearholt, Poe, Pugh, & White, 2007; Stetler, 2001; Titler et al., 2001). In social work and public health, models of EBP emphasize the power of the surrounding sociohistoric, political, economic, organizational, and community context to impede or facilitate positive change (cf. Regehr, Stern, & Shlonsky, 2007). Given the broad-ranging impact of these macrolevel social determinants, the dominant model of EBP in public health focuses on the well-being of the population rather than the individual (Kohatsu et al., 2004). When translating the EBP model to public health, the patient circle becomes the population's needs, values, and preferences. The research circle is retained, but because few RCTs have evaluated policy interventions, there is increased reliance on observational studies, time series analyses, and quasi-experiments. Finally, and very importantly, the third circle in the model of evidence-based public health becomes resources—acknowledging the reality that resource considerations are inescapably front and center in public health decision making. The constraint-ridden world of public health presents the exact quandary that once troubled Archibald Cochrane: an overtaxed system with resources certainly insufficient to meet public health *wants,* and whose constraints require difficult decisions about how to meet population health *needs*.

In 2000, the National Institutes of Health (NIH) Office of Behavioral and Social Sciences Research (OBSSR) and the Society of Behavioral Medicine (SBM) partnered in an effort to improve the evidence base for nondrug, nondevice behavioral interventions to enhance health by upgrading methodological standards for clinical trials and systematic reviews. A new SBM evidence-based behavioral medicine committee advocated for the use of Consolidated Standards of Reporting Trials (CONSORT) guidelines to align standards for the reporting of behavioral clinical trials with those in effect for reporting medical trials (Davidson et al., 2003; Moher et al., 2010). Subsequently, in 2008, OBSSR launched an effort to harmonize the approach to EBP among the diverse health professions that implement behavioral interventions and to create training resources. A Council for Training in Evidence-Based Behavioral Practice (EBBP), led by Bonnie Spring, was constituted to include experts in medicine, nursing, psychology, social work, public health, and information science (Bellamy et al., 2013; Jacobs, Jones, Gabella, Spring, & Brownson, 2012; Newhouse & Spring, 2010; Spring, Ferguson, et al., 2013). The Council issued a white paper that introduced a transdisciplinary three-circles model of EBP and delineated needed competencies (Council for Training in Evidence-Based Behavioral Practice, 2008). The Council also launched *www.ebbp.org,* a free online training resource that includes nine e-learning modules: the EBP practice process, searching for evidence, systematic evidence reviews, RCTs, critical appraisal, shared decision making with individuals, collaborative decision making with communities, stakeholder perspectives, and implementation science.

The Council's transdisciplinary model of EBP appears in Figure 1.1. The model incorporates facets from each member discipline's approach to EBP (Satterfield et al., 2009; Spring & Hitchcock, 2009; Spring & Neville, 2010). From medicine, the transdisciplinary model appropriates its three-circle structure, and from scientific medicine and psychology its prioritization of best available research evidence as the topmost circle. From nursing, social work, and public health comes acknowledgment that health decision making needs to be shared collaboratively to reflect the characteristics, preferences, experiences, and values of individual, family, and community stakeholders who will be affected by the decision. From public health, comes recognition that resource considerations necessarily figure prominently in health decisions, and thus warrant their own circle reflecting financial, logistical, linguistic, and other issues constraining access to care. Finally, from social work comes the insight that clinical and policy decisions about health unfold in an institutional, organizational, and cultural context that inevitably shapes which strategies are likely to be acceptable and effective.

The different training backgrounds that char-

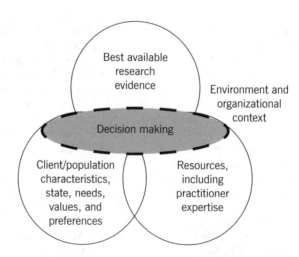

FIGURE 1.1. Transdisciplinary model of EBP. From Spring and Hitchcock (2009). Reprinted with permission from John Wiley & Sons; permission conveyed through Copyright Clearance Center, Inc.

acterize medicine, nursing, social work, psychology, and public health present substantial challenges for transdisciplinary science and integrated practice. Vocabulary, conceptual frameworks, and research methods all differ across these disciplines. However, the need in integrated care to access, critically appraise, and iteratively apply the evidence generated by each discipline requires a common base of training and tools for knowledge acquisition and translation. The transdisciplinary approach to EBP holds the potential to offer such a harmonizing model.

The Five-Step EBP Process

The transdisciplinary model shown in Figure 1.1 may make it appear that integration of the three data strands considered in EBP could occur simultaneously, but this is not the case. After assessing the client, there ensue five clearly defined steps in the EBP process: Ask a question; Acquire the evidence; Appraise the evidence; Apply the evidence; Analyze and Adjust practice. The steps are itemized in Table 1.1 and are performed in the order shown in Figure 1.2. Each step is necessary and represents a skill in which practitioners need to gain competence. Assessment of the patient, other stakeholders, and the surrounding context and resources is assumed to precede the onset of the EBP process and to recur throughout it, rather than being considered a formal step. The EBP process, including initial assessment, is ongoing and cyclical given the dynamic nature of both clients' problems and the research literature. Each step is described below in greater detail, together with a case that illustrates practical application of each stage of the EBP process. Demograph-ics and background information learned during initial assessment of an illustrative client are given in Box 1.1.

Ask: Asking Questions

After initially assessing the patient, the clinician consults the research literature by asking relevant, practical questions that will guide decisions about management or treatment of the presenting problem. Asking effective clinical questions, a competence of EBP, involves formulating queries in a manner that lets them be readily answered. Many types of questions come up in clinical practice:

1. Assessment: questions about best ways to measure, describe, or diagnose a condition.
2. Treatment: questions about interventions to prevent, manage, or improve health problems.
3. Etiology: questions about the influences that cause or predispose one to the onset of illness.
4. Prognosis: questions about the likely course and outcome of a health condition.
5. Harm: questions about potential adverse effects of interventions.
6. Cost-effectiveness: questions about the expense of an intervention relative to clinical outcome.

Because many different questions arise in connection with each patient, the clinician needs to prioritize the most important ones efficiently. When prioritizing questions, two criteria are particularly salient: (1) information that will, in the clinician's judgment, have the greatest impact on the patient's function and quality of life and (2) information that is of

---

TABLE 1.1. Steps of the EBP Process

- *Step 1: Ask.* Ask client-oriented, relevant, answerable questions about the health status and context of individuals or other stakeholders needing help.

- *Step 2: Acquire.* Acquire the best research evidence available to answer the question.

- *Step 3: Appraise.* Critically appraise the evidence for its quality and its applicability to the person, population, context, resources, and problem at hand.

- *Step 4: Apply.* Apply the evidence by engaging in collaborative health decision making with the client and stakeholders.

- *Step 5: Analyze and adjust.* Analyze outcomes and adjust practice accordingly.

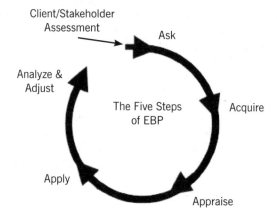

FIGURE 1.2. The five-step EBP process. From Spring and Hitchcock (2009). Reprinted with permission from John Wiley & Sons; permission conveyed through Copyright Clearance Center, Inc.

great perceived significance from the patient's perspective.

The clinician can formulate two different types of questions: background (general) or foreground (specific). The purpose of background questions is to gain general information about a condition or class of clinical tools or treatments. Well-formulated background questions comprise two parts: (1) a question root (*what, who, how,* etc.), including a verb, and (2) a disorder, assessment, treatment, or other health issue. For example, when preparing for a clinical visit with a patient, clinicians may ask overarching background questions to update their general knowledge of a particular health condition, assessment approach, or class of interventions. Once the patient's difficulty has been ascertained, the clinician usually poses more focused foreground questions, seeking information that helps make a choice between

alternative care paths. The acronym used to structure a well-formed foreground question is PICOT, where P designates relevant patient characteristics, I designates the intervention under consideration, C refers to the comparison approach under consideration, O designates the outcome of greatest interest, and T reflects the temporal interval for follow-up. Box 1.2 portrays a background question and a foreground question formulated during the "Ask" step of the case illustration.

Acquire: Acquisition of Evidence

After asking one or more well-constructed clinical questions, the clinician moves to the next step of the EBP process, which is to acquire the evidence to answer his or her questions. To successfully implement this step, the clinician translates the question into an efficient search

---

Box 1.1. Case Illustration: Assessment of Patient, Context, and Resources

The patient is a 27-year-old single, insured, Hispanic heterosexual male who lives with his mother and older sister in a two-bedroom house in the suburbs of a large Midwestern city. He has a 4-year college degree and is currently employed as a stock-worker in a large retail store located near his home. For several years after graduating from college, he was employed as a middle school math teacher at an urban school and was engaged to a music teacher from the same school. After his mother experienced a broken leg 2 years ago, he left teaching and took his current job in order to be able to check on her during the day. During this time, his fiancée ended their engagement. He reports enjoying watching movies and playing video games, but describes increasing isolation, hopelessness, and intrusive thoughts about his mother's health and fears of "going insane." At the time of his self-referral to a community mental health center, he described a prior history of test anxiety during college that was unresponsive to pharmacotherapy and also a history of marijuana abuse.

Box 1.2. Case Illustration: Ask

To prepare for the first clinical visit with the patient, the clinician formulates one background and one foreground question. The background question concerns assessment: "How can I assess whether the patient has obsessive–compulsive disorder (OCD) or psychosis?" The clinician prioritizes this question highly because of the need to determine a diagnosis on which to base treatment and because of the patient's concern that his psychological problem may be severe. She decides to administer the Yale–Brown Obsessive Compulsive Scale (YBOCS) symptom checklist interview and the Structured Clinical Interview for DSM-5 (SCID-5). Having administered the assessments and made the diagnosis of OCD, the clinician then asks a foreground PICOT question about treatment options: "For an adult Hispanic male with OCD, will exposure and response prevention (ERP), as compared to cognitive therapy (CT), reduce symptoms of OCD and improve quality of life at 6-month follow-up?"

---

plan. Relevant learning resources about search strategy can be found at the Web-based tutorial on searching (*www.ebbp.org/training.html*) or through consultation with a librarian or other information science professional. Because the body of primary research is massive and continually growing, most busy practicing clinicians turn first to the secondary, synthesized body of evidence found in systematic reviews (as described by Cuijpers & Cristea, Chapter 5, this volume) and EBP guidelines (as described by Hollon, Chapter 6, this volume) to acquire answers to their questions. The "Acquire" step is portrayed in a case illustration in Box 1.3.

Appraise: Critical Appraisal of Quality and Relevance

The next step in the EBP process is critical appraisal to address how well the acquired research answers the question the clinician posed. The appraisal evaluates the quality of the evidence and its applicability to the patient and current circumstances. A core tenet of EBP is the hierarchy of evidence: the premise that the higher up in a hypothetical evidence pyramid a research design is, the more robust and closer

to the truth its results are as an answer to the clinician's question (Straus, Glasziou, Richardson, & Haynes, 2011). Importantly, there is no single evidence pyramid because there is no single research design equally well equipped to address all of the questions a clinician may pose. Rather, there are multiple evidence pyramids because the highest quality research approach depends on the question being asked. For example, for questions related to etiology or prognosis, a longitudinal cohort research design usually provides the best evidence. In contrast, for questions about the efficacy or effectiveness of treatments, well-conducted RCTs usually provide the best evidence because this research design is least prone to bias or error in allowing clinical change to be attributed causally to the study intervention rather than to extraneous influences.

When appraising evidence quality for questions about whether a treatment works, EBP places primary emphasis on *internal validity,* which is the extent to which the results of a study are true; that is, we can safely conclude that it was the intervention that caused the change in behavior, and not some other extraneous factor, such as differences in assessment

---

Box 1.3. Case Illustration: Acquire

Having diagnosed the patient as having OCD, the clinician translates her foreground PICOT question into an efficient search plan. Using the Cochrane Database of Systematic Reviews (*http://onlinelibrary.wiley.com/cochranelibrary/search*), she types in the following key word search query: "obsessive compulsive disorder" *and* "adult" *and* "exposure response prevention." This search yields zero systematic reviews, so the clinician modifies the search terms to be less restrictive. The clinician enters the following revised key word search query: "obsessive compulsive disorder" *and* "adult." Now, three systematic reviews emerge, one of which, titled "Psychological Treatments versus Treatment as Usual for OCD" (Gava et al., 2007), seems especially relevant. Another systematic review, titled "Second-Generation Antipsychotics for OCD" (Komossa, Depping, Meyer, Kissling, & Leucht, 2010), could be relevant given the patient's stated desire to try psychopharmacological intervention if initial psychological interventions appear ineffective.

---

procedures between intervention and control conditions. Most versions of the evidence hierarchy for treatment questions assign the topmost place to systematic reviews that synthesize the results of multiple RCTs, followed by well-designed, well-implemented single RCTs (Guyatt, Rennie, Meade, & Cook, 2015; IOM, 2011b). Lower down are observational studies without randomization, and at the bottom of the hierarchy are anecdote and opinion.

In contrast to evidence quality, when appraising evidence applicability, the emphasis shifts to external validity. Now the clinician judges whether the research evidence can be generalized to the specific patient, interventionist, and circumstances at hand. For example, were the assessment procedures so onerous that only unusually highly motivated people would have been willing to enroll in the study? Was there high loss to follow-up? If so, then findings may reflect how very conscientious people respond to the treatment rather than how the full population of interest would have responded.

Appraising applicability is challenging because it is rare to have studies that systematically evaluate the broad generalizability of findings. Many population subgroups and settings are understudied. Hence, we lack thorough knowledge about the degree to which most treatments apply universally or have more limitedly utility. To address this challenge, the EBP clinician's best practice when acquiring evidence is to search for evidence of treatment by patient subgroup interaction. If none is found, it cannot be assumed that absence of evidence of interaction equates to evidence that interactions are absent. However, it does warrant that, in the next stage of the EBP process, the clinician may apply the treatment supported by the best available evidence. In so doing, the practitioner proceeds "as if" one size of best nomothetic treatment fits all, meanwhile analyzing the patient's response and adapting accordingly if response is poor. The appraise step is portrayed in the case illustration in Box 1.4.

Most medical school curricula now introduce students to the concepts and methods of EBP, and the IOM (2015) has recommended such training for all health professions. It must be noted that the vast majority of EBP teaching in medicine addresses critical appraisal of published research, reflecting the origins of the field. Between 1993 and 2000, the *Journal of the American Medical Association* introduced the teaching of evidence-based medicine via a series of articles covering the research designs optimally suited to answer clinical questions about therapy, diagnosis, prognosis, and harm. These articles became the basis for the *Users' Guides to the Medical Literature* (Guyatt et al., 2015), critical appraisal companion piece to *Evidence-Based Medicine: How to Practice and Teach It* (Straus et al., 2011), the standard pocket-size EBP textbook in medicine. Such training in library search, science literacy, and critical appraisal has been shown to increase written assessments of EBP knowledge and skills (Hecht, Buhse, & Meyer, 2016). What has not been demonstrated and remains understudied is whether training achieves the intended goal of increasing the use of research evidence in real-time clinical practice.

Apply: Shared Decision Making and Action

Apply is both the most complex step of the EBP process and the one most neglected in evidence-based medicine training. The apply step is portrayed in the case illustration in Box 1.5.

To apply the evidence, the clinician needs to take context into account, while engaging in shared decision making that integrates the three data strands in the model (research evidence, resources, patient characteristics) (Spring, 2008). The term *resources* refers to the skills and infrastructure support needed to provide what research shows to be the most effective practice. Considerations include the availability of physical (e.g., space and time), technological (e.g., information technology support), personnel

---

Box 1.4. Case Illustration: Appraise

In reading the 2007 systematic review by Gava and colleagues, the clinician critically evaluates the quality of the evidence, particularly its internal validity and applicability to the patient's circumstances. The clinician also considers demographic factors, such as race and ethnicity, in determining whether the populations outlined in the review align with the patient's experience. The quality of the systematic review appears high, and the applicability was deemed sufficient, since the RCTs included in the review involved adults with OCD and secondary depressed symptoms without treatment by patient subgroup interactions.

(e.g., trained practitioners), and financial assets needed to deliver empirically supported treatments (ESTs). Few, if any, care delivery systems have resources sufficient to deliver an infinite array of treatments. To be made available to patients, an intervention requires endorsement by higher administration, agreement from other system components (e.g., insurers) and, often, institutional investment in training and quality monitoring.

A recent development in EBP is the formulation of resource-sensitive practice guidelines (cf. Fried et al., 2008). These guidelines review evidence supporting alternative practice recommendations that fit the available infrastructure, human capital, and finances. Administrators and practitioners can utilize the guidelines to gauge whether a complex intervention is feasible to implement with existing assets and in a manner that retains treatment effectiveness. Consider, for example, dialectical behavioral therapy (DBT), an empirically supported treatment for borderline personality disorder that includes four concurrent therapeutic components: individual psychotherapy, group skills therapy, telephone coaching, and a practitioners' consultation group (Linehan et al., 1999). For many facilities, accessing certified DBT practitioners with available time, clinic space for group psychotherapy, and funds for DBT manuals exceeds available resources. Conversely, other settings triangulate their policy decision differently, seeing DBT's resource requirements as being offset by the high burden and cost of managing this patient population.

Evidence-based decision making is the core driving intelligent process that simultaneously integrates consideration of research, resources, and patient preferences (Spring, 2008). One of the first resources the individual clinician needs to appraise is whether his or her training, skills, and competencies are sufficient to offer what the research shows to be a best practice. The clinician also needs to assess whether stakeholders, such as the patient and family members, prefer the treatment supported by best available evidence, or at least find it acceptable. If not, then a collaborative decision may need to be made to select a different clinician who is trained in the best practice, or an alternative second-line treatment that the practitioner is equipped to provide.

The transdisciplinary model of EBP equates practitioner expertise with skills in performing evidence-based decision making and the EBP process. In previous models of EBP, the data strand related to *practitioner expertise* generated substantial controversy due, in part, to the ambiguity of the term (Haynes et al., 1996), which tended to be erroneously perceived as practitioner opinion or unquestioned intuition (Thornton, 2006). The transdisciplinary model operationalizes EBP expertise as competence in the following areas:

1. *Assessment skills* refer to the appraisal of patient characteristics, presenting problems, values, expectations, and environmental context. *Assessment competency* also pertains to the clinician's ability to objectively self-appraise his or her own level of expertise to implement particular treatments and subsequently to assess outcomes of those interventions.

2. *Process skills* involve competence in performing the five steps of EBP: asking well-formulated questions, acquiring best available research evidence, appraising evidence for quality and relevance, applying evidence by engaging in shared decision making with the patient (and other stakeholders who might be affected), and analyzing change and adjusting practice accordingly.

Box 1.5. Case Illustration: Apply

In the apply phase of the EBP process, the clinician makes a collaborative decision that integrates the assessment and research data she has gathered thus far with consideration of her clinical competence and also the patient's preferences and demographics, including race and ethnicity. During his first clinic visit, the patient expressed a clear preference for psychological over pharmacological treatment, despite his willingness to consider medication if nondrug treatment proved unsuccessful. The clinician has 9 years of experience providing psychological treatment for anxiety disorders, including OCD, equipping her with the needed clinical competence. At the second clinic visit, the clinician explains her conceptualization of the patient's difficulty and describes the treatments that research has shown to be effective. After discussing the pros and cons of the different treatment options, the patient and clinician collaboratively form a treatment plan to use ERP.

3. *Communication and collaboration skills* include the capacity to convey information clearly and accurately. These skills designate the ability to listen, observe, adjust, and negotiate as needed in order to achieve understanding and agreement from the patient and other stakeholders on a course of intervention.

4. *Engagement and intervention skills* refer to the practitioner's proficiency at motivating interest, constructive involvement, and positive change from the patient and other stakeholders. The degree of training, experience, and skills required to elicit and sustain interventions varies depending on the complexity, burden, and duration of the intervention.

Training to learn specific research-supported treatments is widely available through workshops or online. For example, SAMHSA and its Center for Mental Health Services provide resource kits for 11 research-supported treatments for psychological disorders and substance abuse (*http://store.samhsa.gov/list/series?name=evidence-based-practices-kits*). Training to learn the EBP process also is available online at *www.ebbp.org/training* and in person. In-person courses on EBP are taught at several locations, including the annual summer workshop titled *How to Teach Evidence-Based Clinical Practice* at McMaster University in Canada and by the Center on Evidence-Based Medicine at Oxford University in the United Kingdom.

Training resources are scarcest for the last two phases of the EBP process (apply and analyze/adjust) that address practical application of EBP. The EBP process module of the *www.ebbp.org* online training tool is one of very few learning resources that illustrates shared decision making to determine whether a research-supported treatment is feasible and appropriate. Chapters 12–22 in Part III of this volume also provide illustrations of the range of ways in which practitioners have carried out these critical steps of apply, analyze, and adjust.

Analyze and Adjust

In the apply step of the EBP process, barring strong contraindications, the patient and clinician select the treatment for the patient's difficulty that is supported by the best available research evidence. Contraindications may emerge if the patient or family strongly opposes the accepted best practice, if the patient previously had an adverse response to the treatment, or if subgroup interactions have been demonstrated to show treatment inefficacy for those who have the patient's cultural, demographic, or biographical characteristics. In choosing the best research-supported treatment, clinician and patient proceed on the assumption that results of the research evaluating the treatment can be generalized to people like the patient. This is a reasonable assumption to make in the absence of more personalized information about the patient's treatment response. On the other hand, generalizability is an assumption that warrants testing once the treatment has been applied and data about the specific patient's response start to become available. Hence, the next EBP process step involves assessing the patient's clinical status on an ongoing basis and adjusting treatment if adaptation is warranted. This analyze and adjust step highlights the iterative nature of EBP and is portrayed in a case illustration in Box 1.6.

Although treatment usually begins with the best "one size fits most" treatment for the average person, progressive adaptation and tailoring is a necessary part of the EBP process. Ordinarily, treatment adaptations are relatively modest and carried out within the scope of core evidence-based transdiagnostic behavior change principles and components that make the treatment effective (Barlow et al., 2011; National

---

Box 1.6. Case Illustration: Analyze and Adjust

Because the patient's initial symptoms were severe, the clinician and patient agreed to assess them weekly in a way that is both empirically and culturally sensitive. Since the outset of treatment, the clinician has analyzed weekly changes in the patient's OCD symptoms, depression, and quality of life. After 6 weeks of treatment, the clinician observes clinically meaningful reductions in the patient's OCD, depression, and quality of life assessment scores. These assessment data align with the patient's subjective appraisal that his socioemotional status and quality of life have improved. In light of this progress, the clinician and patient agree to maintain the current treatment plan, but to shift assessments from weekly to biweekly. If biweekly improvement continues to be evident over the next two months, then assessment will shift to monthly.

Cancer Institute, 2006). However, in some instances, a prolonged lack of improvement or even apparent harm (deterioration of the patient's condition) contraindicates continuing to administer the initially chosen treatment (Lilienfeld, 2007). In that case, clinician and patient together review a new evidence base that now integrates the patient's personalized response to treatment with the aggregate response of many patients, as characterized by research. Together, the patient and stakeholders collaboratively consider alternative intervention strategies.

The Roles of Practitioners in Transdisciplinary EBP

Practitioners have three primary roles they can play in relation to the research evidence in EBP (Figure 1.3). First, as scientists, they create evidence by designing, conducting, analyzing, and reporting primary research. Second, as systematic reviewers, they locate, appraise, and quantitatively synthesize research to make it readily accessible and interpretable by evidence users. Third, as research consumers, they access research evidence, appraise its quality and relevance for their patient's context, and integrate research into their practical decision making. Each of these three ways of relating to research assumes some common base of research knowledge, and each also entails some specialized skills (Spring, 2007). Ideally, learning EBP is an acculturation process begun during professional training that seamlessly integrates research and practice. However, becoming proficient in EBP also is feasible for clinicians who do not acquire the habit during graduate training. As integrated care teams grow increasingly interprofessional and community-engaged, many clinicians function in all three EBP roles. Such boundary spanning helps to ensure that the questions chosen for research investigation are those most relevant to providers and patients. In

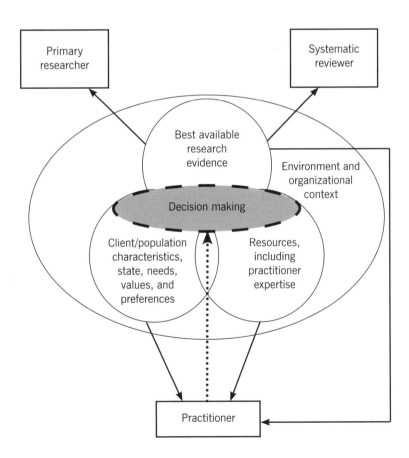

FIGURE 1.3. Three primary relationships of practitioners to evidence-based interventions (*www.ebbp.org*).

turn, active participation of community members in research ensures that study samples are representative and findings are generalizable (Kraemer & Periyakoil, Chapter 4, this volume).

Evidence Creators: Primary Researchers

As scientists, primary researchers design, conduct, analyze, and disseminate research that characterizes the risk factors, course, and causal influences acting on an array of health problems. They validate instruments to assess clinical conditions, and they develop and test interventions whose aim is to prevent or treat health problems. Clinicians translate the evidence base to their practices either by accessing the primary research literature directly or, more often, by applying conclusions drawn from the secondary synthesized literature presented in systematic reviews and treatment guidelines (cf., National Guideline Clearinghouse, 2017).

Evidence Synthesizers: Systematic Reviewers

As systematic reviewers, practitioners aggregate the primary research generated by researchers, and they analyze and interpret the collected research to produce syntheses that can be applied efficiently by clinicians and policymakers. Systematic reviews, which are an increasingly vital part of the infrastructure for EBP implementation, differ from other research reviews in the care allocated to reducing bias while gathering and interpreting primary research.

One tool that systematic reviewers use to reduce bias is the prespecified search protocol, which operationalizes the question to be answered by the systematic review. As described earlier, the question often is phrased in PICOT language, which specifies the target Population, Intervention, Comparison group, study Outcomes (primary and secondary dependent variables), and measurement Time point. Also prespecified to reduce bias are the search key words, as well as clear criteria for study inclusion and exclusion.

Two Web-based learning resources relevant to systematic reviews are available free of charge at *www.ebbp.org/training*. These courses offer an introduction and useful background materials about search and synthesis. The *Search for Evidence Module* provides an overview of how to acquire evidence, including information about search strategies and databases relevant for practicing clinicians. Topics covered in the

Systematic Review Module include evaluating the quality of a review, how and why high-quality reviews can reach different conclusions, and steps in conducting a systematic review. The IOM (2011b) conveyed best practice standards for conducting systematic reviews in a recent volume entitled *Finding What Works in Health Care*. Relatedly, a comprehensive handbook for systematic reviewers is produced by the Cochrane Collaboration (Higgins & Green, 2008).

A useful tool for writing systematic reviews is available from Preferred Reporting Items for Systematic Reviews and Meta-Analyses (PRISMA; Moher, Liberati, Tetzlaff, Altman, & the PRISMA Group, 2009). The PRISMA guidelines, developed in alignment with the Cochrane Collaboration, provide a 27-item checklist and flow diagram to help researchers accurately extract results and write disseminable reviews. Another resource, PROSPERO, is an international database of systematic reviews that were registered prospectively (at inception). Funded by the United Kingdom's NHS, PROSPERO is maintained by the Centre for Reviews and Dissemination at the University of York (*www.crd.york.ac.uk/prospero*). The database now includes more than 10,000 registered protocols and reviews for diverse interventions in health, social care, welfare, public health, education, crime, justice, and international development that have health outcomes.

EBP guidelines take a next step beyond synthesizing primary research data in a systematic review: Guidelines make recommendations about practice or policy. Translating from evidence to practical guidance requires explicitly summarizing the evidence, appraising confidence in the effect size estimate, and judging contextual issues surrounding the translation of findings to practice. Widely implemented guidance about evaluating evidence certainty to support a guideline recommendation is available from the 500-person international collaboration, Grading of Recommendations, Assessment, Development and Evaluation (GRADE) (*www.gradeworkinggroup.org*).

The GRADE group also offers guidance using the DECIDE approach (Developing and Evaluating Communication Strategies to Support Informed Decisions and Practice Based on Evidence) to target communication of evidence-based recommendations to different stakeholders (Treweek et al., 2013). One such strategy is the GRADE Evidence to Decision (EtD) Framework, which can be used to structure clinical recommendations and coverage or policy decisions using the GRADE approach (Neumann et al., 2016) The guideline itself does not emerge directly from the systematic review but is instead developed by an independent panel that includes expert professionals and individuals who have the relevant clinical condition. Accordingly, practice guidelines consider patient preferences when making clinical recommendations of varying strength regarding the potential benefits and harms of alternative clinical courses of action. In its volume on *Clinical Practice Guidelines We Can Trust* (2011a), the IOM conveyed consensual global standards of transparency, rigor, and management of conflict of interests for guidelines. These standards are designed to help clinicians make sound clinical decisions that merit public and professional confidence in health care practice.

Evidence Consumers: Clinicians

The third role in EBP may be the most complex. Only the clinician is required to extract and integrate information from all of the data strands that comprise EBP. Clinicians are research consumers in that they access research evidence and appraise its quality and relevance for their context. As clinicians, practitioners also acquire and analyze information regarding patient characteristics, including developmental course, past and current treatment response, context, values, and preferences. Finally, clinicians assess the institutional, environmental, and social resources that are available to support the patient, and they evaluate their personal training and skills to deliver an appropriate treatment that is both grounded in research and appropriate to the patient's context. They effectively communicate their evaluations to the patient and collaborate on choosing an optimal intervention strategy to which the patient agrees to adhere.

Conclusion and Future Directions

Convergence toward a transdisciplinary approach to EBBP is timely and well aligned with current movement toward increasingly integrated delivery of care. Having diverse health professions team up to provide care makes sense because comorbidity between mental and physical disorders is normative (Druss & Walker, 2011). Of the 25% of the U.S. adult population

with a mental disorder, 68% also have a medical comorbidity. Moreover, among the larger 58% population sector of adults who have a medical condition, 29% also have one or more mental health disorders (Alegria, Jackson, Kessler, & Takeuchi, 2003). Although they were trained to use differing languages, treatment strategies, and conceptual approaches, diverse health professionals on the health care team need to communicate and collaborate effectively to address all of the patient's health needs. The transdisciplinary approach to EBP helps by providing a shared mental model and methodology. Having said this, we must acknowledge that it is still unclear whether implementation of EBP will improve care delivery and health outcomes. Even though findings indicate that use of training tools (e.g., *www.ebbp.org*) increases knowledge, positive attitudes, and self-efficacy about EBP (Steglitz, 2017), the degree to which these gains translate into practice and policy improvement remains unknown.

The main challenges that lie ahead almost certainly will remain those that initially inspired Flexner, Cochrane, and the McMaster group to launch the movement toward EBP. To paraphrase Cochrane, resources for health care will inevitably be limited and insufficient to meet the demand for care. Consequently, it is essential that health care payments be restricted to those treatments that show demonstrated evidence of effectiveness. Moreover, to be sufficient for the population, strategies are needed that allow health resources be allocated across people efficiently in a manner that provides what individuals need but not more and not less.

A very promising development is the emergence of new optimization research methods that allow the development of more efficient behavioral and psychosocial treatments (Collins & Kugler, 2018). Barriers to the uptake of many such treatments have been the intensive multicomponent, multisession nature of many psychosocial interventions, and the need for professionals to deliver them. Also, the heterogeneity of treatment elements included in mental health interventions across different clinical trials has impeded interpretation in meta-analyses. Furthermore, the burden and cost of treatments has been a barrier to widespread scalability and uptake into care delivery systems. Multiphase Optimization Strategy (MOST), adapted from engineering science, addresses these barriers by offering a suite of methods to optimize interventions, making them as efficient as possible before further testing them in an RCT (Collins & Kugler, 2018).

One set of MOST tools involves factorial experiments that assemble (or dismantle) a treatment by determining, for example, the effect size for each of its potential components relative to its cost (Pellegrini, Hoffman, Collins, & Spring, 2014). This allows the developed treatment to be optimized for a criterion such as cost-efficiency (e.g., incorporating only components that achieve the maximum clinical benefit for the least cost). Note that the end goal of this specific MOST approach is to generate a highly efficient treatment that, presumably, will prove effective for the average patient in a subsequent RCT. The aim in developing such a treatment is to produce an intervention whose evidence will fare well upon critical appraisal. In other words, the treatment is likely to be selected in the EBP process as one well supported by available research evidence, and perhaps the most efficient of those. This framework for implementing EBP also is the one adopted in contemporary clinical practice guidelines and lists of ESTs (Chambless & Ollendick, 2001). Beginning treatment with the best research-supported treatment for the "average" patient accords with a nomothetic research tradition and is a reasonably valid, unbiased approach. But, who among us treats only average patients, or patients whose needs remain continuously the same over time?

Here the suite of MOST methods goes further by affording research designs that develop an evidence base for the *rest* of the EBP process—that part of the treatment process that occurs in the face of individual or dynamic response heterogeneity (if a best practice works suboptimally for some patients, or stops working, or even succeeds and warrants timely discontinuation). A critically important contribution of the transdisciplinary model is its reminder that EBP is a process that requires ongoing assessment in order to analyze and adjust treatment over time. Sequential multiphase adaptive randomized trials (SMARTs) support systematic derivation of a research evidence base to guide decisions about how to adapt treatment dynamically over time as a function of incoming data about the patient's response to treatment (Almirall, Nahum-Shani, Sherwood, & Murphy, 2014). Because its five-step process emphasizes dynamic, stepwise adaptation of treatment guided by the patient's response, the transdisciplinary model offers a helpful transition between the single best practice, empirically supported treatment

approach of today and what will likely be the more algorithmically expressed "if–then" decision rules that define the evidence-based dynamic treatment strategies of the future. We can anticipate that mobile digital tools, because of the dense continuous data they collect, will open the door to develop treatments that adapt in even more fine-grained ways to changes in the patient's states of psychological vulnerability and of receptivity to intervention (Nahum-Shani et al., 2018; Spring, Gotsis, Paiva, & Spruijts-Metz, 2013). The future evidence base to emerge from new optimization research designs can be expected to point to not only the best average empirically supported treatment with which to begin treatment but also how to adapt and personalize treatment going forward in increasingly real time.

References

Alegria, M., Jackson, J. S., Kessler, R. C., & Takeuchi, D. (2003). *National Comorbidity Survey Replication (NCS-R), 2001–2003*. Ann Arbor, MI: Inter-university Consortium for Political and Social Research.

Almirall, D., Nahum-Shani, I., Sherwood, N. E., & Murphy, S. A. (2014). Introduction to SMART designs for the development of adaptive interventions: With application to weight loss research. *Translational Behavioral Medicine, 4*(3), 260–274.

American Association of Colleges of Nursing. (2008). AACN "Essentials" Series. Retrieved March 2, 2008, from *www.aacn.nche.edu/education/essentials.htm.*

American Nurses Credentialing Center. (2007). Forces of magnetism. Retrieved March 27, 2009, from *http://198.65.134.123/magnet/programoverview/forcesofmagnetism.aspx.*

American Psychological Association, Presidential Task Force on Evidence-Based Practice. (2006). Evidence-based practice in psychology. *American Psychologist, 61*(4), 271–285.

Baker, T. B., McFall, R. M., & Shoham, V. (2008). Current status and future prospects of clinical psychology: Toward a scientifically principled approach to mental and behavioral health care. *Psychological Science in the Public Interest, 9*(2), 67–103.

Barlow, D. H., Farchione, T. J., Fairholme, C. P., Ellard, K. K., Boisseau, C. L., Allen, L. B., et al. (2011). *Unified Protocol for Transdiagnostic Treatment of Emotional Disorders: Therapist guide.* New York: Oxford University Press.

Beck, A. H. (2004). The Flexner report and the standardization of American medical education. *Journal of the American Medical Association, 291*(17), 2139–2140.

Bellamy, J. L., Mullen, E. J., Satterfield, J. M., Newhouse, R. P., Ferguson, M., Brownson, R. C., et al. (2013). Implementing evidence-based practice education in social work: A transdisciplinary approach. *Research on Social Work Practice, 23*(4), 426–436.

Billroth, T. (1924). *The medical sciences in the German universities: A study in the history of civilization.* Berlin: Macmillan.

Brownson, R. C., Baker, E. A., Leet, T. L., Gillespie, K. N., & True, W. R. (2003). *Evidence-based public health.* New York: Oxford University Press.

Chambless, D. L., & Ollendick, T. H. (2001). Empirically supported psychological interventions: Controversies and evidence. *Annual Review of Psychology, 52,* 685–716.

Chambless, D. L., Sanderson, W. C., Shoham, V., Bennett Johnson, S., Pope, K. S., Crits-Christoph, P., et al. (1996). An update on empirically validated therapies. *The Clinical Psychologist, 49*(2), 5–18.

Cochrane, A. (1972). *Effectiveness and efficacy: Random reflections on health services.* London: Royal Society of Medicine Press.

Collins, L., & Kugler, K. (2018). *Optimization of behavioral, biobehavioral, and biomedical interventions.* New York: Springer.

Cooke, M., Irby, D. M., Sullivan, W., & Ludmerer, K. M. (2006). American medical education 100 years after the Flexner Report. *New England Journal of Medicine, 355,* 1339–1344.

Council for Training in Evidence-Based Behavioral Practice. (2008). Evidence-based behavioral practice. Retrieved February 6, 2016, from *www.ebbp. org.*

Craig, J. V., & Smyth, R. L. (2002). *The evidence-based practice manual for nurses.* London: Churchill Livingstone.

Davidson, K. W., Goldstein, M., Kaplan, R. M., Kaufmann, P. G., Knatterud, G. L., Orleans, C. T., et al. (2003). Evidence-based behavioral medicine: What is it and how do we achieve it? *Annals of Behavioral Medicine, 26*(3), 161–171.

Druss, B. G., & Walker, E. R. (2011). *Mental disorders and medical comorbidity* (Synthesis Report No. 21). Princeton, NJ: Robert Wood Johnson Foundation.

Duffy, T. P. (2011). The Flexner Report—100 years later. *Yale Journal of Biology and Medicine, 84,* 269–276.

Evidence-Based Medicine Working Group. (1992). Evidence-based medicine: A new approach to teaching the practice of medicine. *Journal of the American Medical Association, 268,* 2420–2425.

Flexner, A. (1910). *Medical education in the United States and Canada: A report to the Carnegie Foundation for the Advancement of Teaching* (Bulletin No. 4). New York: Carnegie Foundation for the Advancement of Teaching.

Flexner, A. (1925). *Medical education: A comparative study.* New York: MacMillan.

Fried, M., Quigley, E. M., Hunt, R. H., Guyatt, G., Anderson, B. O., Bjorkman, D. J., et al. (2008). Can global guidelines change health policy? *Nature Clinical Practice Gastroenterology and Hepatology, 5*(3), 120–121.

Gambrill, E. D. (1999). Evidence-based practice: An alternative to authority-based practice. *Families in Society, 80*(4), 341–350.

Gava, I., Barbui, C., Aguglia, E., Carlino, D., Churchill, R., De Vanna, M., et al. (2007). Psychological treatments versus treatment as usual for obsessive compulsive disorder (OCD). *Cochrane Database of Systematic Reviews, 2,* CD005333.

Gibbs, L. E. (2003). *Evidence-based practice for the helping professions: A practical guide with integrated multimedia.* Pacific Grove, CA: Brooks/Cole Thomson Learning.

Greiner, A. C., & Knebel, E. (Eds.). (2003). *Health professions education: A bridge to quality.* Washington, DC: National Academies Press.

Guyatt, G., Rennie, D., Meade, M. O., & Cook, D. J. (2015). *Users' guides to the medical literature: A manual for evidence-based clinical practice* (3rd ed.). New York: McGraw-Hill.

Guyatt, G., Sackett, D., Taylor, D. W., Chong, J., Roberts, R., & Pugsley, S. (1986). Determining optimal therapy: Randomized trials in individual patients. *New England Journal of Medicine, 314*(14), 889–892.

Haynes, R. B., Devereaux, P., & Guyatt, G. H. (2002). Clinical expertise in the era of evidence-based medicine and patient choice. *ACP Journal Club, 136,* A11–A14.

Haynes, R. B., Sackett, D. L., Gray, J. M., Cook, D. J., & Guyatt, G. H. (1996). Transferring evidence from research into practice: 1. The role of clinical care research evidence in clinical decisions. *ACP Journal Club, 125*(3), A14–A16.

Hecht, L., Buhse, S., & Meyer, G. (2016). Effectiveness of training in evidence-based medicine skills for healthcare professionals: A systematic review. *BMC Medical Education, 16,* 103.

Higgins, J. P. T., & Green, S. (2008). *Cochrane handbook for systematic reviews of interventions.* New York: Wiley Cochrane Series.

Institute of Medicine. (2011a). *Clinical practice guidelines we can trust.* Washington, DC: National Academies Press.

Institute of Medicine. (2011b). *Finding what works in health care: Standards for systematic reviews.* Washington, DC: National Academies Press.

Institute of Medicine. (2012). *Primary care and public health: Exploring integration to improve population health.* Washington, DC: National Academies Press.

Institute of Medicine. (2015). *Measuring the impact of interprofessional education (IPE) on collaborative practice and patient outcomes.* Washington, DC: National Academies Press.

Institute of Medicine Committee on Behavioral and Social Sciences in Medical School Curricula. (2004). *Improving medical education enhancing the behavioral and social science content of medical school curricula.* Washington, DC: National Academies Press.

Isaacs, D., & Fitzgerald, D. (1999). Seven alternatives to evidence based medicine. *British Medical Journal, 319,* 1618.

Jacobs, J. A., Jones, E., Gabella, B. A., Spring, B., & Brownson, R. C. (2012). Tools for implementing an evidence-based approach in public health practice. *Preventing Chronic Disease, 9,* Article No. 110324.

Jenicek, M. (1997). Epidemiology, evidenced-based medicine, and evidence-based public health. *Journal of Epidemiology, 7*(4), 187–197.

Johnson, M. G., & Henley, T. (1990). *Reflections on the principles of psychology: William James after a century.* Hillsdale, NJ: Erlbaum.

Kahneman, D., & Klein, G. (2009). Conditions for intuitive expertise: A failure to disagree. *American Psychologist, 64*(6), 515–526.

Kaplan, R. M., Satterfield, J. M., & Kington, R. S. (2012). Building a better physician—The case for the new MCAT. *New England Journal of Medicine, 366,* 1265–1268.

Kohatsu, N. D., Robinson, J. G., & Torner, J. C. (2004). Evidence-based public health: An evolving concept. *American Journal of Preventive Medicine, 27*(5), 417–421.

Komossa, K., Depping, A. M., Meyer, M., Kissling, W., & Leucht, S. (2010). Second-generation antipsychotics for obsessive compulsive disorder. *Cochrane Database of Systematic Reviews, 12,* Article No. CD008141.

Lilienfeld, S. (2007). Psychological treatments that can cause harm. *Perspectives on Psychological Science, 2*(1), 53–70.

Linehan, M. M., Schmidt, H., Dimeff, L. A., Craft, J. C., Kanter, J., & Comtois, K. A. (1999). Dialectical behavior therapy for patients with borderline personality disorder and drug-dependence. *American Journal on Addictions, 8*(4), 279–292.

McKeown, T., & Lowe, C. R. (1966). *An introduction to social medicine.* Philadelphia: Davis.

Moher, D., Hopewell, S., Schulz, K. F., Montori, V., Gotzsche, P. C., Devereaux, P. J., et al. (2010). CONSORT 2010 explanation and elaboration: Updated guidelines for reporting parallel group randomized trials. *British Medical Journal, 340,* c869.

Moher, D., Liberati, A., Tetzlaff, J., Altman, D. G., & the PRISMA Group. (2009). Preferred reporting items for systematic reviews and meta-analyses: The PRISMA statement. *PLoS Medicine, 6*(7), e1000097.

Nahum-Shani, I., Smith, S. N., Spring, B. J., Collins, L. M., Witkiewitz, K., Tewari, A., et al. (2018). Just-in-time adaptive interventions (JITAIs) in mobile health: Key components and design principles for ongoing health behavior support. *Annals of Behavioral Medicine, 52*(6), 446–462.

National Cancer Institute. (2006). *Using what works: Adapting evidence-based programs to fit your needs* (NIH Publication No. 06-5874). Washington, DC: U.S. Department of Health and Human Services.

National Guideline Clearinghouse. (2017). Agency for Healthcare Research and Quality. Retrieved from *www.ahrq.gov/research/findings/factsheets/errors-safety/ngc/national-guideline-clearinghouse.html.*

Neumann, I., Brignardello-Petersen, R., Wiercioch, W., Carrasco-Labra, A. C., Cuello, C., Akl, E., et al. (2016). The GRADE evidence-to-decision framework: A report of its testing and application in 15 international guideline panels. *Implementation Science, 11,* 93.

Newhouse, R. P., Dearholt, S., Poe, S., Pugh, L. C., & White, K. (2007). *Johns Hopkins nursing evidence-based practice model and guidelines.* Indianapolis, IN: Sigma Theta Tau International.

Newhouse, R. P., & Spring, B. (2010). Interdisciplinary evidence-based practice: Moving from silos to synergy. *Nursing Outlook, 58*(6), 309–317.

Okpych, N. J., & Yu, J. L.-H. (2014). A historical analysis of evidence-based practice in social work: The unfinished journey toward an empirically grounded profession. *Social Service Review, 88*(1), 3–58.

Pellegrini, C. A., Hoffman, S. A., Collins, L. M., & Spring, B. (2014). Optimization of remotely delivered intensive lifestyle treatment for obesity using the Multiphase Optimization Strategy: Opt-IN study protocol. *Contemporary Clinical Trials, 38*(2), 251–259.

Regehr, C., Stern, S., & Shlonsky, A. (2007). Operationalizing evidence-based practice: The development of an institute for evidence-based social work. *Research on Social Work Practice, 17*(3), 408–416.

Sackett, D. L. (1969). Clinical epidemiology. *American Journal of Epidemiology, 89,* 125–128.

Sackett, D. L., Rosenberg, W. M., Gray, J. A., Haynes, R. B., & Richardson, W. (1996). Evidence-based medicine: What it is and what it isn't. *British Medical Journal, 312,* 71–72.

Satterfield, J. M., Spring, B., Brownson, R. C., Mullen, E. J., Newhouse, R. P., & Walker, B. B. (2009). Toward a transdisciplinary model of evidence-based practice. *Millbank Quarterly, 87*(2), 368–390.

Spring, B. (2007). Evidence-based practice in clinical psychology: What it is, why it matters; what you need to know. *Journal of Clinical Psychology, 63*(7), 611–631.

Spring, B. (2008). Health decision making: Lynchpin of evidence-based practice. *Medical Decision Making, 28*(6), 866–874.

Spring, B., Ferguson, M., Russell, S., Sularz, A., & Roehrig, M. (2013). Evidence-based behavioral medicine (EBBM). In M. D. Gellman & J. R. Turner (Eds.), *Encyclopedia of behavioral medicine* (pp. 718–725). New York: Springer.

Spring, B., Gotsis, M., Paiva, A., & Spruijt-Metz, D. (2013). Healthy apps: Mobile devices for continuous monitoring and intervention. *IEEE Pulse, 4*(6), 34–40.

Spring, B., & Hitchcock, K. (2009). Evidence-based practice in psychology. In I. B. Weiner & W. E. Craighead (Eds.), *Corsini's encyclopedia of psychology* (4th ed., pp. 603–607). New York: Wiley.

Spring, B., & Neville, K. (2010). Evidence-based practice in clinical psychology. In D. Barlow (Ed.), *The Oxford handbook of clinical psychology* (pp. 128–149). New York: Oxford University Press.

Spring, B., Pagoto, S., Kaufmann, P. G., Whitlock, E. P., Glasgow, R. E., Smith, T. W., et al. (2005). Invitation to a dialogue between researchers and clinicians about evidence-based behavioral medicine. *Annals of Behavioral Medicine, 30*(2), 125–137.

Stavrou, A., Challoumas, D., & Dimitrakakis, G. (2014). Archibald Cochrane (1909–1988): The father of evidence-based medicine. *Interactive Cardiovascular and Thoracic Surgery, 18*(1), 121–124.

Steglitz, J. (2017). *Online tools for evidence-based behavioral practice: A mixed-methods evaluation among graduate students and clinicians.* Doctoral dissertation, Northwestern University, Evanston, IL.

Stetler, C. B. (2001). Updating the Stetler model of research utilization to facilitate evidence-based practice. *Nursing Outlook, 49*(6), 272–279.

Straus, S. E., Glasziou, P., Richardson, W. S., & Haynes, R. B. (2011). *Evidence-based medicine: How to practice and teach it* (4th ed.). London: Churchill Livingstone Elsevier.

Thornton, T. (2006). Tacit knowledge as the unifying factor in evidence based medicine and clinical judgment. *Philosophy, Ethics, and Humanities in Medicine, 1*(1), E2.

Titler, M. G., Kleiber, C., Steelman, V. J., Rakel, B. A., Budreau, G., Everett, L. Q., et al. (2001). The Iowa model of evidence based practice to promote quality care. *Critical Care Nursing Clinics of North America, 13*(4), 497–509.

Treweek, S., Oxman, A. D., Alderson, P., Bossuyt, P. M., Brandt, L., Brozek, J., et al. (2013). Developing and evaluating communication strategies to support informed decisions and practice based on evidence (DECIDE): Protocol and preliminary results. *Implementation Science, 8,* 6.

Weaver, C. A., Warren, J. J., Delaney, C., & International Medical Informatics Association Nursing Informatics Special Interest Group (IMIA-NI, and Evidence-Based Practice Working Group). (2005). Bedside, classroom and bench: Collaborative strategies to generate evidence-based knowledge for nursing practice. *International Journal of Medical Informatics, 74*(11), 989–999.

CHAPTER 2

History and Evolution of the NIH Stage Model

Overcoming Hurdles to Create Behavioral Interventions to Improve the Public Health

LISA S. ONKEN

The NIH Stage Model is an iterative, recursive, and multidirectional model of intervention development conceived as a response to perceived obstacles and needs observed over many decades of research seeking to develop behavioral interventions[1] to alleviate drug abuse, mental health, and other behavioral health problems. Therefore, this chapter has broad relevance to clinical practitioners and scientists irrespective of the particular behavioral intervention approaches used. The Model has been updated over time, evolving as it became clear that the prevailing relatively linear approach to behavioral intervention development, designed to parallel the medications development pipeline, often did not fit or facilitate behavioral intervention development, and often failed to produce potent interventions that could be implemented successfully. It was never intended as prescriptive or restrictive model: On the contrary, it is intended to be used as a tool for intervention developers and practitioners, to help identify where an intervention falls within the full spectrum of the intervention development process, and to help identify the best next steps for successful intervention development.

The NIH Stage Model attempts to define specifically the necessary stages of behavioral intervention research for the benefit of the scientist and the practitioner. It was intended to assist practitioners in choosing which interventions to adopt, learn, and use. This is sometimes readily apparent: When an intervention has not been researched, or it has only been pilot tested, researchers and practitioners alike understand that efficacy has not yet been established and the intervention is not ready for prime time. It may be more difficult to discern whether an intervention is ready for use in practice when the intervention has been researched in full-scale randomized clinical trials, and efficacy has been established. *Efficacy* implies testing under ideal conditions, so it may not always be clear when *real-world* utility has been established, leaving practitioners uncertain about which interventions they should adopt. By fully articulating each of the steps that may be required for moving from research to practice, the NIH Stage Model helps to clarify where an intervention falls within the full spectrum of the behavioral intervention development process, allowing the practitioner to more easily determine its utility and better positioning the scientist to further develop and improve the intervention.

Clinicians may perceive some evidence-based behavioral interventions as more burdensome than helpful. For example, interventions

[1] With regard to the NIH Stage Model, the term *behavioral intervention* is broadly defined to include behavioral, psychological, cognitive, affective, interpersonal and/or psychosocial treatment, and prevention interventions.

may be excessively time-consuming to learn or they may be difficult or time-consuming to administer, or to administer correctly. By building in a focus on the usability of an intervention as early as possible in the intervention development process, the NIH Stage Model supports the development of interventions that are maximally implementable or user-friendly, such that the provider is able to provide the best help for the intervention recipient with the least burden.

If the basic scientific principles underlying an intervention are not known and are therefore not communicated to the practitioner, he or she may be (understandably) hesitant to adopt it. Even if the practitioner does decide to adopt an intervention, without knowing its underlying principles, his or her ability to deliver the intervention faithfully may be impeded, as he or she will have no means of ensuring that those principles are not violated. For the scientist, without information regarding the mechanism of action of an intervention, there may be little to inform scientific "next steps" in the intervention development process. Nonetheless, behavioral intervention clinical trials do not always or even usually examine the mechanism of action of the intervention (i.e., how and why the intervention works). The NIH Stage Model places a heavy emphasis on understanding mechanism of action, or the basic scientific principles underlying an intervention, with the goal of developing principle-driven behavioral interventions for the benefit of the clinician and the scientist.

This chapter provides a historical context for the origins of the NIH Stage Model, with the hope of shedding light on how a well-conceived conceptual framework can facilitate research on behavioral intervention development, and how using a framework that does not address important characteristics of behavioral interventions can impede this goal. The historical context should also help to clarify some of the reasons for the development of this particular conceptual framework and the importance of having a framework for behavioral intervention development that harnesses the power of basic science in pursuit of interventions that can be widely implemented.

Health Problems Linked to Behavior: The Need for Behavioral Interventions

Society always has had to grapple with issues related to human behavior and its relationship to health and the spread of disease. Suboptimal health behaviors, such as sedentary behavior, poor diet, smoking, drinking too much, as well as other poor health behaviors, are linked to many of the diseases human beings experience (Institute of Medicine [IOM], 2015; McGinnis & Foege, 1993; Schroeder, 2007). Some infectious diseases associated with behavior—for example, sexually transmitted diseases such as syphilis—are treatable with medication. However, there was no ready pharmacological solution when the country was confronted with two major epidemics in the 1980s: cocaine and AIDS. Alone, each of these epidemics gave reason for great concern. Taken together, they created a heightened sense of urgency and a demand for solutions that profoundly influenced the development of behavioral interventions.

The Cocaine Epidemic and the War on Drugs

The Drug Enforcement Administration (DEA) was established in 1973 by President Richard M. Nixon to stage "an all-out global war on the drug menace." Cocaine was not initially seen as a concern. In fact, a 1975 White House White Paper explicitly deemed cocaine *not* to be a problem, stating, "Cocaine is not physically addictive . . . and usually does not result in serious social consequences, such as crime, hospital emergency room admissions, or death." Perhaps in part because cocaine was not believed to be particularly dangerous (or even addictive), and was not a central focus of law enforcement efforts, cocaine use increased throughout the 1970s. The DEA reported that by the late 1970s, "a flood of cocaine was entering the country in Miami and being transported north to New York City and to cities and towns all along the East Coast" (*www.dea.gov/index.shtml*). In 1981, *Time* magazine characterized cocaine as a nonaddictive, appealing, and "risk-free" drug with "status," but the host of problems associated with cocaine, including depression, irritability, hallucinations and paranoia, was becoming increasingly evident and the concept of "psychological dependence" on cocaine was introduced (Demarest, 1981), concurrent with reports on the association of cocaine misuse with morbidity and mortality (King, 1981). In 1985, the *New York Times* sounded an alarm regarding a new form of cocaine, crack, that allowed new cocaine users to progress more rapidly from inhaling cocaine powder to smoking the new purified form of cocaine, or "free-basing"

(Gross, 1985). The Director of the National Institute on Drug Abuse (NIDA), Charles Schuster, exclaimed that cocaine is a highly addictive drug, and that what had been viewed as a minor concern had developed over the course of a decade into a "major public health threat" (Schuster & Fischman, 1985).

Use of cocaine had moved quickly from being perceived as relatively benign to become a major public health threat—and one with no treatment. In 1988, at a meeting convened by NIDA, experts in the drug addiction treatment field raised concerns about cocaine users appearing in emergency rooms, often with uncontrollable and even violent behavior. They raised the question: Is cocaine dependence an intractable disorder?

Whereas methadone for opiate addiction had been available for decades (Dole & Nyswander, 1965), there was no such medication available for cocaine addiction (Kleber & Gawin, 1984). High priority was given to pharmacological treatment development for cocaine dependence. In 1990, NIDA established the Medications Development Program, focusing on developing new medications for treating addiction, with a major focus on the development of a medication to treat cocaine dependence (*www.nih. gov/about/almanac/organization/nida.htm*). In 1992, NIDA released a Request for Applications (RFA), "Development of innovative methods to identify medications for treating cocaine abuse" (*http://grants.nih.gov/grants/guide/rfa-files/rfa-da-93-001.html*).

Some drug abuse treatment researchers wondered if, without a medication for cocaine dependence, it would be possible to administer a behavioral treatment to cocaine abusers. The experience with methadone showed that the drug's ability to stop highly unpleasant physical withdrawal symptoms offered some incentive for people addicted to heroin to come to the clinic. When they are receiving methadone, behavioral counseling also can be provided. With no medication for cocaine dependence, what would draw a person addicted to cocaine to the clinic? U.S. Senator Daniel Patrick Moynihan (1989) highlighted the success of methadone and its ability to allow the so-called "talk therapies" to work and argued in support of developing a "methadone clone" that pharmacologically blocks the effects of cocaine. The lack of a cocaine medication, combined with the knowledge that even if a medication were available, medication alone would be insufficient, reinforced the belief that behavioral treatments for cocaine addiction were desperately needed.

The urgent need for a solution to the cocaine epidemic spawned broad support for both a medication and behavioral treatment development for cocaine dependence. NIDA initiated a multisite cooperative agreement to study behavioral treatments for cocaine addiction. The RFA "Research Program to Maximize the Efficacy of Psychotherapy and Drug Abuse Counseling Strategies in the Treatment of Cocaine Abusers" (*http://grants.nih.gov/grants/guide/historical/1990_02_02_vol_19_no_05.pdf*) called for research on the efficacy of psychodynamic psychotherapy, cognitive-behavioral therapy, and drug counseling in the treatment of cocaine abuse. Two million dollars in first-year funds were set aside to support this project, a commitment of funds reflecting strong interest in tackling the cocaine problem, and the realistic concern that it could not be tackled, at least in the near future, with a medication.

The AIDS Epidemic

As the cocaine epidemic was gaining traction, the Centers for Disease Control and Prevention (CDC; 1981) weekly *Morbidity and Mortality Report* described five cases of pneumocystis pneumonia. In December of that same year, an article was published in the *New England Journal of Medicine* on an outbreak of 11 cases of *Pneumocystis carinii* pneumonia (Masur et al., 1981), an infection rarely seen in previously healthy individuals. These were the first publications to report on what was later to be known as the human immunodeficiency virus (HIV) and acquired immune deficiency syndrome (AIDS). Little was known about the cause of the infection, but drug abusers and gay men were identified as potentially at high risk. The IOM (1986) called for $1 billion annually to support research on the treatment and prevention of AIDS. The search for a vaccine or medications to treat the disease had been launched, but it seemed unlikely that an AIDS vaccine would be available soon. The IOM also recommended supporting research on behavioral issues, such as high-risk sexual behavior and drug use related to the spread of HIV, and recommended evaluations of the effectiveness of various "AIDS risk-reduction" interventions.

In 1987, the U.S. Food and Drug Administration (FDA) approved the first antiretroviral medication to prolong the life of individuals with HIV (Molotsky, 1987). Even so, the AIDS epidemic was raging, and by 1992, the estimated number of people age 13 years or older who were newly diagnosed with AIDS had grown from 318 in 1981, to over 75,000 annually (CDC, 2011). Beginning in the early 1980s, gay activists demanded action (Wright, 2013), arguing for, among other things, more federal funding for research and more immediate access to promising medications under development. As time wore on, more and more progress was made in medications development for HIV, and combinations of medications to treat HIV became available (Henkel, 1999). These medication regimens required that pills be taken at specific times of the day, with attention to mealtimes. Moreover, for many, the medications produced unpleasant side effects. These complex medication regimens required an exceedingly high degree of adherence, and not all individuals were able to meet the level required. There was no cure within sight. The lack of a cure for a disease that is transmitted primarily through risky behaviors and the medication adherence issues contributed to the belief that behavioral interventions were needed. They were needed to help prevent HIV, such as interventions to decrease risky behaviors associated with the spread of HIV. Interventions were also needed to encourage people to get tested for HIV and to help people found to be HIV-positive adhere to their HIV medication regimens.

Overlapping Public Health Crises and Initial Treatment and Prevention Efforts

Whereas the earliest cases of AIDS were identified in gay men and in people from Haiti, as the AIDS epidemic progressed, the link between HIV and drug use was increasingly evident. The CDC reported in 1984 that heroin users accounted for 17% of individuals with AIDS (*www.cdc.gov/mmwr/preview/mmwrhtml/00000356.htm*). Moreover, according to the DEA, in the early 1990s, heroin became purer, less expensive, and increasingly trafficked—all of which most likely contributed to a rise in heroin use (*www.dea.gov/about/history/1990-1994.pdf*). Des Jarlais and Friedman (1988) identified intravenous drug use as the second most important risk factor for AIDS in the United States and Europe, and identified an emerging problem beyond heroin use, linking cocaine use with HIV through intravenous drug use and risky sexual behavior associated with cocaine. They also highlighted preliminary studies suggesting that behavior change interventions, such as counseling and interventions in cities like Stockholm to promote testing of individuals for antibodies, might help to slow the spread of the disease. The studies by Des Jarlais and Friedman bolstered the argument that behavioral interventions might be a helpful part of the equation to deal with this deadly epidemic.

The Department of Health and Human Services (DHHS) budget for AIDS prevention and research increased dramatically each year, from $200,000 in 1981 to nearly a $1 billion in 1988 (Johnson & Coleman, 2004). The National Institute of Mental Health (NIMH) funded two Centers in 1986 to focus on HIV and the prevention of its spread. One was the Center for AIDS Prevention Studies (CAPS) at the University of California, San Francisco. The other was the HIV Center for Clinical and Behavioral Studies at the New York State Psychiatric Institute and Columbia University. By 1988, NIMH AIDS expenditures were over $327 million, and NIDA expenditures were approximately $156 million (IOM, 1994). Multiple divisions of the Alcohol, Drug Abuse and Mental Health Administration (ADAMHA) and the NIH and the CDC participated in a Program Announcement titled "Research on Behavior Change and Intervention Programs to Reduce Transmission of HIV" (*http://grants.nih.gov/grants/guide/historical/1988_10_28_Vol_17_no_35.pdf*). A couple of years later (under MH-90-06), NIMH called for a collaborative multisite study to develop behavioral prevention interventions for diverse populations at risk for HIV.

At that time, much of the leading research in behavioral drug abuse treatment development was done at three universities and did not include a focus on minimizing the spread of infectious disease. Rounsaville, Glazer, Wilber, Weismann, and Kleber (1983) at Yale University were studying the effects of interpersonal psychotherapy on methadone-maintained opiate addicts. Researchers at the University of Pennsylvania had just completed a major randomized clinical trial comparing supportive–expressive psychotherapy, a form of psychodynamic therapy developed by Lester Luborksy, with cognitive-behavioral psychotherapy, developed by Aaron Beck (Woody et al., 1983). Stitzer, Bigelow, and Liebson (1980) at Johns Hopkins were pursuing reinforcement-based approaches for treating addiction. The epidemics of AIDS, injection drug use, and cocaine provided a strong impetus for broadening support to include a focus on drug abuse treatment to help to contain the transmission of AIDS. NIDA, with an extraordinary $10 million in funds set aside, released an RFA titled "Research Demonstration Program to Reduce the Spread of AIDS by Improving Treatment for Drug Abuse" (RFA DA-89-01) (*http://grants.nih.gov/grants/guide/historical/1990_04_20_vol_19_no_16.pdf*).

The State of Behavioral Intervention Development Research: Mid-1980s–Early 1990s

By 1980, according to some estimates, over 250 forms of psychotherapy had been developed and were in use (e.g., Herink, 1980). Studies were beginning to test formally the efficacy of such interventions (e.g., Docherty & Parloff, 1984).

Results from the NIMH Treatment of Depression Collaborative Research Program (TDCRP), were first published in 1989 (Elkin et al., 1989). This groundbreaking study was the first collaborative multisite psychotherapy study initiated by the NIMH. There were two primary goals: (1) to test the feasibility and utility of the collaborative clinical trial model, a research design that had been used in the medications development field, and (2) to determine the relative effectiveness of two types of psychotherapy, cognitive-behavioral therapy and interpersonal psychotherapy. Carroll and Rounsaville (1990) argued that the "technology model," a model that "attempts to specify the treatment variable—psychotherapy—in a manner analogous to specification of a drug's formulation in pharmacological trials," as followed within the NIMH TDCRP, was an exemplary model for psychotherapy research and could be a model for the development of psychotherapies for cocaine dependence. The technology model was seen as the "gold standard" for multiple reasons, including clear delineation of the interventions, method of delivery, participants and therapists, outcomes, and so forth. This model thus informed the subsequent multisite NIDA Cocaine Cooperative Agreement (Crits-Christoph et al., 1999) on the efficacy of psychotherapies and counseling approaches for

individuals with cocaine use problems, which was initiated in 1990. And this was to become a prevailing model of psychotherapy research at both NIMH and NIDA for many years to come.

Although the model that guided the TDCRP and the Cocaine Cooperative Agreement was largely welcomed as a positive step forward, putting psychotherapy research on par with pharmacotherapy research, many psychotherapy researchers continued to believe that an important piece of the psychotherapy development process was missing. Specifically, they argued that support for the development of novel approaches had been stymied; that is, there was still no formal support for the pilot work required for the generation of new interventions. Behavioral intervention development researchers were being asked to solve extremely difficult new problems, such as finding a treatment for cocaine dependence, but they were stuck with an impossible "catch-22." Researchers could propose to conduct randomized clinical trials, and such proposals might fare well in review—if they had a compelling rationale, a solid approach, *and* promising pilot data. But how could promising pilot data be obtained without funding?

In response, NIDA convened meetings to explore new directions for behavioral/psychosocial/psychotherapy treatment development research. During these meetings, NIDA researchers consistently expressed a need for a stage of research prior to the type of full-scale efficacy testing in studies like the TDCRP and the Cocaine Cooperative Agreement. The idea was to parallel the three-phase process of medications development (see *Code of Federal Regulations*: 21 CFR 312.21). In this pharmacological model, Phase I studies, the first human studies of a new medication, provide preliminary evidence (usually with small samples) of safety and early evidence of the medication's effects, and are meant to provide enough data to lay the groundwork for a successful Phase II study; Phase II studies provide the first evidence of efficacy in the context of full-scale, highly controlled clinical trials; and Phase III studies are large-scale trials based on positive evidence of efficacy from Phase II studies. Although the psychotherapy research field conducted efficacy clinical trials research analogous to Phase II and effectiveness trials analogous to Phase III, there were no funding opportunity announcements calling for a stage of psychotherapy research analogous to Phase I medication development studies supporting the creation, modification, and pilot testing of interventions.

Mental health treatment researchers experienced the same pressure as drug abuse treatment researchers to generate new interventions for disorders that were complex or inadequately treated. Some problems required new treatments, and some existing treatments required research to identify modifications that could make them even better. Mental health and drug abuse behavioral therapy researchers independently reached the same conclusion: The field needed to generate novel treatment approaches, and federal funding was needed for a stage of research involving the generation of new, innovative approaches prior to clinical trials. This pre-Phase II type research meant that there would be a three-phase intervention development model analogous to the three-phase medication development model.

Thus, fueled by the absence of a medication to combat the cocaine problem or a pharmacological cure for HIV, the methodological advances in psychotherapy and behavioral intervention efficacy testing, and the need for better treatments for mental disorders, enthusiasm was high at NIDA and NIMH for a process of behavioral intervention development mirroring the medication development process. The generation and refinement of interventions were acknowledged as important parts of the behavioral intervention development process, and there was consensus that this early "pre-full-scale clinical trial" phase of research should be supported in addition to efficacy and effectiveness trials.

The First Stage Model

In 1992, NIDA released a program announcement for theoretically based research on the development of new, and the modification of existing, psychosocial therapies for drug dependence (*http://grants.nih.gov/grants/guide/pa-files/PA-92-110.html*). The announcement acknowledged the comparable effort of behavioral intervention development and medication development. For the first time, formal support was provided for an initial stage of behavioral intervention generation, refinement, and pilot testing.

About a year later, with the inception of the Behavioral Therapies Development Program (*http://grants.nih.gov/grants/guide/rfa-files/RFA-DA-94-002.html*), NIDA announced support for three phases[2] of intervention development paralleling the medication development process. The announcement called for a first phase to generate and modify interventions, a second phase to test efficacy, and a third phase to test real-world transferability and effectiveness. NIDA committed $3 million in support for 1994. Later that year, NIDA reaffirmed its commitment to all three necessary parts of the behavioral intervention development process (*http://grants.nih.gov/grants/guide/pa-files/PA-94-078.html*).

This original model of intervention development as described in the NIDA Behavioral Therapies Development program announcements was further described in 1997 by Onken, Blaine, and Battjes. This early NIDA model (described in both the program announcements in Onken et al., 1997) proposed three necessary aspects of intervention development: (1) the need to create, adapt, and pilot-test interventions, along with the linking creation and adaptation to basic science; (2) the efficacy testing of interventions, including testing of mechanisms of behavior change (i.e., how an intervention exerts its effects); and (3) testing of real-world effectiveness, cost-effectiveness, and issues of transportability. Based on a series of workshops convened by NIDA in 1995, 1996, and 1998, Rounsaville, Carroll, and Onken (2001) underscored the parallel process of this model to medication development, and they elaborated on the original model by delineating substages within Stage I, outlining the necessary activities and accomplishments required in Stage I to transition successfully to Stage II.

Rounsaville and colleagues (2001) provided specific guidance to researchers for submitting proposals for each stage. For example, they pro-

---

[2]It should be noted that in the original model, the word *Phase* was used to describe the steps of the behavioral intervention development process, to reinforce the parallel with the medications development pipeline. *Phase* was later replaced with *Stage* to acknowledge that there are indeed inherent differences between medication and behavioral intervention development, and that using the same word to mean different things may bring confusion at best and may foster possible errors in the research process if the intervention development processes are wrongly equated.

vided a checklist indicating what needs to be accomplished during Stage I when submitting a proposal for Stage II research, such as specify the theoretical rationale (theory of the disorder); specify the hypothesized causal chain (theory of change mechanisms); demonstrate feasibility; specify process measures, and so forth. This helped to create some consensus in the field regarding what was necessary to accomplish within Stage I research, and facilitated a common understanding among researchers in the field regarding where along the stages a research project falls.

Successes of the NIDA Stage Model

The NIDA Stage Model arguably played an important role in the evolution of the behavioral treatment research field. It provided a common conceptual framework and language, facilitating communication among scientists, the review of applications, and ultimately the successful development of interventions. The model helped to legitimize the creation of novel approaches as a valuable piece of the behavioral intervention development process. Allowing for Stage I research brought new investigators and new ideas into the field, and facilitated the successful adaptation of existing interventions into efficacious interventions for many behavioral problems.

With formal support for early-stage behavioral intervention development, the quantity of grant applications for early-stage research increased. Early-stage intervention development research was seen as a high-risk, high-reward endeavor. Just as failure is an inherent part of the medication development process, it was generally acknowledged that failure would be an inherent part of the behavioral intervention development process. Many early stage projects were bound to fail, but it was hoped that some would lead to potent new or adapted treatments.

Although there was initial skepticism that cocaine dependence could be successfully treated, efficacious interventions based on behavioral principles were developed to treat cocaine dependence (Carroll & Rounsaville, 1993; Higgins et al., 1993). Many HIV risk-reduction interventions were also shown to be efficacious in randomized clinical trials (Pequegnat & Stover, 2008). Empirically supported behavioral treatments for mental disorders were developed or improved in the early 1990s, including, for example, exposure and response prevention for obsessive–compulsive disorder (Foa, Kozak, Steketee, & McCarthy, 1992). While it cannot be known how many efficacious interventions developed were directly a result of the NIDA Stage Model, the model helped to fuel treatment innovation through the support of Stage I research. The model also appeared to help improve the quality of research proposals, presumably due to the field's mounting consensus regarding when and what stage of research was necessary, and what types of activities were appropriate for that stage. There was a substantial expansion of the range of behavioral interventions being studied, and many successful Stage II efficacy studies ensued.

As noted, much of the initial NIDA Stage Model's impact may have been related to the fact that it put in place a parallel process for behavioral intervention development and medication development. When the model was first created, many believed that this parallel process elevated the visibility and scientific credibility of behavioral intervention development. Indeed, its introduction was associated with an infusion of creativity into the field and the development of many efficacious interventions. But it could take the field only so far. Inherent in the pipeline of create→ efficacy test → effectiveness test (Stage I → Stage II → Stage III) were some striking gaps. Despite the development of efficacious interventions, very few efficacious interventions were making their way through efficacy trials to implementation in the community. One way of solving this problem might be to examine barriers to adoption of evidence-based treatment in the community, and removing those barriers. Another way of solving this problem could involve modifying the interventions to fit into the community. This begs the question: Was the original three-stage model, paralleling the medication development process, sufficient to overcome the efficacy → effectiveness → implementation gap? It was becoming increasingly apparent that the process of intervention development as described in the original three-stage model did not address all of the necessary steps for successful behavioral intervention development. More was needed to bring efficacious interventions to the community. Two things stood out: Existing research did not (1) consistently or sufficiently address the question of the mechanism of action of the intervention and (2) adequately address the ultimate implementability of the intervention, including ease of administration and likelihood of fidelity of delivery. Increased attention to mechanism of action, and to the ultimate implementability of the intervention, was heavily emphasized in the next updated conceptual framework guiding behavioral intervention development within the NIDA Stage Model.

Insufficient Attention to Mechanisms and to Ultimate Implementability

When the original NIDA Stage Model was developed, there existed hundreds of behavioral interventions, but it was not always clear how similar or how different these interventions really were. Furthermore, when it came to the generation of new interventions, it was not always clear how the "novel" ideas for interventions being proposed differed from existing ideas. This is not necessarily a bad thing. If similarities and differences are defined and acknowledged, and the goal is to build on an existing idea, new research may serve to advance the science and improve the potency of an intervention. But what if something is presented as a new and different idea, with a new name, when it is essentially the same as something that already exists? And what if many things are presented as new ideas and given different names, but are essentially the same? Did the advent of Stage I research have the unintended consequence of contributing to the proliferation of treatments that were basically the same? Aside from the obvious scientific questions and the possibility of unintended, undefined, and unclear duplication of effort, the "old wine, new bottle" problem raises practical questions for practicing clinicians. Is it helpful to have numerous versions of basically the same intervention when it has not been clearly established that the interventions are indeed basically the same? Does this leave the clinician in the position of needing to learn five, 10, or 20 different treatments for a particular problem rather than just one or two? Is it even possible for a clinician to learn, and to deliver with fidelity, 20 different treatments for a particular problem, in addition to another 10 or 20 for another problem, and so on?

Perhaps even more troubling was the fact that some treatments, which met widely used criteria for efficacy (Chambless & Hollon, 1998), were decried by some as being based on "pseudoscience" (Herbert et al., 2000). Herbert and colleagues (2000) cited eye movement desensi-

tization and reprocessing (EMDR) as a prominent example of this problem given that many believed it to work because of the principles upon which exposure therapy is based, and not because of the eye movement component, for which there was a lack of evidence. If positive randomized clinical trials alone are sufficient to deem an intervention efficacious, variants of an intervention with new but perhaps clinically unimportant bells and whistles may be deemed efficacious. But even a comparative randomized clinical trial cannot tell us whether something is truly a novel intervention, or an existing intervention in disguise.

What was needed? It became increasingly clear that the field required randomized clinical trials that included a test of the mechanism through which the intervention was purported to work. Such studies would allow the field to more easily ascertain whether something is truly novel. From a practical and scientific perspective, perhaps one of the most important questions raised is whether one intervention operates via the same or different principles as another intervention. Without knowledge gleaned from research about the mechanism responsible for the effects of the intervention, it may be impossible to know what principles underlie the intervention, or if one intervention is actually the same or different than another.

The lack of mechanisms testing is surprising given that the vast majority of early-stage intervention development projects purported to be theoretically based. Nonetheless, most intervention development studies did not explicitly test the theory on which they were based, so there was no basis to conclude that the intervention worked as hypothesized. If several apparently similar but differently named interventions are all hitting the same target and working through the same mechanism, it is probable that they are essentially the same intervention. Confirmation of theoretically derived mechanisms of action is knowledge that a scientific field can build on to produce even more potent interventions. Knowing mechanisms means knowing the principles on which an intervention is working.

In basic behavioral science, studies are designed to confirm or reject theories. They are guided by the scientific goal to understand and to determine basic processes and principles of behavior and behavior change. This perspective can help to offset the situation in which infinite types of interventions are developed, ignoring mechanisms and principles, and then tested in infinite settings and populations. In this situation, one study will not necessarily build on another, and one is left with countless interventions and countless studies. In contrast, with a merging of the practical goals of intervention developers and the scientific goals of basic behavioral scientists, the process of principle-driven behavioral intervention development can be accelerated.

Basic science questions about the mechanisms through which interventions work could be incorporated within clinical trials. It may be possible to understand, for example, that a certain group of 30 interventions affects Factor *A,* causing outcome *X,* whereas another group of 30 interventions may affect outcome *X,* but through different mechanisms, affecting Factor *C.* Now, instead of 60 different interventions, there are two different mechanisms and two different principles of behavior change that can be imparted to clinicians, bringing order to chaos. And there are two confirmed theories of behavior change on which future scientists can build.

Although the original NIDA Stage Model did encourage linking basic science to intervention development and the testing of mechanism, most behavioral intervention studies were not linked to basic science and did not test mechanism. It was becoming increasingly clear that a greater focus on mechanism of action, from the beginning to the end of the behavioral intervention development process, would benefit the treatment developers, practitioners, and ultimate implementability of the intervention. With an understanding of mechanisms, the cacophony of seemingly similar but differently named interventions for a particular problem could be replaced with clear principles of intervention success, serving both scientific and practical goals. An updated model was needed that underscored attention to mechanism as a priority throughout the entire intervention development process.

The second and related limitation that beset the behavioral intervention development field concerned the problems with penetration in routine care settings. In spite of all the progress in generating interventions that were shown to be efficacious, many interventions did not maintain their promise when subjected to larger-scale, real-world effectiveness trials. And even fewer were being successfully disseminated and implemented in the world. For example, Goisman, Warshaw, and Keller (1999) noted that despite research showing efficacy for behavioral and cognitive treatments for depression and anxiety, these treatments were offered less frequently from 1991 to 1996 than was psychodynamic therapy, a treatment that had lacked empirical validation. When treatments did get implemented, McGrew, Bond, Dietzen, and Salyers (1994) described a phenomenon called "program drift," in which intervention programs drifted in fidelity from the original model over time. The decreased positive impact of interventions from the lab to the real world has been termed the "implementation cliff" (Weisz, Ng, & Bearman, 2014).

When focused on real-world implications, one could make the argument (and many did and still do) that it is not necessary to understand mechanism, to know how or why a behavioral intervention works, if indeed the intervention is potent. After all, aspirin was being used successfully for many decades without an understanding of mechanism of action. Aspirin worked, and aspirin worked consistently. But as we have discussed, this was not always the case with behavioral interventions. Many of the behavioral interventions that were being developed, and were being shown to be efficacious, were failing to be implemented successfully in the real world. When there is lack of understanding of mechanism of action of an intervention, it is difficult to understand inconsistent results as interventions are moved into real-world settings, and to understand what the next step might be.

A focus on mechanism of action was seen as being related to implementation, but it was not seen as the sole solution to developing efficacious interventions that were also effective and transportable to the people who need them in the community. In addition, additional steps often were necessary between efficacy and effectiveness trials (e.g., returning to Stage I to improve ultimate implementability, a hybrid efficacy–effectiveness stage) that could to help to close the gap between the two. A new model addressing these issues was needed.

Updating the Model

The updated NIH Stage Model (Figure 2.1; Onken, Carroll, Shoham, Cuthbert, & Riddle, 2014) was created to address some of the problems inherent to the development of behavioral interventions and limitations of the first NIDA Stage Model, with the goals of advancing the science and helping to close the efficacy–effectiveness–implementation gap. Although initially conceived to help develop drug abuse, HIV prevention, alcohol dependence, and mental health interventions, the NIH Stage Model is broadly relevant to any form of behavioral intervention development research. Indeed, it is the conceptual framework that has informed the trans-NIH Common Fund initiative on the Science of Behavior Change (SOBC), as is evident in multiple funding opportunity announcements, such as "Use-Oriented Basic Research: Change Mechanisms of Behavioral Social Interventions" (*http://grants.nih.gov/grants/guide/pa-files/pa-12-119.html*), "Use-Inspired Basic Research to Optimize Behavior Change Interventions and Outcomes" (*http://grants.nih.gov/*

grants/guide/pa-files/pa-16-334.html), and the mechanism-focused cooperative agreement, for example, "Science of Behavior Change: Assay Development and Validation for Self-Regulation Targets (UH2/UH3)" (*http://grants.nih.gov/grants/guide/rfa-files/rfa-rm-14-020.html*). The NIH Stage Model has been adopted by the National Institute on Aging (NIA) (see *www.nia.nih.gov/research/dbsr/stage-model-behavioral-intervention-development*). The NIA is particularly interested in using this model to support research to develop potent, implementable interventions to promote the physical, emotional, and social well-being of individuals as they age. Both SOBC and NIA are also highly interested in infusing a focus on mechanisms of behavior change into the entire intervention development

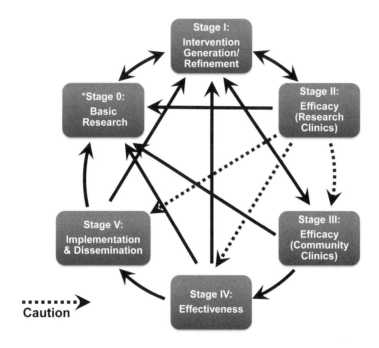

FIGURE 2.1. The updated NIH Stage Model. From Onken et al. (2014). *Stage 0* involves basic science that is presumed to be relevant to intervention development. Research on mechanisms of change is a form of basic science that can be embedded within all other stages of intervention development. *Stage I* encompasses all activities related to the creation, adaptation, and preliminary testing of an intervention. This includes materials and methods to train providers and ensure fidelity of delivery. *Stage II* (pure "efficacy" with high internal validity) research consists of experimental testing of behavioral interventions *in research settings, with research-based providers*. *Stage III* (real-world "efficacy" with high internal validity) research consists of experimental testing (high internal validity) of behavioral interventions *in community settings, with community-based providers*; a hybrid (efficacy–effectiveness) stage. *Stage IV* ("effectiveness" with high external validity) research examines evidence-based interventions in community settings, with community-based providers. *Stage V* ("implementation and dissemination") research examines strategies of implementation and adoption of empirically supported interventions in the real world.

process. This revised model emphasizes several critically important parts of the intervention development process that were not explicit, not emphasized enough, or neglected in the more medication development-like model or considered too late in the behavioral intervention development process. Three are particularly relevant to advancing evidence-based practice (EBP) in real-world settings.

First, the NIH Stage Model strongly emphasizes the infusion of use-inspired basic science wherever possible into every stage of intervention development, such that questions regarding the mechanism of action of the intervention can be addressed and principles underlying interventions can ultimately be imparted to clinicians. Although the first Stage Model did encourage linking basic science and the identification of mechanism of action with intervention development, it was rare when this was done. Moving forward, this integration of use-inspired basic science into clinical and applied intervention development is critical to achieve scientific goals, but it is at least as critical, if not even more critical, to achieve practical goals, such as developing user-friendly, principle-driven interventions.

Second, direct movement from efficacy to effectiveness is rarely successful with behavioral interventions. Though this is the typical path followed in medication development research, modifications to the Stage Model were needed to address the failures that occurred when following this path for behavioral interventions. It was not clear why something would work so well in a research setting, but not in the hands of someone in the community. What was different about the research setting? For one thing, in a rigorous research study in a research setting, providers are exquisitely trained, monitored, and supervised, such that they deliver the intervention with the highest level of fidelity.

To address this challenge, the updated NIH Stage Model requires redefinition of the earliest stage of research when an intervention is created or modified to address this challenge. In the updated model, Stage I work is considered *incomplete* without the inclusion of materials that will maximize the chances that an intervention can be delivered correctly by somebody other than the intervention developer, or his or her research team. In Stage I, researchers should develop materials to ensure adequate training of those who will deliver the intervention and materials to ensure that it be delivered with fidel-

ity. Failure to effectively train can mean failure to show effectiveness of an intervention. This is not something to be dealt with haphazardly, or later in the intervention development process, such as immediately before or during a Stage IV effectiveness trial. Similarly, methods of ensuring adequate fidelity of the intervention are also critical and need to be part of the package as the intervention is being created.

The other emphasis in the updated Stage I is a focus on the earliest possible consideration of the ultimate ease of implementation of the intervention under development. For example, perhaps at least portions of the intervention can be computerized, without negatively impacting the intervention. Or if there is a choice between training instructions in a manual and a Web-based instructional module, one might ask not just whether they are equally instructive but also which one will help more with transportability to the real world. In the updated Stage I, potency of an intervention is still paramount, but ease of implementation is to be considered up front rather than after the fact. Of course, if it would jeopardize the science, or if it is impossible to attend to these issues up front, the idea is to deal with these issues (i.e., return to Stage I) at the earliest possible point that makes sense.

Third, moving directly from Phase II to Phase III may sometimes be successful in medication development, but it simply does not work for most behavioral intervention development (100% technology-based behavioral intervention development may be one prominent exception; see Onken & Shoham, 2015). Moving directly from efficacy testing of a behavioral intervention, with research providers in a research setting, to testing with community providers in a community setting can be an insurmountable obstacle in the absence of adequate training materials for community providers and appropriate measures to ensure fidelity, and so forth.

To help ensure that an intervention can indeed move successfully from efficacy to effectiveness, in addition to defining Stage I to address implementability (which includes addressing ease of delivery, developing adequate training and fidelity materials, etc.), and encouraging the return to Stage I until implementability is sufficiently addressed, an additional type of efficacy research is defined in the updated NIH Stage Model. Stage II is efficacy research in a research setting with research providers. Stage III is efficacy research in a community setting with community providers. Explicitly defining this "hybrid" efficacy–effectiveness stage, and including it in the (albeit multidirectional) pipeline is seen as a necessity for much behavioral intervention development research. We know that it cannot be assumed that a successful Stage II efficacy study will lead to a successful effectiveness (Stage IV) study. We also know that a Stage III efficacy study should shed light on whether an intervention is efficacious in the hands of a community provider. So, in some cases, Stage III work may play a critical role in bridging the efficacy → effectiveness gap. Explicitly including Stage III in the conceptual framework forces the question: For this particular intervention being developed, is Stage III work necessary? If the answer is "yes," but training and fidelity materials have not yet been developed, another question comes up: For this particular intervention being developed, is additional Stage I work necessary (to develop materials to ensure fidelity and to train providers)? The answer to this will almost always be "yes" if training and fidelity materials are necessary but do not exist.

Implications for Contemporary EBP in Action

The focus on mechanism in the updated NIH Stage Model was seen as necessary not only to create a coherent, progressive science of intervention development but also to help with the development of principle-driven and more easily implementable interventions in the context of contemporary EBP. Said another way, an understanding of the underlying principles of behavior change is seen as critical to *both* the scientist developing the intervention and the person who ultimately delivers the intervention. Knowing the mechanism(s) of action of the intervention can help to simplify the intervention. Knowing the mechanism(s) of action can help to increase the potency of an intervention. But also, at least intuitively, it seems plausible that asking someone (e.g., a clinician) to learn a behavioral intervention (e.g., a manualized psychotherapy), without informing him or her how or why the intervention works (i.e., the mechanism of action of the intervention), is a much more difficult request than asking someone to learn that same intervention but telling him or her the important principles behind the approach. In this way, understanding the mechanism or principles of an intervention might not be just a basic science exercise, it may be something that helps

with a clinician's receptivity toward using the intervention, and it also may help with the ability to learn the intervention and deliver it with fidelity. Although this is an empirical question, some of the rationale behind the development of the NIH Stage Model and the emphasis on determining mechanism relates to the argument that knowing the mechanism(s) of action could help clinicians embrace an intervention, learn the intervention, and know just how much they can adapt it and stay true to the principles of the originally tested intervention.

The focus on training and fidelity monitoring materials also was driven by the needs of both scientists and practitioners. For the scientist, how can a randomized controlled trial (RCT) be meaningful if the intervention being tested was not delivered correctly due to inadequate training or fidelity? For the practitioner, how can one be expected to learn and deliver correctly every evidence-based treatment shown to be efficacious in a Stage II study when untested, or inadequate training and fidelity monitoring materials are available? Defining intervention development as incomplete without these materials helps to ensure that scientists work with practitioners in the community to create the most user-friendly and helpful training and fidelity monitoring procedures. In this way, utilizing the NIH Stage Model should help to ensure that practitioners are not placed in the impossible situation of learning and delivering evidence-based treatments in the absence of adequate training and fidelity materials.

Making sense of the literature on behavioral interventions is difficult, but it is even more difficult when different words are used to describe the same thing, or when the same thing is described using different words. The words *efficacy* and *effectiveness* are sometimes used to describe the same type of research, and other times are used to describe different types. A clear, common language facilitates both science and practice. The NIH Stage Model offers a common language and defines efficacy studies as the more rigorously controlled (high internal validity) clinical trials, whereas effectiveness studies have fewer controls and attempt to simulate real-world conditions (high external validity). Furthermore, the NIH Stage Model differentiates two types of efficacy studies, Stage II and Stage III, and it can be useful for the practitioner to know where an intervention is within the intervention development process. For example, if a clinician knows that an "efficacious" treatment has been shown to be efficacious Stage III, he or she might have greater confidence in the treatment than if there was only Stage II evidence. Knowing the "big picture" of where an intervention is in the intervention development process should help to inform practitioners about which interventions are ready for adoption, and which are not.

Knowing the historical context in which the NIH Stage Model evolved helps to explain some of the public health issues for which behavioral interventions were desperately needed, and why the right conceptual framework for behavioral intervention development was so important. Behaviorally related public health emergencies underscored the need for solutions, and the lack of cures for AIDS and cocaine dependence highlighted the need for behavioral interventions. The medication development pipeline was seen as a model for behavioral intervention development (reflected in the original Stage Model), and initially was extremely helpful. The field developed efficacious behavioral interventions not only for cocaine dependence and HIV prevention but also for a variety of other behavioral problems, but a very small percentage of these were implemented in the real world. The model for medication development had limitations as a model for behavioral intervention development due in part to the differences between how behavioral and pharmacological interventions are implemented in the real world. These limitations (characteristic of the original NIDA Stage Model) could only be met by requiring attention to mechanism of action and to training and fidelity monitoring of efficacious interventions throughout the behavioral intervention development process. It became clear that a framework that did not sufficiently address mechanism, fidelity, and training prior to conducting real-world RCTs impedes the transition from efficacy to effectiveness, ultimately paved the way to the implementation cliff. The NIH Stage Model was built on the achievements of the original NIDA Stage Model, incorporating changes that were seen as critical to the goal of developing potent interventions that are successfully transported to and used by the people.

The history of the evolution of the NIH Stage Model not only includes many historical successes in behavioral intervention development research but also reveals some of the stumbling blocks that prevented progress in the field, preventing efficacious interventions from being successfully implemented. The adoption of a medication development-like model, which propelled many successes, ended up impeding the successful transition from efficacy to implementation. Both the failures and successes have shaped the model's evolution. Initially created during major behaviorally related public health epidemics, within the context of skepticism regarding cures, the model has facilitated advances in both science and practice, enabling intervention researchers to develop the best behavioral interventions possible, while building a cumulative and progressive science. Equally important, it enabled clinicians to deliver the best, and most helpful, evidence-based principle-driven interventions to the people who need them most.

Summary

The cocaine epidemic and the AIDS epidemic emerged as two public health emergencies that had no known cures. When these epidemics first arose, there were no medications for cocaine dependence or AIDS. The pressing need for solutions primed the research community to embrace the potential for behavioral intervention development generally and for a specific developmental process that was on equal footing with the medication development process. Early staged models of behavioral intervention development paralleled the medication development process and helped to produce efficacious interventions. However, all too often, these interventions failed to hold up when subjected to large-scale effectiveness testing, and failed to produce actionable research for practicing clinicians. The original, more linear medication development-inspired Stage I (Phase I) → Stage II (Phase II) → Stage III (Phase III) Stage Model was replaced with the more multidirectional, iterative, recursive updated six-stage NIH Stage Model. This model infused basic science questions regarding mechanism of action of the intervention into every stage of intervention development and prioritized practical concerns regarding implementation to have a broad public health impact. Early stage (Stage I) research was defined as incomplete if important issues were left unaddressed regarding the ultimate ease of implementation of an intervention, and the training and the delivery of the intervention with fidelity in the real world. Efficacy research was defined in both research settings (Stage II) and in community settings (Stage III) to emphasize the necessity of ensuring that it is possible for an intervention to work in a community setting, to maximize the chances of success when ultimately conducting a large-scale Stage IV effectiveness study. The ultimate aim of the updated NIH Stage Model is to provide a framework for the field that builds on the successes of the past (while learning from past failures) to create stepping-stones to overcome the efficacy–effectiveness gap, and to create new opportunities for a progressive, cumulative science of behavioral intervention development. The hope is that this model will help to bring into our communities the most useful and most easy-to-administer principle-driven behavioral interventions possible.

References

Carroll, K. M., & Rounsaville, B. J. (1990). *Can a technology model of psychotherapy research be applied to cocaine abuse treatment?* (NIDA Research Monograph Series No. 104, Psychotherapy and Counseling in the Treatment of Drug Abuse, 91-104). Bethesda, MD: National Institute on Drug Abuse.

Carroll, K. M., & Rounsaville, B. J. (1993). History and significance of childhood attention deficit disorder in treatment-seeking cocaine abusers. *Comprehensive Psychiatry, 34*(2), 75–82.

Centers for Disease Control and Prevention. (1981). Pneumocystis pneumonia—Los Angeles. *Morbidity and Mortality Weekly Report, 30*(21), 250–252.

Centers for Disease Control and Prevention. (1984). CDC update on acquired immunodeficiency syndrome (AIDS)—United States. *Morbidity and Mortality Weekly Report, 33*(24), 337–339.

Centers for Disease Control and Prevention. (2011). HIV Surveillance—United States, 1981–2008. *Morbidity and Mortality Weekly Report, 60*(21), 689–693.

Chambless, D. L., & Hollon, S. D. (1998). Defining empirically supported therapies. *Journal of Consulting and Clinical Psychology, 66,* 7–18.

Crits-Christoph, P., Siqueland, L., Blaine, J., Frank, A., Luborsky, L., Onken, L. S., et al. (1999). Psychosocial treatments for cocaine dependence: Results of the NIDA Cocaine Collaborative Study. *Archives General Psychiatry, 56,* 493–502.

Das, G. (1993). Cocaine abuse in North America: A milestone in history. *Journal of Clinical Pharmacology, 33*(4), 296–310.

Demarest, M. (1981, July 6). Cocaine: Middle class high. *Time.* Retrieved from *http://content.time.com/time/covers/0,16641,19810706,00.html.*

Des Jarlais, D. C., & Friedman, S. R. (1988). HIV infection among persons who inject illicit drugs: Problems and prospects. *Journal of Acquired Immune Deficiency Syndrome, 1*(3), 267–273.

Docherty, J., & Parloff, M. (1984). Psychotherapy. *Lancet, 323,* 1074.

Dole, V. P., & Nyswander, M. (1965). A medical treatment of diacetylmorphine (heroin) addiction: A clinical trial with methadone hydrochloride. *Journal of the American Medical Association, 193,* 646–650.

Elkin, I., Parloff, M. B., Hadley, S. W., & Autry, J. H. (1985). NIMH Treatment of Depression Collaborative Research Program: Background and research plan. *Archives of General Psychiatry, 42*(3), 305–316.

Elkin, I., Shea, M. T., Watkins, J. T., Imber, S. D., Sotsky, S. M., Collins, J. F., et al. (1989). National Institute of Mental Health Treatment of Depression Collaborative Research Program: General effectiveness of treatments. *Archives of General Psychiatry, 46,* 971–982.

Foa, E. B., Kozak, M. J., Steketee, G. S., & McCarthy, P. R. (1992). Treatment of depressive and obsessive–compulsive symptoms in OCD by imipramine and behaviour therapy. *British Journal of Clinical Psychology, 31,* 279–292.

Goisman, R. M., Warshaw, M. G., & Keller, M. B. (1999). Psychosocial treatment prescriptions for generalized anxiety disorder, panic disorder, and social phobia, 1991–1996. *American Journal of Psychiatry, 156,* 1819–1821.

Gross, J. (1985, November 29). A new, purified form of cocaine cause alarm as abuse increases. *New York Times.* Retrieved from *www.nytimes.com/1985/11/29/nyregion/a-new-purified-form-of-cocaine-causes-alarm-as-abuse-increases.html?pagewanted=1.*

Henkel, J. (1999, July–August). Attacking AIDS with a "cocktail" therapy: Drug combo sends deaths plummeting. *FDA Consumer Magazine.* Retrieved from *https://permanent.access.gpo.gov/lps1609/www.fda.gov/fdac/features/1999/499_aids.html.*

Herbert, J. D., Lilienfeld, S. O., Lohr, J. M., Montgomery, R. W., O'Donohue, W. T., Rosen, G. M., et al. (2000). Science and pseudoscience in the development of eye movement desensitization and reprocessing: Implications for clinical psychology. *Clinical Psychology Review, 20,* 945–971.

Herink, R. (Ed.). (1980). *The psychotherapy handbook: The A to Z guide to more than 250 different therapies in use today.* New York: New American Library.

Higgins, S. T., Budney, A. J., Bickel, W. K., Hughes, J. R., Foerg, F., & Badger, G. (1993). Achieving cocaine abstinence with a behavioral approach. *American Journal of Psychiatry, 150*(5), 763–769.

Institute of Medicine. (1986). Confronting AIDS: Directions for public health, health care, and research. Retrieved from *www.nap.edu/catalog/938.html.*

Institute of Medicine. (2015). *Measuring the risks and causes of premature death: Summary of a workshops.* Washington, DC: National Academies Press.

Institute of Medicine, Committee on Substance Abuse and Mental Health Issues in AIDS Research. (1994).

AIDS and behavior: An integrated approach. Washington, DC: National Academies Press.

Johnson, J. A., & Coleman, S. (2004). AIDS funding for federal government programs: FY1981–FY2005, CRS Report for Congress. Retrieved from *http://fpc.state.gov/documents/organization/34819.pdf.*

King, W. (1981, June 26). Heavy use of cocaine is linked to surge in death and illnesses. *New York Times.* Retrieved from *www.nytimes.com/1981/06/26/us/heavy-use-of-cocaine-is-linked-to-surge-in-deaths-and-illnesses.html.*

Kleber, H. D., & Gawin, F. H. (1984). The spectrum of cocaine abuse and its treatment. *Journal of Clinical Psychiatry, 45,* 18–23.

Masur, H., Michelis, M. A., Greene, J. B., Onorato, I., Vande Stouwe, R. A., Holzman, R. S., et al. (1981). An outbreak of community-acquired Pneumocystis carinii pneumonia: Initial manifestation of cellular immune dysfunction. *New England Journal of Medicine, 305,* 1431–1438.

McGinnis, J. M., & Foege, W. H. (1993). Actual causes of death in the United States. *Journal of the American Medical Association, 270,* 2207–2212.

McGrew, J. H., Bond, G. R., Dietzen, L., & Salyers, M. (1994). Measuring the fidelity of implementation of a mental health program model. *Journal of Consulting and Clinical Psychology, 62*(4), 670–678.

Molotsky, I. (1987, March 21). U.S. approves drug to prolong lives of AIDS patients. *New York Times.* Retrieved from *www.nytimes.com/1987/03/21/us/us-approves-drug-to-prolong-lives-of-aids-patients.html.*

Moynihan, D. P. (1989, February 26). Yes, we do need a "methadone clone." *New York Times.* Retrieved from *www.nytimes.com/1989/02/26/opinion/yes-we-do-need-a-methadone-clone.html.*

Onken, L. S., Blaine, J. D., & Battjes, R. J. (1997). Behavioral therapy research: A conceptualization of a process. In S. W. Henggeler & A. B. Santos (Eds.), *Innovative approaches for difficult-to-treat populations* (pp. 477–485). Arlington, VA: American Psychiatric Press.

Onken, L. S., Carroll, K. M., Shoham, V., Cuthbert, B. N., & Riddle, M. (2014). Reenvisioning clinical science: Unifying the discipline to improve the public health. *Clinical Psychological Science, 2,* 22–34.

Onken, L. S., & Shoham, V. (2015). Technology and the stage model of behavioral intervention development. In L. Marsch, S. Lord, & J. Dallery (Eds.), *Behavioral healthcare and technology: Using science-based innovations to transform practice* (pp. 3–12). New York: Oxford University Press.

Pequegnat, W., & Stover, E. (2008). Payoff from AIDS behavioral prevention research. In K. H. Mayer & H. Pizer (Eds.), *HIV prevention: A comprehensive approach* (pp. 169–202). London: Elsevier.

Rounsaville, B. J., Carroll, K. M., & Onken, L. S. (2001). NIDA's stage model of behavioral therapies research: Getting started and moving on from Stage 1. *Clinical Psychology: Science and Practice, 8,* 133–142.

Rounsaville, B. J., Glazer, W., Wilber, C. H., Weismann, M. M., & Kleber, H. D. (1983). Short-term interpersonal psychotherapy in methadone-maintained opiate addicts. *Archives of General Psychiatry, 40,* 629–663.

Schroeder, S. A. (2007). We can do better—improving the health of the American people. *New England Journal of Medicine, 357,* 1221–1228.

Schuster, C. R., & Fischman, M. W. (1985). Characteristics of humans volunteering for a cocaine research project. In N. J. Kozel & E. H. Adams (Eds.), *Cocaine use in America: Epidemiologic and clinical perspectives* (NIDA Research Monograph No. 61). Bethesda, MD: National Institute on Drug Abuse.

Stitzer, M. L., Bigelow, G. E., & Liebson, I. (1980). Reducing drug use among methadone maintenance clients: Contingent reinforcement for morphine-free urines. *Addictive Behavior, 5,* 333–340.

Weisz, J. R., Ng, M. Y., & Bearman, S. K. (2014). Odd couple?: Reenvisioning the relation between science and practice in the dissemination-implementation era. *Clinical Psychological Science, 2,* 58–74.

Woody, G. E., Luborsky, L., McLellan, A. T., O'Brien, C. P., Beck, A. T., Blaine, J., et al. (1983). Psychotherapy for opiate addicts: Does it help? *Archives of General Psychiatry, 40,* 639–645.

Wright, J. (2013). Only your calamity: The beginnings of activism by and for people with AIDS. *American Journal of Public Health, 103*(10), 1788–1798.

CHAPTER 3

The Insufficiently Appreciated Raison d'être of Evidence-Based Practice

SCOTT O. LILIENFELD
LORIE A. RITSCHEL
STEVEN JAY LYNN
ROBERT D. LATZMAN

Henry Cotton (1869–1933), superintendent of Trenton State Hospital in New Jersey from 1907 until 1930, was convinced that he had achieved a stunning breakthrough in the treatment of psychotic disorders. When Cotton spoke, many people listened, and for good reason. His academic credentials were impeccable: As a young psychiatrist at Worcester State Psychiatric Hospital in Massachusetts, he was supervised by Adolf Meyer, one of the pioneers of early psychiatry, and later, during a stint in Munich, he studied under two other giants of psychiatry and neurology: Emil Kraepelin and Alois Alzheimer (Davidson, 2016). Inspired by the then recent discovery that general paresis, long presumed to be a mental disorder, was actually caused by the syphilis spirochete (a type of bacterium), Cotton became enamored with the "focal infection" theory. According to this theory, schizophrenia and other serious mental illnesses stem from *chronic sepsis*—a severe and lasting response to bacterial infection—in specific body sites.

Desperate ailments often call for desperate measures. Following the focal infection theory to its logical—or perhaps more accurately, illogical—conclusion, Cotton insisted that the only effective treatment for severe psychopathology was surgical removal of the offending body parts (Scull, 2005). While at Trenton, Cot-ton began by excising his psychiatric patients' teeth. Initially, the psychological outcomes were less than remarkable, so Cotton upped the ante to more directly target the ostensible root causes of his patients' infections, moving on to removing his patients' tonsils. After doing so, he noticed that many of his psychotic patients now began to improve. Encouraged by these seemingly more promising results, he began extirpating other organs, including stomachs, large intestines, spleens, gallbladders, uteruses, ovaries, and testicles (Jones, 2005); he and his surgeons performed 645 colectomies alone. When his radical operations failed to improve his patients' symptoms, Cotton routinely attributed the negative results to the fact that he had not removed enough infected body tissue (Scull, 2005).

Relying exclusively on his clinical judgment and informal observations of what he took to be improvement in patients' symptoms, Cotton reported cure rates approaching 85%. In a 1921 invited address at Princeton University, he described his results as astonishing (Scull, 2005). Many others were equally impressed. In an upbeat appraisal in 1922, the *New York Times* asserted that Cotton's "brilliant leadership" and innovative techniques offered "high hope . . . for the future," and his mentor Adolf Meyer wrote, "He [Cotton] appears to have brought out palpable results not attained by any previous or contemporary attack on the grave problems of mental disorder" (see Cotton, 1922, p. 3361).

Over time, however, Cotton's methods began to receive increasing scrutiny and searing criticism from his psychiatric colleagues. He appeared nonplussed by the fact that his surgeries were associated with a death rate of 30% or higher, contending that these mortality percentages were attributable to the poor baseline physical health of his severely deteriorated patients. Eventually, but all too belatedly, Cotton's star faded as it became glaringly evident that his findings could not be replicated by other surgeons and were based on grossly suboptimal evidence (Charuvastra, 2006). The number of psychiatric patients killed by his barbaric interventions will forever remain unknown.

The Cotton tragedy raises an obvious but painful question: How could so many intelligent scholars have been so disastrously mistaken?

The Enduring Lessons of Henry Cotton

One might be tempted to dismiss Henry Cotton as sadistic, but this interpretation would be too facile. Cotton was a tireless advocate of humane treatment, freeing his patients from physical restraints and providing them with more frequent care from social workers, nurses, and occupational therapists.

More importantly, the tragic tale of Henry Cotton, although gruesome, is hardly isolated. The at times checkered histories of psychiatry and psychology are sobering reminders that intelligent, well-educated, and well-intentioned people can be fooled into believing that ineffective or even harmful treatments work. Many people today forget that the term *snake pit,* a colloquial phrase describing a dilapidated mental hospital, derived from the practice of placing psychiatric patients in pits and tossing snakes at them to terrify them out of their madness (Szasz, 2006). Through the 17th to 19th centuries, blistering, purging, induced vomiting, and bleeding were widely regarded as effective treatments for mental disorders, as were the tranquilizing chair, spinning chair, Utica crib, ice water baths, and a host of other interventions that we today rightly regard as horrifyingly unethical (Grove & Meehl, 1996). For example, the tranquilizing chair, invented by Benjamin Rush, a signer of the U.S. Declaration of Independence, who is often considered the "founder

of American psychiatry," strapped psychiatric patients in a rigid chair, covering their face with a box-like contraption (El-Adl, 2011). The rationale was that immobilizing patients for hours would stabilize their circulatory systems, somehow resulting in improvement. More recently, as we discuss later, prefrontal lobotomy was extensively promoted as a beneficial intervention for schizophrenia and severe depression in the middle decades of the past century despite a virtually wholesale absence of compelling evidence for its effectiveness and troubling indications of disastrous psychological side effects (Valenstein, 1986).

We might assume that such horrific practices were the legacies of bygone and benighted eras, and that we have at long last turned the corner and arrived at a more enlightened age. Although there is a kernel of truth to this sanguine appraisal, this Whiggish depiction of psychiatric history overlooks the fact that the same pitfalls in reasoning that led scores of intelligent mental health experts of the past to be misled by ineffective interventions remain very much a part of our cognitive apparatus today. The heuristics and biases that contributed to the horrific treatment errors of previous generations continue to haunt us, although, fortunately, most of our contemporary missteps are less egregious.

We might also assume that ill-advised treatment decisions are relevant only to somatic interventions, such as prefrontal lobotomy, but not to psychotherapy. This conclusion would again be erroneous. Although many people appear to believe that psychological treatments are at worst innocuous, growing evidence suggests that certain psychological interventions, such as crisis (critical incident stress) debriefing for individuals exposed to potentially traumatic events, suggestive techniques for recovering memories of early child sexual abuse, and Scared Straight interventions for at-risk adolescents, carry a nontrivial risk of harm to many clients (Barlow, 2004; Dimidjian & Hollon, 2010; Lilienfeld, 2007, in press). Yet many of these methods continue to be widely administered despite scientific evidence of potential *iatrogenic* (treatment provider-generated) effects.

Evidence-Based Practice: The Three-Legged Stool

More broadly, the Cotton story, along with other treatment errors in psychiatry and psychology, underscores a crucial but often overlooked point: Without the procedural safeguards afforded by evidence-based practice (EBP), we can *all* be readily deceived by ineffective or harmful interventions. As observed elsewhere in this volume (see Spring, Marchese, & Steglitz, Chapter 1), EBP is a revolutionary concept that originated in Canadian and British medicine in the 1990s (Guyatt et al., 1992; Rosenberg & Donald, 1995; Sackett, Rosenberg, Gray, Haynes, & Richardson, 1996), largely in response to the "recognition that physicians had tended to prioritize tradition and personal experience, giving rise to troubling variation in treatment quality" (Rousseau & Gunía, 2016, p. 671).

Although, to our knowledge, EBP was not directly influenced by psychological research, we can conceptualize it as a logical extension of classic writings on the clinical–statistical debate (Grove & Meehl, 1996; Meehl, 1954). This debate, now long since resolved by large bodies of research evidence, reminds us that statistical predictions of behavior (e.g., client improvement following therapy) derived from preexisting data almost always exceed or, at worst, equal subjective predictions in their accuracy. Hence, treatment selections informed by well-controlled data are more likely to be accurate than those informed by informal clinical observations or clinical intuition, although the latter may sometimes be useful in generating hypotheses to be tested, either formally in controlled studies or informally in therapy sessions.

EBP is commonly regarded as resembling a three-legged stool. This stool consists of (1) the best available research evidence bearing on the *efficacy* (the extent to which an intervention works under controlled conditions) and *effectiveness* (the extent to which an intervention works in real-world settings) of psychological interventions (see Seligman, 1995, for a discussion of the efficacy–effectiveness distinction), (2) clinical expertise, and (3) client preferences and values (Anderson, 2006; Spring, 2007). EBP therefore refers *not* to a body of well-established therapeutic techniques (Thyer & Pignotti, 2011), but rather to a systematic *approach* to appraising research evidence and applying it to clinical work.

EBP traditionally regards research evidence as being arrayed along a hierarchy of evidential certainty, with case study data at the bottom, reflecting more susceptibility to sources of methodological error and therefore greater un-

certainty; correlational and quasi-experimental data toward the middle; and randomized controlled trials (RCTs) and meta-analyses at the top, reflecting less susceptibility to methodological error and therefore greater certainty. Nevertheless, even conclusions derived from rigorous RCTs and meta-analyses should not be regarded as gospel, especially in light of growing evidence that questionable research practices of many kinds exist. For example, selective reporting of data or a variety of "*p*-hacking techniques," including post hoc transformations of variables or exclusion of various outliers until test statistics fall below the sacred $p = .05$ threshold for statistical significance, can contribute to replication failures (for discussion, see John, Lowenstein, & Prelec, 2012; Lilienfeld & Waldman, 2018; Simmons, Nelson, & Simonsohn, 2011). Still, because well-conducted RCTs help to remove more sources of inferential error, such as regression to the mean, spontaneous remission, and placebo effects (see the section "EBP as a Safeguard against Errors in Clinical Inference: Causes of Spurious Therapeutic Effectiveness") than do other research designs, generally they are more likely to yield replicable findings (Ioannidis, 2005).

The three-legged stool of EBP is a reasonable starting point for decision making, although it is conspicuously silent with respect to delineating what constitutes clinical expertise. This omission is problematic given that the association between amount of experience as a therapist and therapeutic effectiveness is at best modest (Dawes, 1994; Tracey, Wampold, Lichtenberg, & Goodyear, 2014). Furthermore, EBP itself is agnostic with respect to which, if any, of the three legs of the stool should be prioritized in treatment decisions. In its delineation of the nature and scope of EBP, the American Psychological Association (2005) Task Force on EBP opted not to adopt an explicit stance on this issue, implying that none of the three legs should be privileged above any other. In contrast, the Canadian Psychological Association (2002) has staked out a decisive position in this regard, asserting that "evidence-based practice relies, first and foremost, on research findings published in the peer-reviewed scientific literature including, at a minimum, treatment process and treatment outcome research" (p. 7).

We side with the CPA in this debate. In our view, what makes EBP distinctive from other approaches to clinical decision making is its research leg. From this perspective, clinical decisions concerning which treatments to administer should ideally be grounded in the best available research evidence regarding therapeutic efficacy and effectiveness.

The past 15 years have witnessed a host of lively debates regarding the proper role of EBP in psychotherapy training and practice. Most of these discussions have centered on the research leg of the EBP stool. Among other things, scholars have differed over whether the current criteria for evidence-based interventions are sufficiently rigorous; whether these criteria are biased in favor of short-term interventions (e.g., behavior therapy), which tend to be easier to investigate, and biased against long-term interventions (e.g., psychoanalysis), which tend to be more challenging to investigate; whether EBP criteria and lists should emphasize underlying principles of change (e.g., inhibitory learning; see Craske et al., 2008) rather than trademarked psychotherapies (e.g., Thought Field Therapy); and whether current operationalizations of the research leg of the EBP stool overemphasize specific therapeutic ingredients, such as cognitive restructuring, at the expense of nonspecific ingredients, such as the therapeutic alliance and induction of expectations for improvement (for a selective sampling of diverse viewpoints on EBP, see Barlow, 2004; Chambless & Ollendick, 2001; Laska, Gurman, & Wampold, 2014; Rosen & Davison, 2003; Shedler, 2015; Wachtel, 2010; Weisz, Weersing, & Henggeler, 2005; Westen, Novotny, & Thompson-Brenner, 2004).

By and large, we regard these lively, albeit at times polemical, debates as healthy for the field. Nevertheless, we do not intend to address, let alone resolve, them here. Instead, in the remainder of this chapter, we aim to address a substantially different, but critical, question that we believe has been accorded insufficient attention: Why is EBP needed in the first place?

Surprisingly, even many otherwise excellent guides to EBP in medicine and other health care domains have accorded short shrift to this question, or have not addressed it all (e.g., Straus, Glasziou, Richardson, & Haynes, 2011). This omission is regrettable. We contend that for students and trainees to grasp EBP adequately, they must first appreciate its core rationale. This rationale, we argue, is that EBP, especially its research leg, affords the best set of tools that clinical scientists have developed to minimize errors in clinical inference and thereby reach more scientifically accurate decisions. These decisions, in turn, should enhance client care.

Eminence-Based Practice versus EBP

With tongues planted firmly in cheek, two authors (Isaacs & Fitzgerald, 1999) distinguished seven alternatives to evidence-based medicine. "There are," they assured readers wary of EBP, "plenty of alternatives for the practicing physician in the absence of evidence" (p. 1618). Among these alternatives are eminence-based medicine, eloquence-based medicine (also known as "elegance-based medicine"), vehemence-based medicine, and confidence-based medicine, with the lattermost jokingly proposed to be specific to surgeons. Continuing to pull gullible readers' legs, the authors proposed "markers" and "measuring devices" for each form of practice. For example, in contrast to evidence-based medicine, for which the typical marker and measuring devices are the RCT and meta-analyses, respectively, for eminence-based medicine, they are "radiance of white hair" and "luminometer" (p. 1618), respectively.

Although the article is satirical, it manages to drive home a serious point: EBP is hardly the only approach to clinical decision making. In particular, one must differentiate EBP from what the authors humorously dubbed eminence-based medicine, more formally and more broadly termed *authority-based practice* (Gambrill, 2001). In this form of practice, pronouncements regarding which treatments to administer are handed down from supervisors to trainees in an *ex cathedra* fashion, much like papal bulls, typically with scant discussion of the scientific quality of the evidence for each treatment or how such evidence was obtained.

The modal approach to teaching EBP in clinical psychology and psychiatry training programs, we suspect, closely approximates eminence-based (authority-based) practice. In the course of their classroom learning and practicum training, students and trainees learn which interventions are best supported by research evidence and are taught how to administer them. A similar approach almost surely applies to the teaching of EBP in most continuing education courses for practicing clinicians. We term this top-down model of psychotherapy education and training the *protocol-based approach* (Lilienfeld, Ritschel, Lynn, Cautin, & Latzman, 2013).

The protocol-based approach is important, even essential, in the education and training of clinical psychologists, psychiatrists, social workers, and other mental health professionals. After all, to help their clients, students and practicing clinicians must learn how to deliver interventions properly. Nevertheless, we maintain that this approach is insufficient, especially if one aims to help students become discerning consumers of the psychotherapy process and outcome literature, who can modify their treatment decisions accordingly in response to novel research evidence. We therefore contend that the protocol-based approach to instruction should be supplemented with a *rationale-based approach* (Lilienfeld et al., 2013). In the rationale-based approach, which we adopt in this chapter, instructors first discuss ubiquitous errors in causal inference to which all people, including experienced clinicians, researchers, and instructors, are prone (see Meehl, 1993), and proceed to explain how EBP helps to compensate for these errors. In addition, in this approach, student concerns and objections regarding EBP are actively elicited and addressed respectfully. In this respect, a rationale-based approach accords broadly with the *activation method* identified in the science education literature as an effective means of dispelling misconceptions (Kowalski & Taylor, 2009). Using this method, misconceptions and other misunderstandings are neither ignored nor dismissed, but instead are actively elicited and respectfully rebutted with accurate information.

Mental Health Professionals' Resistance to EBP: Survey Evidence

A substantial or even exclusive emphasis on a protocol-based approach in clinical training and ongoing professional education programs neglects the point that many students and clinicians appear to be reluctant to embrace the core tenets of EBP. Indeed, survey data on mental health professionals in training, as well as current mental health professionals, suggest that large proportions of professionals are at best ambivalent regarding EBP (see Lilienfeld et al., 2013, for a review).

Admittedly, the evidence on this front is mixed and, at first blush, contradictory. On the one hand, survey data reveal that when asked in the abstract how they feel about EBP, many clinicians are reasonably positive (e.g., Borntrager, Chorpita, Higa-McMillan, & Weisz, 2009; Gray, Joy, Plath, & Webb, 2015). On the other hand, large proportions of clinicians report that they do not view research on psychotherapy

process or outcome to be especially crucial, nor do they regard such research as especially relevant to their clinical decision making or clinical work more broadly.

For example, in a survey of 508 members of American Psychological Association Division 12 (Society of Clinical Psychology), Stewart and Chambless (2007) found that participants agreed only modestly (mean of 3.09 on a 1- to 7-point scale, ranging from 1 = *Strongly Agree* to 7 = *Strongly Disagree*) that controlled research on psychotherapy informs their practice. They rated "current research on treatment outcome" as somewhat influential in their treatment decisions (2.86 on the same scale) but less influential than past clinical experiences (1.53) or colleagues' advice (2.70). Similarly, in a survey of 181 members of American Psychological Association Division 42 (Psychologists in Private Practice), Boisvert and Faust (2006) found that participants expressed moderate agreement (5.05 on a 7-point scale) with the statement that "most therapists learn more about effective therapeutic techniques from their experience than from the research" (p. 712).

In addition, in a study of 400 licensed clinical social workers in the United States, Pignotti (2010) asked practitioners to use a 1- to 7-point scale to rate reasons for selecting treatments. The most highly rated reasons were "Clinical experience with positive results that held up over time" ($M = 6.50$); "Compatibility with your theoretical orientation" ($M = 5.65$); "Compatibility with your personality" ($M = 5.63$); "Clinical experience of fast, positive results with clients" ($M = 5.45$); "Intervention emotionally resonated for you" ($M = 5.20$); "Endorsement by respected professional" ($M = 5.01$); "Your intuition" ($M = 4.95$); and "Colleagues' reports of success" ($M = 4.84$). Receiving a lower rating was "Favorable research in peer-reviewed journals" ($M = 4.74$). A more recent survey of 364 social workers in Australia (Gray et al., 2015) revealed that although 85% of respondents concurred that EBP enhances client care, approximately one-third voiced criticisms regarding EBP. Narrative comments from survey participants pointed to concerns that EBP is based exclusively on RCTs or that subjective clinical judgment and anecdotal observations are often superior to controlled research evidence (see also the section "Widespread Misconceptions Regarding EBP").

Data further point to sizable pockets of resistance toward EBP among graduate students.

Luebbe, Radcliffe, Callands, Green, and Thorn (2007) found that graduate students in U.S. clinical psychology programs were less than enthusiastic when asked whether they desired more integration of EBP within their coursework ($M = 3.13$ on a 1- to 5-point scale) and practicum work ($M = 3.37$). They were more supportive, however, when asked whether they "agree with (the) general principles" of EBP ($M = 3.90$; see also VanderVeen, Reddy, Veilleux, January, & DiLillo, 2012).

On balance, the survey research on mental health professionals' attitudes toward EBP suggests that although most respondents, in principle, appear to be favorably disposed to EBP, they tend to weigh informal sources of evidence, such as clinical experience and clinical intuition, more highly than controlled research data in their treatment decisions. Surprisingly, our field has paid relatively little heed to the reasons for these preferences. Although many of these data derive from studies that are approximately a decade old, there are clear indications that many of these attitudes have persisted over time (Lilienfeld et al., 2013). Although there are multiple sources of resistance to EBP, we focus on two especially important sources here: (1) misconceptions regarding EBP and (2) psychological challenges to accurately appraising and interpreting client change, which in turn predispose mental health professionals and researchers alike to a host of causes of *spurious therapeutic effectiveness,* the latter defined as the inference that treatments work even they do not (Lilienfeld, Ritschel, Lynn, Cautin, & Latzman, 2014).

Widespread Misconceptions Regarding EBP

Much of the resistance to EBP is almost certainly borne of understandable misconceptions concerning this approach. Some of these misunderstandings in turn probably stem in part from the failure of EBP advocates to adequately disseminate the central rationale for EBP. Here, we address 11 prevalent misconceptions regarding EBP (see also Gibbs & Gambrill, 2002; Lilienfeld et al., 2013). As we will discover, several of these misconstruals contain a kernel of truth, although each mischaracterizes EBP in some significant way, shape, or form. We present each statement not in the form of a misconception, but rather in the form of an assertion that dispels it.

EBP Differs from Empirically Supported Therapies

EBP is routinely confused with another three-letter acronym beginning with "E," namely empirically supported therapies (ESTs; see Luebbe et al., 2007, for data demonstrating confusion regarding these concepts among clinical psychology graduate students). Despite their superficial similarity, these concepts are quite different (Westen et al., 2004). Specifically, ESTs, which refer to interventions that have been found to be efficacious for specific psychological disorders in either RCTs or systematic within-in-subject designs, are merely one instantiation of the research leg of the EBP stool (Chambless & Hollon, 1998; Chambless & Ollendick, 2001). One can in principle wholeheartedly embrace EBP while rejecting some or even many of the treatments that are presently classified as ESTs by Division 12 of American Psychological Association or other professional organizations.

EBP Is Agnostic about the Utility of Untested Interventions

EBP, and its research leg in particular, is agnostic regarding whether treatments that have not been subjected to adequate scientific tests will ultimately prove to be efficacious or effective. The often neglected distinction between *invalidated* and *unvalidated* interventions is critical in this regard (Arkowitz & Lilienfeld, 2006). The former treatments have been examined in controlled trials and found not to work; the latter treatments have not been examined, or at least not sufficiently, in controlled trials. The fact that a treatment is currently unvalidated does not mean that it cannot later be assimilated within the research leg of EBP; it means only that its proponents must await adequate scientific evidence before the treatment can be considered for admission into the catalogue of evidence-supported interventions.

EBP Allows for Creativity in Treatment Development

Some critics maintain that EBP stifles innovativeness in the development and testing of novel interventions (Bohart, 2000). To the contrary, EBP places certain constraints only on the administration of treatments, not on their invention. EBP allows practitioners and researchers to create and pilot-test new treatments, with the crucial caveat that clients who receive these interventions should be granted the opportunity to provide full informed consent, including an explicit acknowledgment that these treatments are experimental (Thyer & Pignotti, 2011; see also Blease, 2015; Blease, Lilienfeld, & Kelley, 2016).

EBP Allows for Flexibility in Treatment Administration

Widespread assertions to the contrary, EBP does not necessitate a "cookie-cutter" or "one-size-fits-all" approach to treatment administration (Bohart, 2000). Furthermore, although most ESTs are manualized, the majority of treatment manuals consist of well-delineated guidelines for therapist activities across sessions rather than strict rules for specific therapist behaviors within each session. Indeed, most treatment manuals afford therapists substantial leeway in deciding when and how to deliver interventions (O'Donohue, Ammirati, & Lilienfeld, 2011). In this regard, Kendall, Gosch, Furr, and Sood (2008) proposed "flexibility within fidelity" as a rubric for the administration of evidence-supported treatments. Using this middle-ground approach, practitioners are expected to follow the basic guidelines prescribed by treatment manuals, while avoiding rigid conformity to specific therapeutic protocols. Some evidence suggests that such unbending adherence is linked to poor treatment outcomes (Castonguay, Goldfried, Wiser, Raue, & Hayes, 1996; Owen & Hilsenroth, 2014), although the causal nature of this association is unclear (e.g., less competent therapists may be inclined to hew more rigidly to treatment protocols than are more competent therapists).

EBP Allows for Nonspecific Influences in Psychotherapy

The misconception that EBP focuses largely or entirely on specific therapeutic ingredients (see Messer, 2004) contains a kernel of truth, but it reflects a confusion between EBP and ESTs. ESTs emphasize specific ingredients that differentiate psychotherapies, but at least in principle, EBP incorporates *all* research evidence relevant to therapy outcomes (Thyer & Pignotti, 2011). As a consequence, EBP can subsume evidence concerning the therapeutic alliance, therapist empathy, relationship factors, inculcation of expectancies for improvement, and other nonspecific treatment factors. The research evidence is clear that such variables are important to therapeutic outcomes (Hofmann & Curtis, 2014; Wampold & Imel, 2015) and, for certain conditions (e.g., major depressive disorder), arguably are more predictive of outcomes than specific therapeutic modalities themselves (Cuipers, van Straten, Andersson, & van Oppen, 2008). Moreover, in principle, it is entirely possible to conduct rigorous clinical trials on the efficacy of nonspecific therapeutic approaches.

EBP Is Generalizable

Many authors contend that EBP is likely to generalize only to clients who have been examined in controlled studies. For example, some critics (e.g., Westen et al., 2004) have raised concerns that evidence-supported interventions are unlikely to generalize beyond patients with "pure" conditions (e.g., major depressive disorder) to those with multiple conditions (e.g., major depressive disorder with co-occurring social phobia). To be sure, questions regarding the generalizability of efficacy studies to effectiveness have yet to be conclusively resolved. Nevertheless, in science, including clinical science, at least some reasonable basis for generalization is almost invariably better than none. As psychologist Donald Campbell (1986) observed, generalization from one set of conditions to others inevitably occurs along a "gradient of similarity." Hence, if we have gathered evidence that Treatment X is efficacious for individuals with generalized anxiety disorder, it is almost always more prudent to administer Treatment X to a client with co-occurring generalized anxiety disorder and major depression than to start afresh with an entirely new, untested treatment.

Framing it somewhat differently, clinical science at its best minimizes, although it does not eliminate, uncertainty in our clinical inferences (McFall & Treat, 1999; O'Donohue, Lilienfeld, & Fowler, 2007). Therefore, when selecting treatments, it is almost always better to extrapolate from studies conducted on somewhat similar individuals than to start from scratch. Furthermore, growing evidence suggests that data from rigorously designed efficacy studies do often translate reasonably well to real-world settings (Hans & Hiller, 2013; Hedman et al., 2013; McHugh, Murray, & Barlow, 2009), which motivated the NIH Stage Model (Onken, Chapter 2, this volume).

EBP Includes Evidence Other Than Data Derived from RCTs

Despite what some mental health professionals believe (see Gray et al., 2015), EBP does not neglect research evidence other than RCTs. As discussed earlier, EBP regards research designs as falling along a hierarchy of evidentiary certainty. Although RCTs occupy a higher stratum in this hierarchy than do other sources of research evidence owing to their methodological rigor (see Brush & Halperin, 2016, for a rebuttal of common criticisms of RCTs), other sources of evidence, such as systematic within-subject designs and rigorously conducted quasi-experimental studies, can and often should be considered in EBP. For example, for low-base-rate psychological conditions, large-sample RCTs often are not be feasible, so within-subject designs are frequently a more realistic means of ascertaining treatment efficacy. EBP can also incorporate therapy process data, which can provide helpful information concerning mediators and potential mechanisms of change (Ghaemi, 2009).

The Dodo Bird Verdict Does Not Pose a Serious Challenge to EBP

The Dodo Bird Verdict (Rosenzweig, 1936; see also Wampold et al., 1997), is named after the Dodo Bird in Lewis Carroll's *Alice in Wonderland,* who declared that "everybody has won and all must have prizes." This hypothesis posits that all psychotherapies are equivalent in their effects. A number of authors have invoked the Dodo Bird Verdict to challenge the rationale for EBP (e.g., Duncan, Miller, & Sparks, 2011). If all therapies are equal in their effects, they maintain, the research leg of EBP is unnecessary given that treatment choice does not matter.

An insufficiently appreciated point is that the Dodo Bird Verdict applies to two distinct assertions: (1) Collapsing across all disorders, there is no evidence for differences in efficacy across treatments (namely, no main effects) and (2) there is no evidence that any treatment is more efficacious than any other for any disorder (namely, no statistical interactions). Given that there are at least 600 "brands" of psychotherapy (McKay & Lilienfeld, 2015) and approximately 300 diagnoses in DSM-5 (American Psychiatric Association, 2013), acceptance of the second assertion would necessitate acceptance of the ut-

terly remarkable claim that all 180,000 (600 × 300) treatment-by-disorder combinations yield precisely equal statistical interactions.

Setting aside the exceedingly low a priori likelihood of the equivalence of all treatment-by-disorder interactions, there is ample evidence that the Dodo Bird Verdict, at least when stated boldly in the form of the second assertion, is false (Hunsley & DiGuilio, 2002; Lilienfeld, 2014b; cf. Shedler, 2010). For example, studies demonstrate that behavioral and cognitive-behavioral treatments are more efficacious than other treatments for at least some conditions, such as anxiety disorders (Tolin, 2010), bulimia nervosa (Poulsen et al., 2014), and childhood and adolescent disorders (Chambless & Ollendick, 2001; Weisz, Weiss, Han, Granger, & Morton, 1995).

Furthermore, in either the first or the second assertion, the Dodo Bird Verdict applies only to the minority of psychotherapies that have been examined systematically in controlled trials. Even if all extensively studied psychotherapies turned out to be equally efficacious (for one or all disorders), this would not justify the assumption that an untested therapy can safely be assumed to be as efficacious as are research-supported treatments. Nor would it imply that scientific evidence for this therapy need not be adduced in future studies.

Moreover, both assumptions place the burden of proof to demonstrate that a treatment is ineffective on skeptics rather than on proponents of a treatment. In science, this apportionment of the onus of evidence is often or usually a logical error (Pigluicci & Boudry, 2014), a burden that is amplified considerably when clients' mental health is at stake. Put somewhat differently, we propose that it is up to advocates of an intervention to provide compelling evidence for its efficacy, not up to others to provide compelling evidence against its efficacy.

The Therapeutic Changes Required for EBP Are Quantifiable

Some skeptics object to EBP on the grounds that many of the improvements observed in psychotherapy are too ineffable to be quantified. There is undeniably some truth to the proposition that some client changes in psychotherapy, especially those reflecting subjective emotional and cognitive states, are challenging to measure. Nevertheless, as psychologist E. L. Thorndike (1940) famously observed, "If something exists, then it exists in some quantity. If it exists in some quantity, then it can be measured" (p. 19). If therapists, clients, or both notice an improvement in subjective outcomes (e.g., sense of identity, meaning in life) following treatment, there is no inherent reason why such change cannot be quantified with reasonable reliability and validity. The increasing development of well-validated implicit measures in clinical research (e.g., Nock & Banaji, 2007) suggests that even the outcomes of largely unconscious processes are often amenable to quantification. To the extent that a positive therapeutic outcome suspected by a clinician cannot be measured at all using any available instruments, it is incumbent on proponents of a therapy to temper their claims regarding its efficacy accordingly.

EBP Is Compatible with Complex Higher-Order Interactions

Some skeptics of EBP insist that because clients' behavior cannot be predicted with certainty, the decision-making constraints imposed by EBP are unjustified. For example, Corsini (2008) invoked this logic to defend his decision to exclude scientific evidence bearing on the efficacy of each treatment in his widely adopted psychotherapy textbook. In this context, he approvingly cited Patterson's (1987) argument that to subject psychotherapy to controlled research,

> we would need (1) a taxonomy of client problems or psychological disorders; (2) a taxonomy of client personalities; (3) a taxonomy of therapeutic techniques . . . ; (4) a taxonomy of therapists; and (5) a taxonomy of circumstances. If we did have such a system of classification, the practical problems would be insurmountable. Assuming five classes of variables, each with ten classifications . . . a research design would require 100,000 cells. . . . So, I conclude we don't need complex multivariate analyses and should abandon any attempt to do the crucial, perfect study of psychotherapy. It simply is not possible. (p. 247)

To be sure, the "perfect study of psychotherapy" is indeed probably impossible because all scientific investigations have their limitations. But this caveat does not justify nihilism regarding multivariate analyses of psychotherapy outcome research, let alone regarding scientific conclusions about the efficacy of psychotherapies. The fact that a plethora of variables, such as clients' and therapists' personality traits and other psychological characteristics, may inter-

act statistically in enormously complex ways in predicting treatment outcomes does not exclude the possibility of substantial main effects of certain treatments relative to others.

An example from the medical literature offers an apt analogy in this regard. Individuals with melanoma differ from each another in myriad ways. Some are young and others are old; some are European American and others are African American; some have hypertension and others do not; some have a history of type 2 diabetes and others do not, and so on. Despite these and countless other potential complicating variables, 90% or more of cases of melanoma are essentially curable with early surgery (Berwick, 2010). Similarly, despite enormous heterogeneity in the characteristics of individuals with prostate cancer, this condition has a high cure rate if detected early (Spratt et al., 2013). In the case of psychotherapy, we can similarly make reasonable generalizations regarding overall therapeutic efficacy despite the possibility of complex higher-order interactions (Lilienfeld, 2012).

EBP Is Necessarily Provisional

Some individuals argue that EBP is not feasible because this approach requires knowledge regarding treatment efficacy and effectiveness to be conclusive. Because such knowledge often evolves, the argument continues, EBP will soon become outdated. For example, in response to the question "What scientific idea is ready for retirement?", psychologist Gary Klein (2014) answered, "Evidence-based medicine." He wrote that "we should only trust EBM [evidence-based medicine] if the science behind best practices is *infallible* and *comprehensive,* and that's certainly not the case" (original emphasis).

Nevertheless, the goal of EBP is not to eliminate all potential error; it is to minimize error by turning to the best available current research evidence (Lilienfeld, 2014c). Of course, such evidence may change, but it is far better to draw on today's best data on treatment efficacy and effectiveness than on data collected a decade ago. Furthermore, EBP is not ossified, as demonstrated by continual changes in lists of evidence-based interventions. In keeping with the cardinal principle that science is a provisional, self-correcting process (Sagan, 1995), the research leg of EBP necessarily evolves in response to new scientific evidence. *Contra* Klein, there is no expectation that EBP will or should provide the final word concerning thera-peutic efficacy or effectiveness. These points further underscore the difference between EST and EBP. Whereas the former comprises lists of specific treatments, the latter is a broader approach to evaluating scientific evidence in conjunction with clinical expertise and client values, as well as flexibly incorporating such evidence as it changes over time.

Summary

A host of understandable misconceptions re-garding EBP has arisen, and EBP advocates have often been insufficiently proactive in ad-dressing them. Because EBP emphasizes the scientific evaluation of therapeutic outcome and process, it is inherently provisional and open to correction (cf. Klein, 2014). At the same time, EBP insists that certain sources of research evi-dence concerning client improvement are gen-erally superior to others, as these sources are better suited for ruling out rival hypotheses for therapeutic improvement. We urge practicing clinicians, trainees, instructors, and clinical su-pervisors to address these misconceptions ex-plicitly in a context of lifelong learning, teach-ing, and training. The educational psychology research literature suggests that unless miscon-ceptions are raised proactively and addressed, they will typically persist following instruction (e.g., Winer, Cottrell, Gregg, Foumier, & Bica, 2002). Hence, unless we, as a field, strive to actively dispel misconceptions regarding EBP, such misconceptions are likely to likely to re-main intact.

Ubiquitous Errors in Causal Inference in Clinical Practice

In addition to specific misconceptions regard-ing EBP, a host of psychological factors prob-ably conspire to engender resistance to the no-tion that EBP is essential for clinical decision making. These factors, we suggest, can contrib-ute to erroneous observations concerning client improvement, as well as erroneous inferences concerning the causes of such improvement. In addition, they may lead some therapists to overestimate their success rates and underes-timate their failure rates. Walfish, McAlister, O'Donnell, and Lambert (2012) found that therapists estimated that, on average, only 3.7% of clients in their caseloads became worse fol-

lowing treatment (see also Hannan et al., 2005). Yet the research literature consistently suggests that the rate of client deterioration following psychotherapy hovers around 10% (Boisvert & Faust, 2003). Here, we address three overarch-ing sources of erroneous observations and in-ferences regarding client improvement: naive realism, confirmation bias, and the illusion of control.

Naive Realism

We propose that a key impediment to evaluat-ing change in treatment accurately is what psy-chologists, following philosophers, have termed *naive realism*: the erroneous belief that we can always trust the raw data of our sensory impres-sions (Ehrlinger, Gilovich, & Ross, 2005; Ross & Ward, 1996). A host of phrases in our lan-guage attest to the ubiquity of naive realism in our everyday thinking: "I saw it with my own eyes," "I'll believe it when I see it," "Seeing is believing," and "What you see is what you get." As that astute trio of esteemed psychologists, the Marx Brothers (1933), famously quipped, "Who are you gonna' believe, me or your own eyes?" Naive realists, of course, trust their eyes over the omniscient Groucho—never a wise idea.

How Naive Realism Can Fool Us

Naive realism overlooks the crucial point that although we see reality in part as it is, our per-ceptions of the world are shaped by our hypoth-eses, hunches, and biases. In many respects, the saying "Believing is seeing" may be at least as accurate as the inverse (Gilovich, 1991). Fur-thermore, naive realism can predispose us to neglect alternative explanations for change, in-cluding client change, especially when these ex-planations are not immediately apparent. Nobel Prize-winning psychologist Daniel Kahneman (2011) described the heuristic of "What you see is all there is"—WYSIATI—as a core mental shortcut in daily life. Because of the WYSIATI principle, we often neglect to consider causal variables that do not fall within our current men-tal radar screens. For example, if while watch-ing the evening news we see a house crumble to the ground during a powerful summer storm, we may mistakenly attribute the collapse entire-ly to the impact of the torrential wind and rain. In fact, the bad weather may have only been the last straw; perhaps the house was poorly constructed or maintained, and was on the verge of falling apart anyway.

Naive Realism and Unsupported Psychological Interventions

Naive realism probably helps to explain why Henry Cotton and many of his fellow psychiatrists were certain that his bogus surgical techniques were effective. Presumably, they compared his patients' clinical status—or at least their recollections of their clinical status—at Time 2 (postintervention) with those at Time 1 (preintervention), and they perceived what they believed to be improvement. They then concluded that the surgical intervention must have been responsible for this perceived change, neglecting to consider a host of rival explanations for this change that we will soon examine (see also Lilienfeld, Lohr, & Olatunji, 2008; Rousseau & Gunía, 2016).

Naive realism was almost surely a central player in the popularity of prefrontal lobotomy among countless mental health professionals during the middle decades of the past century. In referring to the effectiveness of lobotomy for severe psychiatric illness, the most prominent American advocate of this technique, neurosurgeon Walter Freeman, boasted, "I am a sensitive observer, and my conclusion is that a vast majority of my patients get better as opposed to worse after my treatment" (see Dawes, 1994, p. 28). In all likelihood, Freeman and others either perceived change when it did not occur or misinterpreted it when it did. Incidentally, it was not merely Freeman who was duped by his myriad clinical observations. In 1949, the Nobel committee awarded Egas Moniz, the Portuguese neurologist who pioneered the application of prefrontal lobotomy to humans, the Nobel Prize in Physiology or Medicine for his surgical contributions. They did so in spite of the fact that Moniz's conclusions regarding the effectiveness of lobotomy were based exclusively on his qualitative and descriptive accounts of patients' behavior before and after surgery (Tierney, 2000).

As we discuss in a later section ("EBP as a Safeguard against Errors in Clinical Inference: Causes of Spurious Therapeutic Effectiveness"), naive realism can also foster erroneous inferences of the sources of improvement in psychotherapy (Lilienfeld et al., 2008, 2014). For example, a therapist may conclude incorrectly that because a depressed client improved

substantially across a 3-month period following a psychological intervention, the intervention must have produced the improvement. To be certain, it *may* have, or at least it may have played a major role. But without knowledge of the *hypothetical counterfactual* (Dawes, 1994)—information about how well the client would have fared without treatment—there is no way to know with any degree of certainty.

Naive Realism and Ambiguity Surrounding the Concept of "Evidence"

The concept of naive realism brings us to a final fraught issue: the meaning of the word *evidence.* This familiar word would seem to be straightforward enough, but it in fact lends itself to misunderstandings (Stuart & Lilienfeld, 2007). Perhaps owing to the scientific cachet of EBP, many proponents of unsupported, questionable, or downright pseudoscientific techniques have been eager to claim the mantle of "evidence-based treatment." For example, one website claims that the technique of "group therapeutic drumming," a treatment that has never been subjected to controlled trials, makes use of a set of "evidence-based rhythmic interactive activities" (*http://www.positiverepercussions. com/#!group-therapeutic-drumming/edefz*). The website of the Therapeutic Touch International Association, which promotes Therapeutic Touch®, a trademarked method premised on the dubious notion that the manipulation of invisible energy fields by moving hands at a distance from the body can heal physical and psychological disorders, touts it as "a holistic, evidence-based therapy that incorporates the intentional and compassionate use of universal energy to promote balance and well-being" (*http://therapeutic-touch.org*). It perhaps goes without saying that the premise underpinning Therapeutic Touch is unsubstantiated: Its practitioners cannot even discern the presence or absence of patient energy fields at better than chance levels (Rosa, Rosa, Sarner, & Barrett, 1998).

Are the proponents of these techniques being deliberately dishonest in professing evidence-based status? We doubt it. Instead, we suspect that, like many advocates of scientifically questionable therapies, they are interpreting the word *evidence* very differently than the founders of EBP intended. For proponents of Group Therapeutic Drumming and Therapeutic Touch, the "evidence" to which they are referring is largely, if not entirely, the data of their informal clinical observations. They repeatedly "see" people improve following their intervention of choice, and they regard this evidence as sufficient for concluding that the treatment worked. In contrast, EBP advocates, ourselves included, would contend that that such evidence is far too fallible and open to rival explanations to provide a firm foundation for inferences of treatment efficacy or effectiveness.

Another way of framing the difference between these two means of evidence is to distinguish *naive empiricism* from *systematic empiricism*. Naive empiricism, much like the allied concept of naive realism, posits that raw sensory observations comprise a sufficient basis for drawing valid scientific inferences. Inherent in this view is "the assumption that observations can be unbiased" (Strong, 1991, p. 206), an assumption that decades of psychological research (see Dawes, Faust, & Meehl, 1989) have demonstrated to be, well, naive. In contrast, systematic empiricism posits that although raw sensory observations are essential sources of initial information, they are subject to a plethora of potential biases and other errors in inference (Stanovich, 2012), such as confirmation bias and illusory correlation, both of which we discuss later. Hence, such preliminary observations, although potentially useful, must be refined and honed by research methods, which we can conceptualize as partial safeguards against human error (Lilienfeld, Ammirati, & David, 2012).

Confirmation Bias

Some scholars have dubbed confirmation bias the "mother of all biases" (Gilovich & Ross, 2015), as it is arguably the most pervasive bias in everyday life. It is also the core bias that scientific methodology is designed to counteract (Lilienfeld, 2010; Tavris & Aronson, 2007). *Confirmation bias* is the deeply ingrained propensity to seek out evidence consistent with our hypotheses, and to deny, dismiss, or distort evidence that is not (Nickerson, 1998). As a consequence of this bias, clinicians, clients, and researchers may be inclined to unconsciously "cherry-pick" outcomes that are consistent with improvement and to explain away ("She's somewhat more depressed now than she was before treatment, but she needs to get worse before she gets better") or neglect outcomes that are inconsistent with improvement (Casarett, 2016; Garb, 1998; Lilienfeld et al., 2013). Confirmation bias

almost certainly contributes to another cognitive error, *illusory correlation,* the tendency to perceive statistical associations between variables in their objective absence (Chapman & Chapman, 1967; Lilienfeld, Watts, Robinson, & Smith, 2016). Because therapists naturally tend to seek out evidence that supports their hypotheses of client improvement and to ignore or underweight evidence that does not, they may sometimes perceive erroneous associations between their therapeutic ministrations and subsequent client improvement.

The Illusion of Control

A large body of evidence drawn from social psychology demonstrates that most or all of us are prone to experiencing a sense of control over random events (Langer, 1975; Matute, Yarritu, & Vadillo, 2011), a phenomenon known as the *illusion of control*. For example, when they have the opportunity to acquire money, most people prefer to a roll a die or flip a coin rather than to leave these actions to others, even though doing so does not enhance the odds of winning. The same illusion probably helps to account for the popularity of scratch-off lottery tickets, which may leave purchasers with the misleading sense that they somehow possess a measure of control over the winning numbers. As applied to psychotherapy, practitioners may at times develop an erroneous perception that their actions are responsible for generating positive changes in their clients, when in fact this association may not necessarily be causal (Casarett, 2016). For example, laboratory data suggest that when frequent spontaneous remissions in clients occasionally overlap with the timing of specific therapeutic interventions, individuals may conclude that these interventions are producing the spontaneous remissions, even when the link is merely coincidental (Blanco, Barberia, & Matute, 2014; Matute et al., 2011).

EBP as a Safeguard against Errors in Clinical Inference: Causes of Spurious Therapeutic Effectiveness

In fascinating but troubling research on *medical reversals,* Prasad and his colleagues (Prasad & Cifu, 2015; Prasad, Cifu, & Ioannidis, 2012) canvassed the growing literature on widely used medical procedures that have been demon-

strated to be highly questionable or outright ineffective. According to their estimates, perhaps
40% of established medical practices have been
overturned by subsequent research evidence.
For example, coronary angioplasty for stable
coronary artery disease, arthroscopic knee surgery, vertebroplasty for bone fractures, and hormone replacement therapy for postmenopausal
women have been all been shown to be no more
efficacious than placebo control conditions in
multiple, large RCTs. Strikingly, many of the
nearly 150 cases of demonstrably ineffective
procedures identified by Prasad and colleagues
continue to be widely used despite clear-cut
data to the contrary (Zuger, 2015). Furthermore,
even for beneficial medical procedures, such as
cancer chemotherapy, data suggest that physicians tend to overestimate their effectiveness
(Casarett, 2016).

The ubiquity of such examples highlights one
of the foremost challenges to the provision of effective psychological treatment, the *therapeutic
illusion,* which refers to the tendency to perceive
an ineffective intervention as effective (Casarett, 2016). Although we have reviewed broad
cognitive predispositions to the therapeutic illusion, there is a host of more specific causes
of this illusion in the case of psychotherapies;
we have elsewhere referred to these sources as
causes of spurious therapeutic effectiveness
(CSTEs; Lilienfeld et al., 2013).

In a previous publication, we described 26
potential CSTEs and proposed that CSTEs provide perhaps the most compelling rationale for
EBP (Lilienfeld et al., 2014). Specifically, without the inferential safeguards afforded by the research leg of EBP, all of us—clinicians, clients,
researchers, and consumers of the psychotherapy literature—can readily fall victim to CSTEs
and, in the process, to erroneous inferences
concerning therapeutic efficacy and effectiveness. Readers should bear in mind that many
informal inferences of client improvement in
psychotherapy by therapists, clients, and other
observers are surely correct and should not be
reflexively discarded. Nevertheless, CSTEs
remind us that such inferences can sometimes
be erroneous and need to be corroborated by
systematic data. Here we focus on nine of the
aforementioned 26 CSTEs that are especially
important, well researched, and problematic in
clinical decision making and the ways in which
EBP affords protection for clients, clinicians,
and the public.

Regression to the Mean

As the old saw "What goes up must come
down" reminds us, regression to the mean is
a statistical fact of life, although it should also
be extended to the phrase "What goes down
must come up." Mathematically, unless pre-
and posttest scores are perfectly correlated, extreme scores tend to become less extreme upon
retesting (Kruger, Savitsky, & Gilovich, 1999;
Streiner, 2001). Although the phenomenon of
regression to the mean was recognized as far
back as the 19th century by Sir Francis Galton,
Charles Darwin's cousin (Galton (1886) termed
it "regression towards mediocrity"), it remains
insufficiently appreciated as a CSTE. Regression to the mean can fool therapists and patients
alike into believing that a useless treatment is
effective (Gilovich, 1991). Although we have
no formal data to support this conjecture, we
suspect that *regression to the mean* accounts
for more mistaken inferences concerning psychotherapy improvement than any other source.
As Campbell and Kenny (1999) observed, "It
seems likely that regression toward the mean
leads people to believe in the efficacy of scientifically unjustified regimens. . . . Many a
quack has made a good living from regression
toward the mean" (p. 48). Exacerbating regression to the mean is the fact that many patients
seek out treatment when their symptoms are at
their worst, thereby maximizing the chances
that they will improve even without intervention (Lilienfeld, 2014a).

Fortunately, randomization of clients to conditions, a key feature of the research prong of
EBP, helps to control for regression to the mean.
To be clear, randomization does not eliminate
regression effects, but it helps to eliminate regression effects as *explanations* for between-
group differences. In adequately sized samples,
the likelihood of regression effects should be
approximately equalized in both experimental
and control groups.

The Placebo Effect

The ubiquitous *placebo effect* ("placebo" derives from the Latin for "I shall please") is
commonly conceptualized as improvement resulting from the mere expectation of improvement (Steer & Ritschel, 2010; also see Shapiro
& Shapiro, 1997, for a broader definition). The
placebo effect should not be confused with
other nonspecific treatment effects (Kienle &

Kienle, 1997), including other CSTEs, because it is specific to expectancy effects. By instilling hope and the belief that one can conquer life's challenges, virtually any credible treatment can be at least somewhat helpful for alleviating demoralization (Frank & Frank, 1991), which is a central element of distress-related psychopathology (Tellegen et al., 2003).

In psychotherapy outcome research, attention placebo control groups are designed to control for expectancy effects and other nonspecific effects, such as improvement arising from contact with a caring professional (Paul, 1966). Systematic comparisons of attention placebo control groups with wait-list control groups have typically yielded a small to medium average weighted effect size ($d = 0.40$; Lambert & Ogles, 2004). This effect size amounts to approximately half of the overall mean effect of psychotherapy. It is debatable, however, whether placebo effects should be regarded as "artifacts" in psychotherapy research given that some of the genuine effects of psychological treatment almost certainly stem from the restoration of hope (Frank & Frank, 1991; Wampold, Frost, & Yulish, 2016).

Spontaneous Remission

The term *spontaneous remission* originated in medicine to describe instances in which disorders resolve without intervention (Beyerstein, 1997). For some psychological disorders, such as major depressive disorder, spontaneous remissions are extremely common (Cuijpers & Cristea, 2015). Because the fields of psychology and psychiatry have until recently underestimated individuals' resilience in the face of stressors (Bonanno, 2004), they have very likely also underestimated clients' capacity to draw on their coping mechanisms to recover from adversity. In other cases, spontaneous remission probably results from fortuitous changes in clients' lives, such as starting a fulfilling job or embarking on a supportive romantic relationship. As neo-Freudian theorist Karen Horney (1945) wisely noted, "Life itself remains a very effective psychotherapist" (p. 240). As in the case of regression effects, randomization to conditions minimizes spontaneous remission as a CSTE because the likelihood of such remission should be approximately equated in experimental and control groups given sufficiently large samples.

Maturation

Another source of erroneous inferences of therapeutic effectiveness is *maturation*: improvement owing to naturally occurring emotional or cognitive development (Cook & Campbell, 1979). For example, children and adolescents with high levels of what some scholars regard as prepsychopathic features, such as poor impulse control, callousness, low frustration tolerance, and defiance, may get better without treatment because these features sometimes diminish with the passage of time (Edens, Skeem, Cruise, & Cauffman, 2001). Maturation can be a CSTE even for adult clients. For example, burgeoning evidence suggests that some patients with borderline personality disorder display substantial improvements in adulthood, perhaps even in the absence of treatment (Gunderson et al., 2011; Shea et al., 2009). As is the case for many other CSTEs, randomization controls for maturation by ensuring that it is equated across treatment and no-treatment groups.

Effort Justification

Because clients often invest a great deal of time, energy, effort, and money in treatment, they may feel a psychological need to justify this commitment, a phenomenon called *effort justification* (Cooper, 1980). Effort justification may account for some of the improvement following psychological treatments, especially those that are demanding or arduous (Freijy & Kothe, 2013). In a classic study, undergraduates with marked snake phobic symptoms benefited just as much from engaging in strenuous physical exercises (e.g., running quickly in place) as from exposure therapy (Cooper & Axsom, 1982), presumably because the former "treatment" induced them to psychologically justify their intense effort expenditure. Effort justification can be challenging to control for in studies of psychotherapy, although it can be minimized as an explanation for between-group differences by comparing the active treatment with an intervention that is approximately equated in the time, energy, and effort expended by clients.

Multiple Treatment Interference

When clients finally decide to enroll in treatment, they often obtain other interventions simultaneously (Kendall, Butcher, & Holmbeck, 1999), a confound known as *multiple treatment interference* or *co-intervention bias*. These interventions may be formal treatments, such as other psychotherapies, but they may also be informal "treatments," such as confiding in a valued friend or a priest, consulting self-help books, or taking a long-overdue retreat in a bucolic setting. In any or all of these cases, multiple treatment interference can render it difficult or impossible to confidently attribute client change to the intervention of choice. Randomization of clients to conditions again helps to minimize the confound of multiple treatment interference, as it decreases the likelihood that clients assigned to the active treatment will differ from those assigned to the control treatment in their use of adjunctive interventions.

Retrospective Rewriting of One's Pretreatment Level of Functioning

Clients' implicit causal narratives and expectations of change probably shape their impressions of improvement. Specifically, their beliefs that they should get better following treatment may influence their memories of their psychological adjustment. Some clients may persuade themselves that they have improved following treatment by misremembering their preintervention level of functioning as worse than it was (Ross, 1989). In one study, researchers randomly assigned undergraduates to either a study skills course intended to improve their grades or to a no-intervention control condition, and measured their grades before and after the intervention. Although the class failed to improve students' study skills or grades, students in the experimental condition perceived it to be effective. Why? Data showed that they had misremembered their initial study skills as worse than they were (Conway & Ross, 1984). This CSTE can be eliminated as an explanation for spurious treatment effects by administering symptom measures at both pretest and posttest.

Absence of Knowledge of the Hypothetical Counterfactual

One major reason for erroneous inferences of therapeutic effectiveness is the inevitable absence of information regarding the *hypothetical counterfactual* (Dawes, 1994): our inability to know what would have occurred in the absence of treatment. Because clinicians in routine practice settings of necessity are unaware of how their clients would have fared in a control condition, they cannot gauge the extent to which the observed improvement in their clients would have occurred without intervention.

For example, research indicates that critical incident stress debriefing (CISD), which is used to diminish the risk of posttraumatic stress symptoms among trauma-exposed victims, is ineffective and perhaps iatrogenic (Litz, Gray, Bryant, & Adler, 2002; McNally, Bryant, & Ehlers, 2003). Counterintuitively, however, many people who have received this treatment believe that it helped them (Carlier, Voerman, & Gersons, 2000). A study by Mayou, Ehlers, and Hobbs (2000) helps to explain why. In their investigation of car accident victims, they reported that patients with high levels of posttraumatic stress disorder (PTSD) symptoms who received CISD improved across a 3-year period, superficially suggesting that the treatment had worked. Yet patients with equally high levels of PTSD symptoms who received no treatment at all improved considerably more, indicating that CISD had actually harmed them, perhaps by impeding natural coping mechanisms.

By definition, the use of control groups removes this CSTE. It ensures that the hypothetical counterfactual becomes reality, thereby allowing us to compare people exposed to the intervention with those who were not.

Selective Attrition

Finally, clients who drop out of therapy are rarely a random subsample of all clients, a phenomenon known as *selective attrition*. In contrast to other CSTEs, which operate at the level of individual clients, selective attrition operates at the level of a therapist's caseload. Research demonstrates that clients who are not improving in psychotherapy are especially likely to drop out of treatment (Garfield, 1994; Tehrani, Krussel, Borg, & Munk-Jørgensen, 1996; see also Swift & Greenberg, 2015); in addition, the presence of personality disorders, which itself is a risk factor for poor therapy outcome, may be a harbinger of early termination (Brorson, Arnevik, Rand-Hendriksen, & Duckert, 2013). As a consequence of these selection biases, therapists may conclude mistakenly that their treatments are effective merely because their remaining clients are those that have improved. Fortunately, a variety of statistical methods, including intent-to-treat analyses, are available to handle the problem of selective attrition in psychotherapy outcome research (e.g., Little & Yau, 1996).

Summary

A plethora of CSTEs, a mere nine of which we have summarized here, can predispose individuals, including therapists, independent observers, and clients themselves to conclude that ineffective psychotherapies are effective (Lilienfeld et al., 2014; see also Casarett, 2016). The existence of CSTEs offers perhaps the most compelling rationale for EBP, especially its research leg. Without the procedural safeguards afforded by research techniques, such as randomization of clients to conditions, blinding of observers, attention placebo control groups, and standardized observations of client change, even highly intelligent and well-educated individuals can draw erroneous inferences of treatment effectiveness. Because these methodological refinements are hardly infallible, EBP, along with it associated lists of evidence-based treatments, will necessarily be an imperfect instrument for clinical decision making. But as a self-correcting approach to such decisions, it is ultimately our best hope for overcoming biases and other errors in judgment, and our best guide to treatment selection under conditions of uncertainty. Moreover, CSTEs can also inform and ideally enhance routine clinical care. By becoming more cognizant of CSTEs, therapists can thoughtfully monitor and evaluate alternative explanations for client improvement throughout treatment (see Lilienfeld et al., 2014, for concrete examples).

Closing Thoughts: EBP and Error Correction

The stories of Henry Cotton's surgeries, prefrontal lobotomy, tranquilizing chairs, and other tragic errors in mental health treatment convey invaluable lessons that should be imparted anew to every generation of mental health professionals. Remembering the history of clinical errors that gave rise to EBP underscores the reality that scientific progress is a long and bumpy road of gradually corrected mistakes (Wood & Nezworski, 2005). As a field, we have thankfully come a long way from the days of Henry Cotton.

At the same time, we must be vigilant against the temptations of smugness or complacency. Cotton, after all, performed his surgeries less than a century ago, and was invited by prestigious academic institutions to share the fruits of his medical "discoveries." We must continually remind ourselves that we are all vulnerable to the same ubiquitous mistakes in thinking that afflicted Cotton and his psychiatric colleagues. EBP, particularly its research leg, although by no means a panacea, is an essential set of bulwarks against commonplace reasoning glitches that can predispose to serious inferential errors. EBP therefore affords us our best chance of minimizing decision-making mistakes and enhancing client care. In the words of Nobel Prize-winning physicist Richard Feynman (1974), in science "the first principle is that you must not fool yourself, and you are the easiest person to fool" (p. 12). The same credo, we maintain, holds for clinical practice.

Fortunately, knowledge of CSTEs can be a valuable inferential bulwark for practitioners, as awareness of these cognitive errors can help to immunize them against thinking traps in their everyday work. Such knowledge should be reinforced by continuing education, ongoing reminders of the crucial role of EBP in helping to counteract CSTEs, and ideally both. Specifically, the knowledge that one's clinical observations and inferences are fallible can be a helpful check against epistemic certainty and a reminder to seek out alternative explanations for apparent client improvement. For example, an awareness of regression effects can remind clinicians to consider the possibility that at least some client changes could reflect naturally occurring shifts in symptoms that are unrelated to treatment; an awareness of placebo effects and effort justification can remind clinicians to consider the possibility that at least some client changes reflect nonspecific effects; and an awareness of multiple treatment interference can remind clinicians to ask clients about additional interventions that they may be receiving (see also Lilienfeld et al., 2014). In this way, practitioners can operate effectively as scientific thinkers in the clinical setting.

References

American Psychiatric Association. (2013). *Diagnostic and statistical manual of mental disorders* (5th ed.). Arlington, VA: Author.

American Psychological Association. (2005). *Report of the 2005 Presidential Task Force on Evidence-Based Practice*. Washington, DC: Author.

Anderson, N. B. (2006). Evidence-based practice in psychology. *American Psychologist, 61,* 271–285.

Arkowitz, H., & Lilienfeld, S. O. (2006). Psychotherapy on trial. *Scientific American Mind, 17*(2), 42–49.

Barlow, D. H. (2004). Psychological treatments. *American Psychologist, 59,* 869–884.

Berwick, D. (2010). Nature or nurture—which is responsible for melanoma? Retrieved from *www.skincancer.org/nature-or-nurturewhich-is-responsible-for-melanoma.html.*

Beyerstein, B. L. (1997). Why bogus therapies seem to work. *The Skeptical Inquirer, 21,* 29–34.

Blanco, F., Barberia, I., & Matute, H. (2014). The lack of side effects of an ineffective treatment facilitates the development of a belief in its effectiveness. *PLOS ONE, 9*(1), e84084.

Blease, C. R. (2015). Talking more about talking cures: Cognitive behavioural therapy and informed consent. *Journal of Medical Ethics, 41,* 750–755.

Blease, C. R., Lilienfeld, S. O., & Kelley, J. M. (2016). Evidence-based practice and psychological treatments: The imperatives of informed consent. *Frontiers in Psychology, 7,* 1170.

Bohart, A. C. (2000). Paradigm clash: Empirically supported treatments versus empirically supported psychotherapy practice. *Psychotherapy Research, 10,* 488–493.

Boisvert, C. M., & Faust, D. (2003). Leading researchers' consensus on psychotherapy research findings: Implications for the teaching and conduct of psychotherapy. *Professional Psychology: Research and Practice, 34,* 508–513.

Boisvert, C. M., & Faust, D. (2006). Practicing psychologists' knowledge of general psychotherapy research findings: Implications for science–practice relations. *Professional Psychology: Research and Practice, 37,* 708–716.

Bonanno, G. A. (2004). Loss, trauma, and human resilience: Have we underestimated the human capacity to thrive after extremely aversive events? *American Psychologist, 59,* 20–28.

Borntrager, C. F., Chorpita, B. F., Higa-McMillan, C., & Weisz, J. R. (2009). Provider attitudes toward evidence-based practices: Are the concerns with the evidence or with the manuals? *Psychiatric Services, 60,* 677–681.

Brorson, H. H., Arnevik, E. A., Rand-Hendriksen, K., & Duckert, F. (2013). Drop-out from addiction treatment: A systematic review of risk factors. *Clinical Psychology Review, 33,* 1010–1024.

Brush, J. E., & Halperin, J. L. (2016). A baby in the bathwater: Preserving evidence-based medicine. *Journal of the American College of Cardiology, 68*(2), 214–216.

Campbell, D. T. (1986). Relabeling internal and external validity for applied social scientists. *New Directions for Program Evaluation, 31,* 67–77.

Campbell, D. T., & Kenny, D. A. (1999). *A primer on regression artifacts.* New York: Guilford Press.

Canadian Psychological Association. (2002). Evidence-based practice of psychological treatments: A Canadian perspective. Retrieved from *www.cpa.ca/docs/file/practice/report_of_the_ebp_task_force_final_board_approved_2012.pdf.*

Carlier, I. V., Voerman, A. E., & Gersons, B. P. (2000). The influence of occupational debriefing on post-traumatic stress symptomatology in traumatized police officers. *British Journal of Medical Psychology, 73,* 87–98.

Casarett, D. (2016). The science of choosing wisely—overcoming the therapeutic illusion. *New England Journal of Medicine, 374,* 1203–1205.

Castonguay, L. G., Goldfried, M. R., Wiser, S., Raue, P. J., & Hayes, A. M. (1996). Predicting the effect of cognitive therapy for depression: A study of unique and common factors. *Journal of Consulting and Clinical Psychology, 64,* 497–504.

Chambless, D. L., & Hollon, S. D. (1998). Defining empirically supported therapies. *Journal of Consulting and Clinical Psychology, 66,* 7–18.

Chambless, D. L., & Ollendick, T. H. (2001). Empirically supported psychological interventions: Controversies and evidence. *Annual Review of Psychology, 52,* 685–716.

Chapman, L. J., & Chapman, J. P. (1967). Genesis of popular but erroneous psychodiagnostic observations. *Journal of Abnormal Psychology, 72,* 193–204.

Charuvastra, A. (2006). Madhouse: A tragic tale of megalomania and modern medicine. *Journal of Nervous and Mental Disease, 194,* 553–554.

Conway, M., & Ross, M. (1984). Getting what you want by revising what you had. *Journal of Personality and Social Psychology, 47,* 738–748.

Cook, T. D., & Campbell, D. T. (1979). *Quasi-experimentation: Design and analysis for field studies.* Skokie, IL: Rand McNally.

Cooper, J. (1980). Reducing fears and increasing assertiveness: The role of dissonance reduction. *Journal of Experimental Social Psychology, 16,* 199–213.

Cooper, J., & Axsom, D. (1982). Effort justification in psychotherapy. In G. Weary & H. Mirels (Eds.), *Integrations of clinical and social psychology* (pp. 98–121). New York: Oxford University Press.

Corsini, R. J. (2008). Introduction to 21st century psychotherapies. In R. J. Corsini & D. Wedding (Eds.), *Current psychotherapies* (pp. 1–14). Pacific Grove, CA: Brooks/Cole.

Cotton, H. A. (1922). Infection of the gastrointestinal tract in relation to systemic disorders: Neurological viewpoint: Special relation of clinical symptoms to regional distribution of focal infection. *American Journal of the Medical Sciences, 164,* 329–337.

Craske, M. G., Kircanski, K., Zelikowsky, M., Mystkowski, J., Chowdhury, N., & Baker, A. (2008). Optimizing inhibitory learning during exposure therapy. *Behaviour Research and Therapy, 46,* 5–27.

Cuijpers, P., & Cristea, I. A. (2015). What if a placebo effect explained all the activity of depression treatments? *World Psychiatry, 14,* 310–311.

Cuijpers, P., van Straten, A., Andersson, G., & van

Oppen, P. (2008). Psychotherapy for depression in adults: A meta-analysis of comparative outcome studies. *Journal of Consulting and Clinical Psychology, 76,* 909–922.

Davidson, J. (2016). Bayard Holmes (1852–1924) and Henry Cotton (1869–1933): Surgeon–psychiatrists and their tragic quest to cure schizophrenia. *Journal of Medical Biography, 24,* 550–559.

Dawes, R. M. (1994). *House of cards: Psychology and psychotherapy build on myth.* New York: Free Press.

Dawes, R. M., Faust, D., & Meehl, P. E. (1989). Clinical versus actuarial judgment. *Science, 243,* 1668–1674.

Dimidjian, S., & Hollon, S. D. (2010). How would we know if psychotherapy were harmful? *American Psychologist, 65,* 21–33.

Duncan, B. L., Miller, S. D., & Sparks, J. A. (2011). *The heroic client: A revolutionary way to improve effectiveness through client-directed, outcome-informed therapy.* New York: Wiley.

Edens, J. F., Skeem, J. L., Cruise, K. R., & Cauffman, E. (2001). Assessment of "juvenile psychopathy" and its association with violence: A critical review. *Behavioral Sciences and the Law, 19,* 53–80.

Ehrlinger, J., Gilovich, T., & Ross, L. (2005). Peering into the bias blind spot: People's assessments of bias in themselves and others. *Personality and Social Psychology Bulletin, 31,* 680–692.

El-Adl, M. (2011). Early intervention in psychiatry: Challenges and opportunities. In L. L'Abate (Ed.), *Mental illnesses: Understanding, prediction, and control* (pp. 373–384). London: InTech.

Feynman, R. P. (1974). Cargo cult science. *Engineering and Science, 37,* 10–13.

Frank, J. D., & Frank, J. B. (1991). *Persuasion and healing.* Baltimore: Johns Hopkins University Press.

Freijy, T., & Kothe, E. J. (2013). Dissonance-based interventions for health behaviour change: A systematic review. *British Journal of Health Psychology, 18,* 310–337.

Galton, F. (1886). Regression towards mediocrity in hereditary stature. *Journal of the Anthropological Institute of Great Britain and Ireland, 15,* 246–263.

Gambrill, E. (2001). Social work: An authority-based profession. *Research on Social Work Practice, 11,* 166–175.

Garb, H. N. (1998). *Studying the clinician: Judgment research and psychological assessment.* Washington, DC: American Psychological Association.

Garfield, S. (1994). Research on client variables in psychotherapy. In A. E. Bergin & S. Garfield (Eds.), *Handbook of psychotherapy and behavior change* (4th ed., pp. 190–228). Oxford, UK: Wiley.

Ghaemi, S. N. (2009). *A clinician's guide to statistics and epidemiology in mental health: Measuring truth and uncertainty.* Cambridge, UK: Cambridge University Press.

Gibbs, L., & Gambrill, E. (2002). Evidence-based practice: Counterarguments to objections. *Research on Social Work Practice, 12,* 452–476.

Gilovich, T. (1991). *How we know what isn't so: The fallibility of human reasoning in everyday life.* New York: Free Press.

Gilovich, T., & Ross, L. (2015). *The wisest one in the room: How you can benefit from social psychology's most powerful insights.* New York: Simon & Schuster.

Gray, M., Joy, E., Plath, D., & Webb, S. A. (2015). What supports and impedes evidence-based practice implementation?: A survey of Australian social workers. *British Journal of Social Work, 45,* 667–684.

Grove, W. M., & Meehl, P. E. (1996). Comparative efficiency of informal (subjective, impressionistic) and formal (mechanical, algorithmic) prediction procedures: The clinical–statistical controversy. *Psychology, Public Policy, and Law, 2,* 293–323.

Gunderson, J. G., Stout, R. L., McGlashan, T. H., Shea, M. T., Morey, L. C., Grilo, C. M., et al. (2011). Ten-year course of borderline personality disorder: Psychopathology and function from the Collaborative Longitudinal Personality Disorders study. *Archives of General Psychiatry, 68,* 827–837.

Guyatt, G., Cairns, J., Churchill, D., Cook, D., Haynes, B., Hirsh, J., et al. (1992). Evidence-based medicine: A new approach to teaching the practice of medicine. *Journal of the American Medical Association, 268,* 2420–2425.

Hannan, C., Lambert, M. J., Harmon, C., Nielsen, S., Smart, D. W., Shimokawa, K., et al. (2005). A lab test and algorithms for identifying clients at risk for treatment failure. *Journal of Clinical Psychology, 61,* 155–163.

Hans, E., & Hiller, W. (2013). A meta-analysis of nonrandomized effectiveness studies on outpatient cognitive behavioral therapy for adult anxiety disorders. *Clinical Psychology Review, 33,* 954–964.

Hedman, E., Ljótsson, B., Rück, C., Bergström, J., Andersson, G., Kaldo, V., et al. (2013). Effectiveness of Internet-based cognitive behaviour therapy for panic disorder in routine psychiatric care. *Acta Psychiatrica Scandinavica, 128,* 457–467.

Hofmann, S. G., & Curtis, J. (2014, September 21). The strawman debate continues. *PsycCritiques, 60*(38).

Horney, K. (1945). *Our inner conflicts.* Oxford, UK: Norton.

Hunsley, J., & DiGiulio, G. (2002). Dodo bird, phoenix, or urban legend?: The question of psychotherapy equivalence. *Scientific Review of Mental Health Practice, 1,* 11–22.

Ioannidis, J. A. (2005). Contradicted and initially stronger effects in highly cited clinical research. *Journal of the American Medical Association, 294,* 218–228.

Isaacs, D., & Fitzgerald, D. (1999). Seven alternatives to evidence based medicine. *British Medical Journal, 319,* 1618.

John, L. K., Loewenstein, G., & Prelec, D. (2012). Measuring the prevalence of questionable research practices with incentives for truth telling. *Psychological Science, 23,* 524–532.

Jones, A. H. (2005). The cautionary tale of psychiatrist Henry Aloysius Cotton. *Lancet, 366,* 361–362.

Kahneman, D. (2011). *Thinking, fast and slow.* New York: Macmillan.

Kendall, P. C., Butcher, J. N., & Holmbeck, G. N. (Eds.). (1999). *Handbook of research methods in clinical psychology* (2nd ed.). New York: Wiley.

Kendall, P. C., Gosch, E., Furr, J. M., & Sood, E. (2008). Flexibility within fidelity. *Journal of the American Academy of Child and Adolescent Psychiatry, 47,* 987–993.

Kienle, G. S., & Kiene, H. (1997). The powerful placebo effect: Fact or fiction? *Journal of Clinical Epidemiology, 50,* 1311–1318.

Klein, G. (2014). Evidence-based medicine. Retrieved from *www.edge.org/response-detail/25433.*

Kowalski, P., & Taylor, A. K. (2009). The effect of refuting misconceptions in the introductory psychology class. *Teaching of Psychology, 36,* 153–159.

Kruger, J., Savitsky, K., & Gilovich, T. (1999). Superstition and the regression effect. *Skeptical Inquirer, 23,* 24–29.

Lambert, M. J., & Ogles, B. M. (2004). The efficacy and effectiveness of psychotherapy. In M. J. Lambert (Ed.), *Bergin and Garfield's handbook of psychotherapy and behavior change* (5th ed., pp. 139–193). New York: Wiley.

Langer, E. J. (1975). The illusion of control. *Journal of Personality and Social Psychology, 32,* 311–328.

Laska, K. M., Gurman, A. S., & Wampold, B. E. (2014). Expanding the lens of evidence-based practice in psychotherapy: A common factors perspective. *Psychotherapy, 51,* 467–481.

Lilienfeld, S. O. (2007). Psychological treatments that cause harm. *Perspectives on Psychological Science, 2,* 53–70.

Lilienfeld, S. O. (2010). Can psychology become a science? *Personality and Individual Differences, 49,* 281–288.

Lilienfeld, S. O. (2012). Public skepticism of psychology: Why many people perceive the study of human behavior as unscientific. *American Psychologist, 67,* 111–129.

Lilienfeld, S. O. (2014a). Beware the regression fallacy. Retrieved from *www.psychologytoday.com/blog/the-skeptical-psychologist/201401/beware-the-regression-fallacy.*

Lilienfeld, S. O. (2014b). The Dodo Bird verdict: Status in 2014. *Behavior Therapist, 37,* 91–95.

Lilienfeld, S. O. (2014c). Evidence-based practice: The misconceptions continue. Retrieved from *www.psychologytoday.com/blog/the-skeptical-psychologist/201401/evidence-based-practice-the-misunderstandings-continue.*

Lilienfeld, S. O. (in press). Potentially harmful psychological treatments. In J. G. Beck (Ed.), *Oxford research encyclopedia of psychology.* New York: Oxford University Press.

Lilienfeld, S. O., Ammirati, R., & David, M. (2012). Distinguishing science from pseudoscience in school psychology: Science and scientific thinking as safeguards against human error. *Journal of School Psychology, 50,* 7–36.

Lilienfeld, S. O., Lohr, J. M., & Olatunji, B. O. (2008). Encouraging students to think critically about psychotherapy: Overcoming naive realism. In D. S. Dunn, J. S. Halonen, & R. A. Smith (Eds.), *Teaching critical thinking in psychology: A handbook of best practices* (pp. 267–271). Malden, MA: Wiley-Blackwell.

Lilienfeld, S. O., Ritschel, L. A., Lynn, S. J., Cautin, R. L., & Latzman, R. D. (2013). Why many clinical psychologists are resistant to evidence-based practice: Root causes and constructive remedies. *Clinical Psychology Review, 33,* 883–900.

Lilienfeld, S. O., Ritschel, L. A., Lynn, S. J., Cautin, R. L., & Latzman, R. D. (2014). Why ineffective psychotherapies appear to work a taxonomy of causes of spurious therapeutic effectiveness. *Perspectives on Psychological Science, 9,* 355–387.

Lilienfeld, S. O., & Waldman, I. D. (2018). *Psychological science under scrutiny: Recent challenges and proposed solutions.* New York: Wiley.

Lilienfeld, S. O., Watts, A. L., Robinson, B. A., & Smith, S. F. (2016). Scientific research in forensic samples. In M. Cima (Ed.), *The handbook of forensic psychopathology and treatment* (pp. 49–91). New York: Routledge.

Little, R., & Yau, L. (1996). Intent-to-treat analysis for longitudinal studies with drop-outs. *Biometrics, 52,* 1324–1333.

Litz, B. T., Gray, M. J., Bryant, R. A., & Adler, A. B. (2002). Early intervention for trauma: Current status and future directions. *Clinical Psychology: Science and Practice, 9,* 112–134.

Luebbe, A. M., Radcliffe, A. M., Callands, T. A., Green, D., & Thorn, B. E. (2007). Evidence-based practice in psychology: Perceptions of graduate students in scientist–practitioner programs. *Journal of Clinical Psychology, 63,* 643–655.

Marx Brothers. (1933). Duck Soup script: Dialogue transcript. Retrieved from *http://www.script-o-rama.com/movie_scripts/d/duck-soup-script-transcript-marx.html.*

Matute, H., Yarritu, I., & Vadillo, M. A. (2011). Illusions of causality at the heart of pseudoscience. *British Journal of Psychology, 102,* 392–405.

Mayou, R. A., Ehlers, A. A., & Hobbs, M. M. (2000). Psychological debriefing for road traffic accident victims: Three-year follow-up of a randomised controlled trial. *British Journal of Psychiatry, 176,* 589–593.

McFall, R. M., & Treat, T. A. (1999). Quantifying the information value of clinical assessments with signal detection theory. *Annual Review of Psychology, 50,* 215–241.

McHugh, R. K., Murray, H. W., & Barlow, D. H. (2009). Balancing fidelity and adaptation in the dissemination of empirically-supported treatments: The promise of transdiagnostic interventions. *Behaviour Research and Therapy, 47,* 946–953.

McKay, D., & Lilienfeld, S. O. (2015, September 9). Therapy: The effective kind. *Psychology Today.*

Retrieved from *www.psychologytoday.com/us/blog/ your-fears-and-anxieties/201509/therapy-the-effective-kind.*

McNally, R. J., Bryant, R. A., & Ehlers, A. (2003). Does early psychological intervention promote recovery from posttraumatic stress? *Psychological Science in the Public Interest, 4,* 45–79.

Meehl, P. E. (1954). *Clinical versus statistical prediction: A theoretical analysis and a review of the evidence.* Minneapolis: University of Minnesota Press.

Meehl, P. E. (1993). Philosophy of science: Help or hindrance? *Psychological Reports, 72,* 707–733.

Messer, S. B. (2004). Evidence-based practice: Beyond empirically supported treatments. *Professional Psychology: Research and Practice, 35,* 580–588.

Nickerson, R. S. (1998). Confirmation bias: A ubiquitous phenomenon in many guises. *Review of General Psychology, 2,* 175–220.

Nock, M. K., & Banaji, M. R. (2007). Prediction of suicide ideation and attempts among adolescents using a brief performance-based test. *Journal of Consulting and Clinical Psychology, 75,* 707–715.

O'Donohue, W. T., Ammirati, R., & Lilienfeld, S. O. (2011). The quality healthcare agenda in behavioral healthcare reform: Using science to reduce error. In W. T. O'Donohue (Ed.), *Understanding the behavioral healthcare crisis: The promise of integrated care and healthcare reform* (pp. 203–226). New York: Routledge.

O'Donohue, W. T., Lilienfeld, S. O., & Fowler, K. A. (2007). Science is an essential safeguard against human error. In W. T. O'Donohue & S. O. Lilienfeld (Eds.), *The great ideas of clinical science: 17 principles that every mental health professional should understand* (pp. 3–27). New York: Routledge.

Owen, J., & Hilsenroth, M. J. (2014). Treatment adherence: The importance of therapist flexibility in relation to therapy outcomes. *Journal of Counseling Psychology, 61,* 280–288.

Patterson, C. H. (1987). Comments. *Person-Centered Review, 1,* 246–248.

Paul, G. L. (1966). *Insight vs. desensitization in psychotherapy: An experiment in anxiety reduction.* Stanford, CA: Stanford University Press.

Pigliucci, M., & Boudry, M. (2014). Prove it!: The burden of proof game in science vs. pseudoscience disputes. *Philosophia, 42,* 487–502.

Pignotti, M. (2010). The use of novel unsupported and empirically supported therapies by licensed clinical social workers. *Dissertation Abstracts International Section A,* 71.

Poulsen, S., Lunn, S., Daniel, S. I., Folke, S., Mathiesen, B. B., Katznelson, H., & Fairburn, C. G. (2014). A randomized controlled trial of psychoanalytic psychotherapy or cognitive-behavioral therapy for bulimia nervosa. *American Journal of Psychiatry, 171,* 109–116.

Prasad, V. K., & Cifu, A. S. (2015). *Ending medical reversal: Improving outcomes, saving lives.* Baltimore: Johns Hopkins University Press.

Prasad, V., Cifu, A., & Ioannidis, J. P. (2012). Reversals of established medical practices: Evidence to abandon ship. *Journal of the American Medical Association, 307,* 37–38.

Rosa, L., Rosa, E., Sarner, L., & Barrett, S. (1998). A close look at therapeutic touch. *Journal of the American Medical Association, 279,* 1005–1010.

Rosen, G. M., & Davison, G. C. (2003). Psychology should list empirically supported principles of change (ESPs) and not credential trademarked therapies or other treatment packages. *Behavior Modification, 7,* 300–312.

Rosenberg, W., & Donald, A. (1995). Evidence based medicine: An approach to clinical problem-solving. *British Medical Journal, 310,* 1122–1126.

Rosenzweig, S. (1936). Some implicit common factors in diverse methods in psychotherapy. *American Journal of Orthopsychiatry, 6,* 412–415.

Ross, L., & Ward, A. (1996). Naive realism in everyday life: Implications for social conflict and misunderstanding. In T. Brown, E. Reed, & E. Turiel (Eds.), *Values and knowledge* (pp 103–135). Hillsdale, NJ: Erlbaum.

Ross, M. (1989). Relation of implicit theories to the construction of personal histories. *Psychological Review, 96,* 341–357.

Rousseau, D. M., & Gunía, B. C. (2016). Evidence-based practice: The psychology of EBP implementation. *Annual Review of Psychology, 67,* 667–692.

Sackett, D. L., Rosenberg, W. M., Gray, J. M., Haynes, R. B., & Richardson, W. S. (1996). Evidence based medicine: What it is and what it isn't. *British Medical Journal, 312,* 71–72.

Sagan, C. (1995). *The demon-haunted world: Science as a candle in the dark.* New York: Random House.

Scull, A. (2005). *Madhouse: A tragic tale of megalomania and modern medicine.* New Haven, CT: Yale University Press.

Seligman, M. E. (1995). The effectiveness of psychotherapy: *The Consumer Reports* study. *American Psychologist, 50,* 965–974.

Shapiro, A. K., & Shapiro, E. (1997). *The powerful placebo: From ancient priest to modern physician.* Baltimore: Johns Hopkins University Press.

Shea, M., Edelen, M. O., Pinto, A. A., Yen, S. S., Gunderson, J. G., Skodol, A. E., et al. (2009). Improvement in borderline personality disorder in relationship to age. *Acta Psychiatrica Scandinavica, 119*(2), 143–148.

Shedler, J. (2010). The efficacy of psychodynamic psychotherapy. *American Psychologist, 65,* 98–109.

Shedler, J. (2015). Where is the evidence for "evidence-based" therapy? *Journal of Psychological Therapies in Primary Care, 4,* 47–59.

Simmons, J. P., Nelson, L. D., & Simonsohn, U. (2011). False-positive psychology undisclosed flexibility in data collection and analysis allows presenting anything as significant. *Psychological Science, 21,* 1359–1366.

Spratt, D. E., Pei, X., Yamada, J., Kollmeier, M. A.,

Cox, B., & Zelefsky, M. J. (2013). Long-term survival and toxicity in patients treated with high-dose intensity modulated radiation therapy for localized prostate cancer. *International Journal of Radiation Oncology, Biology, Physics, 85,* 686–692.

Spring, B. (2007). Evidence-based practice in clinical psychology: What it is, why it matters; what you need to know. *Journal of Clinical Psychology, 63,* 611–631.

Stanovich, K. (2012). *How to think straight about psychology* (10th ed.). Boston: Pearson.

Steer, R. Y., & Ritschel, L. A. (2010). Placebo. In I. Weiner & W. E. Craighead (Eds.), *Corsini encyclopedia of psychology* (pp. 1252–1254). Hoboken, NJ: Wiley.

Stewart, R. E., & Chambless, D. L. (2007). Does psychotherapy research inform treatment decisions in private practice? *Journal of Clinical Psychology, 63,* 267–281.

Straus, S. E., Glasziou, P., Richardson, W. S., & Haynes, R. B. (2011). *Evidence-based medicine: How to practice and teach it* (4th ed.). Edinburgh, UK: Elsevier.

Streiner, D. L. (2001). Regression towards the mean: Its etiology, diagnosis, and treatment. *Canadian Journal of Psychiatry, 46,* 72–76.

Strong, S. R. (1991). Theory-driven science and naive empiricism in counseling psychology. *Journal of Counseling Psychology, 38,* 204–210.

Stuart, R. B., & Lilienfeld, S. O. (2007). The evidence missing from evidence-based practice. *American Psychologist, 62,* 615–616.

Swift, J. K., & Greenberg, R. P. (2015). *What is premature termination, and why does it occur?* Washington, DC: American Psychological Association.

Szasz, T. (2006). Mental illness as brain disease: A brief history lesson. *Ideas on Liberty, 56,* 24–25.

Tavris, C., & Aronson, E. (2007). *Mistakes were made (but not by me): Why we justify foolish beliefs, bad decisions, and hurtful actions.* Boston: Houghton-Mifflin.

Tehrani, E. E., Krussel, J. J., Borg, L. L., & Munk-Jørgensen, P. P. (1996). Dropping out of psychiatric treatment: A prospective study of a first-admission cohort. *Acta Psychiatrica Scandinavica, 94*(4), 266–271.

Tellegen, A., Ben-Porath, Y. S., McNulty, J. L., Arbisi, P. A., Graham, J. R., & Kaemmer, B. (2003). *MMPI-2 Restructured Clinical (RC) scales: Development, validation, and interpretation.* Minneapolis: University of Minnesota Press.

Thorndike, E. L. (1940). *Human nature and social order.* New York: Macmillan.

Thyer, B. A., & Pignotti, M. (2011). Evidence-based practices do not exist. *Clinical Social Work Journal, 39,* 328–333.

Tierney, A. J. (2000). Egas Moniz and the origins of psychosurgery: A review commemorating the 50th anniversary of Moniz's Nobel Prize. *Journal of the History of the Neurosciences, 9,* 22–36.

Tolin, D. F. (2010). Is cognitive-behavioral therapy more effective than other therapies?: A meta-analytic review. *Clinical Psychology Review, 30,* 710–720.

Tracey, T. J., Wampold, B. E., Lichtenberg, J. W., & Goodyear, R. K. (2014). Expertise in psychotherapy: An elusive goal? *American Psychologist, 69,* 218–229.

Valenstein, E. S. (1986). *Great and desperate cures: The rise and decline of psychosurgery and other radical treatments for mental illness.* New York: Basic Books.

VanderVeen, J. W., Reddy, L. F., Veilleux, J. C., January, A. M., & DiLillo, D. (2012). Clinical PhD graduate student views of their scientist-practitioner training. *Journal of Clinical Psychology, 68,* 1048–1057.

Wachtel, P. L. (2010). Beyond "ESTs": Problematic assumptions in the pursuit of evidence-based practice. *Psychoanalytic Psychology, 27,* 251–272.

Walfish, S., McAlister, B., O'Donnell, P., & Lambert, M. J. (2012). An investigation of self-assessment bias in mental health providers. *Psychological Reports, 110,* 639–644.

Wampold, B. E., Frost, N. D., & Yulish, N. E. (2016). Placebo effects in psychotherapy: A flawed concept and a contorted history. *Psychology of Consciousness: Theory, Research, and Practice, 3*(2), 108–120.

Wampold, B. E., & Imel, Z. E. (2015). *The great psychotherapy debate: The evidence for what makes psychotherapy work.* New York: Routledge.

Wampold, B. E., Mondin, G. W., Moody, M., Stich, F., Benson, K., & Ahn, H. N. (1997). A meta-analysis of outcome studies comparing bona fide psychotherapies: Empirically, all must have prizes." *Psychological Bulletin, 122,* 203–215.

Weisz, J. R., Weersing, V. R., & Henggeler, S. W. (2005). Jousting with straw men: Comment on Westen, Novotny, and Thompson-Brenner (2004). *Psychological Bulletin, 131,* 418–426.

Weisz, J. R., Weiss, B., Han, S. S., Granger, D. A., & Morton, T. (1995). Effects of psychotherapy with children and adolescents revisited: A meta-analysis of treatment outcome studies. *Psychological Bulletin, 117,* 450–468.

Westen, D., Novotny, C. M., & Thompson-Brenner, H. (2004). The empirical status of empirically supported psychotherapies: Assumptions, findings, and reporting in controlled clinical trials. *Psychological Bulletin, 130,* 631–663.

Winer, G. A., Cottrell, J. E., Gregg, V. R., Foumier, J. S., & Bica, L. A. (2002). Fundamentally misunderstanding visual perception: Adults' belief in visual emissions. *American Psychologist, 57,* 417–424.

Wood, J. M., & Nezworski, M. T. (2005). Science as a history of corrected mistakes: Comment. *American Psychologist, 60,* 657–658.

Zuger, A. (2015, October 30). Book review: "Ending medical reversal" laments flip-flopping. *New York Times.* Retrieved from *www.nytimes.com/2015/11/03/science/book-review-ending-medical-reversal-laments-flip-flopping.html.*

PART II

CORE COMPONENTS OF EVIDENCE-BASED PRACTICE

CHAPTER 4

Doing Right by Your Patients

What Do Clinicians Need to Know about Randomized Clinical Trials?

HELENA CHMURA KRAEMER
VYJEYANTHI S. PERIYAKOIL

Evidence-based practice (EBP) requires that clinicians use the results of clinical research to make decisions for the individual patients whom they treat. Within the hierarchy of clinical research, a randomized clinical trial (RCT) is often placed at the pinnacle (see Spring, Marchese, & Steglitz, Chapter 1, this volume). In an RCT, participants are randomly assigned to either the treatment group or the control group, and other rules are followed to ensure validity of the conclusions. This approach contrasts with other types of clinical trials, such as those that are uncontrolled (i.e., there is no comparison group or historical controls are used) or nonrandom (e.g., when participants are assigned to the intervention or control arm by a nonrandom process, for example, by patient or clinician preference). A well-designed and implemented RCT that minimizes bias and has a higher likelihood of leading to robust and reproducible conclusions about treatment effects is thus considered to be a "gold standard" approach in evaluating a treatment. There are perhaps hundreds of books written to guide researchers on conducting RCTs, and perhaps thousands of RCTs in the literature; however, our focus in this chapter is on what clinicians need to know about RCTs for the sake of their patients and the integrity of their fields.

Both of us are researchers, one a clinician (Periyakoil), the other a biostatistician (Kraemer). We both have been patients, with loved ones who also have been patients. The issues we address here try to reconcile what we know as researchers with what we know as clinicians and patients, in the hope of convincing clinicians to be more willing to use the scientific literature that reports RCTs and to participate in RCTs. Conversely, we address these issues in the hope of convincing researchers to make RCTs more relevant to the needs of clinicians and patients.

We aim to reconcile some of the inherent tensions between clinical research and practice by explaining to clinicians the key elements of an RCT, why the criteria for conducting an RCT are as they are, why these criteria are necessary to guard against erroneous results, and how to distinguish valid RCTs from flawed ones. (Not infrequently, researchers need these reminders as well!) We point out strategies sometimes used in RCTs that compromise their relevance to clinical decision making. We also discuss the various roles a clinician might play in an RCT, in collaboration with the clinical researchers who design, execute, analyze, and report the results. We argue that clinicians have important roles to play with respect to RCTs, to guide the best possible care for their own patients and to improve the quality of RCTs, strengthen the relationship between clinical research and practice, and potentially lead to robust and relevant clinical research that improves overall quality of clinical care for all patients.

Inherent Tensions

Feinstein (1985) discussed the ethical challenges for clinicians related to RCTs. He pointed out that there are two sets of viewpoints for clinicians with regard to RCTs, each completely justifiable, but the two are often irreconcilable: the "societal" versus the "samaritan."

From the "samaritan" viewpoint, clinicians "are obligated to do their best for individual patients" (Feinstein, 1985, p. 704). Thus, the concern of the clinician is to promote the best possible care and avoid error, one patient at a time. From the "societal" viewpoint, clinicians who conduct RCTs (hereafter, only for simplicity, called "researchers," for many are also clinicians) are "obliged to find and demonstrate worthwhile agents of therapy" (p. 704). Thus, the concern of the researcher is to design, conduct, and report clinical trials that improve how *other* clinicians deal with *their* future patients. Their ethical responsibility is not merely to protect those patients who actually participate in the trial, but to ensure that the trial does not result in incorrect conclusions that might harm patients whom the researchers might never meet. Frequently, what needs to be done in the trial to protect future patients and clinicians ("societal" mode) may not align with what the researcher would have done had he or she been acting as that patient's clinical decision maker ("samaritan" mode). With the emphasis on EBP (Sackett, Strauss, Richardson, Rosenberg, & Haynes, 2000), clinicians are urged to base decision making for each patient on the results of clinical trials, thus making the success of the "samaritan" mode dependent on the success of the "societal" mode, and vice versa. Yet the tensions between these two viewpoints continue, often to the detriment of patients' well-being.

An interesting and dismaying fact: In the "samaritan" viewpoint, clinicians can be sued for malpractice (and often are) for harming *one* patient, while in the "societal" viewpoint, clinicians can (and do) publish highly misleading studies at no personal risk, even if these studies ultimately may harm *thousands* of patients

(Ioannidis, 2005a, 2005b). Consequently, this reality places a burden on all clinicians to understand the issues related to RCTs, in order to assess whether any particular RCT is both valid and relevant to their patients' needs, and to ignore those that are not. This is also motivation for all clinicians to become involved in RCTs in some capacity, so that their voices will be heard. Their voices can clarify which questions require answers and can encourage the highest quality of research to answer those questions.

Yet, as we have noted, clinicians are often uncertain about how to access and interpret the reports of RCTs. Often, they also are reluctant to participate in RCTs, and to encourage their patients to do so. Thus, patients participating in RCTs may not be representative of the patients whom clinicians see, the questions to which clinicians need answers are ignored, or the answers provided are not clearly interpretable by clinicians. At the same time, errors occur in RCTs that might have been avoided had the voices of clinicians been heard in designing, executing, or reporting the results of RCTs. In our view, the resolution of these inherent tensions begins with understanding the key elements and rationale for an RCT, then, building on this foundation of knowledge, embodying three critical roles that clinicians have an opportunity to fill (i.e., as audience/interpreter of RCTs for individual patients, as consultant to the researchers conducting the RCT, and as ambassador for the RCT).

Why an RCT, and What Is It?

The purpose of an RCT is to evaluate the impact of choosing one of two treatments, the as yet unproved treatment of interest (T) and a control/comparison treatment (C), based on clinical outcome in a particular population of patients, to inform clinicians who may face the choice for their patients as to which is better. Often an RCT may involve more than two treatments, but the goal would still be to compare any pair of these treatments and decide between them. For simplicity, then, we focus on RCTs that compare only two treatments. The rationale and justification for the hypothesis that T and C differ in whatever the primary outcome is, must be a priori (i.e., stated before the RCT is underway). This is usually required in any proposal for funding of the RCT. In the United States, clinicians can check by looking up the RCT registration on *clinicaltrials.gov*. We define the essential criteria of an RCT and the rationale for these criteria, all of which need to be interpreted to determine the relevance and value of any RCT for a clinical practice.

Control/Comparison Group

If we are interested in the effect of T, why not just give T to a series of patients and see whether they improve? In research design "terms," this would mean conducting a simple pretreatment–posttreatment design, with no control group. A major problem with this strategy is that the decision to treat is usually based on an observation of high symptom burden in the patient. Since such an observation is not completely reliable, those patients with a false "high" (those who, because of error of measurement, register much higher than their true value) will be included, but those with a false "low" (those who register much lower than their true value) will be excluded. Then, even when there is absolutely no overall change in clinical status of the patients, the group as a whole will appear to improve because the false "highs" will subsequently revert to their true lower response, and the others included will remain at more or less the same response. This phenomenon is known as *statistical regression to the mean* (Campbell & Kenny, 1999).

Statistical regression to the mean is one case of a statistical artifact, but it is by no means the only one. A *statistical artifact* is some pattern seen in a dataset that is due not to patient behavior or response but to measurement, design, or analysis errors. Let's consider some other key potential statistical artifacts in a simple pretreatment–posttreatment design.

First, initiation of a treatment often inspires expectation effects. As Yogi Berra was quoted as saying: "If I hadn't believed it, I wouldn't have seen it!" Such expectation effects (on the part of the patients, as well as the treatment evaluators) often result in the appearance of improvement when there is none. Second, secular trends also may impact a simple pretreatment–posttreatment design. For example, as evaluators become more and more comfortable with measurement techniques, there are often drifts in measurement of patient response even when patients are completely stable. Alternatively, patients replying to the same questions over and over become less thoughtful about response, simply repeating what they have said before, or

responding the way they think the researchers want them to respond. All such effects can present a false impression of improvement when there is none.

For these reasons, it is important to be skeptical of treatments whose effectiveness is not based on RCTs. A simple pretreatment–posttreatment design cannot overcome the potential biases that are introduced by the statistical artifacts that we have reviewed. In contrast, *it is an RCT criterion that a control or comparison treatment (C) is required to determine which the treatment of interest (T) is to be compared.* Since, under RCT "rules," statistical artifacts equally affect both treatment (T) and control or comparison (C) groups, the difference in response between the groups then indicates the true effect of T. The RCT therefore provides the type of evidence that can allow one to have more confidence in the effect of the treatment. In reading the published reports of an RCT, it is important to pay attention to the comparison between the T and C. It occasionally happens that researchers, unable to demonstrate that the two treatments differ, then report on each treatment separately, claiming that both produced improvement. Be warned: This improvement is usually primarily statistical artifact! Only the comparison between two treatments is meaningful.

Randomization

It is clear, now, why *comparing* T and C is important, but why *randomize* patients to them? Why not take a series of patients from clinic records given T and another series of patients given C, and simply compare their response to treatment? Well, clinicians rarely make important decisions—such as whether to use T versus C—randomly. Instead, clinicians tend to try to pick the treatment most likely to benefit the patient. This makes good sense from the "samaritan" viewpoint; clinicians want to use the interventions they believe will be most helpful for a given patient. It is a problem, though, from the "societal" viewpoint in planning a research study. Those patients in clinic records who were given T and those who were given C often (perhaps usually) are not comparable to each other; those given T would not likely respond to C as did those given C, and vice versa.

Thus, to ensure that the two groups are comparable to start with, they should be randomly assigned from the same population. *Conse-*

quently, it is an RCT criterion that a sample is drawn from the population to which the conclusions are meant to apply, then randomly assigned to the treatment (T) and control/comparison (C) conditions.

It should be noted that randomization to T and C results not in two *matched* samples, but in two *random* samples from the same population. Usually, the first table in a report of the results of the RCT is a list of descriptive statistics of baseline characteristics of those assigned to T and to C (age, gender, ethnicity, race, socioeconomic status, clinical history, severity, etc.). This is valuable information for clinicians reading the report, who can then assess how the population sampled compared with the patients they see. With randomization, each baseline characteristic has a 5% chance of significantly differentiating the T and C groups (reported as $p < .05$). If there are multiple baseline measurements, one should always expect some significant differences between T and C. Problems arise when, seeing such differences, researchers then amend the a priori hypothesis they designed the RCT to test, to one that "adjusts for" or "controls for" the baseline differences seen (Kraemer, 2015). This is post hoc testing; it changes the rules and goals of the game while the game is under way by changing the focus from the a priori hypothesized effect of T versus C in the total population, to the effect of T versus C for the subpopulation of patients matched on whatever variable(s) was "controlled for/matched on," hence post hoc. This is a bit like offering to place a bet at prerace odds on a horse, as the horses approach the finish line. Often the conclusions based on such testing prove to be nonreplicable in future testing, for, of course, different baseline characteristics will be "statistically significant" in any future studies. Thus, if an RCT proposes a priori to "adjust for" some baseline variable, providing rationale and justification for that hypothesis, and the study is designed adequately to address that question, it is valid to "adjust," but, if the decision is based on examining the data from the RCT, all bets are off. Unfortunately, such "adjustment" is rather common practice.

However, after an RCT is completed and conclusions drawn on the hypothesis that the RCT was designed to test, it is good research practice to explore the RCT dataset to develop hypotheses for future studies, or to better understand the results of this RCT. Researchers might explore

whether any baseline characteristics moderated the treatment effect, that is, identify subpopulations of eligible patients who have different responses to T versus C (Kraemer, Frank, & Kupfer, 2006). This is true regardless of whether any particular baseline characteristic significantly differentiated the T and C groups in that RCT. However, any results of such exploration should be reported separately from the conclusions based on the RCT, and reported as tentative hypotheses to be tested in future RCTs.

Of the various criteria defining an RCT, randomization often seems particularly concerning to clinicians. However, this wariness seems to arise not so much from the randomization per se but from what is used as the C condition. We would propose (even if many disagree), that if there is effective treatment already available, the patients participating in a RCT should never be given less than that effective treatment, that anything less is essentially withholding treatment. Thus, if clinicians already have access to effective treatments and would not consider (in the "samaritan" mode) taking a "wait and see" approach with such a patient (sometimes called a *nocebo*), or using a placebo (an intervention known to have no effect), then (in the "societal" mode) a wait list, placebo, or nocebo control is not the best choice for C. The ideal choice of control group for clinicians is what would have been used for patients had T not been available: the current "standard of treatment" or "treatment as usual" (i.e., asking clinicians to make decisions as they would ordinarily do, with response evaluated by "blinded" evaluators in the RCT).

At the very earliest stages of development of a new treatment, for example, RCTs done for U.S. Food and Drug Administration (FDA) approval, a placebo might be the first choice simply because it is easier to find that T is more effective than placebo than it is to find that T is more effective than the best already available treatment. If a newly developed treatment cannot be shown to be better than doing nothing, it would seem foolhardy to further pursue evaluation of that treatment. But, as a consequence, treatments described in advertisements or by pharmaceutical company representatives as "approved by the FDA" may be less effective and/or have more side effects that other treatments previously "approved by the FDA."

Finally, if patients being considered for an RCT know that the treatment they will receive is unlikely to be less (and likely to be more) effective than what they would receive if they choose not to participate in the RCT, they are more likely to agree to participate (resulting in a more representative sample from the population of interest), and they are less likely to drop out (helping with the "intention to treat" problem in analysis that we describe below).

Choice of a C group is a difficult choice for researchers. It often seems that, whatever choice researchers make, and however careful and thoughtful their choice, someone will criticize! The message to clinicians is to consider whether the choice between T and whatever C is selected applies to their own decision making. If a RCT uses an inert placebo in a situation in which you, the clinician, would never consider an inert placebo over the treatment you usually choose and believe effective, this RCT might be one you would choose to ignore.

Population and Sampling

It is a criterion for an RCT that the population sampled be well described, for the results of the RCT are unlikely to generalize beyond the limits of the population sampled. If the study focuses on males over age 50, the results cannot be presumed to apply to younger men or to women. This was a major problem with cardiology studies that were conducted before about 1990. All the RCTs on which one of us (Kraemer) was then consulted sampled male populations, which led her naively to believe that women rarely had heart attacks! Yet the cardiac event then and now is a major killer of women, and the presentation of coronary disease, as well as its treatment, for women is not the same as that for men. Generalizing from RCTs involving only men to the general population was a major error. The population is defined both by the sampling frame (i.e., how the patients were recruited) and by the baseline description usually reported in the first table of an RCT report. As a clinician, it is important to pay attention to the recruitment methods and the sample characteristics to determine the relevance of the population to the patients one treats.

It also must be remembered that a study done at a single site may not generalize to other sites because of sociodemographic differences between the populations accessible at any one site, or differences in medical practices, or idiosyncrasies of the clinicians or research staff (Kraemer & Robinson, 2005). It has been our experience, for example, that having office staff members who are personable, kind and patient, makes a big difference to the success of any treatment in an RCT, and the different staff members at different sites may explain some site differences. This is why multisite RCTs are particularly valuable: They can investigate the generalizability of the RCT conclusion to the wider population of sites represented by those in the RCT, and they can provide clues about potentially important factors that can be tested in future RCTs (e.g., the warmth of office staff members).

The inclusion–exclusion criteria are often set too stringently, very often in RCTs conducted by pharmaceutical companies in seeking approval for licensing a new medication by the FDA. In such trials, patients whom the researchers anticipate will be hard to treat, resistant to treatment, uncooperative, and so forth, are likely to be excluded in order to have the best possible chance of finding T effective. Wouldn't you, if you were in that position? In some cases, the majority of patients with the indication to be treated are excluded from participation (Humphreys & Weisner, 2000). Since the results of an RCT apply only to the population sampled in the RCT, the results of such RCTs will not apply to many, perhaps most, of a clinician's patients. The results of such RCTs should be taken with the proverbial grain of salt.

The RCTs of greatest applied clinical value take "all comers," thus seeking to cover the full spectrum of patients for whom clinicians might be faced with the decision between T and C. These trials are often called *effectiveness* or *pragmatic* RCTs (Glasgow, Magid, Beck, Ritzwoller, & Estabrooks, 2005; Hoagwood, Hibbs, Brent, & Jensen, 1995; March et al., 2005; Tunis, Stryer, & Clancy, 2003). Clearly, any patient with the indication to be treated, who is likely to be harmed by T1 or T2 (e.g., pregnant women in drug studies), who could not possibly benefit (e.g., non-English speakers in a group therapy program delivered in English), or who is unwilling to participate, must ethically be excluded from participation. Otherwise, pragmatic trials prioritize enrolling a broad and representative sample, keeping the inclusion and exclusion criteria minimal. When one reads RCTs, it is important to pay close attention to the recruitment methods and inclusion and exclusion criteria, and to ask oneself: "How closely do the patients included in the trial resemble the patients I treat in my practice?"

Treatment Protocols

Since the end product of an RCT is a recommendation to clinicians as to which of T and C is to be preferred for the patients in the population sampled, *it is a criterion for an RCT that the protocols for both T and C be defined and described,* carefully and completely enough that clinicians, in their practices, can reproduce what researchers did in the study. Moreover, valuable information in the report of RCT results includes whether the researchers assessed whether the T and C were delivered as intended (fidelity), and to what extent patients followed the instructions they were given (compliance). It does not suffice, for example, to say that a certain drug was used for T: Dosage, timing, what concomitant treatments were allowed or disallowed, and so forth, must all be specified to give a clinician any hope that the results reported in the RCT may be relevant to his or her own patients. Defining treatment protocols for nonpharmacological treatments (e.g., psychotherapy) is a particular challenge, for the protocols must delineate what the therapists must do, what they must not do, and the manner or style with which these actions must be undertaken (Arean & Kraemer, 2013). Although some have objected to the use of treatment protocols for psychotherapy, concerned that they oversimplify the process of psychotherapy, such protocols are essential to guide clinicians as to how to reproduce the treatment in their practices. It is possible to create both standardized and flexible manuals (Chambless & Ollendick, 2001). For example, protocol-driven manuals standardize what the clinician does session by session (Craske & Barlow, 2007). Principle-driven manuals articulate the core strategies of a psychotherapy and the theory that guides the clinician in the flexible application of these strategies

Blinding Procedures

One general ethical issue in conducting RCTs is what has been called *clinical equipoise.* It is not ethical to randomize patients to two treatments if the researchers are already sure that T is better than C. That constitutes a deliberate exposure of patients to a treatment known by the researchers to be inferior. The researchers conducting the RCT must each have reasonable doubt as to which, T or C, is better before randomization becomes ethical, and the design must be such that the results will likely shake that reasonable

doubt. There are ethical reasons for this (Freedman, 1987), but from a practical point of view, the matter is straightforward. If the researcher already "knows" the "right" answer, he or she will almost inevitably bias the design, measurements, analysis, or reporting of the results in the direction of that "right" answer. Those doing RCTs are always motivated by a hope or belief that T may be better than C, but in the conduct of the RCT, each must be as willing to prove that as its opposite: reasonable doubt.

Blinding is one critical way to protect against bias. If the assessment of outcome is influenced by prior knowledge of which individual patients were assigned to T and which to C, the outcomes are likely to be biased. Because the motivation to do an RCT, at least an ethical RCT, is rooted in some rationale and justification to believe that T may be preferable to C for the patients in the population sampled (the a priori hypothesis), researchers are vulnerable to bias. If those doing assessment of outcome believe or hope that T is preferable to C, they may be more sensitive to improvement in the T group and less in the C group, thus increasing the risk of a self-fulfilling prophecy. Then, even if T is less effective than C, it may look better because of the (implicit or explicit) biases of the evaluators. *Consequently, it is a criterion of an RCT that the assessment of treatment outcome should be protected from the biases of evaluators: "blinding" of outcome.*

Ideally, there would be triple blinding; that is, the clinicians delivering the treatments, the patients receiving the treatments, and the researchers evaluating response to treatment are all kept unaware of which treatment is being received by which patient. Practically, however, it is often difficult, if not impossible, to "blind" everyone. Certainly, if the treatment is psychotherapy, those delivering the treatment cannot be blinded, even if the patients receiving the treatment may not be aware of the protocol guiding that treatment. The minimal requirement, then, is that those evaluating treatment outcome be kept as "blinded" as possible, which is to say that those delivering the treatment should not be evaluators of treatment outcome, and wherever possible, treatment outcome measures should be objective ones.

Analysis by Intention to Treat

Finally, once a patient is randomized into a RCT, that patient's outcome must be included in analyzing the RCT results. Thus, analysis by intention to treat, or ITT, as is often called in the research literature, means that all patients who were randomized are included in the analyses. This RCT rule preserves the representativeness of the sample, and the randomness of assignment to T and to C. *Analysis by ITT is also a criterion of a valid RCT.* Randomization results in two random (not matched) samples from the same population (whatever that population is). If those who drop out after randomization are omitted from analysis, the advantage of randomization is lost, for treatment response and reaction are often part of the reasons for such dropouts. For example, it is not unusual to see an RCT evaluating a psychotherapy intervention that requires weekly meetings for several weeks, to propose to limit analysis only to those patients who attend at least, say, three meetings. This criterion often is uncomfortable for researchers, who may often prefer to ignore those who drop out after randomization or who do not comply, in order to make T appear as effective as possible. Why, they ask, should the results of those not fully exposed to T be used to evaluate T? The answer is that dropout often represents patients "voting with their feet" (i.e., expressing their dissatisfaction with their assigned treatment by dropping out). Thus, dropout itself may be an outcome of treatment choice. Researchers are required to report how much dropout there was (usually in the Consolidated Standards of Reporting Trials [CONSORT] diagram), and if the percentage is high in either the T or C group, clinicians reading the results should become somewhat leery. The RCT report is also required to convey how missing data are handled, but, even for other researchers and biostatisticians, assessment of whether the assumptions made and the mathematical methods applied are correct is a difficult task.

Choice of Outcome Measures

The decision to recommend T versus C in an RCT is based on which has the better outcome. T may be better than C in reducing symptoms but have a far worse side effects profile. Which outcome is chosen as "primary," or which outcomes are reported, have a major influence on the decision, as well as on a clinician's decision to use T rather than C (Zimmerman et al., 2006). The choice of outcomes in a study should be relevant to patient preferences and include patient-reported outcomes to the extent possible. Thus, a study might report depression improvement as the primary outcome, but a patient might be equally interested in improvement in occupational functioning (perhaps even more so), making it important for clinicians to identify information that is relevant to what patients want. Also, patients might have different views about what constitutes success of a treatment. This is also a component of research design that can benefit from input of clinicians, who may be able to use their clinical experiences to identify factors important to patients.

The choice of the primary outcome is always a difficult one. Every individual patient may experience change, for the better or for the worse, in symptom level, quality of life, functional status, side effects (e.g., rash, headaches), change in risk of heart attacks, or in libido. How much preferable T is to C for an individual patient in the population sampled depends on which benefits and which harms he or she experiences and how the benefits counterbalance the harms. However, the pattern of benefits and harms differs from one patient to another, and what value a patient places on each benefit and harm also differs. Thus, in the societal mode, the task is to choose a single outcome (or very few or a composite; Kraemer, Frank, & Kupfer, 2011; Wallace, Frank, & Kraemer, 2013) likely to be important to the majority of those in the population. Whatever the choice, it will not satisfy each individual patient or clinician.

Moreover, the analysis of any single outcome may be based on various different measures of the same outcome. For example, in a trial of a drug for major depressive disorder, one might use the Hamilton Depression Rating Scale (HDRS; Hamilton, 1960) score at the end of treatment, or the change in the HDRS over the treatment period, or the slope of the HDRS over time in treatment, or an indicator of whether there was a 50% decrease in the HDRS over the treatment period or any of a number of others. Or one might use a completely different depression scale with all such variations.

The reliability and validity of which measure is used has a major impact on the RCT results. The crucial question for the clinician is whether a differential response on whatever the outcome measure chosen by the researchers would be convincing evidence for choosing T over C. For example, if the primary measure selected in an RCT in a population of patients with major depressive disorder were a change in some brain function, however scientifically interesting and important such a result might be, would that convince you to use it on your depressed patients? On the other hand, if it could be shown that symptoms were reduced, quality of life improved, functional ability was enhanced, and risk of suicide was reduced, such measures are more relevant to the goals of clinical practice. Once a clinician accepts the primary outcome as relevant to his or her decision making, the primary task is to evaluate how much difference is reported between T and C patients (effect sizes) and to decide whether that difference is convincing enough to apply T rather than C to his or her patients. A highly "statistically significant" result may be of little or no clinical significance, and a nonstatistically significant result, while indicating an inconclusive result, may prove highly clinically significant in future, better-designed RCTs.

The sensitivity of the measure to individual differences in a patient's response also is critical. For example, a binary outcome (e.g., Is there a 50% decrease in the HDRS over the treatment period?) will often require doubling or tripling the sample size to detect any treatment effects, and the effect of the treatment will appear smaller. On the other hand, a trajectory measure (the slope of HDRS over repeated measured during the treatment period) will often result in much greater power to detect treatment effects and a larger impact. As a rule of thumb, if the sample size necessary to detect a treatment effect in an RCT is inversely proportional to its reliability coefficient, then the greater the reliability of the outcome measure, the smaller the sample size necessary to detect a T versus C difference. For this reason, if the RCT result is reported as "statistically significant," the question for clinicians is whether the effect size is big enough to convince them to use T rather than C. However, if the RCT result is reported as "not statistically significant," this is essentially a "hung jury," most likely due to poor choices in measurement, design, or analysis.

An important consideration for clinicians is the harm–benefit balance for individual patients. Thus if 50% of patients are better off with T than with C in terms of symptom reduction, but the same 50% experience major disabling side effects, the fact that T is better than C for symptom reduction may not be relevant. Although researchers of psychotherapy studies often have not reported information about adverse effects, this information is essential for

clinicians to know, so that they can weigh the harm–benefit balance.

The bottom line is that clinicians considering an RCT should critically evaluate the outcome chosen, and the measure of that outcome, to see whether this would provide convincing (to them) evidence of the effectiveness of the treatments under evaluation.

Fidelity

It is the task of the researchers to define the population of interest, to sample that population, to randomize to T and to C, to follow the treatment protocols for the delivery of treatments, and to follow the research protocol for the measurement of outcome. The term used to describe how researchers follow the rules they themselves set up for the RCT is *fidelity*. It is a remarkable fact how often, after RCT onset, researchers begin to fiddle with the inclusion–exclusion criteria, with rules for delivery of treatment, or evaluation of outcome. Any deviations from protocol, planned or accidental, during an RCT, compromise the validity of the RCT results. This is like changing the rules and conditions of the game after the game is under way! It is possible for clinicians to check the ways in which studies are described in the literature against the preregistration information on websites such as *clinicaltrials.gov*. Any study results in which the study has low fidelity must be interpreted with caution.

Roles a Clinician Might Play in an RCT

Three roles are essential for clinicians with respect to RCTs:

1. In the first role, the clinician works in the "samaritan" mode and acts as the *audience* to whom the results of RCTs are reported, and the *interpreter* of those results for his or her own patients as a basis of clinical decision making. In the second and third roles, the clinician works in the "societal" mode.
2. In the second role, the clinician serves as *consultant* to the researchers who conduct RCTs, or as an "ambassador" linking the researchers in an RCT with patient participants in the RCT.
3. In the third role, the clinician has the important task of serving as *champion* of RCTs, engaging with researchers to ensure that

they are asking questions that are meaningful to patient care and encouraging patients to participate in RCTs.

The Clinician as Audience and Interpreter of the RCT

We have outlined the key elements of the RCT and the rationale for each of these elements. Carefully reviewing the results of RCTs and being judiciously guided by the results in the care of the individual patient is the heart of EBP. The overall question for a clinician is first: Given the previously discussed RCT rules, is this a study that produced results I can trust? Table 4.1 summarizes the key RCT rules and questions for clinicians to ask of published reports to evaluate how well the RCT followed each rule. Evaluating these key elements is important to inform the clinician in deciding whether the results are worth consideration at all.

For example, a study (Stamfer et al., 1991) published in 1985 based on a survey of 121,964 female nurses between ages 30 and 55 years, with longitudinal follow-up, compared two groups: those who did (T) and did not (C) use hormone replacement therapy (HRT), with a comparison in the occurrence of heart disease in the two groups as the outcome. There were a number of statistical problems with what was reported, but fundamentally this was *not* a RCT, valid or not. It was an observational study. The conclusion suggesting HRT for women of a certain age (in absence of strong counterindication), in order to reduce the incidence of coronary disease, should not have motivated *any* clinician to use HRT for that purpose. Nevertheless, many clinicians did exactly that over approximately the next 15 years. Motivated by an apparent increased risk of breast cancer and no major change in risk for heart disease, the Women's Health Initiative Investigators (2002) conducted an RCT. They found that with HRT (compared to placebo), there was a slight increase in risk of heart disease, but a major increase in the risk of breast cancer and of cognitive decline. In fact, that RCT had to be brought to an early close because the increased risks with HRT were apparent quite soon in the planned RCT.

There are statistical methods to bring the conclusions drawn from observational studies more in line with what would have resulted from an RCT (Jo & Stuart, 2009; Rosenbaum & Rubin, 1983), but the methods are complicated and based on assumptions that often are not met. Observational studies serve important purposes, particularly as the motivation and basis of RCTs, but as a basis of clinical decision making between treatments, they remain inferior to RCTs. If there are serious departures from any of the RCT criteria listed in Table 4.1, the validity of the conclusions become questionable, and the clinician should be wary of adopting recommendations based on those conclusions.

Once the clinician is reasonably assured that the study is a valid RCT, the next question concerns what conclusions were warranted. Clinicians often are intimidated by the "results sec-

---

TABLE 4.1. Crucial Questions for Clinicians to Ask in Considering Use of RCT Results in Clinical Decision Making

1. Is the sampled population described well-enough, so that you can determine whether a patient belongs?

2. Is there an appropriate control or comparison treatment (C) against which the treatment is evaluated (T)?

3. Are the protocols for T and C described clearly enough to emulate in your practice?

4. Are sampled patients RANDOMLY assigned to T or C?

5. Is the outcome measure one that would motivate you to use T rather than C?

6. Was there suitable protection against bias (e.g., "blinding")?

7. Did the RCT result in a recommendation for T or C (i.e., was there a "statistically significant" difference between outcomes of T and C)?

8. Was the size of the differential effect of T versus C reported strongly enough to motivate you to use T rather than C?

Note. Items 1–6 are determined from the Materials and Methods section of the report, 7 and 8 from the Results.

tion" of an RCT report and uncertain about how to interpret what is written. A number of excellent resources exist for explaining specific statistical tests in accessible, commonsense terms. Wikipedia is a good place to start, but there are also dictionaries in different fields (e.g., Last, 1995).

Here, we focus on the logical steps that are necessary in reading the results of RCTs. First, it is important to realize that a "statistically significant result at the 5% level" ($p < .05$) means that the sample size was large enough to detect some deviation from the null hypothesis that T and C were absolutely equivalent. Thus "statistical significance" is a comment about the design, not about the effectiveness of T versus C. A "nonstatistically significant result" means that the sample size was not large enough to detect any deviation from the null hypothesis, an inconclusive result. Such nonstatistically significant results are usually the result of inadequate sample size, unreliable outcome measures, poor design, or because the hypothesis was not adequately justified or was misled by what was already in the research literature. While valid but nonstatistically significant results should be published so as to avoid publication bias in meta-analyses (Cooper & Hedges, 1994) that would ultimately determine whether a consensus has been reached, such RCTs individually should *not* be the basis of any conclusions. The clinician should choose to wait for further better-designed studies, or meta-analyses of multiple studies documenting statistical significance.

Second, it is important to remember that statistical significance does not mean clinical significance. Every RCT report should include an effect size that clinicians can interpret either in addition to, or in place of, the p-value (Kraemer & Kupfer, 2006). There are several such effect sizes (Cumming, 2011). Our favorite for clinical use is number needed to treat (NNT) (Bogarty & Brophy, 2005; Cook & Sackett, 1995; Wen, Badgett, & Cornell 2005). If one sampled pairs of patients from the population, and treated one of each pair with T, the other with C, and considered one individual a "success" and the other a "failure" depending on which had a clinically preferable outcome (tossing a fair coin in case of a tie), how many pairs would one have to draw to expect to find one more "success" among those given T? Answer: NNT. The ideal number NNT is 1, in which case every patient given T has an outcome preferable to that of every patient given C. That never happens!

The larger the NNT, the more patients would be treated unnecessarily with T; they would have done just as well with C. Now, considering how serious the diagnosis is, the consequences of inadequate treatment, the costs of T and of C, how many patients would you, as a clinician, be willing to treat with T unnecessarily to have one success you would not have had with C? If the reported NNT falls much above that limit, the result may be statistically significant but not clinically significant, and you might consider T and C clinically equivalent. If the reported NNT falls below that limit, the result then is both statistically and clinically significant, and worth consideration in decision making. No one can tell a clinician what his or her critical value of NNT should be. Different clinicians may therefore interpret the same result differently. This is as it should be. For us, for prevention (e.g., preventing heart disease, cancer, polio) in which most in the sample will not have onset with or without adequate treatment, an NNT of around 200 would be acceptable; for acute treatment of existing disorders, an NNT of around 4 would be preferable.

There are also other effect sizes that might be reported: success rate difference, Cohen's *d*, odds ratio, and so forth (Kraemer & Kupfer, 2006). Some are simply the result of rescaling the NNT. Success rate difference, for example, equals 1/NNT, and, while obviously equivalent to NNT, is much easier to use in computations. Cohen's *d* is meant only for special circumstances, and in those circumstances, is also a rescaling of NNT. Odds ratio (OR) is often used in the RCT literature to compare success rates. However, the OR is only an indicator of nonrandomness (Kraemer, 2004; Kraemer et al., 1999; Newcombe, 2006; Sackett, 1996). When equal to 1, OR indicates no treatment effect (NNT infinite). When equal to any value greater than 1, it puts a lower limit on NNT: $NNT > (\sqrt{(OR)} + 1)/(\sqrt{(OR)} - 1)$. When OR = 4 is reported, for example, this means that NNT is somewhere between 3 and infinity, and that does not help clinical decision making. OR is unfortunately widely used, and widely misinterpreted. In reading such results, clinicians should try to find the two success rates being compared in the computation of OR. Then NNT = 1/difference in success rates.

Third, once the clinician is reasonably assured that the study is a valid RCT, and the result is clinically meaningful, the next questions must move to the level of the individual patient.

Does the population sampled in the RCT include this particular patient? If not, the conclusions are irrelevant for this patient (but perhaps not for others). Is the outcome measure one of clinical importance to the clinician and to this patient? For example, in a RCT of treatment for major depressive disorder, we personally would be more impressed with an increase in a valid and reliable quality of life (QOL) measure than with a decrease in a HDRS (Hamilton, 1960), which measures only symptom levels. Decrease of symptoms, as reflected in the HDRS, would certainly be picked up in the QOL measure, but the QOL scores would also reflect serious side effects and discomfort associated with the treatment, and would therefore more closely mirror the benefit–harm balance for an individual patient, like me. Other patients may feel differently. That is as it should be.

A complex consideration occurs with, for example, antipsychotics for treatment of schizophrenia. In one study (Lieberman et al., 2005), one drug was significantly more effective in reducing symptoms than another, but it was also associated with significant weight gain. If one were the parent of a teenager with schizophrenia, a child totally unable to attend school, often in trouble with the law, unable to interact with peers, one would be delighted to see a 10-pound weight gain, were one's child then able to function at close to normal levels. How one balances reduction of symptoms versus weight gain may well vary from one patient (or parent) to another. Thus, if an RCT reports only reduction of symptoms, or only weight gain, or does not balance one against the other in individual patients, it may leave the question of conclusions for this patient unclear.

There is, of course, the problem of whether the statistical analyses results are done correctly or not. It is the function of an institutional review board (IRB) to assess ethical issues and the overall viability of a RCT proposal. It is the function of reviewers of a proposal also to assess what is proposed for ethics and viability, as well as issues such as whether the tests proposed are valid and optimal or whether the RCT proposed has adequate power. It is the function of reviewers of research papers for publication to assess what was done in the RCT, which statistical tests are used, and what is reported, both its completeness and credibility. Thus, there are multiple levels of protection to prevent incorrect conclusions from entering the research literature. It is not the responsibility of the clinicians reading those reports, nor given the space limitations in publications, is it possible to do so. However, clinicians do have to be aware that some invalid analyses do slip through. This is one reason that independent validation or confirmation of the conclusions through meta-analysis (Cooper & Hedges, 1994; as described by Cuijpers & Cristea, Chapter 5, this volume) is always necessary to document a "scientific fact."

The Clinician as Consultant

When an author proofreads his or her own manuscript, he or she frequently cannot detect even some obvious errors. One tends to develop a sort of functional blindness to errors in materials one has worked hard to produce. In the same way, clinical researchers, having worked long and hard on developing the rationale and justification for an RCT, focusing on the myriad design, measurement and analytic issues, develop a functional blindness to what are sometimes errors in the proposal for an RCT, in conducting the RCT or in the interpretation and presentation of the results of an RCT, that are glaring to others. Clinicians as consultants can serve an important role as the "proofreaders" of proposals and papers and as ethical guides for researchers.

An amusing example: In a study of adolescents, it was proposed to study physical and behavioral changes expected to occur during the pubertal years. Well into the design phase, an outside observer of the discussion wondered what possible measurement instrument could be appropriately used for both boys and girls. Were boys to be faced with questions about menarche and breast development, and girls with questions about erections and wet dreams? Clearly, two separate instruments were needed, one for boys and the other for girls, which also meant that separate analyses would have to be done for boys and girls. In short, the study had to be redeveloped as two separate, parallel studies, one of adolescent boys and one of adolescent girls. It is remarkable how often a discerning clinician, caring for patients in the real world, can spot this kind of problem, one that seems to elude the most rigorous researchers because of their focus on more esoteric issues. Having clinicians hear or read the research questions and the proposal of how the researchers hope to address those questions can often prevent major errors.

To take a more serious, personal (Kraemer), and still controversial example: In one RCT, it was proposed that there would be a blood draw at entry to the study for genotyping and that the cell lines would be immortalized, so that possible genetic moderators of treatment response could be explored (a good and valid goal). The informed consent form stated this, as required, but also stated that the immortalized cell lines could thereafter be used for any purpose the geneticists desired, including being sold to a commercial company for medical development, and that the patient renounced any right to remuneration should that happen. Being well aware of past abuses in research based on genetics, I objected on ethical grounds to that informed consent form, even though the IRB had approved it. Personally, I cannot see how it constitutes "informed" consent when the patient is not told exactly what can or will happen to his or her data, and have the right to object to certain uses. Rather than participating in a study about which I had ethical qualms, I resigned. It is important to understand that no biostatistician, no researcher, no clinician (as well as no patient), is required to participate in any research study. Each has the right to refuse participation for any reason, good or bad. Whether I was right or wrong here is not the issue, and I accept that many think there is nothing wrong with such informed consent. If a clinician acting as consultant to any RCT has any doubt as to the ethics of a proposed study, it is incumbent on that clinician to bring the matter to the attention of those proposing the study, and if the situation is not remedied to his or her satisfaction, to resign from participation. Ethics is a personal matter.

Clinicians as consultants are also valuable in anticipating the questions other clinicians are likely to have about the RCT. For example, in one multisite RCT on low birthweight (<37 weeks gestation), premature babies (<2,500 grams), an instrument was used at the time of birth to ascertain the gestational age for determination of eligibility. If the mothers had early prenatal care, it was relatively easy to obtain a reliable and valid estimate of gestational age. However, low birthweight and prematurity are associated with low socioeconomic status, poverty, and lack of access to good medical care. Many of the mothers had no prenatal care. For those mothers, an assessment was proposed that examined the physical and neurological developmental signs of the newborn and thereby estimated gestational age. Clinicians involved in

the study protested strongly that in their experience, this instrument overestimated gestational age in high-stress pregnancies, which would result in excluding many infants from the study who should have qualified. Their concerns motivated a pilot study on this issue, which verified the experience of the clinicians (Constantine et al., 1987). The criteria for inclusion were accordingly modified (Infant Health and Development Program, 1990).

Clinicians as consultants are also valuable in anticipating whether the burden placed on patients by the treatment and evaluation protocols will be acceptable to their patients. Finding out, after the RCT is under way, that patients are not willing to undergo certain tests, to answer certain questions, to tolerate 4–6 hours of testing, or weekly test sessions, is a disaster. Clinicians often have a better sense of what patients will or can do.

Finally, clinician input on the papers reporting RCT results is often particularly valuable. Every field develops a jargon that is often confusing, if not incomprehensible, to those not in the field. This is true, too, of researchers. They use a certain language and take certain things for granted. The result is that the way RCT results are reported may become incomprehensible to the clinicians reading those reports. To have clinicians as consultants who will ask for clarification for certain statements, or point out the ways in which what is said may be misinterpreted by other clinicians reading those reports, improves the clarity and value of RCT reports.

The Clinician as Ambassador

In many cases, clinicians are invited not merely to act as consultants but to be involved in an RCT, to recruit their patients into the RCT, to deliver the treatment protocols defined by the RCT, and/or to evaluate the outcomes for the RCT. There is a particular advantage to this, since the treatment is then being delivered and/ or evaluated in the exact milieu and for the exact type of patients who would ultimately be affected by the RCT conclusions. Implementing the RCT in this context increases the *ecological validity* (i.e., the extent to which what is found in a research study demonstrates what would be found in clinical applications).

Once again, ethical considerations become primary. If a clinician questions the ethical basis (e.g., use of a placebo as a control), or the validity of what is being proposed, he or she should inform the researchers proposing the study and opt out of participation. Each clinician, as well as each researcher, is responsible for the ethical conduct of research.

But then, once involved, it is incumbent on each clinician who is a participant in the RCT to follow the rules (fidelity!), for if different clinicians were to exclude eligible patients or include ineligible patients, to overcall the assigned randomization, to deviate from the treatment protocols, or to modify the outcome measures, that would undermine the validity of the RCT. In short, the clinician must move from the "samaritan" viewpoint to the "societal" viewpoint for the duration of the RCT. If this is not possible for the clinician, he or she should not participate in the RCT.

Having clinicians involved in the RCT has several advantages (beyond ecological validity). One challenge inherent to any RCT is the fact that patients are recruited because they have an illness, likely with distressing consequences. Patients who serve as study subjects in an RCT often feel overwhelmed by the addition of the burden of study participation to the burden of their illness and may consider dropping out of the study. In situations like these, the clinician caring for the patient is in a unique and trusted position to support the patient, to carefully assess his or her symptoms, and to counsel the patient about whether or not to continue in the study. In many cases, the patient's disquiet resolves with assurance and support, and he or she is able to complete the study, thereby decreasing dropout rates. If the disquiet reflects limiting side effects, the clinicians may be able to provide relief without deviating from the study protocol, again preventing dropout. Otherwise, if the patient's concern cannot be dealt with within the study protocol, the clinician can support the patient's decision in his or her communication with the researchers. Whatever the case, if the protocol requires "blinding" of the clinician, the clinician remains "blinded" to whether the patient is receiving the T or C.

At the end of an RCT, the clinician often has the important role of debriefing patients. While the study outcome measures will likely measure issues that are pertinent to the research question, there may be other positive experiences or burdensome side effects the patient may have experienced and about which the researchers did not ask. For example, sildenafil, a selective 5-phosphodiesterase inhibitor that dilates cardiac vessels by acting on cyclic guanosine monophosphate (GMP), was originally tested to study its effects on angina. Although it was ineffective in relieving angina, clinicians noticed that penile erections were induced in some patients. The drug has since been utilized to treat erectile dysfunction (Ballard et al., 1998; Campbell, 2000).

In Conclusion

In this chapter, we have discussed the perils and pearls of RCTs. Designing, conducting, analyzing, and publishing an RCT, then implementing appropriate practice changes based on the results is a long and intense process. However, in order for us to constantly improve clinical care and to innovate more effective treatments, we need extensive empirical research in which clinicians and researchers partner to identify the toughest and most relevant questions and conduct studies that involve diverse patients.

RCTs developed and implemented by pharmaceutical companies often involve clinicians, who are remunerated for each patient entered into the RCTs. Clinicians need to be aware of the RCT issues raised here. Before agreeing to participation in such a RCT, clinicians should review the rationale and justification for the RCT, the design of the RCT, and decide whether their participation is ethical and wise. Otherwise, many RCTs are still conducted largely in academic medical centers largely not informed by clinicians in practice. In fact, clinicians may refuse to engage in the design and implementation of an RCT because they are disinterested, extremely busy, or wary of researchers. Researchers may not value clinicians' input in the research design, or worse, they may see the clinician as a silent and mindless consumer of their research. Researchers, too, may not be willing to have clinicians join the research team, or they may exclude them from the products of research (publications and presentations). This lack of trust leads to extremely expensive, publicly funded research being conducted in academic centers in which the results may not be particularly relevant to the real-world clinical environment.

It is important that funding agencies and professional organizations encourage every research team to include clinicians as members of the investigative team and engage them in every stage of the research, and encourage clinicians to be willing to take on such roles.

To do EBP requires clinicians to read and use the RCT literature to provide the best care for their patients. In this chapter, we have provided concrete and specific guidelines for clinicians in this critical activity. We have argued that using the RCT literature in this way is essential from the "samaritan" viewpoint of ethical clinical practice. At the same time, we have argued that from the "societal" viewpoint, it is essential that clinicians be engaged in the design, conduct, and interpretation of RCTs to increase the chance that the trials do not result in incorrect conclusions that might harm patients in the future. EBP provides a framework for linking inextricably the success of the "samaritan" and "societal" modes, making one dependent on the success of the other in order to promote the best possible care for patients now and in the future.

References

Arean, P. A., & Kraemer, H. C. (2013). *High-quality psychotherapy research.* Oxford, UK: Oxford University Press.

Ballard, S. A., Gingell, C. J., Tang, K., Turner, L. A., Price, M. E., & Naylor, A. M. (1998). Effects of sildenafil on the relaxation of human corpus cavernosum tissue in vitro and on the activities of cyclic nucleotide phophodiesterase isozymes. *Journal of Urology, 159*(6), 164–171.

Bogarty, P., & Brophy, J. (2005). Numbers needed to treat (needlessly?). *Lancet, 365,* 1307–1308.

Campbell, D. T., & Kenny, D. A. (1999). *A primer on regression artifacts.* New York: Guilford Press.

Campbell, S. F. (2000). Science, art and drug discovery: A personal perspective. *Clinical Science (London), 99*(4), 255–260.

Chambless, D. L., & Ollendick, T. H. (2001). Empirically supported psychological interventions: Controversies and evidence. *Annual Review of Psychology, 52*(1), 685–716.

Constantine, N. A., Kraemer, H. C., Kendall-Tackett, K. A., Bennett, F. C., Tyson, J. E., & Gross, R. T. (1987). Use of physical and neurologic observations in the assessment of gestational age for low birthweight infants. *Journal of Pediatrics, 110,* 921–988.

Cook, R. J., & Sackett, D. L. (1995). The number needed to treat: A clinically useful measure of treatment effect. *British Medical Journal, 310,* 452–454.

Cooper, H., & Hedges, L. V. (1994). *The handbook of research synthesis.* New York: Russell Sage Foundation.

Craske, M. G., & Barlow, D. H. (2007). *Mastery of your anxiety and panic* (4th ed.). New York: Oxford University Press.

Cumming, G. (2011). *Understanding the new statistics: Effect sizes, confidence intervals, and meta analysis.* New York: Routledge.

Feinstein, A. R. (1985). *Clinical epidemiology: The architecture of clinical research.* Philadelphia: Saunders.

Freedman, B. (1987). Equipoise and the ethics of clinical research. *New England Journal of Medicine, 317,* 141–145.

Glasgow, R. E., Magid, D. J., Beck, A., Ritzwoller, D., & Estabrooks, P. A. (2005). Practical clinical trials for translating research to practice: Design and measurement recommendations. *Medical Care, 43*(6), 551–557.

Hamilton, M. (1960). A rating scale for depression. *Journal of Neurology, Neurosurgery, and Psychiatry, 23,* 56–62.

Hoagwood, K., Hibbs, E., Brent, D., & Jensen, P. (1995). Introduction to the special section: Efficacy and effectiveness in studies of child and adolescent psychotherapy. *Journal of Consulting and Clinical Psychology, 63*(5), 683–687.

Humphreys, K., & Weisner, C. (2000). Use of exclusion criteria in selecting research subjects and its effect on the generalizability of alcohol treatment outcome studies. *American Journal of Psychiatry, 157,* 588–594.

Infant Health and Development Progam. (1990). Enhancing the outcomes of low birth weight, premature infants: A multisite randomized trial. *Journal of the American Medical Association, 263,* 3035–3042.

Ioannidis, J. P. A. (2005a). Contradicted and initially stronger effects in highly cited clinical research. *Journal of the American Medical Association, 294*(2), 218–228.

Ioannidis, J. P. A. (2005b). Why most published research findings are false. *PLoS Medicine, 2*(8), 696–791.

Jo, B., & Stuart, E. E. (2009). On the use of propensity scores in principal causal effect estimation. *Statistics in Medicine, 28,* 2857–2875.

Kraemer, H. C. (2004). Reconsidering the odds ratio as a measure of 2×2 association in a population. *Statistics in Medicine, 23*(2), 257–270.

Kraemer, H. C. (2015). A source of false findings in published research studies: Adjusting for covariates. *JAMA Psychiatry, 72*(10), 961–962.

Kraemer, H. C., Frank, E., & Kupfer, D. J. (2006). Moderators of treatment outcomes: Clinical, research, and policy importance. *Journal of the American Medical Association, 296*(10), 1–4.

Kraemer, H. C., Frank, E., & Kupfer, D. J. (2011). How to assess the clinical impact of treatments on patients, rather than the statistical impact of treatments on measures. *International Journal of Methods in Psychiatric Research, 20*(2), 63–72.

Kraemer, H. C., Kazdin, A. E., Offord, D. R., Kessler, R. C., Jensen, P. S., & Kupfer, D. J. (1999). Measuring the potency of a risk factor for clinical or policy significance. *Psychological Methods, 4*(3), 257–271.

Kraemer, H. C., & Kupfer, D. J. (2006). Size of treatment effects and their importance to clinical research and practice. *Biological Psychiatry, 59*(11), 990–996.

Kraemer, H. C., & Robinson, T. N. (2005). Are certain multicenter randomized clinical trials structures misleading clinical and policy decisions? *Controlled Clinical Trials, 26*(5), 518–529.

Last, J. M. (1995). *A dictionary of epidemiology.* New York: Oxford University Press.

Lieberman, J. A., Stroup, T. S., McEvoy, J. P., Swartz, M. S., Rosenheck, R. A., Perkins, D. O., et al. (2005). Effectiveness of antipsychotic drugs in patients with chronic schizophrenia. *New England Journal of Medicine, 353*(12), 1209–1223.

March, J. S., Silva, S. G., Compton, S., Shapiro, M., Califf, R. M., & Krishnan, R. (2005). The case for practical clinical trials in psychiatry. *American Journal of Psychiatry, 152*(5), 836–846.

Newcombe, R. G. (2006). A deficiency of the odds ratio as a measure of effect size. *Statistics in Medicine, 25,* 4235–4240.

Rosenbaum, P. R., & Rubin, D. B. (1983). The central role of the propensity score in observational studies for causal effects. *Biometrika, 70*(1), 41–55.

Sackett, D. L. (1996). Down with odds ratios! *Evidence-Based Medicine, 1,* 164–166.

Sackett, D. L., Strauss, S., Richardson, W. S., Rosenberg, W., & Haynes, R. B. (2000). *Evidence-based medicine.* London: Churchill Livingstone.

Stampfer, M. J., Colditz, G. A., Willett, W. C., Manson, J. E., Rosner, B., Speizer, F. E., et al. (1991). Postmenopausal estrogen therapy and cardiovascular disease: Ten-year follow-up from the Nurses' Health Study. *New England Journal of Medicine, 325*(11), 756–762.

Tunis, S. R., Stryer, D. B., & Clancy, C. M. (2003). Practical clinical trials: Increasing the value of clinical research for decision making in clinical and health policy. *Journal of the American Medical Association, 290*(12), 1624–1632.

Wallace, M. L., Frank, E., & Kraemer, H. C. (2013). A novel approach for developing and interpreting treatment moderator profiles in randomized clinical trials. *JAMA Psychiatry, 70*(11), 1241–1247.

Wen, L., Badgett, R., & Cornell, J. (2005). Number needed to treat: A descriptor for weighing therapeutic options. *American Journal of Health-System Pharmacy, 62*(1), 2031–2036.

Women's Health Initiative Investigators. (2002). Principal results from the Women's Health Initiative randomized controlled trial. *Journal of the American Medical Association, 288*(3), 321–333.

Zimmerman, M., McGlinchey, J. B., Posternak, M. A., Friedman, M., Attiullah, N., & Boerescu, D. (2006). How should remission from depression be defined?: The depressed patient's perspective. *American Journal of Psychiatry, 163*(1), 148–150.

CHAPTER 5

Systematic Reviews in Mental Health

PIM CUIJPERS
IOANA A. CRISTEA

Every year, hundreds of thousands of biomedical articles are published, including more than 16,000 randomized controlled trials (RCTs) examining the effects of treatments (Cuijpers, 2016), and these numbers increase every year. With such large numbers of randomized trials, it becomes more and more difficult to maintain an overview of a field of interventions. Both clinical practitioners and researchers who want to stay "on top" of the latest empirical findings find that it is not possible to do so, despite the best of intentions. Consequently, reviews are needed to help clinicians and researchers make good use of the clinical intervention literature in their work. Reviews also help to inform clinical practice guidelines, which are the focus of Hollon (Chapter 6, this volume).

There are different types of reviews. *Traditional (narrative) reviews* are written by experts in a specific field, and they rely very much on the authority of the author, as well as the author's own perspective on what counts as relevant and how data should be interpreted. It is usually not clear how the studies included in the review were selected, whether all relevant outcomes for all studies are described, and how the quality of the studies was assessed. It is difficult, therefore, to verify the conclusions of such reviews. Also, the author's own biases and allegiance can play a significant role in influencing the conclusions of the review. In contrast, *systematic reviews* have a clear objective and try to answer a precise research question. Based on that question, the criteria for which studies should be included are defined, and orderly searches for these studies are conducted using a systematic and reproducible methodology. These reviews also assess the quality, the characteristics of the included studies, and the outcomes of the studies in a systematic way. *Meta-analyses* are a specific type of systematic review. The only difference with other systematic reviews is that the findings of the included studies are statistically integrated into estimates of the effects of the interventions being tested, and these are accompanied by an assessment of their statistical significance.

In this chapter, we focus mostly on traditional meta-analyses of outcome studies examining the effects of interventions. What we say about meta-analyses is also true for systematic reviews, except the parts about the statistical integration of the results. Meta-analyses, in principle, can integrate all outcomes of studies that have a standard error; therefore, they are not limited to studies about effects of intervention; for example, meta-analysis can be used to integrate the findings of longitudinal prospective studies that examine risk factors for a specific disorder. Many of the principles that we describe are also true for such meta-analyses, although some issues may differ, such as the formulation of the research question or the assessment of the validity of the included studies.

The results of meta-analyses are used by all stakeholders in mental health care. Policymakers use meta-analyses to decide about treatments that are included in health care programs and the financial coverage to be provided for such treatments. Patients use the results of meta-analyses to make decisions about whether they want a treatment or not. Researchers use meta-analyses to generate new research questions, to examine methodological limitations of existing trials, and to estimate sample sizes for future trials. Clinicians use meta-analyses for the development of decision-making tools and treatment guidelines, and they may use them to direct them to key individual studies (e.g., specific RCTs that may be particularly informative for some of their patients). Given the importance of meta-analyses in delivering (and improving) evidence-based practice, it is critical to develop the skills to interpret and make use of meta-analyses. This chapter is designed to serve as your guide. We lead you, step by step, through the process of conducting a meta-analysis, so that you can get a detailed look "behind the scenes." We also highlight core questions to ask and dimensions to evaluate along the way, so that you can determine how much you can trust a meta-analysis to guide your clinical practice and research.

Advantages and Problems of Meta-Analyses

Integrating the results of multiple trials in a meta-analysis has several advantages (Cuijpers, 2016). First of all, because the results of many studies are combined into one effect size, the precision and accuracy with which an effect can be estimated is much better than each of the included trials. This precision is better because the number of included participants is much larger, or in technical terms, *the statistical power is higher*. Also, meta-analyses can address questions that require large samples and would be hard to address with individual trials, including questions about moderators of treatment effects.

There are, however, also several *problems* with meta-analyses. One is often referred to as the "garbage in, garbage out" problem. This means that if the studies that are included in the meta-analysis are of low quality, the results of the meta-analysis also will be of low quality (al-

though the meta-analysis in itself may be done very well). So a meta-analysis can never be better than the sum of the studies it summarizes.

Another problem is that meta-analyses "combine apples and oranges." Especially in mental health care, there are usually considerable differences between studies. For example, the exact inclusion criteria for participants, the recruitment methods, the characteristics of the participants, the manuals for the treatments, and the therapists delivering the intervention all may vary. Also, rarely are trials examining one intervention exact replications of another. Consequently, some critics say that the results of these studies cannot be integrated in a single meta-analysis.

A third problem of meta-analyses is researcher allegiance, or "agenda-driven" bias of the researchers who conduct the meta-analyses. Meta-analyses are often written by researchers who are strong supporters the interventions they examine, and they may be inclined to stress the positive effects of the interventions they examine.

Fortunately, there are ways to address these potential problems, which we explore in detail in this chapter. This is good news because systematic reviews and meta-analysis form the foundation of clinical guidelines, which are presented Hollon (Chapter 6, this volume). Together, these types of publications are powerful tools for researchers and practitioners who want to use the existing evidence base to shape future studies or the care that they deliver in their clinical practices.

Formulating Research Questions for Meta-Analyses with the PICO Acronym

Every study starts with a good research question. That is also true for meta-analyses. Research questions for meta-analyses are typically formulated with the use of the *PICO* acronym (although some investigators also recommend attention to "time" and "setting" and propose using the *PICOTS* framework). PICO stands for *P*articipants, *I*nterventions, *C*omparisons, and *O*utcomes. A research question for a meta-analysis could be, for example, "What is the efficacy of cognitive-behavioral therapy (CBT) on sleep diary outcomes, compared with control, for the treatment of adults with chronic insomnia?" (Trauer, Qian, Doyle, Rajaratnam, & Cunnington, 2015). All four elements of the PICO are in there: *P,* adults with chronic insomnia; *I,* CBT; *C,* control groups; *O,* sleep diary outcomes.

Just like randomized trials, meta-analyses focus on a contrast between an intervention and a comparator. Effect sizes and outcomes of trials and meta-analyses typically describe the difference between the intervention and the comparator after treatment. However, some meta-analyses also compare the difference between baseline and posttest within one group of participants receiving an intervention. In both of these cases, however, there is a comparison—either between two groups or two moments in time.

Identifying Trials in Bibliographical Databases

Once a good research question has been articulated, the next step in conducting a meta-analysis is to identify trials in a systematic, reproducible way. The goal is to include all studies that are relevant and meet the inclusion criteria.

Included studies are identified most often through searches in bibliographical databases. For meta-analyses in mental health, at least three of these bibliographical databases should be searched. *PubMed* is a website that provides free access to Medline, life science journals, and online books. Medline is the National Library of Medicine's database of citations and abstracts in the fields of medicine, nursing, dentistry, veterinary medicine, health care systems, and preclinical sciences. Pubmed now has 25 million citations and abstracts from more than 5,600 biomedical journals, and it is free for any user (*www.ncbi.nlm.nih.gov/pubmed*). *PsycInfo* is a bibliographical database from the American Psychological Association with almost 4 million bibliographic records from more than 2,500 scientific journals, books, and theses on the behavioral and social sciences. Unfortunately, it is not freely accessible. The *Cochrane Central Register of Controlled Trials* (CENTRAL) is the database from the Cochrane Collaboration and contains only randomized trials in the biomedical sciences. The Cochrane database identifies trials by searching other bibliographical databases and by hand-searching the contents of about 2,400 scientific journals. *Clinicaltrials.gov* also is a very useful source for identifying clinical trial protocols.

In addition to these core databases, there are many others that may be relevant to mental health. Embase (another general biomedical bibliographical database) includes many journals that are not included in PubMed. There are also many *subject-specific databases,* such as CINAHL (nursing science), BiblioMap (health promotion research), ERIC (education), and AgeLine (aging issues). Other databases include citation databases (e.g., ISI Web of Knowledge, Scopus, and Google Scholar), national and regional databases (e.g., LILACS from Latin Amerca, IndMED from India, and several Chinese databases (Xia, Wright, & Adams, 2008).

Relevant studies can also be identified using other methods, such as checking the references of included trials, identifying earlier meta-analyses to see which studies were included, hand-searching the contents of major journals of the field, searching conference proceedings, or contacting key experts in the field to check whether you missed studies. Often, articles that appear outside of published journals are referred to as the "grey literature," and there are differences of opinion regarding the pros and cons of including such articles in a meta-analysis. As a reader of meta-analyses, what is critical is that the meta-analysis clearly describes the search strategy and decisions about what types of studies are and are not included. In addition, it is helpful if the meta-analysis is registered, so that one can determine that these basic methods were applied consistently throughout the meta-analytic process; one can check for the preregistration of systematic reviews through the database PROSPERO (*www.crd.york.ac.uk/prospero*), which is an international registry of health-related systematic reviews and meta-analyses.

Searching in Bibliographical Databases

Based on PICO research question, inclusion and exclusion criteria for the trials that are the object of the meta-analysis are formulated. So they typically describe the characteristics of the participants for the trials they will include, the interventions, the comparator, and the outcomes.

The PICO terms are also used to develop search strings to identify studies in the bibliographical databases. In these searches, a balance has to be found between sensitivity and precision. Broad searches generate large amounts of records, but the chance of missing trials that meet inclusion criteria is small. Narrow searches result in a smaller number of records, but the chance that trials are missed is greater. The identification of search terms, based on the inclusion and exclusion criteria, that adequately filter is an extremely important part of the meta-analytic process. The search terms help to ensure the quality and similarity of included studies.

When searching in bibliographical databases, it is important to search for not only text words in the title and abstract but also key words. Every bibliographical database has a system of attaching key words to records using a thesaurus, and these key words are hierarchically structured into a taxonomy. For example, in PubMed, these key words are called MeSH terms (Medical Subject Headings).

Searches in bibliographical databases make intensive use of Boolean operators (like AND, OR, and NOT). Brackets can help with defining such search strings. Suppose, for example, that you want to conduct a meta-analysis on psychological treatment for generalized anxiety disorder and you need to do a search of individual RCTs. In that case, you could develop a search string combining terms for generalized anxiety disorder and treatment, and it might look like this: *("generalized anxiety" OR "worry*") AND (psychotherapy or "cognitive behavior therapy" OR "interpersonal psychotherapy").* In this example, you can also see how truncation may be used. *Truncation* is a searching technique used in databases in which a word ending is replaced by a symbol, usually the asterisk (*). For example, if you use "worry*" as a search term in PubMed, you will find records with not only "worry" but also "worrying." Apart from truncation, *wildcards* ("?") can be used to replace the letter of a word. For example, the term "m?n" will identify records with the term "man," "men," "min," "mun," and so forth.

Search filters are often used in searches in bibliographical databases (see the website from the "InterTASC Information Specialists' Sub-Group Search Filter Resource" [*www.york. ac.uk/inst/crd/intertasc*] for a useful overview of search filters for many different types of studies). When conducting meta-analyses of randomized trials, search filters for trials are often used. For example, PubMed has a useful MeSh term for randomized trials ("Randomized Controlled Trial"[Publication Type]).

As a reader of meta-analytic reviews, what this means is that it is critical to pay attention to the search terms used by the authors. The use of search terms determines what studies are included or excluded. Knowing this helps one to

determine how useful a meta-analysis will be in guiding one's clinical practice given the types of patients and problems with which one works.

Selection of Studies

A published meta-analysis should have a Preferred Reporting Items for Systematic Reviews and Meta-Analyses (PRISMA) flowchart, which delineates the process of selecting studies from bibliographical databases up until the inclusion of the studies in the meta-analysis. The PRISMA flowchart requires that the exact number of records found in bibliographical databases be reported, as well as the total number of full-text papers that are retrieved, the number of trials that meet inclusion criteria, and the reasons why full text papers were excluded. This is to ensure that an independent researcher has all the necessary information to reproduce the search. As a reader of meta-analytic reviews, one might have cause for concern if one does not find a PRISMA diagram. It is challenging to assess the search and inclusion–exclusion process without this information. Also, it might indicate that the authors are not adhering to other generally accepted standards in the field.

Moreover, preferably the records resulting from the searches should be read by two independent researchers. During this process, those records possibly meeting inclusion criteria are selected, and the full texts of these records are retrieved. It is not required in this phase to indicate reasons why records are not selected. It is usually only reported that they were excluded based on the title and the abstract. After retrieval of the full-text papers, these should be read in order to see if they meet inclusion criteria. This should again be done by two independent reviewers. This selection process results in a first list of studies to be included in the meta-analysis. The first list of studies probably is not the definite list of studies because often during the extraction of the data from the individual trials, it turns out that one of the inclusion criteria is not met after all, or, for example, that it is not possible to calculate effect sizes because essential information is missing.

Data Extraction: Study Characteristics

When the decisions about the inclusion of studies has been made, the data extraction can begin. There are three types of data that have to be extracted from each included study: characteristics of the studies, risk of bias (or quality assessment), and the data that are needed for the calculation of effect sizes.

The characteristics of the studies are always summarized in a table in the paper describing the included studies. These descriptions typically follow the PICO of the meta-analyses and illustrate the key characteristics of the participants, the intervention that is examined, and the comparators. The outcomes are not always included in the descriptive table because these are also converted to the effect sizes and are reported in the results of the paper. There are no straightforward rules by which characteristics of the included studies are extracted. That depends on the subject of the meta-analysis, the included studies, and the exact research question.

Quality and Risk of Bias

Assessment of risk of bias is an essential part of any meta-analysis. It is directly related to the need to address concerns about the "garbage in, garbage out" problem. A meta-analysis can never be better than the sum of its parts, that is, the set of studies that it summarizes. If the original studies have high risk of bias, no meta-analysis, regardless of how sophisticated it is, can solve this problem.

There is a difference between quality and risk of bias, although the two concepts overlap. *Quality* indicates how well a study has been designed and conducted. What is good quality, however, is not so easy to define. There are many rating scales of study quality, but it is often not clear which concepts these scales measure; therefore, these scales vary considerably. In fact, a recent analysis (Armijo-Olivo, Fuentes, Ospina, Saltaji, & Hartling, 2013) of tools of evaluating methodological qualities of RCTs revealed inconsistencies among themselves, and between the items in these tools and the Cochrane Collaboration Risk of Bias (RoB; Higgins et al., 2011).

Defining and assessing risk of bias is more straightforward than methodological quality. *Bias* is a systematic error in a study, or deviation from the true or actual outcomes, in results or inferences. *Risk of bias* can be seen as denoting "weak spots" of randomized trials, where the researchers (usually without intention or even

awareness) can influence the outcomes of the study. These weak spots do not automatically imply that there is bias; hence, it is more correct to talk about "risk of bias" instead of bias. Many meta-analyses use the Cochrane RoB assessment tool (described in the *Cochrane Handbook for Systematic Reviews of Interventions* [Higgins & Green, 2011], which gives an excellent overview of the different types of risk of bias [*http://handbook.cochrane.org*]). There are different kinds of bias; here, we discuss five important areas of risk of bias: selection bias, detection bias, attrition bias, reporting bias, and allegiance bias.

Selection bias refers to systematic differences between the groups that were randomized in the trial. If the random assignment to conditions in trials (as reviewed by Kraemer & Periyakoil in Chapter 4, this volume) has not been done well, there may be systematic differences between participants in the intervention and, respectively, the comparison group. Selection bias can be caused by errors in the randomization process. There are two "weak spots" in this process. The first "weak spot" is the generation of the order in which participants are assigned to conditions. This is called *sequence generation*. Using a random numbers table, a computerized random number generator, throwing dice, or tossing a coin are all valid ways of generating random numbers. Assigning participants by date of birth, the date of admission, patient record number, or by the judgment of a clinician, however, are not valid methods of randomizing. The second "weak spot" is *allocation concealment*. This means that the researchers and the participants cannot foresee the assignment because this could allow them to influence the process of randomization. The allocation to conditions should therefore be concealed as much as possible from researchers and participants. Some strategies for doing so include asking an independent person, who is not involved in the trial, to do the assignment to conditions, or making sequentially numbered, opaque, and sealed envelopes containing the condition to which the participant is assigned. In mental health research, the method of randomization was not described in most studies on mental health problems at all until about 10 years ago, and it was usually only reported that participants were randomized (Chen et al., 2014; Cuijpers, van Straten, Bohlmeijer, Hollon, & Andersson, 2010).

Another "weak spot" of randomized trials is *detection bias,* which refers to systematic differences between groups in how outcomes are assessed. Detection bias can be prevented by blinding (or masking) of participants, the personnel involved in the study, and outcome assessors. In trials testing the effects of drugs, it is possible to blind patients who participate. Patients receive a pill that may contain the medication that is tested or a placebo pill. This placebo pill is exactly the same as the medication, but without the active substance. In psychological interventions, blinding of participants is usually not possible because participants and clinicians delivering the intervention typically know whether they are assigned to the intervention or to a control condition. It is therefore very possible that effects of interventions are (partly) caused by the participant's expectations about the intervention. Unfortunately, there is no solution for this problem. It is nonetheless possible in trials on psychological interventions to blind assessors of outcome. If assessors are not blinded, they are inclined to assume that the participants who did receive the intervention are better off than the ones who did not and therefore overrate the outcomes of the intervention (Higgins & Green, 2011). In many psychological interventions, outcomes of a trial are assessed with self-report measures, and not through interviews with (blinded) assessors. Self-assessment of outcome is also not blinded and may therefore result in bias, too.

Attrition bias refers to the bias that is caused by the participants who drop out of the trial. Trials should include *intent-to-treat analyses,* which means that all participants who were randomized are included in the analyses of the outcome, regardless of whether they dropped out of the trial. Missing data from participants who dropped out should be imputed. There are good methods for imputation of missing data available, such as using the last observation that is available (the last observation carried forward), multiple imputation techniques, or mixed models for repeated measurements (Crameri, von Wyl, Koemeda, Schulthess, & Tschuschke, 2015; Siddiqui, Hung, & O'Neill, 2009). There is, however, no consensus about whether any of these methods are better or whether there are differences between results. Earlier trials on psychological interventions rarely used these methods.

Another type of bias in randomized trials is *reporting bias.* It often happens that more than one primary outcome is used to measure the effects of an intervention. If one of these outcomes shows better effects of the intervention than another outcome, researchers are sometimes inclined to report only the outcome showing the most favorable effects for the intervention. But that is wrong because it results in an overestimation of the effects when the study is included in a meta-analysis. In recent years, many trials are registered in trial registries or the design of the study is published in protocol papers before the study has started (see, e.g., *clinicaltrials.gov*). In these protocols, it can be verified whether the planned outcome measures were indeed used in the analyses.

These four types of bias can be assessed with the Cochrane RoB Assessment Tool, which has clear criteria for each of these types of risk of bias, which are scored as low risk of bias (when the paper clearly describes that the type bias was handled well), high risk of bias (when the paper describes a procedure that indicates that the risk of bias is present), or unclear risk of bias (when the paper does not give enough information to say whether there was risk of bias or not). Again, it is again important that these assessments of the risk of bias are done by two independent researchers in conducting the meta-analysis.

A final type of bias that is not included in the RoB Assessment Tool but is very important for psychological interventions is *researcher allegiance.* This can be defined as a researcher's "belief in the superiority of a treatment [and] . . . the superior validity of the theory of change that is associated with the treatment" (Leykin & DeRubeis, 2009, p. 55). There is considerable evidence that researcher allegiance is associated with better outcomes for the preferred treatment (Dragioti, Dimoliatis, Fountoulakis, & Evangelou, 2015; Munder, Brütsch, Leonhart, Gerger, & Barth, 2013). This may be because treatments are implemented with better fidelity by investigators who have allegiance to those treatments; however, the impact of researcher allegiance is not well understood or measured in the literature.

One's confidence in the findings reported by a meta-analytic review should be based, in part, on the extent to which the authors have attended consistently, accurately, and transparently to questions of study quality and risk of bias. These considerations are protections for authors, readers, and the field at large when it comes to concerns about the "garbage in, garbage out" problem.

Calculating Effect Sizes

In meta-analyses, the effects of an intervention are statistically integrated. In order to do this, an effect size has to be calculated for each study that is included in the meta-analysis. The effect size is a way of quantifying the difference between groups. This effect size for each study has to be standardized in some way to make it comparable to the effect sizes of the other studies; otherwise, they cannot be integrated. In mental health research, usually Cohen's d or Hedges' g are used as effect sizes. These effect sizes are based on continuous outcomes (that can take any value in a given range) and indicate the difference between the means of the two groups, in terms of the standard deviations of the two groups. An effect size of 0.5 means that the two groups differ from each other by 0.5 standard deviation.

Cohen's d can be calculated as the difference between the means of the two groups, divided by their pooled standard deviation. Hedges' g is calculated with the same formula, but then a somewhat different method to calculate the pooled standard deviation. For small samples, Hedges' g gives a more accurate estimate of the effect size. In order to calculate an effect size, the mean, standard deviation, and the number of participants for each group is needed. If the mean and standard deviation are not given in one of the original studies to be included in a meta-analysis, other statistics, such as the t-value or the p-value can be used to calculate the effect size.

One of the big advantages of effect sizes is that they allow us to see how large effects are. Significance testing of the difference between a group that received an intervention and a control group only indicates whether that difference is statistically significant, not how large that difference is. In contrast, an effect size says something about the size of the effects. Usually effect sizes of 0.20 are considered to be small, 0.50 are moderate, and 0.80 are large. Based on several hundred meta-analyses in the educational and psychological interventions, Lipsey and Wilson (1993) estimated that effect sizes less than $d = 0.32$ are small, those that are 0.33 to 0.55 are moderate, and those greater than 0.56 are large.

It is important to remember, however, that the effect size is still a statistical concept and does not directly say something about the clinical relevance of the effects of an intervention. For example, an effect size of $d = 0.1$ would be considered very clinically relevant for an intervention aimed at improving survival, but this same effect size may not be considered clinically meaningful for an intervention aimed at improving social skills or knowledge about a mental health problem.

A big disadvantage of effect sizes is that they are difficult to explain to participants, clinicians, and policymakers. They also say very little about the chance that a patient will be free from a mental health problem after receiving a treatment. One common way to solve that is to transform effect sizes into the *number needed to treat* (NNT), which indicates the number of patients that have to be treated in order to generate one additional positive outcome (Laupacis, Sackett, & Roberts, 1988). The NNT is much easier to understand than effect sizes. Although the NNT is based on dichotomous outcomes of trials (see below), it can still be estimated from effect sizes (based on continuous outcomes). There are several ways of converting an effect size to the NNT, all of which assume that the mean scores follow a normal or near normal distribution (da Costa et al., 2012; Furukawa & Leucht, 2011).

Although most meta-analyses in mental health care focus on continuous outcomes, such as depressive or anxiety symptom severity, and effect sizes such as Cohen's d and Hedges' g, many important mental health outcomes are dichotomous, for example, the number or proportions of responders to treatment, and the number of patients who relapse or number of participants dropping out of an intervention are dichotomous outcomes. Dichotomous outcomes are much easier to understand for patients and clinicians, as a patient either responds to a treatment or not or has a relapse or not.

Dichotomous effects of treatments in trials are usually expressed in terms of *relative risks* (RRs) or *odds ratios* (ORs). The RR is the "risk" of participants for an outcome in the intervention group, divided by the risk in the comparison group. The exact formula for the RR is given in Table 5.1. In other words, the RR is the proportion of participants with an outcome in the intervention group, divided by the proportion in the comparison group. So if there is no difference between the two groups, the RR is 1 and if the 95% confidence interval (CI) around RR does not include 1, the RR is significant (significantly different from 1).

The OR is more difficult to understand. The OR is the "odds" that an event will occur in

TABLE 5.1. Possible Dichotomous Outcomes in an RCT

	Event (success)	No event (fail)	Total
Therapy	A	C	(A + C)
Control	B	D	(B + D)
Odds ratio (OR) =	$\dfrac{(A*D)}{(C*B)}$	=	Odds of success in the treatment group / Odds of success in the comparison group
Relative risk (RR) =	$\dfrac{A /(A + C)}{B /(B + D)}$	=	Risk of success in treatment group / Risk of success in comparison group
Risk difference (RD) =	[A /(A + C)] – [B/B + D)]	=	Risk in therapy group – risk in control group
Number needed to treat	(NNT) = 1/RD		= 1 divided by the risk difference

the treatment, compared to the "odds" occurring in the comparison group. The "odds" itself is the ratio of the probability that a particular event will occur to the probability that it will not occur. Because the OR is so difficult to understand, it is often advised not to use it as an outcome in trials and meta-analyses. The *risk difference* (RD) is the risk for the event in the intervention group minus the risk for the event in the comparison group. The NNT is 1 divided by the RD.

Pooling of Effect Sizes and Heterogeneity as a Key Concept in Meta-Analyses

The strength of a meta-analysis is that the effect sizes for each individual study can be "pooled" by calculating the mean of these effect sizes. This pooled effect size is the best estimate of the "true" effect size for that intervention that is available. However, it is not adequate to simply calculate the mean of these effect sizes across the studies because, in that case, small studies would have the same "weight" as large studies. It is important that in calculating the pooled effect size, large studies get more weight than small studies.

A key issue for the pooling of effect sizes is *heterogeneity,* which is the variability among studies. It refers directly to the problem of comparing "apples and oranges" in meta-analyses that we mentioned earlier. *Statistical heterogeneity* refers to the variability across the effect sizes that are found for the included studies. If there is statistical heterogeneity, this means that the observed effect sizes are more different

from each other than what would be expected due to chance (random error) alone. *Clinical heterogeneity* refers to the variability among the participants, interventions, and outcomes across the studies included in the meta-analysis. *Methodological heterogeneity* refers to variability in study design and risk of bias. If there is too much clinical and methodological heterogeneity, a meta-analysis is not useful. Statistical heterogeneity is caused by clinical and methodological heterogeneity. In a meta-analysis, the term *heterogeneity* usually indicates statistical heterogeneity.

Heterogeneity is a key issue in understanding the results of a meta-analysis. Heterogeneity in meta-analyses in mental health is often high, and this is true for both statistical and clinical heterogeneity. It is therefore very important in meta-analyses with high levels of heterogeneity to examine sources of heterogeneity. We explain below how that can be done. If (statistical) heterogeneity is high and the causes of this cannot be identified, this means that there is variability among the effect sizes of this intervention that cannot be explained. This further implies that we in fact do not know under which conditions an intervention is effective and how large these effects are.

Basically, there are two methods for pooling effect sizes in meta-analyses. The *fixed effect model* assumes that all studies are exact replications of each other and share a common (true) effect size (Borenstein, Hedges, Higgins, & Rothstein, 2009). All variables that may have an effect on the outcomes of the interventions are identical across all trials. Because these trials estimate exactly the same effect size, the effect sizes found in the trials only vary due to random error inherent in each study. In the *random effects model,* it is not assumed that all trials are exact replications of each other. Each trial can introduce its own underlying variance because of the differences between the trials. So effect sizes differ from each other not only because of random error, as in the fixed effects model, but also because of the true differences between the studies.

In mental health, research trials can hardly ever be considered to be exact replications of each other, and it is recommended that researchers use the random effects model and not the fixed effect model. Sometimes researchers let the choice for the fixed or the random effects model depend on the level of heterogeneity found (see below), but that is wrong. If there are differences between the studies (clinical and methodological heterogeneity) the random effects model should always be used.

The Forest Plot as the Core of a Meta-Analysis

The *forest plot* is a good summary of a meta-analysis and in many ways its core. Any paper reporting the results of a meta-analysis has (or should have) such a forest plot. It provides a graphical representation of the effect size for each study, as well as the 95% CI around that effect size and the pooled effect size (with 95% CI). The 95% CI of the effect size is given as a line through the effect size. The longer that line is, the broader the 95% CI and the smaller the sample size. So if an effect size has a short line through it, that means it is a large study. And large studies should be closer to the mean effect size (because they estimate the effect size more precisely) than smaller studies. If large studies still deviate much from the pooled effect size, this indicates probable heterogeneity. If the 95% CI of the effect size of a study does not overlap with the 95% CI of the pooled effect size for all studies together, that study could be an "outlier." If a study is an outlier, it is important to examine whether there are characteristics of that study that could explain why this is the case. If there are many outliers in a meta-analysis, heterogeneity is probably also high. Hollon (Chapter 6, this volume) provides an example of a forest plot and additional explanation about how to interpret such a plot in a meta-analysis.

Although the forest plot can provide a first indication as to whether there is heterogeneity (many studies, especially large ones, with effect sizes diverting from the pooled effect size; many outliers), a much better way to examine heterogeneity is to calculate it in term of percentages. The I^2 statistic indicates heterogeneity in percentages or, in other words, the percentage of the variability in effect sizes that can be attributed to heterogeneity rather than chance (Higgins, Thompson, Deeks, & Altman, 2003). A percentage of 25% is considered low heterogeneity; 50% is moderate, and 75% is high.

It is important to calculate not only the I^2 for a meta-analysis but also the 95% CI around I^2 (Ioannidis, Patsopoulos, & Evangelou, 2007). Especially with smaller numbers of studies and small numbers of participants, the uncertainty around I^2 can be considerable. For example, it is very well possible that I^2 is zero, but that the 95% CI goes from 0 to 75%. In that case, the 0% heterogeneity is not very meaningful.

There is also a formal test for significance of heterogeneity, based on what is called Q (a χ^2 statistic). This tests whether observed differences between effect sizes can be explained by chance alone. If this is the case, then there is no significant heterogeneity. However, this test should be interpreted with caution because it has low power, and this is a problem when there are small numbers of studies and small sample sizes per study. So, the I^2 statistic is more informative when it comes to assessing heterogeneity.

If heterogeneity is very high, it may be advisable not to perform or publish a meta-analysis at all because a pooled effect size may mislead and suggest that this pooled effect size is meaningful when it is not.

Examining Sources of Heterogeneity

When a meta-analysis finds heterogeneity, it is important to examine possible sources of this. It may be true that a characteristic of the participants, the intervention, or the study is related to the effect size and that subgroups of studies exist with effect sizes that differ very much from each other. This results in high levels of heterogeneity, but it is in fact related to the different effect sizes for these subgroups of studies.

There are different ways of examining sources of heterogeneity. We discussed the first one already, namely, checking whether there are outliers. *Outliers* are studies that differ considerably from the rest of the studies. Outliers usually result in an increase in heterogeneity. If the characteristics of these studies are really different from the other studies, then this may explain why these studies result in such different effect sizes.

Another way of examining possible sources of heterogeneity is by *subgroup analyses.* In these analyses, the set of included studies is divided into two or more subgroups. Then researchers test whether the effect sizes differ significantly from each other, and whether heterogeneity is lower in each of the subgroups compared to the overall group of studies. Usually, researchers perform these subgroup analyses using a mixed effects model in which the effect sizes within the subgroups are pooled with a random effects model, then test the effect sizes between the subgroups with a fixed effect model.

Metaregression analyses may also be used to examine heterogeneity in meta-analyses. In a bivariate metaregression analysis, the association between a continuous characteristic of the studies and the effect sizes is computed. For example, the association between the effect size and the number of sessions in an intervention might be examined in a metaregression analysis. In multivariate metaregression, more than one predictor is examined at the same time in one model. In these analyses, continuous outcomes (e.g., number of sessions, number of participants per condition, year of publication) and categorical variables may be examined at the same time, just as is done in a "normal" regression analysis.

It is important to note that subgroup and metaregression analyses are useful for examining possible sources of heterogeneity, but the results should always be interpreted with caution. A significant predictor is *not* evidence for a causal association between this predictor and outcome. For example, suppose that a meta-analysis of a therapy compared with care-as-usual control groups shows that individual treatment has significantly higher effect sizes than group treatments. This finding cannot be considered as causal evidence that individual treatments are indeed more effective than group treatments. It is very well possible that this difference in effect size is caused by another variable that is not measured. The best way to show that there is a difference between individual and group treatments is to focus on trials that directly randomize patients to individual or group treatments. A meta-analysis of such studies does result in the best evidence for a possible difference. Subgroup analyses can only result in indirect evidence for such differences.

Publication Bias

One problem of meta-analyses is that not all the studies conducted are actually published. Authors, editors, and journals are inclined to favor publication of studies that show significant effects for interventions. If a study shows no or only small effects, such studies often are not published. And this is a problem for meta-analyses because these are based on published studies; if negative studies are not published, this may considerably overestimate the true effect of an intervention. But if a study is not published, how can we solve this problem? We do not know what the effect size of these unpublished studies are, so we also do not know what the true effect size is.

Sometimes direct estimates of unpublished studies can be made, for example, by checking the trials on drugs submitted to the U.S. Food and Drug Administration (Turner, Matthews, Linardatos, Tell, & Rosenthal, 2008) or by checking whether funded grants for trials on psychotherapy led to published studies (Driessen, Hollon, Bockting, Cuijpers, & Turner, 2015). However, usually such direct estimates of publication bias are not possible.

It is possible nonetheless to get indirect estimates of publication bias. These estimates are based on the assumption that large studies (with many participants) can make a more precise estimate of the effect size, while the effect sizes found in smaller studies can divert more from the pooled effect size because they are less precise in their estimates of the effect size. Random variations of the effect sizes are larger in studies with relatively fewer participants compared to those with many participants. This difference can be represented graphically in a *funnel plot,* in which the effect size is represented on the horizontal axis and the size of the study on the vertical axis. When the size of the study is smaller, the effect sizes can divert more from the mean effect size, and when the study has more participants, its effect size should be closer to the pooled effect size across all studies. So when small studies divert more from the pooled effect size, they should be found in both in the positive and the negative direction. If they are found in the positive direction but not in the negative direction, this can be seen as an indication for publication bias. This "asymmetry of the funnel plot" can be tested with formal statistical tests (e.g., Egger's regression intercept test or Begg and Mazumdar's rank correlation test), but the missing studies can also be imputed, using Duval and Tweedie's trim and fill procedure (Duval & Tweedie, 2000), which estimates how many studies are missing due to publication bias and also calculates the pooled effect size after adjustment for publication bias. Hollon (Chapter 6, this volume) provides an example of a funnel plot and its interpretation.

Other Types of Meta-Analyses

We have focused most of this chapter on "traditional" meta-analyses. However, two othertypes of meta-analyses are worthy of brief mention.

In *network meta-analyses,* different comparisons may be included at the same time. In traditional meta-analyses, only one comparison can be examined at a time. The PICO describes only one comparison between an intervention and a comparison group. In network meta-analyses, more comparisons may be examined at the same time. Suppose, for example, that there are two treatments for one mental disorder, and both treatments have been tested in trials that have compared them with control groups, and other trials have directly compared these two treatments with each other. In a traditional meta-analysis, three separate analyses should be done, two for each treatment compared with a control group and one for the direct comparisons between the two treatments. In a network meta-analysis, all these comparisons may be examined at once in the same analysis. The network meta-analysis is also called a *multiple treatment comparison meta-analysis* or a *mixed treatment meta-analysis.*

In *"individual patient data" meta-analyses,* the primary data of trials from a systematic review are collected and analyzed (Riley, Lambert, & Abo-Zaid, 2010). The advantage of this type of meta-analysis is that all analyses may be done in the same way across trials and in that way make a better estimate of the true effect size. There is also enough statistical power to examine moderators of outcome. "Individual patient data" meta-analyses are also sometimes called *mega-analyses.*

Conclusion

In this chapter we have discussed the methods of meta-analyses in mental health care and have presented a guide for readers on how to interpret the methods and results of meta-analyses. We have discussed the methods that researchers use for identifying relevant studies, extracting data from studies that meet the inclusion criteria, analyzing the results of these studies, and statistically integrating the results of these studies into pooled effect sizes.

Many resources exist for learning more about meta-analyses, including more extensive books on the methods of meta-analyses, such as the Cochrane handbook (Higgins & Green, 2011). We also encourage readers to familiarize themselves with the PRISMA Statement (Moher, Liberati, Tetzlaff, Altman, & the PRISMA Group, 2009). PRISMA is a guide for authors of meta-analyses about what should be reported. The PRISMA statement, which contains an evidence-based minimum set of items for reporting in systematic reviews and meta-analyses, has been accepted by most journals in the biomedical field. Authors of meta-analyses are advised to use PRISMA to improve the reporting of systematic reviews and meta-analyses.

Meta-analyses have become indispensable tools for integrating the results of the thousands of randomized trials in health care, including mental health care. The results of meta-analyses are used by patients, clinicians, and policymakers in mental health care. In order to use meta-analyses well, it is necessary to understand how they are conducted and reported, and to bring a critical lens to the findings.

References

Armijo-Olivo, S., Fuentes, J., Ospina, M., Saltaji, H., & Hartling, L. (2013). Inconsistency in the items included in tools used in general health research and physical therapy to evaluate the methodological quality of randomized controlled trials: A descriptive analysis. *BMC Medical Research Methodology, 13,* 116.

Borenstein, M., Hedges, L. V., Higgins, J. P. T., & Rothstein, H. R. (2009). *Introduction to meta-analysis.* Chichester, UK: Wiley.

Chen, P., Furukawa, T. A., Shinohara, K., Honyashiki, M., Imai, H., Ichikawa, K., et al. (2014). Quantity and quality of psychotherapy trials for depression in the past five decades. *Journal of Affective Disorders, 165,* 190–195.

Crameri, A., von Wyl, A., Koemeda, M., Schulthess, P., & Tschuschke, V. (2015). Sensitivity analysis in multiple imputation in effectiveness studies of psychotherapy. *Frontiers in Psychology, 6,* 1042.

Cuijpers, P. (2016). Meta-analyses in mental health research: A practical guideline. Retrieved from *http://bit.do/meta-analysis.*

Cuijpers, P., van Straten, A., Bohlmeijer, E., Hollon, S. D., & Andersson, G. (2010). The effects of psychotherapy for adult depression are overestimated: A meta-analysis of study quality and effect size. *Psychological Medicine, 40*(2), 211–223.

da Costa, B. R., Rutjes, A. W. S., Johnston, B. C., Reichenbach, S., Nüesch, E., Tonia, T., et al. (2012). Methods to convert continuous outcomes into odds ratios of treatment response and numbers needed to treat: Meta-epidemiological study. *International Journal of Epidemiology, 41*(5), 1445–1459.

Dragioti, E., Dimoliatis, I., Fountoulakis, K. N., & Evangelou, E. (2015). A systematic appraisal of allegiance effect in randomized controlled trials of psychotherapy. *Annals of General Psychiatry, 14,* 25.

Driessen, E., Hollon, S. D., Bockting, C. L. H., Cuijpers, P., & Turner, E. H. (2015). Does publication bias inflate the apparent efficacy of psychological treatment for major depressive disorder?: A systematic review and meta-analysis of US National Institutes of Health-funded trials. *PLOS ONE, 10*(9), e0137864.

Duval, S., & Tweedie, R. (2000). Trim and fill: A simple funnel-plot-based method of testing and adjusting for publication bias in meta-analysis. *Biometrics, 56*(2), 455–463.

Furukawa, T. A., & Leucht, S. (2011). How to obtain NNT from Cohen's *d*: Comparison of two methods. *PLOS ONE, 6*(4), e19070.

Higgins, J. P. T., Altman, D. G., Gotzsche, P. C., Juni, P., Moher, D., Oxman, A. D., et al. (2011). The Cochrane Collaboration's tool for assessing risk of bias in randomised trials. *British Medical Journal, 343*(2), d5928.

Higgins, J. P. T., & Green, S. (Eds.). (2011). Cochrane Handbook for Systematic Reviews of Interventions Version 5.1.0 [updated March 2011]. Retrieved from *www.cochrane-handbook.org.*

Higgins, J. P. T., Thompson, S. G., Deeks, J. J., & Altman, D. G. (2003). Measuring inconsistency in meta-analyses. *British Medical Journal, 327,* 557–560.

Ioannidis, J. P. A., Patsopoulos, N. A., & Evangelou, E. (2007). Uncertainty in heterogeneity estimates in meta-analyses. *British Medical Journal, 335,* 914–916.

Laupacis, A., Sackett, D. L., & Roberts, R. S. (1988). An assessment of clinically useful measures of the consequences of treatment. *New England Journal of Medicine, 318*(26), 1728–1733.

Leykin, Y., & DeRubeis, R. J. (2009). Allegiance in psychotherapy outcome research: Separating association from bias. *Clinical Psychology: Science and Practice, 16*(1), 54–65.

Lipsey, M. W., & Wilson, D. B. (1993). The efficacy of psychological, educational, and behavioral treatment: Confirmation from meta-analysis. *American Psychologist, 48*(12), 1181–1209.

Moher, D., Liberati, A., Tetzlaff, J., Altman, D. G., & the PRISMA Group. (2009). Preferred reporting items for systematic reviews and meta-analyses: The PRISMA Statement. *PLoS Medicine, 6*(7), e1000097.

Munder, T., Brütsch, O., Leonhart, R., Gerger, H., & Barth, J. (2013). Researcher allegiance in psychotherapy outcome research: An overview of reviews. *Clinical Psychology Review, 33*(4), 501–511.

Riley, R. D., Lambert, P. C., & Abo-Zaid, G. (2010). Meta-analysis of individual participant data: Rationale, conduct, and reporting. *British Medical Journal, 340,* c221.

Siddiqui, O., Hung, H. M. J., & O'Neill, R. (2009). MMRM vs. LOCF: A comprehensive comparison based on simulation study and 25 NDA datasets. *Journal of Biopharmaceutical Statistics, 19*(2), 227–246.

Trauer, J. M., Qian, M. Y., Doyle, J. S., Rajaratnam, S. M. W., & Cunnington, D. (2015). Cognitive behavioral therapy for chronic insomnia: A systematic review and meta-analysis. *Annals of Internal Medicine, 163*(3), 191–204.

Turner, E. H., Matthews, A. M., Linardatos, E., Tell, R. A., & Rosenthal, R. (2008). Selective publication of antidepressant trials and its influence on apparent efficacy. *New England Journal of Medicine, 358*(3), 252–260.

Xia, J., Wright, J., & Adams, C. E. (2008). Five large Chinese biomedical bibliographic databases: Accessibility and coverage. *Health Information and Libraries Journal, 25*(1), 55–61.

CHAPTER 6

Clinical Practice Guidelines

STEVEN D. HOLLON

Clinical practice guidelines (CPGs) are intended to provide a guide to the best and most efficacious practices for mental and physical health. In the best of all possible worlds, CPGs serve the public interest; they provide guidance to the consumer with respect to what works best and the possible harms associated with the various treatment options. They also provide guidance to the practitioner as to the pros and cons of the various treatment options and what new skills can be learned to update one's quality of practice. Both trainees and established practitioners can benefit from such guidance as they seek to allocate limited time and resources for initial learning and maintaining skills over time. Finally, they provide guidance to the administrator regarding the costs and benefits of the various treatment options and quality assurance efforts to evaluate the extent to which routine services are aligned with best practice guidelines. The sections to follow consider how CPGs are best constructed and the quality of guidelines that already exist.

What Are CPGs?

Evidence-based CPGs represent a systematic approach to translating the best available research evidence into clear statements regarding treatments for people with various health conditions. Some have described psychotherapy as an art, but no one would submit to surgery with a physician who operated solely in the basis of whim or prior expertise. As discussed by Spring, Marchese, and Steglitz (Chapter 1, this volume), there is a general consensus in medicine and mental health that CPGs should be based on (1) the *best available research evidence* (2) as filtered through the prism of *practitioner expertise* (3) to arrive at the best decisions consistent with *patient preferences and values*. Note that in this definition, the best available research evidence is privileged; it is the starting point for all subsequent decisions. We have 70 years of accumulated research evidence regarding what works best and for whom, and it would be foolish to throw that away. Note also that practitioner expertise is not ignored; clinical experience does come into play in helping to individuate the various options based on what practitioners have observed in their past work and what they are most competent to do. Finally, note too that the patient is accorded final control in terms of choosing what is to be done from among the various options available. The simple fact that a given treatment may have a higher expected rate of success than another (on average) does not mean that treatment must be chosen; the patient has the ultimate right to weigh the benefits and harms and to make the choice most consistent with his or her preferences. Good CPGs do not dictate; rather, they simply guide.

A Brief History of CPGs

In the mental health fields, CPGs are widely used in many regions of the world, as discussed in detail below. In the United States, the American Psychiatric Association has published CPGs since 1992. In contrast, other bodies, such as the American Psychological Association, have long resisted CPGs on the grounds that they constrain their members' practice (most dues-paying members are practicing clinicians). (Throughout the rest of this chapter, I use the designation "psychiatric APA" to refer to that organization and refer to the psychological organization simply as "APA.") In 2010, however, the APA decided that it was in the best interest of its members to not leave the process to other professions, and it formed a steering committee to advise it on the generation of such CPGs. I served as the first Chair of this Advisory Steering Committee (ASC), and much of what is presented in the rest of this chapter describes my experiences in that process.

The United States is unique among the western democracies in not having some independent governmental agency generate CPGs. That was not always the case. Back in the early 1990s the Agency for Health Care Policy and Research (AHCPR) produced a series of high-quality treatment guidelines, including one on the treatment of depression in primary care (Muñoz, Hollon, McGrath, Rehm, & VandenBos, 1994). However, a subsequent guideline concluded that there was little evidence to support the use of surgery for back pain, and the orthopedic surgeons lobbied Congress to kill the agency. The AHCPR has been resurrected (in part) in the form of the Agency for Health Care Research and Quality (AHRQ), which is allowed to conduct systematic reviews of the empirical literature but not to turn them into CPGs. That is left to the various professional guilds, and the CPGs they produce tend to reflect the biases and predilections of those professional organizations. As George Bernard Shaw once said, all professions are "conspiracies against the laity" and it is only human nature that they tend to confuse the interests of their members with the interests of the public. The sole exceptions in this country are the guidelines produced by the Veterans Administration/Department of Defense (VA/DOD), which tend to be high quality in their implementation and recommendations. However, these guidelines tend to be specific to a military population and do not necessarily generalize to civilians.

Most other upper middle- and high-income countries have independent governmental organizations that generate treatment guidelines, especially those with socialized medicine or other single-payer system. In the United Kingdom, the National Health Service (NHS) commissions the National Institute for Health and Clinical Excellence (NICE) to generate CPGs for both medicine and mental health, and the guidelines it produces are marvels of scientific rigor and economic savvy. We spent considerable time consulting with the people who oversee the NICE guidelines with respect to mental health (Steve Pilling in particular) and much that we advised the APA to do was drawn from those consultations. When NICE constructs a guideline, it does an exhaustive search of the empirical literature with respect to the treatment of a given disorder, giving priority to randomized clinical trials (RCTs); it then presents that guideline to a multidisciplinary guideline panel that includes nonprofessional patient care representatives or actual current or former patients, who weigh the benefits and harms of the respective interventions and make recommendations that are then implemented within the NHS. The process is based on the best available research evidence as filtered through expert clinical judgment and leavened with the perspective of actual patients or their advocates.

This is the process that the APA sought to emulate. Our efforts were greatly facilitated by the publication of standards by the Institute of Medicine (IOM, 2011a) for generating guidelines that the public could trust, based on independent and comprehensive systematic reviews of the empirical literature (IOM, 2011b). These standards represented a compilation of the current best practices in guideline generation (heavily influenced by NICE) and have been largely adopted by the Guideline International Network (GIN) across both medicine and mental health. The sections that follow describe the processes recommended by the IOM (and largely practiced by NICE) that the advisory steering committee recommended to the APA for CPGs.

Generating CPGs: NICE and the IOM Standards

Both the IOM and NICE recognize that the decision-making process is too complex to rest solely on empirically based prescriptive recommendations and too consequential to rely solely on clinical consensus. The process of generating CPGs typically is based on two sequential steps: (1) a comprehensive systematic review of the empirical literature (giving greatest weight to well-conducted RCTs) and (2) evaluation of the findings from that systematic review by a guideline development panel (GDP) that considers the quality of the evidence and the relative benefits and harms associated with the various clinical practices reviewed. The GDP, which comprises practitioners, scientists, methodologists, and patient representatives, is then asked to generate recommendations that are informed by the empirical literature but that take clinical experience into account, as depicted in Figure 6.1. As a consequence, CPGs are based on the best available research evidence as filtered through expert clinical judgment and taking patient preferences into account. The process is not unlike a jury trial in which the best of

the available forensic evidence is presented to a jury charged with arriving at final decision regarding guilt or innocence.

Several years ago, I had the opportunity to sit in with a GDP charged by NICE with updating their CPG on depression, and it was most instructive. The GDP comprised nearly 20 individual members (an odd number is always recommended in the event that votes are taken) representing an array of different professions (psychology, psychiatry, general practice, social work, and nursing) involved in the treatment of depression and different theoretical orientations (dynamic–interpersonal, cognitive-behavioral, humanistic–experiential, and pharmacological–somatic). The patient care representatives played an important role in keeping the professionals honest in terms of focusing on what was in the best interests of the public. A systematic review had already been conducted, and the day that I was there, the GDP went over the evi-

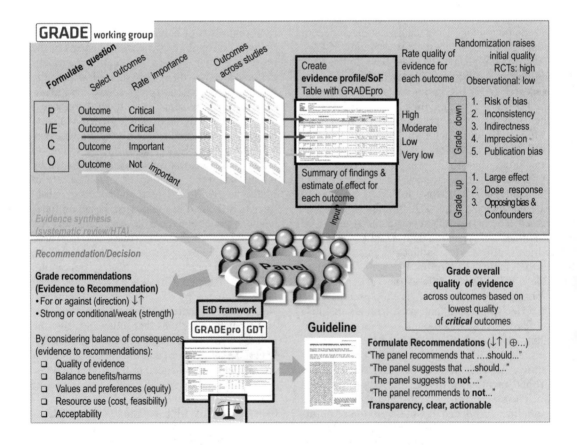

FIGURE 6.1. Systematic reviews used to inform GDPs. From Falck-Ytter and Schünemann (2009). Reprinted by permission.

dence with respect to several different types of treatment, with the effect sizes of the individual studies graphically displayed on forest plots and the influence of publication bias assessed in the form of funnel plots (both described in greater detail below).

At various points, the GDP asked for additional information about particular studies or different reconfigurations of the comparisons between different interventions or controls, and this information the representative of the team that conducted the SR was usually able to provide within less than an hour or so, often based on additional analyses of the extracted database. What I found particularly interesting was the effect that the evidential displays had on members of the GDP from different theoretical perspectives. It is hard to argue for one's preferred modality when confronted with real data that suggest a lack of efficacy or greater efficacy for another treatment. It is harder still to do so with patient representatives in the room. Hard data generate consensus.

Guideline Development Panels

The IOM (2011a) recommends following eight standards when constructing a CGP. Each is discussed briefly in turn:

Standard 1: Establishing Transparency

Transparency means that sufficient information is provided to allow guideline users to understand the way the recommendations were derived. NICE posts the process that they follow in guideline development on a public website (*www.nice.org.uk/about/what-we-do/our-programmes/nice-guidance/nice-guidelines/how-we-develop-nice-guidelines*) and the APA does the same. In particular, information is provided regarding how the respective CGP members were recruited and any potential conflicts of interest (COIs) are posted on that site.

Standard 2: Management of COIs

COIs are defined as any "set of circumstances that creates a risk that professional judgment or actions regarding a primary interest will be unduly influenced by a secondary interest" (IOM 2011a, p. 46). This includes not only opportunity for financial gain or professional advancement but also the "intellectual passions" of the panelists. In essence, although I have long been

tenured and derive no financial gain as a consequence, I regard myself as having a COI with respect to cognitive therapy.

COIs themselves can be handled in a number of ways. Since expertise is to be represented on our panels and expertise often goes hand in hand with intellectual passion, we did not exclude potential members on those grounds but relied instead on disclosure. In most instances, we passed over investigators who developed an intervention and chose instead others with that orientation who did not have "ownership" of the intervention. For example, Myrna Weissman, who developed interpersonal psychotherapy, had volunteered to serve on the panel and she would have been terrific, but for appearances' sake, we elected to go instead with her colleague Laura Mufson, who shared her expertise but was not one of the original developers.

Financial ties are somewhat trickier to manage when physicians come on board, since so many of them accept funding from the pharmaceutical industry. This somewhat newer development goes back to the deregulation started by Reagan in the early 1980s. Before that time, the medical profession saw its role as that of protecting the public from unsubstantiated claims of corporate interests that put profits before patients (pharmaceutical companies are in business to do well not to do good), but that has changed over the subsequent decades. The United States in one of only two countries in the world that allows direct to consumer advertising of prescription medications (New Zealand being the other), and it is no accident that we lead the world in the use of psychiatric medications. That being said, there are members of the medical community who are known for their approbation in that regard and a subset of whom who do not accept monies from pharmaceutical companies. These were the physicians that we tried to choose for inclusion on the guideline panels.

Standard 3: Guideline Development Panel Composition

The IOM recommends forming multidisciplinary panels (as NICE routinely does), and this is something with which I strongly agree. Multidisciplinary panels are less likely to be biased in their recommendations than panels drawn from a single discipline, since the latter tend to be swayed by guild considerations. Members of the public often have to choose between multiple competing interventions for a given disorder, and it is helpful to have panel members who know the relative strengths and harms of each to formulate those recommendations. What we have done is to follow the principle that cognitive psychologists refer to as *adversarial collaboration,* in which competing biases are dealt with by mutual offsetting inclusion rather than exclusion (Mellers, Hertwig, & Kahneman, 2001).

I have collaborated with some truly first-rate biological psychiatrists throughout my career, and I know from experience that patients are more likely to see the advantages of medication treatment after talking with one of them, and more likely to see the advantages of cognitive therapy after talking with me, despite the fact that both my psychiatric colleagues and I try our best not to oversell our respective therapies. This is one of those instances when good intentions are not enough to overcome implicit biases. We simply must have professionals with competing perspectives contributing to the recommendations in order for them to be unbiased.

We also try to balance our guideline panels with respect to theoretical orientation across the different types of psychosocial interventions (dynamic, interpersonal, behavioral, cognitive, experiential, and family) and professional activity (research, practice, and administration). Each panel typically includes at least one research methodologist with expertise in meta-analysis, and every effort is made to be diverse with respect to gender, race, and ethnicity. Our preference has been to follow the IOM recommendations (as does NICE) and include patients and patient representatives on the panels. Including consumers on the panels helps to focus the professionals on the real-life meaning of the work at hand and of the commitment to the public interest rather than narrow self-interest or guild concerns.

Standard 4: Interaction between the GDP and the Systematic Review Team

The IOM describes several models of interaction between the GDP and the systematic review team, ranging from complete isolation to full interaction. We prefer something closer to the latter. While you do not want the preconceptions of the GDP biasing the systematic review, it is helpful for the panel to play a role in shaping the questions that are asked, so that evidence that is reviewed speaks to the most salient issues. When I sat in with the NICE GDP several years ago, the panelists were able to send questions through an intermediary to the systematic review team and get evidence-based responses throughout the day.

Standard 5: Rating Strength of Recommendations

Several systems are available for rating the strength of the recommendations. The most widely used is Grading of Recommendations, Assessment, Development and Evaluation (GRADE; Schünemann, Brożek, & Oxman, 2009). However, it is somewhat cumbersome, and we have adopted a more streamlined version (Guyatt et al., 2006). Strong recommendations indicate that the benefits clearly outweigh the harms (or vice versa), whereas weak recommendations indicate a less clear balance of the two types of outcomes. It is important to note that the strength of the recommendations is not the same thing as the strength of the evidence (discussed below). Treatments that produce harms are likely to be discouraged, even when the strength of the evidence is not all that extensive (Dimidjian & Hollon, 2010).

Standard 6: Articulation of Recommendations

Guideline panels need to be clear about just what actions they are recommending. We ask our guideline panels to generate key action statements that recommend specific behaviors for the clinician to follow. Following the IOM, we use specific language to separate strong from weak recommendations ("We recommend" vs. "We conditionally recommend"), then provide specifics regarding what should be done (e.g., "We recommend that providers encourage patients to relive and work through their traumas").

Standard 7: External Review

Once the guideline is in draft form, we make it available to both selected external reviewers and the general public for comment prior to publication. There are experts in the field from whom we want to be sure to solicit comments, and the larger public can provide valuable input for improving the recommendations. The IOM recommends keeping authorship of the critiques confidential so as to encourage free expression, but we do plan to make available to the public a written record of each critique and the response that it elicited.

Standard 8: Updating

The IOM recommends updating the guidelines whenever there are significant changes in (1) benefits and harms, (2) important outcomes, (3) available interventions, (4) evidence that current practice is optimal, (5) the value placed on different outcomes, or (6) resources available for health care. These are the most sensible recommendations, and they clearly serve the public interest. That being said, they may be hard to implement and likely require posting changes on the same website where the existing guideline resides. We plan to follow recent guidelines from the AHRQ (Newberry et al., 2013).

Conducting Systematic Reviews

The IOM standards for conducting systematic reviews represent a succinct and helpful summary of current best practices in the field (IOM, 2011b). These practices that are largely followed by NICE and other leading guideline generators tend to dominate what is done in medicine. The standards represent the four major stages in conducting a systematic review: (1) initiating the review, (2) finding and assessing individual studies, (3) synthesizing the body of evidence, and (4) reporting the results. The process of conducting a systematic review is reviewed in detail by Cuijpers and Cristea (Chapter 5, this volume), but the IOM standards are summarized briefly here given the importance of systematic reviews for the work of CPGs.

Standard 1: Initiating the Systematic Review

The IOM specifies the importance of using a team with the requisite skills in information search and quantitative methods, and soliciting input from guideline users and stakeholders. NICE maintains its own cadre of personnel with the necessary expertise, who move from one systematic review to the next, and in the United States, the AHRQ develops contracts with university-associated or freestanding evidence-based practice centers (EPCs) to actually conduct the reviews. The IOM provides standards for developing the systematic review protocol that is submitted for independent peer review by outside experts. The protocol is then made publicly available by placing it in a regis-

try specified by the Preferred Reporting Items for Systematic Reviews and Meta-Analyses (PRISMA; Liberati et al., 2009).

The first key step in this process is formulating the topic for the systematic review, also known as *scoping*. This is accomplished by developing an *analytic framework* that provides a conceptual overview of the questions of interest. This conceptual road map usually includes specification of patient and contextual factors that might influence the outcomes of interest (moderators) and the causally active treatment processes and patient mechanisms by which those effects are produced (mediators). Figure 6.2 provides an example of an analytic framework for depression.

The second key step in this process is to generate a set of structured questions to operationalize the analytic framework. Most systematic reviews adopt the widely used PICOTS format that incorporates populations (P), interventions (I), comparisons (C), outcomes (O), time (T), and settings (S). An example of a PICOTS question might be as follows: For patients with major depressive disorder (P), is behavioral activation (I) superior to treatment as usual (C) in reduction of acute distress (O) across the course of acute treatment (T) in general medical settings in rural India (S) (see, e.g., Patel et al., 2017). Specific PICOTS questions may be generated for different subtypes of depression (or different demographic groups), different types of treatments (including other types of psychosocial interventions or medication treatment), different types of comparisons (ranging from no treatment through alternative active interventions), different outcomes (including functional indices and quality of life), different temporal intervals (ranging from acute response to long-term follow-ups), and different kinds of settings (ranging from general practice to inpatient settings). We prefer to have the GDP involved in generating the analytic framework and formulating the PICOTS so as to provide a focus for the systematic review team to follow in their search.

Organizing the information search around the PICOTS questions can structure the literature search, but it also has a downside. I recently served as a key informant on a systematic review commissioned by the Association of Internal Medicine that was funded by the AHRQ and executed by the Research Triangle Institute (RTI), one of the currently funded EPCs. The basic conclusion was that the second-generation

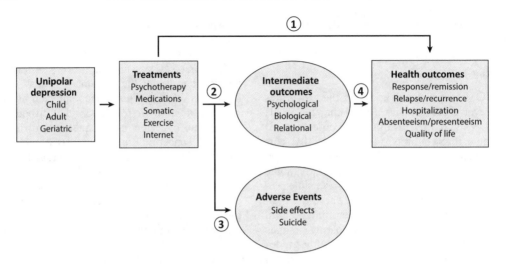

FIGURE 6.2. Example of an analytic framework. From Hollon et al. (2014). Reprinted by permission of Annual Reviews; permission conveyed through Copyright Clearance Center, Inc.

antidepressants and cognitive therapy did not differ with respect to acute response and remission or treatment dropout (Amick et al., 2015). The review itself was very nicely implemented but did not include any comparisons to interpersonal psychotherapy (IPT), one of the most efficacious psychosocial interventions, because its efficacy was largely established before the introduction of the second-generation antidepressants. This is not a criticism of the review that was conducted, just that the literature covered provided no specific comparisons between two of the most efficacious interventions in the literature. This is an issue that network analyses were designed to address (see Mayo-Wilson et al., 2014).

What PICOTS questions can do is to facilitate identification of factors that moderate or mediate response to treatment, but only to the extent that the existing literature provides answers to those questions. Individuals within a larger population (P) differ in a number of different ways, and any number of characteristics can be explored to see if they predict differential response to treatment (moderation). Unfortunately, much of the published literature reports only main effects and does not test for moderation. This is in part due to an overabundance of caution on the part of statisticians who warn against testing for subgroup differences on a post hoc basis (Pocock, Assmann, Enos, & Kasten, 2002). This is a reasonable concern, since any large dataset will yield a number of

significant interactions solely on the basis of chance, and testing for differences within subsets of patients in the absence of interactions magnifies that risk. At the same time, not testing for moderation can slow the identification of important subgroup differences, since if we do not know what we do not know, then we would not know to test for moderation in an a priori fashion. Initial severity provides an example. It was considered controversial when first reported as a moderator on a post hoc basis in the National Institute of Mental Health (NIMH) Treatment of Depression Collaborative Research Program (Elkin et al., 1989). Nonetheless, numerous subsequent studies replicated the effect once investigators knew to look for it (Dimidjian et al., 2006; Fournier et al., 2010). Tests for moderation based on metaregressions in the context of meta-analyses do not necessarily solve the problem, since the variance between studies is often not as great as the variance between individuals within a given study (Driessen, Cuijpers, Hollon, & Dekker, 2010). Individual patient-level meta-analyses largely resolve this issue, since they capture that individual variability (Weitz et al., 2015).

Even more exciting are recent efforts to generate algorithms based on multiple indices that identify the optimal treatment for a given patient (Cohen & DeRubeis, 2018). The personalized advantage index (PAI) represents one recent example (DeRubeis et al., 2014). The PAI is constructed by generating separate algorithms that predict how a given individual would do in each condition based on the response of all other patients in those conditions except the target patient. Each patient then receives a score predicting response to each condition (the "factual" one received and the "counterfactual" one not received) and the difference between those scores (if large enough) indicates the optimal condition that that patient should have received. The PAI is less susceptible to shrinkage than more conventional multivariate approaches because it does not capitalize on chance based on idiosyncratic variation in the scores of individual patients. Applying the PAI to patients randomized to cognitive therapy versus antidepressant medications in a trial that found no differences between the two approaches (DeRubeis et al., 2005) indicated that about 30% of the patients would have done better with cognitive therapy than with medications and another 30% of the patients would have done better with medications than with cognitive therapy. Assigning patients to their optimal intervention (only about half were so assigned) would have improved response by as much as the difference between either active treatment and the pill-placebo control (DeRubeis et al., 2014). In essence, being able to identify the best treatment for a given patient can improve overall response even without doing anything to improve the treatments. More recent versions of this approach have relied on machine learning (a form of pattern recognition) to identify higher-order interactions between potential indices and can accommodate nonlinear relations (Kessler, 2018).

Whereas identifying moderation can improve the efficiency of treatment by virtue of getting the right treatment to the right patient, identifying mediation can improve the efficacy of treatment by allowing the therapist to do more of those things that make the treatment work. This is most directly relevant to treatment processes (what the therapist does) but also indirectly to treatment mechanisms (the processes within the client that transmit the effect of treatment to the outcome). Every treatment is a complex package of different components, and knowing which of those components most influences outcome can allow a therapist to do more of those things and less of others. For example, if posttraumatic stress disorder (PTSD) is best treated by encouraging clients to relive their traumatic experience(s), then focusing on that component will generate the best results. If what is going on within the patient is that trau-

matic memories are accessed instead of being avoided and that accessing those memories allows them to be put into some larger perspective (or at least degraded before they are sent back into storage), then taking steps to enhance that perspective taking (or that degradation) should make treatment more efficacious.

Mediation is harder to detect than moderation (it is easier to detect an effect than it is to explain it) but ultimately more valuable. When the analytic framework is constructed in such a way as to facilitate the search for mediation, the whole enterprise is enhanced; as the great social psychologist Kurt Lewin (1943, p. 118) once said, "There is nothing as practical as a good theory." Nonetheless, efforts to test for mediation are even less likely to be reported in the literature than tests of moderation, so that each is largely promissory at this point in time. However, commenting on the dearth of such information in the existing literature can increase the likelihood that future investigators will try to conduct just such tests. In that fashion, CPGs can improve the quality of the literature by pointing out its current limitations. One final point is that moderation and mediation do not operate in isolation. Whenever you have moderation, you have differential mediation (Kazdin, 2007). If different patients respond differentially to different treatments, this means that they are adhering to different causal mechanisms. Moreover, mediation ought only apply for those patients who respond differentially to a given treatment. In effect, detecting moderation can work to improve the sensitivity of our tests of mediation and increase the odds of detecting an effect.

PICOTS questions also can be used to explore other aspects of treatment response. Therapist effects can be examined in terms of differences between therapists or as interactions (moderators) within the context of the interventions (I). Specificity can be explored within the context of the different types of comparisons (C). Any treatment that is better than its absence can be said to be *efficacious* (that is the minimum that we expect an intervention to do), and any treatment that exceeds a nonspecific control (like a pill-placebo or supportive therapy) can be said to be *specific* (Chambless & Hollon, 1998). If a treatment is better than other alternative interventions, it can be said to be *superior*. This requires comparisons to alternative (and presumably) specific interventions. This is the whole reason for constructing CPGs. It is not sufficient that a treatment is efficacious to be recommended; "energy field therapy" is more efficacious than its absence for largely non-specific reasons and is based on a theory that represents a physical impossibility. Lilienfeld (2011) has argued that theoretical plausibility must also be considered. Pseudoscience dates to Mesmer, and it is never wise to fool the public.

Different kinds of outcomes (O) can be examined in different sets of questions and often go beyond purely symptomatic change. Cognitive therapy was more likely to get patients with moderate to severe depression back to work than medication treatment (Fournier et al., 2015), and a culturally adapted version of behavioral activation not only reduced depression more than enhanced usual care in a general medical setting in rural India but also reduced rates of intimate partner violence (Patel et al., 2017). Different temporal factors (T) often differentiate between different treatments; patients treated to remission with cognitive therapy are only about half as likely to relapse following treatment termination as patients treated to comparable remission with medications (Cuijpers et al., 2013). Contextual factors such as setting (S) can be explored as moderators as well. It is clear that PICOTS questions can help organize the literature search.

Standard 2: Finding and Assessing Individual Studies

The IOM recommends working with a research librarian and other information specialists to conduct a comprehensive search based on explicit inclusion and exclusion criteria. It can be particularly important to search the "gray" literature: studies that were conducted but never got published. Turner, Matthews, Linardatos, Tell, and Rosenthal (2008) found that the newer antidepressant medications (from fluoxetine on) failed to separate from pill-placebo in nearly half the studies registered with the U.S. Food and Drug Administration (FDA) to win marketing approval. However, few of those negative trials were ever published, and those that were typically were "spun" to make it appear that they were positive. As a consequence, the published literature inflated the effect of the newer antidepressant medications by about 25%. *Publication bias* (selective publication of positive findings) and *outcome reporting bias* (selective presentation of positive findings) can skew a literature, and efforts are needed to protect the field from both kinds of bias, whether intended or otherwise. This problem is not just limited to industry-funded trials. A recent review found that nearly one-fourth of the grants for studies of psychosocial treatments for depression produced no publications; exclusion of the data from those unpublished trials inflated the apparent efficacy of psychotherapy by about as much as was the case for medications (Driessen, Hollon, Bockting, Cuijpers, & Turner, 2015). Publication bias is a sociological phenomenon that inflates the apparent efficacy of all different kinds of treatments.

There are several other points that need to be made. The IOM recommends using two or more independent reviewers to determine whether a study meets criteria for inclusion, and two or more independent reviewers to extract the data from it. This increases the cost of the systematic review but has been shown to reduce errors in the screening process by up to one-third (Edwards et al., 2002). The IOM also recommends rating each study for risk of bias using predefined criteria like the one developed by the Cochrane Collaboration (Higgins et al., 2011). While I endorse both recommendations, I would note that most existing datasets were extracted prior to the call for independent reviewers and that the assessment for risk of bias largely focuses on factors that affect internal validity, such as lack of adequate concealment of randomization, as discussed in detail by Kraemer and Periyakoil (Chapter 4, this volume). While the IOM notes that it is important to assess the fidelity of treatment implementation, it provides no guidance for how to do so. Investigator allegiance is one of the most powerful determinants of outcome in the treatment literature (Luborsky et al., 1999), and differences in competence to implement a given modality likely represents the biggest sources of uncontrolled variability in outcomes for the same treatment (Leykin & DeRubeis, 2009). Our inability to quantify variability in the quality of execution of the same treatment across different studies is one reason I want an expert panel to review the findings, since they tend to know who is competent to implement the respective modalities.

Standard 3: Synthesizing the Body of Evidence

The IOM recommends using a prespecified method like GRADE to systematically assess the strength of a body of evidence. It also recommends conducting a qualitative synthesis of the body of evidence as a whole that includes descriptions of the clinical and methodological characteristics of the studies and the strengths and limitations of the studies as a whole. This is a good and useful thing to do so long as it does not tie the hands of the GDP. A good systematic review team should be expert in search methodology but is not necessarily expert in the content area that they are searching, whereas members of the GDP are usually chosen because of their expertise in a particular area of research. For example, the recent systematic review of second generation antidepressants previously cited (Amick et al., 2015) initially failed to detect that an Iranian study that found behavioral activation superior to antidepressant medications fol-

lowed medical practice in Tehran that capped the medication dosage at about half maximum dosage that is typically used elsewhere (Moradveisi, Huibers, Renner, Arasteh, & Arntz, 2013). Treating this study as an efficacy trial skewed the summary (to some extent) in favor of the psychosocial intervention. This was an error that a multidisciplinary GDP likely would not have made.

Forest plots are an invaluable way to represent variability in outcome as part of the effort to synthesize a literature. This was one of the things that most struck me when I sat in with the depression GDP for NICE. Figure 6.3 presents a pair of forest plots from a recently published meta-analysis comparing prior ex-

a

Study name	Statistics for each study			
	Odds ratio	Lower limit	Upper limit	p-value
Blackburn, 1986	9,60	0,85	108,72	0,07
Dobson, 2008	3,25	0,88	12,01	0,08
Evans, 1992	9,00	0,81	100,14	0,07
Hollon, 2005	2,86	0,94	8,71	0,07
Jarret, 2000	0,50	0,04	6,68	0,60
Kovacs, 1981	2,88	0,73	11,38	0,13
Shea, 1992	1,66	0,65	4,21	0,29
Simons, 1986	3,15	0,67	14,86	0,15
	2,61	1,58	4,31	0,00

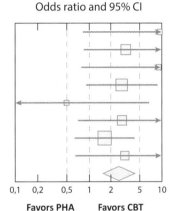

b

Study name	Statistics for each study			
	Odds ratio	Lower limit	Upper limit	p-value
David, 2008	1,50	0,70	3,22	0,30
Dobson, 2008	2,80	0,88	8,91	0,08
Evans, 1992	2,00	0,15	26,19	0,60
Hollon, 2005	1,64	0,59	4,57	0,34
Jarret, 2000	0,25	0,02	2,76	0,26
	1,62	0,97	2,72	0,07

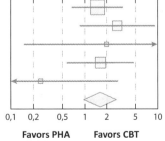

FIGURE 6.3. Example of a forest plot. *Top:* Long-term effects of cognitive-behavioral therapy (CBT) (without continuation during follow-up) compared with pharmacotherapy (*discontinued* during follow-up): Forest plot of odds ratio of response. *Bottom:* Long-term effects of CBT (without continuation during follow-up) compared with pharmacotherapy (*continued* during follow-up): Forest plot of odds ratio of response. From Cuijpers et al. (2013). Reprinted by permission of BMJ Publishing Group Ltd.

posure to cognitive therapy to prior exposure to antidepressant medications (Cuijpers et al., 2013). The eight studies included in that literature are tabled on the left and odds ratios (as an estimate of effect sizes) are presented on the right. What can be seen is that the majority of the studies in the literature show an enduring effect for prior cognitive therapy; in aggregate, patients treated to remission with that approach are less than half as likely to relapse following treatment termination than patients treated to comparable levels of remission with medications with an odds ratio of 2.61. What it also does is provide a graphic display of the outliers in the literature and especially the one study that goes the other way. In that trial, patients treated to remission on medications were less likely to relapse following treatment termination than patients treated to remission with cognitive therapy (Jarrett et al., 2000). While there is no obvious explanation for that disparity, the fact that it was the smallest sample in the cohort (as denoted by the size of the square) and listed as a pilot study in the title of the article both contribute to the notion that it was a true outlier in the set. As the great 20th-century philosopher and catcher for the New York Yankees Yogi Berra once said, "You can see a lot by just looking."

Figure 6.4 depicts another type of graphical presentation that can be of great assistance in understanding a literature. Funnel plots graph effect sizes as a function of the standard error or some other metric indicating the size of the sample. If we assume that there is a "true" effect for a given intervention, then samples taken (effect sizes generated from individual studies) should be normally distributed around that "true" mean; that is, the distribution of effect sizes should be normally distributed, with larger studies falling closer to the mean and smaller studies showing greater variability. The top panel in Figure 6.4 displays the funnel plot for comparisons of psychotherapy to control in the treatment of depression (Cuijpers, Smit, Bohlmeijer, Hollon, & Andersson, 2010). As can be seen, the data in Figure 6.4 are anything but symmetrical, exactly what one would expect if small studies with weak effects were systematically excluded from the literature due to publication bias. The bottom panel depicts the number of studies that would have to be imputed to make the distribution symmetrical. Imputing studies to correct for publication bias decreases the estimated effect of psychotherapy

by about one-fourth, a reduction virtually identical to what was found when unpublished data from grant-funded studies were included in the calculations. This is impressive convergence for two different methodological approaches and increases our confidence in the use of funnel plots to estimate and correct for publication bias in a literature.

My experience sitting in with the NICE depression GDP convinced me that presenting carefully crafted systematic reviews of the empirical literature in graphical form to a multidisciplinary panel of experts who differ in their expertise and orientation provides the best way currently available to arrive at fair and balanced recommendations based on the best available scientific evidence. The different panel members kept each other honest, and the presence of the patient representatives kept things focused on the public interest. Errors and omissions in the evidence presented (and there were few) literally leapt off the screen, and biases and preconceptions were hard to maintain in the face of the graphic presentation of the data.

Standard 4: Reporting the Systematic Review

Finally, the IOM provides explicit recommendations for how to present the systematic review that includes an abstract, an executive summary, and a summary written for the lay public. It also recommends including the rationale and objectives of the systematic review, a method section that describes the search protocol, including the analytic framework and the PICOTS questions, and discussion section and conclusions for each key question, as well as gaps in the evidence and future research needs. The IOM also suggests sending the resulting document out for independent review perhaps as part of publication.

This is all very reasonable and should be done, but the published review is not the same as the actual guidelines themselves. As I described earlier, there is wisdom to filtering systematic reviews through expert guideline panels that can bring clinical expertise and patient preferences to bear in crafting the treatment recommendations. It is the expertise of the SR team that makes sure that nothing is overlooked in the empirical literature, but it is the judgment of the guideline panel that turns that empirical evidence into actionable clinical recommendations.

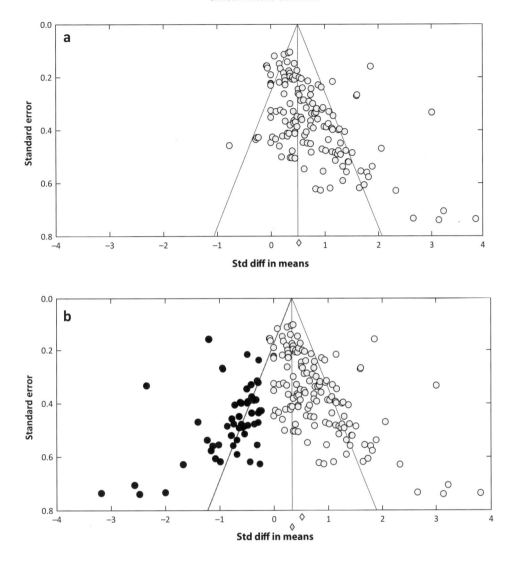

FIGURE 6.4. Funnel plot of the mean effect size and standard error. *Top:* Unadjusted for publication bias. *Bottom:* Adjusted for publication bias. From Cuijpers, Smit, Bohlmeijer, Hollon, and Andersson (2010). Reprinted by permission of Cambridge University Press.

Using CPGs to Inform Mental Health Care

What CPGs Currently Exist That Are Relevant to Mental Health Care?

Several organizations already generate CPGs. NICE is not only the most prolific of the guideline generators but, as previously noted, it generates the highest quality guidelines in the field. It has generated over 20 high-quality guidelines relevant to the various mental health disorders and updates them at periodic intervals. The Scottish Intercollegiate Guidelines Network

also generates guidelines of its own, although it is not clear why it does so, since they tend to overlap with those generated by NICE. Other Western democracies such as Canada and Australia also generate guidelines, but with fewer resources than is the case for NICE. The Netherlands updates its guidelines on an ongoing basis. It is not entirely clear why different countries feel the need to generate separate guidelines, since they all look to the same empirical literature, but the rationale usually given is that health care systems differ in different locales.

My own sense is that NICE sets the standard and that health care delivery systems should be adapted to provide the most efficacious treatments rather than the other way around.

In the United States, the VA/DOD has generated several high-quality guidelines, although they are few in number and focus on those disorders most relevant to a military population. The psychiatric APA and the American Academy of Child and Adolescent Psychiatry (AACAP) have been almost as prolific as NICE, but in the past have eschewed conducting systematic reviews or constructing multidisciplinary guideline panels. That is likely to change in the wake of the publication of the IOM guidelines and the APA plans to do the next guideline on oppositional defiant disorder (ODD) in collaboration with the AACAP (and are in talks with leaders of the psychiatric APA to do the same with respect to adult disorders). It is clear that the AHRQ wants the various professional organizations to work together to staff the guideline panels, and what is likely to develop is a process in which the professions come together to request that the AHRQ fund an EPC to conduct a systematic review that a multidisciplinary GDP uses to construct a CPG. That would be good for the disciplines and even better for the public. No country depends as heavily on medications as we do in the United States. For the psychotic disorders, treatment starts with medications, but there is no nonpsychotic disorder that is not better treated with one of the empirically supported psychotherapies that has enduring effects than with medications.

An even more satisfying solution would be to recognize that the treatment literature is truly international and that disorders are more similar around the globe than health care systems. There already exists an international organization, GIN, whose mission is to pool resources across nations in an effort to improve the efficiency of guideline generation. It simply makes no sense for different organizations to duplicate each other's efforts in extracting data from existing studies and conducting systematic reviews. Our advisory steering committee had arranged informally with the people who oversee NICE to gain access to the data they had extracted from the previous 40 years of RCTs in depression in exchange for making available to them the data we extracted from studies conducted since the time of their last review. For reasons that I still do not understand our psychological APA turned down the offer. The greatest part of the expense in generating a CPG is conducting the systematic review, and there is no reason to duplicate that expense. The literature needs to be updated, but there is no reason not to pool the data already extracted from existing trials and to make that available to all in return for adding to the corpus with respect to extractions from the newest studies. Pim Cuijpers at the Vrije University in Amsterdam maintains a set of extracted data, updated regularly from all the psychosocial RCTs published in English, that is freely available at *www.evidencebased-psychotherapies.org* (Cuijpers, van Straten, van Oppen, & Andersson, 2008). There is no reason why this cannot be done at the behest of governmental agencies under the coordination of GIN.

How to Access Updated CPGs

The best way to access the highest quality CPGs currently available is to go to the NICE website (*www.nice.org.uk/guidance*). Over a dozen such guidelines are currently listed under various mental health disorders (several are like the anxiety disorders, broken down into several subdisorders), and they are updated on a periodic basis. Each guideline provides an overview and executive summary, a clinical flow chart describing key decision points, and extended sections describing the various clinical interventions currently used in treatment. Best of all, the evidentiary basis for the recommendations in the guidelines is fully documented, and the interested reader can see exactly what studies were considered and their characteristics in the appendices. The guidelines and evidence on which they were based are fully transparent, and it is possible to see exactly what studies went into the deliberations and how they were evaluated. We have nothing like it in this country, although the VA/DOD guidelines come close (*www.healthquality.va.gov/guidelines/mh*).

How to Evaluate CPGs: Are Their Recommendations Worth Following?

Although the guidelines themselves have not been evaluated empirically, it is possible to evaluate their quality rationally based on the processes that were followed in their generation. NICE and the VA/DOD guidelines adhered most closely to the recommendations laid out by the IOM and it shows in the quality of the guidelines they developed. Again, transparency is a key, and it is reassuring to be able to see exactly what literature was reviewed and what decisions formed the basis for the recommendations. Guidelines that are well developed (e.g., NICE and the VA/DOD) are based on systematic reviews of the literature as interpreted by multidisciplinary panels of experts (and patient representatives), and they provide an audit trail regarding exactly how they arrived at their recommendations. Moreover, those recommendations are presented in terms of actionable statements: "For patients with the following disorders, choose among these first-line treatments . . . ." The recommendations are based on the empirical literature as processed through clinical expertise and consistent with patient preferences. It is hard to imagine better.

This does not mean that the recommendations necessarily need to be followed. There may be reasons to prefer secondary or tertiary options. This is especially likely to be the case when the patient is reluctant to pursue a first-line option. Exposure is the most potent of the interventions for most of the anxiety disorders (including obsessive–compulsive disorder [OCD] and the phobias), and reliving traumatic memories (trauma-focused treatments) are the most potent interventions for PTSD (Ehlers et al., 2010). The major problem with these interventions is that many patients (and not a few clinicians) find them frightening. The risk of harm is remarkably low, but going through them is distressing. No clinician should ever force a treatment on a patient who is unwilling, but that clinician does have an obligation to inform the patient about the available treatment options, and the benefits and harms. Patient choice always trumps clinical judgment, and each trumps the research evidence. Similarly, it is also important to consider the other domains of evidence-based practice (EBP): the expertise of the clinician; the extent to which the patient's comorbidity, complexity, and sociodemographic characteristics are represented by the literature; and the setting in which the treatment is delivered. That being said, the clinician does at least have an obligation to inform the patient with respect to what the research evidence says and to make a referral, if indicated.

Potential Contributions and Limitations of CPGs

Well-constructed CPGs (e.g., NICE and the VA/DOD guidelines) represent the highest level of evidence currently available, precisely because they incorporate the most complete and systematic reviews of the empirical literature (including meta-analyses when appropriate) as interpreted by a multidisciplinary panel of experts from different theoretical orientations, with input from patients and patient representatives. The data do not interpret themselves, and opinions regarding individual studies and meta-analyses are open to multiple interpretations. I am a big fan of meta-analyses, but I do not think that they alone are sufficient to guide clinical practice. For example, most meta-analytic reviews of the depression literature show that all treatments work, and that they work equally well (Cuijpers et al., 2008). However, psychodynamic psychotherapy has rarely been tested and has never beaten a nonspecific control in any RCT. IPT, on the other hand, has been shown to be as efficacious as antidepressant medications in trials when each was superior to nonspecific controls. That is why most treatment guidelines (e.g., NICE) recommend IPT as a first-line treatment for depression but not dynamic psychotherapy. The effects sizes are comparable, but the quality of the evidence supporting IPT is simply more impressive. This is where expert judgment comes into play.

Another limitation of CPGs is that they are only as comprehensive as the studies that have been conducted; however, *absence of evidence is not evidence of absence.* Just because a treatment has not been tested does not mean that it does not work. That said, in a single-payer system like that in the United Kingdom (and like what we may be moving toward in the United States), absence of evidence is likely tantamount to absence of reimbursement. If there are interventions that are known to be efficacious, then it is unlikely that some third party (the government or an insurer) will pay for treatments of unknown efficacy. It just makes no economic sense. Individuals will still be free to pay out of pocket for untested treatments, but the number of potential patients who are willing and able to do so will only decline over time.

Promoting Guideline Adoption

Barriers to Adoption

The major barrier to adoption of CPG recommendations is that most experienced clinicians were trained in interventions that have garnered little empirical support. Most clinicians do what they were trained to do and are reluctant to adopt new practices. This is a problem in all branches of health care, but it is especially a problem in mental health, where adherence to a particular theoretical perspective almost becomes an article of faith. Dynamic therapists are steeped in an ideology, and the same is true of behaviorists and experiential therapists. Although I have known clinicians who are exceptions, my own sense is that change in practice is largely generational. There are reasons why practicing clinicians have faith in the procedures that they use, but they have more to do with the lack of exposure to evidence-based treatments in graduate training. Moreover, all of us are subject to information-processing biases and heuristics that lead us to attribute positive change to what we do, and lack of change to patient characteristics (Lilienfeld, Ritschel, Lynn, Cautin, & Latzman, 2014). No self-respecting oncologist would continue to rely on practices that were learned decades earlier, but this is what most experienced psychotherapists do. This proclivity has until recently been fully supported by the psychological APA, which for years opposed any effort to generate CPGs (Hollon et al., 2014). Within the last decade the governing Council of the psychological APA issued a major statement that all psychotherapies work and all work equally well, despite the lack of empirical support.

The psychological APA recently completed its first CPG (on the treatment of PTSD), and it essentially gave its strongest recommendations to several different kinds of trauma-focused exposure therapies. Although the initial guideline passed the psychological APA Council easily enough (on an 80/20 margin), by the subsequent year there was considerable consternation among the clinical community and over 45,000 signatures of a petition to rescind. How much of that was due to the less enthusiastic recommendation for eye movement desensitization and reprocessing (EMDR), which has never gotten the respect that it deserves from the scientific community, as opposed to the tendency of many practicing clinicians to be avoidant when it comes to helping their clients relive the trauma was difficult to discern, but the point remains that the guideline was not well received by the clinical community. After a very heated debate, the motion to rescind was defeated by a 70/30 margin, so the guideline remains in place, but it does suggest that change will not be easy. Subsequent guidelines were less controversial, but largely because of the nature of the topic (childhood obesity rarely involves direct services by independent practitioners) or the breadth of the recommendations (depression responds to most widely practiced psychotherapies). Uptake by the professional community remains in question.

Facilitators to Adoption

There is a saying at the NIMH that "you cannot herd cats, but you can move their food." The United Kingdom has invested over £700 million pounds to train therapists in those treatments that NICE finds to have empirical support. Practitioners in the United Kingdom are still free to provide whatever treatments they want, but if one wants to work for the National Health Service (NHS), one has to provide treatments that have been shown to work. In the United Kingdom, the "food" has been moved.

This program is called Increasing Access to Psychological Treatments (IAPT), and it is changing the very nature of the treatment that is provided in the United Kingdom (Clark, 2011). The architects of this approach did not work through the existing professional organizations to produce buy-in; rather, they went directly to the treasury officials that oversee the NHS and made the case that the government would save money if it provided efficacious treatments that were known to have enduring effects (Layard & Clark, 2015). Progress in that direction in the United States slowed when the Affordable Care Act (ACA) was put in jeopardy by the 2016 election, but given that the ACA survived, we may again start moving toward a situation that resembles that in the United Kingdom, in which (for the first time) it will be in the interest of the taxpayer to direct federally funded reimbursement to those treatments that actually work. Depending on the outcome of the next election, reimbursement in the United States may once again be on the move.

Conclusions

There is an emerging consensus that CPGs should be based on the best available empirical evidence as filtered through clinical expertise and leavened by patient preference. There also is an emerging clinical science that the best way to generate such CPGs is to construct multidisciplinary panels of experts and patient representatives, and have them generate treatment recommendations based on systematic reviews of the empirical literature. The IOM recommends that guidelines be developed by multidisciplinary panels of experts from diverse theoretical orientations, joined by patients or their representatives working from carefully crafted systematic reviews of the best available science funded by dispassionate government agencies. This is the approach that NICE has adopted, and it is wholly consistent with the kind of adversarial collaboration that cognitive psychologists recommend to deal with ingrained biases (Mellers et al., 2001). Professional guilds are intended to protect the interests of their members (not the public), and proprietary organizations by their very nature put profits over patients. Human nature being what it is, it would be foolish to do anything else. The use of multidisciplinary panels to generate CPGs is a methodology that has served the public well in the rest of medicine, and it should be applied to mental health.

References

Amick, H. R., Gartlehner, G., Gaynes, B. N., Forneris, C., Asher, G. N., Morgan, L. C., et al. (2015). Comparative benefits and harms of second generation antidepressants and cognitive behavioral therapies in initial treatment of major depressive disorder: Systematic review and meta-analysis. *British Medical Journal, 351,* h6019.

Chambless, D. L., & Hollon, S. D. (1998). Defining empirically supported therapies. *Journal of Consulting and Clinical Psychology, 66,* 7–18.

Clark, D. M. (2011). Implementing NICE guidelines for the psychological treatment of depression and anxiety disorders: The IAPT experience. *International Review of Psychiatry 23,* 375–384.

Cohen, Z. D., & DeRubeis, R. J. (2018). Treatment selection in depression. *Annual Review of Clinical Psychology, 14,* 15.1–15.28.

Cuijpers, P., Hollon, S. D., van Straten, A., Bockting, C., Berking, M., & Andersson, G. (2013). Does cognitive behavior therapy have an enduring effect that is superior to keeping patients on continuation pharmacotherapy? *BMJ Open, 3*(4), e002542.

Cuijpers, P., Smit, F., Bohlmeijer, E., Hollon, S. D., & Andersson, G. (2010). Efficacy of cognitive-behavioural therapy and other psychological treatments for adult depression: Meta-analytic study of publication bias. *British Journal of Psychiatry, 196,* 173–178.

Cuijpers, P., van Straten, A., van Oppen, P., & Andersson, G. (2008). Are psychological and pharmacologic interventions equally effective in the treatment of adult depressive disorders?: A meta-analysis of comparative studies. *Journal of Clinical Psychiatry, 69,* 1675–1685.

DeRubeis, R. J., Cohen, Z. D., Forand, N. R., Fournier, J. C., Gelfand, L. A., & Lorenzo-Luaces, L. (2014). The Personalized Advantage Index: Translating research on prediction into individualized treatment recommendations: A demonstration. *PLOS ONE, 9,* e83875.

DeRubeis, R. J., Hollon, S. D., Amsterdam, J. D., Shel-

ton, R. C., Young, P. R., Salomon, R. M., et al. (2005). Cognitive therapy vs. medications in the treatment of moderate to severe depression. *Archives of General Psychiatry, 62,* 409–416.

Dimidjian, S., & Hollon, S. D. (2010). How would you know if psychotherapy was harmful? *American Psychologist, 65,* 21–33.

Dimidjian, S., Hollon, S. D., Dobson, K. S., Schmaling, K. B., Kohlenberg, R. J., Addis, M. E., et al. (2006). Behavioral activation, cognitive therapy, and antidepressant medication in the acute treatment of major depression. *Journal of Consulting and Clinical Psychology, 74,* 658–670.

Driessen, E., Cuijpers, P., Hollon, S. D., & Dekker, J. J. M. (2010). Does pretreatment severity moderate the efficacy of psychological treatment of adult outpatient depression?: A meta-analysis. *Journal of Consulting and Clinical Psychology, 78,* 668–680.

Driessen, E., Hollon, S. D., Bockting, C. L. H., Cuijpers, P., & Turner, E. H. (2015). Does publication bias inflate the apparent efficacy of psychological treatment for major depressive disorder?: A systematic review and meta-analysis of US National Institutes of Health-funded trials. *PLOS ONE, 10*(9), e0137864.

Edwards, P., Clark, M., DiGuiseppi, C., Pratap, S., Roberts, I., & Wentz, R. (2002). Identification of randomized controlled trials in systematic reviews: Accuracy and reliability of screening records. *Statistics in Medicine, 21,* 1635–1640.

Ehlers, A., Bisson, J., Clark, D. M., Creamer, M., Pilling, S., & Richards, D., et al. (2010). Do all psychological treatments really work the same in posttraumatic stress disorder? *Clinical Psychology Review, 30,* 269–276.

Elkin, I., Shea, M. T., Watkins, J. T., Imber, S. D., Sotsky, S. M., Collins, J. F., et al. (1989). National Institute of Mental Health Treatment of Depression Collaborative Research Program: General effectiveness of treatments. *Archives of General Psychiatry, 46,* 971–982.

Falk-Ytter, Y., & Schunemann, H. J. (2009). *Rating the evidence: Using GRADE to develop clinical practice guidelines.* Slide presentation at the Agency for Healthcare Research and Quality conference, Rockville, MD.

Fournier, J. C., DeRubeis, R. J., Amsterdam, J. A., Shelton, R. C., & Hollon, S. D. (2015). Gains in employment status following antidepressant medication or cognitive therapy for depression. *British Journal of Psychiatry, 206*(4), 332–338.

Fournier, J. C., DeRubeis, R. J., Hollon, S. D., Dimidjian, S., Amsterdam, J. D., Shelton, R. C., et al. (2010). Antidepressant drug effects and depression severity: A patient-level meta-analysis. *Journal of the American Medical Association, 303,* 47–53.

Guyatt, G., Gutterman, D., Bauman, M. H., Addrizzo-Harris, D., Hylek, E. M., Phillips, B., et al. (2006). Grading strength of recommendations and quality of evidence in clinical guidelines: Report from an

American College of Chest Physicians task force. *Chest, 129,* 174–181.

Higgins, J. P. T., Altman, D. G., Gotzsche, P. C., Juni, P., Moher, D., Oxman, A. D., et al. (2011). The Cochrane Collaboration's tool for assessing risk of bias in randomised trials. *British Medical Journal, 343*(2), d5928.

Hollon, S. D., Areán, P. A., Craske, M. G., Crawford, K. A., Kivlahan, D. R., Magnavita, J. J., et al. (2014). Development of clinical practice guidelines. *Annual Review of Clinical Psychology, 10,* 213–241.

Institute of Medicine. (2011a). *Clinical practice guidelines we can trust.* Washington, DC: National Academies Press.

Institute of Medicine. (2011b). *Finding what works in health care: Standards for systematic reviews.* Washington, DC: National Academies Press.

Jarrett, R. B., Kraft, D., Schaffer, M., Witt-Browder, A., Risser, R., Atkins, D. H., et al. (2000). Reducing relapse in depressed outpatients with atypical features: A pilot study. *Psychotherapy and Psychosomatics, 69,* 232–239.

Kazdin, A. E. (2007). Mediators and mechanisms of change in psychotherapy research. *Annual Review of Clinical Psychology, 3,* 1–27.

Kessler, R. C. (2018). The potential of predictive analytics to provide clinical decision support in depression treatment planning. *Current Opinion in Psychiatry, 31*(1), 32–39.

Layard, R., & Clark, D. M. (2015). *Thrive: How better mental health care transforms lives and saves money.* Princeton, NJ: Princeton University Press.

Lewin, K. (1943). Psychology and the process of group living. *Journal of Social Psychology, 17,* 113–131.

Leykin, Y., & DeRubeis, R. J. (2009). Allegiance in psychotherapy outcome research: Separating association from bias. *Clinical Psychology: Science and Practice, 16*(1), 54–65.

Liberati, A., Altman, D. G., Tetzlaff, J., Mulrow, C., Gøtzsche, P. C., Ionnanidis, J. P., et al. (2009). The PRISMA statement for reporting systematic reviews and meta-analyses of studies that evaluate health care interventions: Explanation and elaboration. *Annals of Internal Medicine, 151*(4), W65–W94.

Lilienfeld, S. O. (2011). Distinguishing scientific from pseudoscientific psychotherapies: Evaluating the role of theoretical plausibility, with a little help from Reverend Bayes. *Clinical Psychology: Science and Practice, 18*(2), 105–112.

Lilienfeld, S. O., Ritschel, L. A., Lynn, S. J., Cautin, R. L., & Latzman, R. D. (2014). Why ineffective psychotherapies appear to work: Taxonomy of causes of spurious therapeutic effectiveness. *Perspectives on Psychological Science, 9,* 355–387.

Luborsky, L., Diguer, L., Seligman, D. A., Rosenthal, R., Krause, E. D., Johnson, S., et al. (1999). The researcher's own therapy allegiances: A "wild card" in comparisons of treatment efficacy. *Clinical Psychology: Science and Practice, 6*(1), 95–106.

Mayo-Wilson, E., Dias, S., Mavranezouli, I., Kew, K.,

Clark, D. M., Ades, A. E., et al. (2014). Psychological and pharmacological interventions for social anxiety disorder in adults: A systematic review and network meta-analysis. *Lancet Psychiatry, 1,* 368–376.

Mellers, B., Hertwig, R., & Kahneman, D. (2001). Do frequency representations eliminate conjunction effects?: An exercise in adversarial collaboration. *Psychological Science, 12*(4), 269–275.

Moradveisi, L., Huibers, M. J. H., Renner, F., Arasteh, M., & Arntz, A. (2013). Behavioural activation v. antidepressant medication for treatment depression in Iran. *British Journal of Psychiatry, 202,* 204–211.

Muñoz, R. F., Hollon, S. D., McGrath, E., Rehm, L. P., & VandenBos, G. R. (1994). On the AHCPR depression in primary care guidelines: Further considerations for practitioners. *American Psychologist, 49,* 42–61.

Newberry, S. J., Ahmadzai, N., Motala, A., Tsertsvadze, A., Maglione, M., Ansari, M. T., et al. (2013). *Surveillance and identification of signals for updating systematic review: Implementation and early experience* (Methods Research Report, AHRQ Publication No. 13-EHC088-EF). Rockville, MD: Agency for Healthcare Research and Quality.

Patel, V., Weobong, B., Nadkarni, A., Weiss, H. A., Anand, A., Naik, S., et al. (2014). The PREMIUM randomised controlled trials of the effectiveness and cost-effectiveness of lay counsellor-delivered psychological treatments for harmful and dependent drinking and moderate to severe depression in primary care in India. *Trials, 15,* 101.

Patel, V., Weobong, B., Weiss, H. A., Anand, A., Bhat, B., Katti, B., et al. (2017). The Healthy Activity Program (HAP), a lay counsellor delivered brief psychological treatment for severe depression, in primary care in India: A randomised controlled trial. *Lancet, 389*(10065), 176–185.

Pocock, S. J., Assmann, S. E., Enos, L. E., & Kasten, L. E. (2002). Subgroup analysis, covariate adjustment and baseline comparisons in clinical trial reporting: Current practice and problems. *Statistics in Medicine, 21,* 2917–2930.

Schünemann, H. J., Brožek, J., & Oxman, A. D. (2009). GRADE handbook for grading quality of evidence and strength of recommendations. Retrieved from *www.who.int/hiv/topics/mtct/grade_handbook.pdf.*

Spring, B., & Hitchcock, K. (2009). Evidence-based practice in psychology. In I. B. Weiner & W. E. Craighead (Eds.), *Corsini's encyclopedia of psychology* (4th ed., pp. 603–607). New York: Wiley.

Turner, E. H., Matthews, A. M., Linardatos, E., Tell, R. A., & Rosenthal, R. (2008). Selective publication of antidepressant trials and its influence on apparent efficacy. *New England Journal of Medicine, 358,* 252–260.

Weitz, E. S., Hollon, S. D., Twisk, J., van Straten, A., Huibers, M. J. H., David, D., et al. (2015). Does baseline depression severity moderate depression outcomes between CBT versus pharmacotherapy?: An individual patient data meta-analysis. *JAMA Psychiatry, 72*(11), 1102–1109.

CHAPTER 7

Moving Beyond "One Size Fits All"

ZACHARY D. COHEN
YONI K. ASHAR
ROBERT J. DeRUBEIS

Half a century ago, Gordon Paul (1967) reviewed psychotherapy outcome research and concluded that "in all its complexity, the question towards which all outcome research should ultimately be directed is the following: *What* treatment, by *whom,* is most effective for *this* individual with *that* specific problem, and under *which* set of circumstances?" (p. 111, original emphasis). Paul's article has been extensively cited, and the previous passage has often been invoked or abbreviated to "What works for whom?" The idea is a good one, recognizing that no single approach is likely to be best for every person who presents with a mental health problem.

Improving outcomes across mental health treatments is imperative (Holmes et al., 2018). The predominant approach has been to develop new treatments, such as novel neurological (e.g., deep brain stimulation: Mayberg et al., 2005), pharmacological (e.g., ketamine: McGirr et al., 2015), and psychological treatments (e.g., positive affect treatment: Craske, Meuret, Ritz, Treanor, & Dour, 2016). However, this approach on its own is likely to be insufficient. Depression, which is the world's leading cause of disability (World Health Organization, 2017), provides an example. Numerous evidence-based interventions for major depressive disorder (MDD) have been developed, but the average treatment response rate remains at about 50% (Luty et al.,

2007; National Health Service, 2016; Papakostas & Fava, 2010). In this chapter we describe an alternative approach—*treatment selection,* which aims to identify for each person the treatment that is best for him or her.

Treatment selection focuses on the role of "individual differences"—the idea that individuals respond differently to treatment, and that these differences can be studied and characterized. It responds directly to the principle that therapists "attend to the individual person to make the complex choices necessary to conceptualize, prioritize, and treat multiple symptoms," as described by the American Psychological Association (2006, p. 279) and as highlighted by other evidence-based practice models (see Spring, Marchese, & Steglitz, Chapter 1, this volume).

The treatment selection approach has been applied profitably in medicine (Ashley, 2016; National Research Council, 2011), where it has been termed *precision* medicine (Hamburg & Collins, 2010) or *personalized* medicine (Katsnelson, 2013; Schleidgen, Klinger, Bertram, Rogowski, & Marckmann, 2013). For example, in oncology, the choice of anticancer drug can be tailored to match genetic mutations detected in a particular patient's tumor, leading to improved outcomes (Paez et al., 2004; Rosell et al., 2012). Could similar approaches help improve outcomes in mental health? This is the question that motivates this chapter.

Traditionally, results from clinical trials have been analyzed and reported in terms of *average treatment response across all individuals*. In a typical study, researchers compare responses to treatments *A, B,* and *C,* and declare the treatment with the greatest average response the "winner." This approach has been described as a "horse race" approach to psychotherapy research. And, in lumping patients together, it obscures the very information that could best guide personalized clinical decision making.

In reality, each treatment produces a wide distribution of treatment responses. In treatment selection, it is the distribution of response scores that is of interest rather than the average treatment response. To analyze and report treatment effects at the level of individual patients, rather than treatment-average effects, new methods are needed. The third section of this chapter provides an accessible introduction to these emerging methods.

In the next section, we describe treatment selection as practiced by mental health clinicians today. In doing so, we review the empirical support for the kinds of treatment selection decisions clinicians make every day.

Treatment Selection as Practiced by Clinicians Today

Most clinicians seek to move beyond the "one size fits all" approach and to prioritize the *person* sitting across the room. They realize the importance of recognizing differences in diagnostic presentations and the specific problems with which clients struggle, as well as the importance of the client's personality and other sociodemographic and cultural considerations. For example, a client with social anxiety may be struggling primarily with low self-esteem, poor social skills, a history of scarring social interactions, or a combination of these factors. A client also might present with a range of comorbid diagnoses, such as substance abuse problems or eating disorders, all of which might influence clinical decision making. Clinicians also frequently prioritize the problems the client most wants to address. For example, a depressed woman might want to focus on interpersonal issues or, alternatively, on how to make progress toward employment goals. Most clinicians also attend to features of the client's environment relevant to treatment. A young man who is homeless and estranged from his parents might require a different approach than would a father with three children who is stressed at work and in his marriage.

A clinician who attends to information about a specific client's presentation will generate hypotheses about the client's expected response to a given treatment (Lorenzo-Luaces, De Rubeis, & Bennett, 2015; Raza & Holohan, 2015). Here is an example from one of our intake reports in our training clinic (modified to protect the client's anonymity), which exemplifies such a line of reasoning:

> Given the client's difficulty with emotion tolerance and impulsivity, and in light of her history of self-injury and dissociation, the imaginal exposure interventions in prolonged exposure for posttraumatic stress disorder (PTSD) might prove especially difficult at this time. To minimize the risk of self-harm, it will be important to provide interventions that target emotion regulation and coping skills to help her engage productively, with a subsequent focus on imaginal exposure.

Such a conclusion may draw on a variety of sources, including a clinician's history with clients with similar features, his or her experiences in training and supervision, reasoning based on theory, and the empirical literature on treatment response (Cook, Dinnen, Simiola, Thompson, & Schnurr, 2014; Raza & Holohan, 2015). In fact, gathering and integrating such relevant information to inform recommendations about treatment are key tasks that clinicians do every day.

Unfortunately, the gap that has existed between clinical practice and clinical research has left clinicians with limited empirical guidance for this process. As a result, most clinicians (ourselves included) have tended to use an approach consistent with what Perlis (2016) has dubbed *artisanal medicine*.

Artisanal and Actuarial Medicine

Artisanal medicine refers to the practice of making treatment decisions in an idiosyncratic or unsystematic manner, or in a manner guided by theory and experience, but largely uninformed by the empirical evidence. Given the historical paucity of statistical approaches that could inform clinical decision making, artisanal approaches are typically the only option available for tailoring treatment to the individual.

Artisanal approaches are hobbled by several limitations that limit the validity and utility of such approaches for decision making (Dawes, 1979, 2005; Dawes, Faust, & Meehl, 1989; Perlis, 2016; Tversky & Kahneman, 1983). For example, when a clinician notes improvements in a patient's life, it is tempting to conclude that the improvement resulted from treatment, when it in fact could have been driven by factors in the patient's life unrelated to treatment. Hannan and colleagues (2005) examined clinicians' ability to predict their own clients' response to treatment and found that clinicians only predicted deterioration in .01% of their clients, in contrast to the 7.3% who actually deteriorated. Clinicians are also unreliable when assessing their own skills and outcomes: For example, when a large sample of mental health professionals were asked to compare their own clinical skills and performance to those of their peers, 25% indicated their skill was at the 90th percentile or higher, and none viewed themselves as being below average (Walfish, McAlister, O'Donnell, & Lambert, 2012). Clinicians also overestimated their clients' rates of improvement and underestimated their rates of deterioration (Walfish et al., 2012). A meta-analysis of 75 studies on clinician judgment accuracy revealed that clinicians with more experience or education were only modestly more accurate in their predictions compared to less experienced clinicians (Spengler et al., 2009). The factors, findings, and examples we described earlier do not mean that clinicians are especially bad at those kinds of judgments. It simply means they are human. The limitations of human judgment, which influence all of us, have been well described by Tversky and Kahneman (1974) and by Lilienfeld and colleagues (Lilienfeld, Ammirati, & David, 2012; Lilienfeld, Ammirati, & Landfield, 2009).

Actuarial decision making—defined as making predictions in a statistical, algorithmic, and reproducible way (Grove, Zald, Lebow, Snitz, & Nelson, 2000)—can overcome some of the difficulties inherent in human judgment (e.g., Dawes et al., 1989; Pauker & Kassirer, 1980). Research on this approach suggests that decision making via actuarial processes is more efficient than clinical judgment (Grove & Meehl, 1996). In practice, clinicians rarely are able to observe the counterfactuals that would be needed to assess the validity of their decisions. Consider the following example: If a clinician believes that a given client would be better off in psychodynamic therapy than in behavioral activation therapy, the clinician will likely attempt to ensure that the patient receives psychodynamic therapy. If the clinician is successful, then the only outcome that can be observed for that client is how he or she actually fares in psychodynamic therapy. The clinician does not have the opportunity to learn how the client *would have done* had he or she received behavioral activation; thus, the clinician is missing crucial information to evaluate the validity of his or her judgment. Given the complexity of each patient, it is unlikely that any one clinician has the opportunity to treat and observe the outcomes of enough similar patients to construct a valid decision rule. Of course, it is possible that some clinicians possess implicit models to guide treatment selection that produce better predictions than others; however, there have been few (if any) studies identifying and characterizing these individuals or their implicit models. Given the lack of data regarding clinicians who are "good" at treatment allocation, new clinicians cannot be trained in this important ability.

The case for using actuarial methods to personalize treatment in mental health was made forcefully over 60 years ago by Paul Meehl (1954). The field of mental health treatment has only just begun to apply Meehl's line of thinking. Some treatment selection decisions in clinics today do use features of actuarial decision making, in that they use measurable variables that have been the focus of empirical research. Clinicians who value evidence-based practice (EBP) can make treatment selection decisions guided by data regarding (1) diagnosis, (2) the client's treatment preferences, (3) the client's self-reported response to previous treatments, and (4) symptom severity. How good is the evidence base that guides such decisions? We answer this question in the following sections.

Using Diagnosis to Guide Treatment Selection

For much of the 20th century, scientific efforts focused on characterizing the core pathologies of the DSM-defined diagnostic categories and developing related treatments. This was the most relevant research available for a clinician who sought empirical guidance in tailoring treatment to the client sitting in front of him or her. Successes in these efforts included evidence for specific treatments for specific disorders (e.g., cognitive-behavioral therapy [CBT] for MDD [Beck, Rush, Shaw, & Emery, 1979]). These interventions have been evaluated in randomized clinical trials (RCTs; see Kraemer & Periyakoil, Chapter 4, this volume), in which active treatments have been compared to control conditions or to other active treatments. Based on findings from such studies, these treatments have been considered to be "empirically supported" for clients with the associated diagnosis (Chambless & Hollon, 1998). Similarly, specific classes of psychiatric drugs have been investigated under the assumption that they are best suited for specific disorders (Fineberg, Brown, Reghunandanan, & Pampaloni, 2012). Thus, clinicians were provided a resource for tailoring treatments by attending to the diagnostic status of the client.

It makes sense that treatment recommendations would follow from accurate diagnosis. For example, antibiotic treatment is appropriate for bacterial but not viral infection. The same is true in some mental health contexts. For example, CBT for bulimia nervosa has been shown to be superior to other forms of psychotherapy (Linardon, Wade, de la Piedad Garcia, & Brennan, 2017). Thus, a clinician working with a patient whose primary problem is bulimia nervosa has a clear first-line treatment recommendation. Similarly, when treating a patient with the diagnosis of bipolar disorder, clinical practice guidelines, based on substantial evidence, recommend mood stabilizers (e.g., lithium) or second-generation antipsychotics (Connolly & Thase, 2011). However, for many mental health diagnoses, especially depression, there exist an abundance of empirically supported treatments (ESTs) that have roughly similar efficacy. Thus, a depression diagnosis is not particularly informative for treatment selection. Moreover, many clients present with more than one disorder (Hirschfeld, 2001; Kessler, Chiu, Demler, & Walters, 2005; Kircanski, LeMoult, Ordaz, & Gotlib, 2017), requiring clinicians to use the artisanal approach to sequence and combine different ESTs for clients. In summary, for some conditions (e.g., bulimia nervosa, mania), a clear diagnosis guides a clear treatment recommendation. But for many other conditions and comorbidities, diagnosis often cannot point us toward a preferred treatment.

Using Client Preference to Guide Treatment Selection

EBP guidelines also specify the importance of attending to clients' preferences. This recommendation is based on not only respect for the client's autonomy and dignity but also an assumption that a treatment preferred by a client will outperform a nonpreferred treatment. Surprisingly, studies examining the relationship between client preference and treatment outcomes include findings that are positive (Kocsis et al., 2009; Mergl et al., 2011; Swift & Callahan, 2009; Swift, Callahan, & Vollmer, 2011), mixed (Dunlop et al., 2017; McHugh, Whitton, Peckham, Welge, & Otto, 2013; Preference Collaborative Review Group, 2008), and even negative (Dunlop et al., 2012, Leykin, DeRubeis, et al., 2007; Renjilian et al., 2001; Winter & Barber, 2013). One reason for this is that a patient in an RCT, by virtue of agreeing to randomization, is indicating that he or she does not have a *strong* preference for one treatment or another. Another reason is that a patient may not have a good sense of what to expect in a particular treatment, resulting in a relatively uninformed preference. More research is needed on patient preferences in typical clinical (nonrandomized) treatment contexts and on the value of providing patients with more information about treatment options prior to decision making. In summary, although respecting a patient's preference is an integral part of ethical clinical practice, its utility for guiding what will work best for an individual patient is unclear.

Using Previous Treatment Experience to Guide Treatment Selection

Numerous outcome studies have found that treatment history is associated with future response for pharmacological treatments. For example, prior exposure to and history of nonresponse to antidepressant medications (ADMs) have each been found consistently to predict poor outcome to future courses of antidepressants (Amsterdam, Lorenzo-Luaces, & DeRubeis, 2016; Amsterdam & Shults, 2009; Amsterdam et al., 2009; Byrne & Rothschild, 1998). Moreover, there is evidence that the number of prior ADM exposures predicts response differentially across ADM and cognitive therapy (CT): Leykin, Amsterdam, and colleagues (2007) found that multiple previous ADM-exposures predicted a poorer response to ADM, but not to CT, such that patients with two or more prior exposures to ADMs were more likely to benefit from CT than from ADM. Clearly, assessing pharmacological treatment history is important and could be used to inform treatment selection.

Very little research exists on the relationship between prior psychotherapy and future response to treatment (Boswell, McAleavey,

Castonguay, Hayes, & Locke, 2012). In addition to the difficulty of accurately assessing prior psychotherapy, this research is complicated by the correlation between factors that are independently associated with reduced likelihood of response to treatment (e.g., recurrent, chronic, and treatment-resistant forms of depression) and treatment history. Grenyer, Deane, and Lewis (2008) found no relationship between prior psychotherapy and response to supportive–expressive dynamic psychotherapy for depression. However, Boswell and colleagues (2012) found that prior psychotherapy (as well as prior psychotropic medication) were associated with decreased response to counseling. These findings stand in contrast to recent work by Blau and DiMino (2018), who found that college students with prior counseling experience had more favorable outcomes relative to never-counseled students. Additional research is needed in this area, with increased focus on assessing the type and dosage of prior psychotherapy, and on the distinction between prior positive response and prior exposure. At this point, the utility of this information for guiding what will work best for an individual patient is unclear.

Using Symptom Severity to Guide Treatment Selection

Many clinicians assign patients with less severe symptoms to less intensive treatments, and patients with more severe symptoms to more intensive treatments (Lorenzo-Luaces et al., 2015). There is evidence to support this practice. Active treatments (e.g., ADMs, CBT) have greater efficacy relative to control treatments (e.g., pill-placebo, psychological control treatment) at higher levels of pretreatment depression severity, indicating that more severely depressed patients need more intensive treatment (Barbui, Cipriani, Patel, Ayuso-Mateos, & van Ommeren, 2011; Driessen, Cuijpers, Hollon, & Dekker, 2010; Fournier et al., 2010; Khan, Leventhal, Khan, & Brown, 2002; Kirsch et al., 2008). Similarly, most practice guidelines use symptom severity as an indicator that stronger treatments or combination treatments (e.g., ADMs and psychotherapy) are preferred over lower-intensity interventions (American Psychiatric Association, 2010; National Institute for Health and Clinical Excellence, 2009). However, in comparisons of two active treatments of similar intensity levels for major depression, baseline severity does not moderate treatment outcomes (Vittengl et al., 2016; Weitz et al., 2015).

In contrast, a common view among clinicians who work with patients diagnosed with PTSD is that stronger treatments (e.g., trauma-focused CBTs such as prolonged exposure [PE] or cognitive processing therapy [CPT]) are contraindicated for more patients with more severe symptoms or more complex presentations. Consistent with this view, there is some evidence that the superiority of stronger over weaker treatments in PTSD is greater among patients whose presentations are less severe (Wiltsey Stirman et al., 2019). Many clinicians see complex patients as being "unready" to engage with more intensive interventions (Cook et al., 2014; Rosen et al., 2016). Empirical support for this belief, which is reinforced by practice guidelines, has been mixed (Cook, Simiola, Hamblen, Bernardy, & Schnurr, 2017; Osei-Bonsu et al., 2017). Thus, at the present moment, the literature does not provide a clear treatment recommendation for patients with PTSD with higher levels of symptom severity.

Relatedly, many clinicians assume that patients with higher symptom severity need medication and not psychotherapy (*www.webmd. com/depression/guide/understanding-depression-treatment#3*), a belief that is reinforced by some practice guidelines (*http://psychiatry-online.org/pb/assets/raw/sitewide/practice_ guidelines/guidelines/mdd.pdf*). Studies, reviews, and meta-analyses have not supported such assumptions belief: Psychotherapy and ADMs are equally effective across the range of baseline severity (DeRubeis et al., 2005; Furukawa et al., 2017; Simon & Perlis, 2010; Weitz et al., 2015), at least in outpatient contexts.

Summary

The existing evidence does not provide a clear guide for clinicians who value EBP. Data are available to support the use of diagnosis, client preference, treatment history, and symptom severity for some clients but not for others. For this reason, the field has moved to focus more heavily on multivariable approaches to treatment selection.

Interpreting Results of Treatment Selection Research

In this section, we provide an overview of treatment selection methodology, with an eye toward helping the reader interpret findings reported in the treatment selection literature. We first describe the difference between prescriptive and prognostic variables, then discuss the interpretation of treatment selection research results.

Prescriptive and Prognostic Variables

Treatment selection approaches largely[1] rely upon variables that can be measured prior to treatment and that predict treatment outcomes reliably. Such variables can be considered as either prescriptive or prognostic. *Prescriptive variables* indicate which treatment is better for a patient, among several treatment options. Prescriptive variables have often been referred to as *moderators* in the research literature. They affect the direction or strength of the differences in outcome between two or more treatments (Baron & Kenny, 1986). For example, Fournier and colleagues (2008) found that the presence of a comorbid personality disorder among depressed patients predicted better response to ADM relative to CT, while the absence of a personality disorder predicted a better response to CT than to ADM.

A variable is *prognostic* if it predicts response regardless of which treatment is delivered. For example, higher baseline depression severity is a prognostic variable: It is associated with worse outcomes, for both medications and CT (Weitz et al., 2015). Prognostic information can be used to provide realistic expectations to the treating clinician, as well as the client and family, regardless of the treatment chosen. Additionally, prognostic variables can identify patients who are unlikely to respond, and such patients can be monitored more closely (Lutz et al., 2014). Prognostic variables do not provide the kind of information that is needed to optimize the choice between two or more treatment options, as they indicate the responsiveness of the patient to treatment in general.

Whether a variable is prognostic or prescriptive can depend on the context of treatment options being considered. For example, baseline depression severity predicts outcomes similarly for CT and medication treatments (Weitz et al., 2015), making it *prognostic* in this context. However, higher baseline severity predicts a larger advantage of medication over placebo

and of psychotherapy over nondirective supportive counseling, making baseline severity *prescriptive* in these contexts (Ashar, Chang, & Wager, 2017; Driessen et al., 2010; Fournier et al., 2010).

Interpreting Prognostic Variables

A common misinterpretation of a prognostic finding is to infer that clients found to have a poor prognosis in a given treatment will fare better with a different treatment (Simon & Perlis, 2010). For example, consider the finding that in CT, patients with chronic depression have lower recovery rates than those with nonchronic depression (Fournier et al., 2009). One might be tempted to conclude that other interventions such as ADM treatment or psychological treatments specifically targeting chronic depression (e.g., CBASP; McCullough, 2003) should be preferred to CT for individuals with chronic depression. Alternatively, it could be that CT is as effective as other available treatments for chronic depression (Cuijpers, Huibers, & Furukawa, 2017). This alternative hypothesis is supported by an RCT that compared CT to ADM and found that chronicity was *prognostic*: It was associated with similarly lower response rates in both treatments (Fournier et al., 2009). Likewise, an RCT comparing CBASP to ADM in individuals with chronic depressions found no difference in response rates (Nemeroff et al., 2003). Thus, prognostic findings do not necessarily provide good information on which to base a preference between two or more evidence-based treatments.[2]

Interpreting Prescriptive Variables

Prescriptive variables can be difficult to interpret correctly. In this section, we focus on single prescriptive variables, often called *moderators,* which have been the main focus of research to date. Moderator research has been attractive in part because of the relative simplicity of research designs and statistical analyses when

---

[1] Some proposed treatment selection approaches rely on "early response" indicators. These approaches cannot answer the question about which treatment to recommend at the initiation of treatment and thus are beyond the focus of this chapter.

[2] Two prognostic models validated within the same sample could be used together to make treatment recommendations for an individual. For example, one model would predict response to treatment *A,* the other model would predict response to treatment *B,* and the two predictions would be compared to select a treatment. This approach was proposed by Kessler and colleagues (2017) and adapted by Deisenhofer and colleagues (2018) for the purpose of guiding treatment decisions in PTSD.

analyzing a single variable. However, making sense of findings from such studies and applying results to clinical practice is often not straightforward.

Consider the following scenario. A clinician is presented with a depressed patient and must choose between CBT or ADM treatment. The clinician finds a paper that concludes that "clients with a greater number of prior ADM exposures fare worse in ADM treatment." Should the clinician use this finding to select a treatment for the patient?

In fact, this simple description of the research finding is insufficient to inform a decision, since it is consistent with several different patterns of relationship between prior ADM exposures and treatment outcomes. We depict six hypothetical relationships in Figure 7.1. Critically, without knowing which of these six is the true relationship, a treatment recommendation cannot be made.

If the data are as depicted in Figure 7.1a, the clinician should prescribe ADMs only if the client has had 0 or 1 prior ADM exposures. If data are as depicted in Figure 7.1b, the clinician should opt for CT for all patients except those with no prior ADM exposures, for whom no difference is predicted between CT and ADM. If the data are as depicted in Figure 7.1f, either CT or ADM is indicated because clients with prior ADM exposures fare worse in both treatments. In fact, the findings on which the statement is based is depicted in Figure 7.1e (Leykin, Amsterdam, et al., 2007).

This example illustrates one of the many ways in which the same statement—"clients with a greater number of prior ADM exposures fared worse in ADM treatment"—can refer to importantly different patterns, which is why such statements by themselves are insufficiently detailed to inform treatment selection decisions.

In empirical reports, the distinctions are rarely made between the different types of prescriptive relationships depicted in Figure 7.1. When the details of these relations are only implied rather than precisely stated, they lead to inconsistent, misleading, or simply incorrect interpretations. We offer this as a warning to readers wading into the treatment moderator literature.

The Source of the Data

In addition to paying careful attention to the specific results, it is critical to consider the source of the data. To date, most prediction have utilized data from randomized trials. This has inherent limitations when attempting to generalize to the typical (nonrandomized) treatment context. Future efforts, exemplified by the ongoing work of Gillan and Daw (2016) to collect mental health treatment outcome data online also incorporate naturalistic (nonrandomized) data (Kessler, 2018), such as large treatment databases that can be generated from electronic medical records (EMR; Perlis et al., 2012). However, the potential influence of unknown confounds (i.e., third variable problems) is a limitation of treatment selection efforts outside the context of RCT data. The bias in predictions in such studies can derive from the "selection effects" that result when clients with a given feature (e.g., history of nonresponse to ADMs) are preferentially provided a given treatment (e.g., CT). A full discussion of the potential risks of using nonrandomized data is beyond the scope of this review, but a recent analysis by Agniel, Kohane, and Weber (2018) highlights the complexity of such efforts. The authors reviewed hospital EMR data from more than 600,000 patients on 272 common laboratory tests and found that for 68% of the tests, the *timing* of when the labs were ordered were more predictive of patient survival than the results of the tests. Despite these obstacles, the promise of EMR or electronic health record (EHR) data is compelling; Simon and colleagues (2018) used demographic and clinical EHR data from 3 million patients seen in primary care and mental health specialty clinics to develop a 90-day suicide risk index. Their model relied on information about prior suicide attempts, mental health and substance use diagnoses, responses to the suicide question from a commonly used depression questionnaire, and prior inpatient or emergency mental health treatment. Individuals in the top 5% of their risk index accounted for almost half of all subsequent suicide attempts and deaths by suicide. Predictive tools of this kind have great promise in helping to inform and improve clinical decision making.

Another key issue in interpreting findings rests with characteristics of the research sample and research treatment. It is risky to generalize research findings to a population outside the one from which the research sample was drawn. For example, findings regarding one treatment may not hold for a treatment believed to be similar, as evidenced by many reports that sets of variables and models found to predict treatment response to one ADM have failed to generalize to a different ADM (Chekroud et al., 2016; Ini-

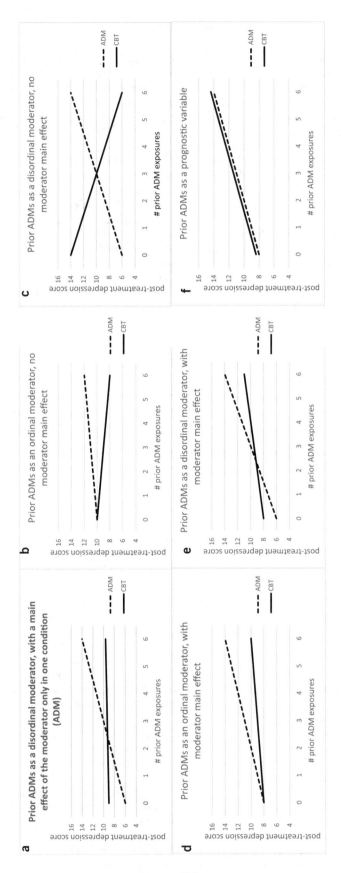

FIGURE 7.1. Six hypothetical relationships that could support the finding "clients with a greater number of prior ADM (antidepressant) exposures fared worse in ADM treatment." The dashed line represents expected posttreatment depression score in ADM, and the solid line represents expected outcome in cognitive-behavioral therapy (CBT).

esta et al., 2018; Iniesta, Malki, et al., 2016; Perlis, Fijal, Dharia, Heinloth, & Houston, 2010). Clinicians seeking to apply research findings must consider to what extent they can have confidence that (1) the client in front of them comes from the same population as that in which the research was conducted and (2) the treatment being considered is similar to the treatment delivered in the study.

Finally, a finding is only a finding until it is replicated. Statistical relationships reported from a lone research investigation should be used with great caution. This is especially true of findings in the prediction literature (relative to, for example, findings from experimental manipulations), as these often arise from exploratory analyses that are at higher risk for false positives.

Statistical and Clinical Significance

Reliance on tests of significance can result in misleading impressions about the importance of predictive variables (Nuzzo, 2014; Wasserstein & Lazar, 2016). This can happen in at least two ways. First, statistical significance testing typically applies arbitrary thresholds (e.g., $p < .05$) to determine which variables matter. However, the difference in the predictive utility of an excluded variable that "just missed" the threshold (e.g., $p = .06$) and one that is "barely" significant (e.g., $p = .04$) is trivial (Mickey & Greenland, 1989). As Rosnow and Rosenthal (1989, p. 1277) noted: "Dichotomous significance testing has no ontological basis. . . . Surely, God loves the .06 nearly as much as the .05." Further complicating the matter is that most clinical trials do not have sufficient statistical power to detect moderators at conventional statistical thresholds (i.e., $p < .05$), such that moderators will not be detected unless they are unusually strong.

Second, statistically significant results should be interpreted in context of their clinical significance. In large sample sizes, statistically significant results associated with small effect sizes can be of negligible clinical significance (Lo, Chernoff, Zheng, & Lo, 2015; Meehl, 1978). If a variable predicts a difference of 0.2 points on an anxiety scale with treatment A instead of B, does this really matter?[3] Janes, Pepe,

Bossuyt, and Barlow (2011) proposed a series of questions, none of which invoke statistical significance, to use when evaluating treatment selection markers:

1. Does the marker help patients choose amongst treatment options?
2. If the marker is measured as a continuous variable, how should information from it be used to inform treatment decisions?
3. What is the expected impact on the population of using the marker to select treatment?
4. For what proportion of patients is a change in the treatment recommendation likely if the marker is measured and patients' values on it are used in decision making?

Moving beyond statistics, consideration of factors such as cost, feasibility, and client burden should be weighed against the additive predictive power provided by variables that must be collected specially for treatment selection (Perlis, Patrick, Smoller, & Wang, 2009).

Furthermore, outcomes for evaluating the benefits of data-informed treatment selection should include more than reductions in the scores obtained on disorder-specific symptom questionnaires, although the vast majority of treatment selection models have been constructed using only such data (cf. Wallace, Frank, & Kraemer, 2013). Outcome indices that combine symptom change with measures of side effects, social and occupational functioning, and quality of life will support a more informative, holistic approach to treatment selection (Kraemer & Frank, 2010).

Multivariate Models for Treatment Selection

Development of the Personalized Advantage Index

The vast majority of research on the prediction of treatment response in mental health has focused on the role of one predictor, considered in isolation. This is understandable: If a single predictive variable associated with clinically meaningful differences can be identified in a treatment context, application to practice is likely to be straightforward (despite all the caveats and cautions we have described). Moreover, if a single variable can account for how well one treatment will perform relative to another for any given individual, it is likely that the variable reflects an important mechanism of one or both treatments. However, as we discuss

---

[3] Although small effects may not be clinically significant on the individual level, they can often have meaningful impacts when considered at the population level.

in more detail later in the chapter, this "univariate" approach has largely failed to generate powerful predictions and has therefore had little impact on mental health practice (Simon & Perlis, 2010). This has led researchers to pivot to multivariate predictive approaches in recent years (Cohen & DeRubeis, 2018). Multivariate models integrate information from *multiple* predictors jointly (e.g., age, severity, employment status, social support) to generate a treatment recommendation. Multivariable models are likely to yield more powerful predictions (Chekroud et al., 2016; Delgadillo, Huey, Bennett, & McMillan, 2017; Iniesta, Malki, et al., 2016; Koutsouleris et al., 2016; Kraemer, 2013; Perlis, 2013), and they comport with our understanding of psychopathology and treatment response as complex, multiply determined phenomena (Drysdale et al., 2017).

We began to explore the possibility that multivariable linear modeling or machine learning[4] (Iniesta, Stahl, & McGuffin, 2016; Passos, Mwangi, & Kapczinski, 2016) approaches could be brought to bear on precision medicine problems in mental health in 2011. This quest was initiated with a specific goal in mind: to find or develop an approach that could identify clients with MDD for whom ADMs are likely to be more beneficial than CT, and vice versa. Two of our own findings prompted this interest. First, in a sample of clients with moderate to severe MDD, ADM and CT had produced nearly identical group-average effects on depressive symptoms over the course of a 16-week RCT (DeRubeis et al., 2005). Second, five variables (marital status, employment status, personality disorder [PD] comorbidity, antidepressant treatment history, and the number of recent stressful life events) had been identified that independently served as moderators of symptom change in this sample (Fournier et al., 2009). However, none of these five variables were powerful enough to separate those for whom one of the treatments was likely to produce greater symptom change relative to the other (Fournier et al., 2009).

Moreover, the five variables were relatively uncorrelated with each other, suggesting that they reflected different dimensions of treatment response. The variables acted like vectors, such that a patient's value on one variable could point to a slight advantage for ADM, while his or her value on another variable might point in the direction of CT. For example, as noted earlier, clients who were unemployed improved more in CT than in ADM (Fournier et al., 2009). It was also the case that clients with comorbid PD improved more with ADM than they did in CT, whereas clients without comorbid PD improved more in CT than in ADM (Fournier et al., 2008). But what recommendation should be made for a client with comorbid PD (indicating ADM) who was unemployed (indicating CT)? How does the clinician integrate this conflicting information along with the other three variables when forming a treatment recommendation? Multivariable models are needed to recommend a treatment in such situations.

Another important concept was that effective guidance for clinicians and clients would be unlikely to be best described in binary terms. Instead, for some clients, the difference in outcome between treatments might be quite substantial, while for others it would be negligible, and for still others in between. To address these challenges, DeRubeis, Cohen, and colleagues (2014) developed the personalized advantage index (PAI) approach, which has been the foundation for recent efforts by several different research teams (Cohen, Kim, Van, Dekker, & Driessen, 2019; Deisenhofer et al., 2018; Huibers et al., 2015; Keefe et al., 2018; Vittengl, Clark, Thase, & Jarrett, 2017; Webb et al., 2018; Zilcha-Mano et al., 2016).

The PAI approach to treatment selection involves the generation of a prediction of the expected differential benefit (in graded terms) of one intervention over one or more alternative treatment options. This begins with the identification of pretreatment variables in a dataset that predict differential response to two or more treatments. Once these predictors (moderators) are identified, a multivariable statistical model is constructed, comprising main effects of predictors as well as interaction terms representing the prescriptive variables' interaction with treatment.[5] An individual's PAI derives from the difference between his or her predicted out-

---

[4] "Machine-learning (essentially synonymous with 'data-mining' or 'statistical learning') refers to a class of approaches that focus on prediction rather than interpretation or mechanism" (Gillan & Whelan, 2017, p. 35).

[5] Some of the machine-learning models we have constructed do not include interaction terms per se, but they perform the same task of modeling differential response. For examples of this approach, see Deisenhofer and colleagues (2018) or Schweizer and colleagues (2019).

comes in two treatments (TxA and TxB). The sign of the difference indicates which of the two treatments is expected to be preferred for that patient. The magnitude of the difference reflects the magnitude of the predicted advantage of the indicated treatment over the nonindicated treatment. If a PAI is large, one might strongly advise a client to pursue a specific treatment. However, if the predicted advantage is small (e.g., a PAI close to zero), then one's recommendation might be more tempered (Cohen & DeRubeis, 2018).

We also have extended our use of the PAI to characterize and utilize patient subtypes in treatment selection decision processes. Some patients do equally well or equally poorly in all treatments, while for others, the particular treatment matters. The prototype clients (adapted from Cohen & DeRubeis, 2018; DeRubeis, Gelfand, German, Fournier, & Forand, 2014) described in Figure 7.2 aim to help in better understanding the types of clients for whom treatment selection might be relevant. For easy patients, any level of active treatment (from the highest to lowest strength) would result in high levels of improvement. For the challenging patients at the other end of the spectrum, little to no improvement would be expected at any but the highest level of therapy strength. *Pliant patients* are defined as those whose improvement would vary as a function of therapy quality, such that with very poor quality therapy or no therapy, little to no improvement would be expected, and with the highest quality therapy possible, significant improvement would result. The pliant patient category may be broken down further into two subgroups: individuals who would improve if they received quality treatment of any type versus other individuals who would improve only if "matched" to the specific treatment they receive (see Figure 7.2, types 2 and 2a/2b). These latter individu-

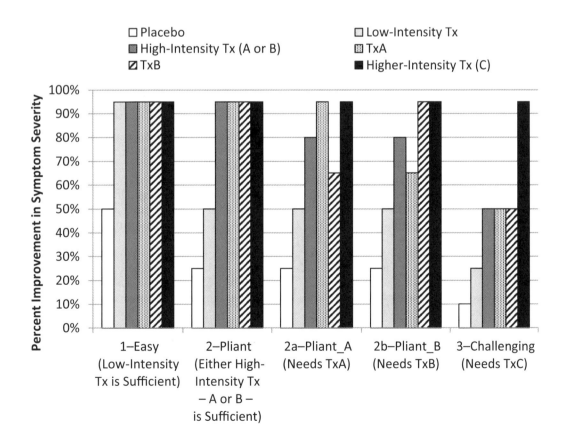

FIGURE 7.2. Depiction of expected improvement for five patient prototypes in different treatment contexts. *Note.* Tx, treatment.

als (type 2a/2b), who respond well but only to a *specific* treatment, are the individuals for whom treatment selection will be most important.

This insight can be leveraged in a stratified care context. Patients who respond equally well or equally poorly to all treatments could be given the cheapest/safest treatment. However, ethical considerations arise in prescribing a weak treatment to a severely ill patient, simply because the patient is statistically unlikely to respond to a stronger treatment. On the other hand, "pliant" patients could be matched to the treatment of appropriate strength/cost/risk.

Lorenzo-Luaces, DeRubeis, van Straten, and Tiemens (2017) implemented such an approach as a proof of concept, with data from a randomized comparison of a high-intensity treatment (CT) with low-intensity treatment (brief therapy [BT]) and treatment as usual (TAU). On average, the differences between the high-intensity treatment and each of the two comparison conditions were small (van Straten, Tiemens, Hakkaart, Nolen, & Donker, 2006). The reasonable interpretation given by the authors was that high-intensity treatment was no more effective in this population than low-intensity treatment (van Straten et al., 2006). However, when Lorenzo-Luaces and colleagues fit a multivariable model that arrayed patients from those with the poorest to the best prognoses, those with poor prognoses evidenced significantly higher rates of recovery in CT (60%) than in BT (44%) or TAU (39%). In contrast, patients with model-predicted better prognoses evidenced nearly identical recovery rates across the three treatments. These findings represent an example of how treatment selection principles may be applied in stratified medicine in a way that might increase substantially the efficiency of mental health treatment systems.

The approach used to construct PAI models described earlier can be adapted to inform stratified medicine decisions for stepped care, where the choice is often between a high- versus low-intensity treatment. When the high-intensity treatment is more effective, on average, the goal is usually to differentiate between individuals who are likely to benefit much more from the high-intensity treatment than the low-intensity treatment and individuals for whom the expected differential benefit is small. In this case, patients can be arrayed along a continuum, at one end of which are patients who would be expected to evidence a poor response to a weak treatment, but who might benefit sub-stantially from a strong treatment, especially if it is one that is suited to them. At the other end of the continuum are patients who are predicted to experience a positive response irrespective of the quality of the treatment. These are patients for whom a minimal treatment is expected to produce as much or nearly as much benefit as a strong, intensive treatment.

Other Multivariable Prescriptive Approaches

Other approaches to multivariate modeling also have been proposed in the mental health context. Barber and Muenz's (1996) reanalysis of data from the Treatment of Depression Collaborative Research Program (TDCRP; Elkin et al., 1989) provided one of the earliest examples of multivariable prediction of treatment response in mental health. Using data from the comparison of CT to interpersonal psychotherapy (IPT) for MDD, the authors built a "matching factor" that combined the prescriptive value of several moderators (marital status, avoidance, obsessiveness, and baseline severity) in a linear regression model predicting symptom change. The authors also explored the prescriptive value of two PD diagnoses, avoidant PD and obsessive–compulsive PD, and proposed that models including these factors could be used to match patients to CT or IPT.

Since this early work, many different analytic approaches have been taken to develop multivariate models. Drawing on a novel statistical technique, Lutz and colleagues (2006) used the "nearest neighbor" modeling approach to predict differential outcomes between two variations of CBT. This approach was adapted from methods used to predict avalanches in the Swiss Alps. Each client's outcome in each treatment is predicted from the outcomes of a group of clients who are most similar to the index client, and who have undergone either of the treatments. Here, similarity is defined by calculating the Euclidean distance between two clients' values on a vector of factors (i.e., the square root of the sum of the squared differences in values for each of the standardized variables). Within this group of "neighbors," the average outcome in each of the two interventions is calculated. These averages are considered the best predictions of outcome for the index client in each of the two treatments.

Kraemer (2013) proposed a statistical approach to treatment selection that involves the creation of a single variable (termed M^*, and most often referred to as *M Star*) that represents a weighted combination of multiple moderators. Using data from a randomized comparison of IPT versus the antidepressant escitalopram, Wallace and colleagues (2013) demonstrated the approach, creating a combined moderator that comprised eight predictors: baseline depression severity, psychomotor activation, medical reassurance, number of depressive episodes, age, gender, anxiety, employment status. Recently, other groups have used the M^* approach to analyze studies of treatment-resistant late-life depression (Smagula et al., 2016) and anxiety disorders (Niles, Loerinc, et al., 2017; Niles, Wolitzky-Taylor, Arch, & Craske, 2017).

The evolution from single- to multivariable treatment selection is also exemplified by a series of papers by Iniesta, Uher, and colleagues (Iniesta, Malki, et al., 2016; Iniesta et al., 2018; Uher et al., 2012). The authors used data from the Genome-based Therapeutic Drugs for Depression (GENDEP) study (Uher et al., 2009), in which participants were randomized to either a tricyclic antidepressant or a serotonin selective reuptake inhibitor. Initially, they tested the prognostic and prescriptive utility of each of nine variables is isolation (six symptom dimensions and three symptom cluster factors derived from those symptoms), and only found evidence for the anxiety symptom dimension as a moderator of antidepressant response (Uher et al., 2012). Recognizing the limitations of the single-variable approach, they then explored an expanded set of potential variables using a multivariable approach (Iniesta, Malki, et al., 2016). They found that models simultaneously including the effects of multiple variables predicted differential response to antidepressants with clinically meaningful accuracy, thus demonstrating the potential of multivariable approaches for treatment selection. Recently, they reanalyzed the GENDEP sample and combined genetic data with clinical and demographic variables to create drug-specific predictive models for antidepressant response that they validated in a held-out test sample (Iniesta et al., 2018).

Finally, other groups have used variants of the methods already described to address treatment selection questions (Cloitre, Petkova, Su, & Weiss, 2016; Westover et al., 2015). A recent review by Cohen and DeRubeis (2018) described over two dozen recent treatment selection efforts and revealed significant methodological heterogeneity, which can contribute to difficulties in detecting consistencies and inconsistencies in predictors, and creates a barrier to identifying "best practices" (Doove, Dusseldorp, Van Deun, & Van Mechelen, 2014).

Selection between Treatments Differing in Costs, Harms, and Other Dimensions

Treatments differ in terms of strength, cost, availability, and risk. While we have focused primarily on efficacy, it is but one consideration for treatment selection. Many health care systems follow a form of stratified care, the goal of which is to make best use of scarce treatment resources by organizing treatment options hierarchically. Briefer and less costly treatments are accessed first by many clients, so that more intensive options are available for those who are deemed to need them (Bower & Gilbody, 2005). Here, the more relevant question might be "What is the best way to allocate the stronger/costlier/less available/riskier (hereafter 'stronger') treatment?" Predictive modeling in a stratified care context should aim to enhance the efficient allocation of limited or costly resources, as well as to minimize patients' unnecessary exposure to treatments that require significant time commitments or are associated with increased side effect risk (Hingorani et al., 2013).

There are two ways in which the "stronger" treatments might produce superior group average change. One possibility is that individuals may vary in regard to the degree to which they benefit more from the stronger treatment versus the weaker one. In such cases, the identification of client characteristics that predict differential response between the stronger and the weaker interventions is of paramount importance. Alternatively, all clients might be expected to benefit more from the stronger treatment, and by similar amounts. In such cases, although allocation to the stronger treatment could not be based on differences in expected improvement, it could depend on prognosis in the weaker treatment. For example, the stronger treatment could be allocated to those with the worst prognoses in the weaker treatment. This would fit well within a stepped care model, based on the idea that those predicted to fare poorly in the weaker treatment would, eventually, be more likely to be given the stronger treatment as the next step.

Recently published efforts that use data from the National Health Service (NHS) Improving

Access to Psychological Therapy (IAPT) program highlight ways in which multivariable models may be used to guide stratified medicine in mental health. IAPT follows a hybrid stepped care/stratified care model, in which the majority of clients start with lower-intensity psychological interventions, and those who do not respond are stepped-up to higher intensity psychotherapy. Saunders, Cape, Fearon, and Pilling (2016) used latent profile analysis to create eight profiles that defined patient clusters, each of which described sets of baseline demographic data and symptom features that tended to co-occur. They successfully identified subsets of clients (those with profiles similar to each other) for whom outcomes were different in high-intensity treatment versus low-intensity psychological treatment. This model could be used to identify patients to send directly to the more intensive care, rather than having all patients start with the low-intensity treatment option. In a different sample, Delgadillo, Moreea, and Lutz (2016) created an index that generated predictions as to which clients were likely to achieve reliable and clinically significant reductions in depression or anxiety symptoms. Follow-up work using an index of case complexity yielded similar results in a separate sample of IAPT patients (Delgadillo et al., 2017). This case complexity index aimed to create treatment selection recommendations that clinicians can readily understand and interpret, and its utility is currently being tested in a clinical trial.

A relevant consideration in stepped care contexts is whether treatment selection decisions optimize patient outcomes, the efficient allocation of clinic resources, or a combination of these two concerns. A more intensive treatment might provide only marginal benefit for a patient, but at a high cost. From a population or clinic perspective, treatment selection decisions should weigh expected patient improvement versus expected cost. For example, a 5-point improvement may be worth a marginal cost of $5,000, but not $50,000.

Some work has examined the integration of expected harms into treatment selection decisions. For example, Kraemer and colleagues asked hypothetical patients to choose between profiles of expected improvements and side effects of two different drugs (Kraemer & Frank, 2010; Kraemer, Frank, & Kupfer, 2011). They were then able to quantify how patients valued the harms–benefit trade-off. Is 5 points of expected benefit worth twice as many side effects,

or a 40% increased likelihood of a serious adverse event? Ultimately, this might be a personal decision for each patient. Information about patient harms must be presented to patients in informing treatment decisions.

In an analogous manner, a CT clinic that aims to increase its rate of success could use the findings from a prognostic study to inform the selection of patients for the clinic by taking preferentially those patients with good scores on a prognostic index. *But* the practical prediction question, from the patient's point of view, parallels the "placement" issue: "Which treatment is best for me?"

Future Directions

Evidence-based treatment selection in mental health today lags far behind where we need it to be. Few clinics or clinicians employ treatment selection algorithms, and few treatment selections algorithms have been robustly supported by multiple independent studies in independent samples. Clinicians need to be confident integrating these data and such approaches into their daily work. One conclusion from research to date is that single-variable models are unlikely to be valuable sources of information for strong recommendations about treatment selection for individual patients. Multivariable models represent a promising new direction, as we have argued, though validation studies are needed to establish the utility of emerging multivariable models.

Moreover, the pretreatment assessments that inform the treatment selection models of tomorrow will likely include biomarkers and other measures that promise to reveal prescriptive relationships, in addition to the self-report, environmental, demographic, and clinical variables that have been used in most treatment selection studies reported to date. Recent work has shown promise for neurobiological (Gabrieli, Ghosh, & Whitfield-Gabrieli, 2015; Jollans & Whelan, 2016; Pizzagalli, 2011; Stephan et al., 2017), and neurocognitive and behavioral variables (Webb et al., 2018), as well as measures of immune function (Uher et al., 2014). Several recent studies have been designed specifically to generate knowledge relevant to outcome prediction in depression treatment (Dunlop et al., 2012; Green et al., 2017; Grieve et al., 2013; Lam et al., 2016; Trivedi et al., 2016; Williams, 2017). They feature potential biomarkers, including information from neuroimaging (McGrath et al., 2013; Pizzagalli et al., 2018) and genetic tests (Iniesta et al., 2018; Lam et al., 2016; Ward et al., 2018).

Research aiming to identify biological predictors of mental health outcomes is still in its infancy. Although many promising findings have been reported (Drysdale et al., 2017), very few of these have been replicated in independent samples (Woo, Chang, Lindquist, & Wager, 2017). Additionally, biological measures can be costly and difficult to collect in routine clinical settings. As our understanding and awareness of these variables increases, it will be important to demonstrate the added value of more expensive predictors, or to link them to more easily assessible variables that can serve as "proxies" until such times as the cost of measurement decreases.

Moreover, for treatment selection to be effective, clinicians and clients must have available different treatment options from which to choose. For example, treatment selection at the level of intervention "packages" (i.e., ADM vs. CBT vs. IPT) would not be useful in some rural locations where evidence-based psychotherapy is unavailable, and the majority of mental health treatment is delivered by family medicine doctors who prescribe antidepressants. Similarly, a psychotherapist who is trained only to provide CBT might not be open to a recommendation that his or her client would be better suited for IPT. In the United States, the Veterans Administration health care system is an excellent candidate for treatment selection, as it has established an infrastructure for training and delivery of a variety of evidence-based treatments for PTSD, including CPT, PE, PCT, and eye movement desensitization and reprocessing (EMDR).

Another context ripe for treatment selection is the NHS IAPT system in the United Kingdom, which treats over 560,000 patients per year, collects a standard set of baseline predictive variables, and offers different forms of psychotherapy at different levels of intensity (Clark, 2018). Both stratified medicine (determining for whom low-intensity treatment is sufficient and who should begin with high-intensity treatment) and treatment selection between equivalent treatments (selecting which psychotherapy among a set of equally effective interventions would be best for an individual) would be possible within IAPT. We are currently running a prediction tournament in which 13 teams have been given a large sample of anonymized patient data that include the set of universally collected baseline variables and treatment outcomes. If the models that are developed prove useful, they could be instantiated in IAPT clinics across the United Kingdom and could provide individualized outcome predictions that could be used by clinicians and clients in a shared decision-making process to improve the way in which treatments are allocated. The potential impact that treatment selection could have at this scale should not be underestimated. If model-informed treatment allocation could improve IAPT's current 50% recovery rate by even 5%, it could result in 28,000 more individuals recovering each year.

Conclusions

Moving beyond "one size fits all" (the title of this chapter) has been a goal of both clinicians and researchers for many decades. Recognizing that unique individuals will respond differently to treatment, clinicians have long attempted to personalize or adapt treatments to their clients. Recent successes in precision medicine in other areas have inspired new research efforts in clinical psychology.

Although we have not yet addressed with confidence the question that Paul asked so many decades ago—what works for whom?— we are getting closer to a time when research will inform the questions that clinicians and clients are asking. We have recognized that efforts to guide treatment selection based on a single feature of the client are misguided. Despite the appealing simplicity of such studies, they have had limited impact on client care (Simon & Perlis, 2010). There is great value for clinicians in knowing when and why to be skeptical of the research literature, and simple single-variable prediction results should invite such caution. Similarly, many of the more complex multivariate approaches used today are limited by the exploratory nature of the models. Again, clinicians and clients are wise to demand that this work continue, so that promising findings are put to the test of validation and replication. Despite these cautions, the PAI and many of the other multivariable treatment selection approaches we have reviewed are on the cutting edge of efforts to integrate science and practice.

This knowledge matters. Clinicians want to provide individuals struggling with mental health problems with treatments that work. Reducing the number of ineffective treatments to which individuals are exposed will reduce their suffering and will benefit communities through reducing the loss of work productivity associated with mental illness (Layard, Clark, Knapp, & Mayraz, 2007). We all will benefit from an improved understanding of what will work for whom.

References

Agniel, D., Kohane, I. S., & Weber, G. M. (2018). Biases in electronic health record data due to processes within the healthcare system: Retrospective observational study. *British Medical Journal, 361*, k1479.

American Psychiatric Association. (2010). *Practice guideline for the treatment of patients with major depressive disorder.* Arlington, VA: Author.

American Psychological Association. (2006). Evidence-based practice in psychology: APA presidential task force on evidence-based practice. *American Psychologist, 61*(4), 271–285.

Amsterdam, J. D., Lorenzo-Luaces, L., & DeRubeis, R. J. (2016). Step-wise loss of antidepressant effectiveness with repeated antidepressant trials in bipolar II depression. *Bipolar Disorders, 18*, 563–570.

Amsterdam, J. D., & Shults, J. (2009). Does tachyphylaxis occur after repeated antidepressant exposure in patients with bipolar II major depressive episode? *Journal of Affective Disorders, 115*, 234–240.

Amsterdam, J. D., Williams, D., Michelson, D., Adler, L. A., Dunner, D. L., et al. (2009). Tachyphylaxis after repeated antidepressant drug exposure in patients with recurrent major depressive disorder. *Neuropsychobiology, 59*, 227–233.

Ashar, Y. K., Chang, L. J., & Wager, T. D. (2017). Brain mechanisms of the placebo effect: An affective appraisal account. *Annual Review of Clinical Psychology, 13*, 73–98.

Ashley, E. A. (2016). Towards precision medicine. *Nature Reviews Genetics, 17*, 507–522.

Barber, J. P., & Muenz, L. R. (1996). The role of avoidance and obsessiveness in matching patients to cognitive and interpersonal psychotherapy: Empirical findings from the Treatment for Depression Collaborative Research Program. *Journal of Consulting and Clinical Psychology, 64*, 951–958.

Barbui, C., Cipriani, A., Patel, V., Ayuso-Mateos, J. L., & van Ommeren, M. (2011). Efficacy of antidepressants and benzodiazepines in minor depression: Systematic review and meta-analysis. *British Journal of Psychiatry, 198*, 11–16.

Baron, R. M., & Kenny, D. A. (1986). The moderator–mediator variable distinction in social psychological research: Conceptual, strategic, and statistical considerations. *Journal of Personality and Social Psychology, 51*, 1173–1182.

Beck, A. T., Rush, A. J., Shaw, B. F., & Emery, G. (1979). *Cognitive therapy of depression.* New York: Guilford Press

Blau, G., & DiMino, J. (2018). Impact of brief counseling on nonurgent prior- versus never-counseled samples. *Journal of College Student Psychotherapy.* [Epub ahead of print]

Boswell, J. F., McAleavey, A. A., Castonguay, L. G., Hayes, J. A., & Locke, B. D. (2012). Previous mental health service utilization and change in clients' depressive symptoms. *Journal of Counseling Psychology, 59*, 368–378.

Bower, P., & Gilbody, S. (2005). Stepped care in psychological therapies: Access, effectiveness and efficiency. *British Journal of Psychiatry, 186*, 11–17.

Byrne, S. E., & Rothschild, A. J. (1998). Loss of antidepressant efficacy during maintenance therapy: Possible mechanisms and treatments. *Journal of Clinical Psychiatry, 59*, 279–288.

Chambless, D. L., & Hollon, S. D. (1998). Defining empirically supported therapies. *Journal of Consulting and Clinical Psychology, 66*, 7–18.

Chekroud, A. M., Zotti, R. J., Shehzad, Z., Gueorguieva, R., Johnson, M. K., & Trivedi, M. H. (2016). Cross-trial prediction of treatment outcome in depression: A machine learning approach. *Lancet Psychiatry, 3*, 243–250.

Clark, D. M. (2018). Realizing the mass public benefit of evidence-based psychological therapies: The IAPT Program. *Annual Review of Clinical Psychology, 14*, 159–183.

Cloitre, M., Petkova, E., Su, Z., & Weiss, B. (2016). Patient characteristics as a moderator of post-traumatic stress disorder treatment outcome: Combining symptom burden and strengths. *British Journal of Psychiatry Open, 2*, 101–106.

Cohen, Z. D., & DeRubeis, R. J. (2018). Treatment selection in depression. *Annual Review of Clinical Psychology, 14*, 209–236.

Cohen, Z. D., Kim, T. T., Van, H. L., Dekker, J. J., & Driessen, E. (2019). A demonstration of a multimethod variable selection approach for treatment selection: Recommending cognitive–behavioral versus psychodynamic therapy for mild to moderate adult depression. *Psychotherapy Research.* [Epub ahead of print]

Connolly, K. R., & Thase, M. E. (2011). The clinical management of bipolar disorder: A review of evidence-based guidelines. *Primary Care Companion to CNS Disorders, 13*, 10r01097.

Cook, J. M., Dinnen, S., Simiola, V., Thompson, R., & Schnurr, P. P. (2014). VA residential provider perceptions of dissuading factors to the use of two evidence-based PTSD treatments. *Professional Psychology: Research and Practice, 45*, 136–142.

Cook, J. M., Simiola, V., Hamblen, J. L., Bernardy, N., & Schnurr, P. P. (2017). The influence of patient readiness on implementation of evidence-based PTSD treatments in Veterans Affairs residential programs. *Psychological Trauma: Theory, Research, Practice, and Policy, 9*, 51–58.

Craske, M. G., Meuret, A. E., Ritz, T., Treanor, M., & Dour, H. J. (2016). Treatment for anhedonia: A neuroscience driven approach. *Depression and Anxiety, 33,* 927–938.

Cuijpers, P., Huibers M. J., & Furukawa, T. A. (2017). The need for research on treatments of chronic depression. *JAMA Psychiatry, 74,* 242–243.

Dawes, R. M. (1979). The robust beauty of improper linear models in decision making. *American Psychologist, 34,* 571–582.

Dawes, R. M. (2005). The ethical implications of Paul Meehl's work on comparing clinical versus actuarial prediction methods. *Journal of Clinical Psychology, 61,* 1245–1255.

Dawes, R. M., Faust, D., & Meehl, P. E. (1989). Clinical versus actuarial judgment. *Science, 243,* 1668–1674.

Deisenhofer, A. K., Delgadillo, J., Rubel, J. A., Böhnke, J. R., Zimmermann, D., Schwartz, B., et al. (2018). Individual treatment selection for patients with posttraumatic stress disorder. *Depression and Anxiety, 35,* 541–550.

Delgadillo, J., Huey, D., Bennett, H., & McMillan, D. (2017). Case complexity as a guide for psychological treatment selection. *Journal of Consulting and Clinical Psychology, 85,* 835–853.

Delgadillo, J., Moreea, O., & Lutz, W. (2016). Different people respond differently to therapy: A demonstration using patient profiling and risk stratification. *Behaviour Research and Therapy, 79,* 15–22.

DeRubeis, R. J., Cohen, Z. D., Forand, N. R., Fournier, J. C., Gelfand, L. A., & Lorenzo-Luaces, L. (2014). The Personalized Advantage Index: Translating research on prediction into individualized treatment recommendations: A demonstration. *PLOS ONE, 9,* e83875.

DeRubeis, R. J., Gelfand, L. A., German, R. E., Fournier, J. C., & Forand, N. R. (2014). Understanding processes of change: How some patients reveal more than others—and some groups of therapists less—about what matters in psychotherapy. *Psychotherapy Research, 24,* 419–428.

DeRubeis, R. J., Hollon, S. D., Amsterdam, J. D., Shelton, R. C., Young, P. R., Salomon, R. M., et al. (2005). Cognitive therapy vs medications in the treatment of moderate to severe depression. *Archives of General Psychiatry, 62,* 409–416.

Doove, L. L., Dusseldorp, E., Van Deun, K., & Van Mechelen, I. (2014). A comparison of five recursive partitioning methods to find person subgroups involved in meaningful treatment–subgroup interactions. *Advances in Data Analysis and Classification, 8,* 403–425.

Driessen, E., Cuijpers, P., Hollon, S. D., & Dekker, J. J. (2010). Does pretreatment severity moderate the efficacy of psychological treatment of adult outpatient depression?: A meta-analysis. *Journal of Consulting and Clinical Psychology, 78,* 668–680.

Drysdale, A. T., Grosenick, L., Downar, J., Dunlop, K., Mansouri, F., Meng, Y., et al. (2017). Resting-state connectivity biomarkers define neurophysiological subtypes of depression. *Nature Medicine, 23,* 28–38.

Dunlop, B. W., Kelley, M. E., Aponte-Rivera, V., Mletzko-Crowe, T., Kinkead, B., Ritchie, J. C., et al. (2017). Effects of patient preferences on outcomes in the Predictors of Remission in Depression to Individual and Combined Treatments (PReDICT) study. *American Journal of Psychiatry, 174,* 546–556.

Dunlop, B. W., Kelley, M. E., Mletzko, T. C., Velasquez, C. M., Craighead, W. E., & Mayberg, H. S. (2012). Depression beliefs, treatment preference, and outcomes in a randomized trial for major depressive disorder. *Journal of Psychiatric Research, 46,* 375–381.

Elkin, I., Shea, M. T., Watkins, J. T., Imber, S. D., Sotsky, S. M., Collins, J. F., et al. (1989). National Institute of Mental Health treatment of depression collaborative research program: General effectiveness of treatments. *Archives of General Psychiatry, 46,* 971–982.

Fineberg, N. A., Brown, A., Reghunandanan, S., & Pampaloni, I. (2012). Evidence-based pharmacotherapy of obsessive–compulsive disorder. *International Journal of Neuropsychopharmacology, 15,* 1173–1191.

Fournier, J. C., DeRubeis, R. J., Hollon, S. D., Dimidjian, S., Amsterdam, J. D., Shelton, R. C., et al. (2010). Antidepressant drug effects and depression severity: A patient-level meta-analysis. *Journal of the American Medical Association, 303,* 47–53.

Fournier, J. C., DeRubeis, R. J., Shelton, R. C., Gallop, R., Amsterdam, J. D., & Hollon, S. D. (2008). Antidepressant medications v. cognitive therapy in people with depression with or without personality disorder. *British Journal of Psychiatry, 192,* 124–129.

Fournier, J. C., DeRubeis, R. J., Shelton, R. C., Hollon, S. D., Amsterdam, J. D., & Gallop, R. (2009). Prediction of response to medication and cognitive therapy in the treatment of moderate to severe depression. *Journal of Consulting and Clinical Psychology, 77,* 775–787.

Furukawa, T. A., Weitz, E. S., Tanaka, S., Hollon, S. D., Hofmann, S. G., Andersson, G., et al. (2017). Initial severity of depression and efficacy of cognitive-behavioural therapy: Individual-participant data meta-analysis of pill-placebo-controlled trials. *British Journal of Psychiatry, 210,* 190–196.

Gabrieli, J. D., Ghosh, S. S., & Whitfield-Gabrieli, S. (2015). Prediction as a humanitarian and pragmatic contribution from human cognitive neuroscience. *Neuron, 85,* 11–26.

Gillan, C. M., & Daw, N. D. (2016). Taking psychiatry research online. *Neuron, 91,* 19–23.

Gillan, C. M., & Whelan, R. (2017). What big data can do for treatment in psychiatry. *Current Opinion in Behavioral Sciences, 18,* 34–42.

Green, E., Goldstein-Piekarski, A. N., Schatzberg, A. F., Rush, A. J., Ma, J., & Williams, L. (2017). Personalizing antidepressant choice by sex, body mass index, and symptom profile: An iSPOT-D report. *Personalized Medicine in Psychiatry, 1,* 65–73.

Grenyer, B. F., Deane, F. P., & Lewis, K. L. (2008). Treatment history and its relationship to outcome in psychotherapy for depression. *Counselling and Psychotherapy Research, 8,* 21–27.

Grieve, S. M., Korgaonkar, M. S., Etkin, A., Harris, A., Koslow, S. H., Wisniewski, S., et al. (2013). Brain imaging predictors and the international study to predict optimized treatment for depression: Study protocol for a randomized controlled trial. *Trials, 14,* 224.

Grove, W. M., & Meehl, P. E. (1996). Comparative efficiency of informal (subjective, impressionistic) and formal (mechanical, algorithmic) prediction procedures: The clinical–statistical controversy. *Psychology, Public Policy, and Law, 2,* 293–323.

Grove, W. M., Zald, D. H., Lebow, B. S., Snitz, B. E., & Nelson, C. (2000). Clinical versus mechanical prediction: A meta-analysis. *Psychological Assessment, 12,* 19–30.

Hamburg, M. A., & Collins, F. S. (2010). The path to personalized medicine. *New England Journal of Medicine, 363,* 301–304.

Hannan, C., Lambert, M. J., Harmon, C., Nielsen, S. L., Smart, D. W., Shimokawa, K., et al. (2005). A lab test and algorithms for identifying clients at risk for treatment failure. *Journal of Clinical Psychology, 61,* 155–163.

Hingorani, A. D., van der Windt, D. A., Riley, R. D., Abrams, K., Moons, K. G., Steyerberg, E. W., et al. (2013). Prognosis research strategy (PROGRESS) 4: Stratified medicine research. *British Medical Journal, 346,* e5793.

Hirschfeld, R. M. (2001). The comorbidity of major depression and anxiety disorders: Recognition and management in primary care. *Primary Care Companion to the Journal of Clinical Psychiatry, 3,* 244–254.

Holmes, E. A., Ghaderi, A., Harmer, C. J., Ramchandani, P. G., Cuijpers, P., Morrison, A. P., et al. (2018). The Lancet Psychiatry Commission on psychological treatments research in tomorrow's science. *Lancet Psychiatry, 5,* 237–286.

Huibers, M. J., Cohen, Z. D., Lemmens, L. H., Arntz, A., Peeters, F. P., Cuijpers, P., et al. (2015). Predicting optimal outcomes in cognitive therapy or interpersonal psychotherapy for depressed individuals using the Personalized Advantage Index approach. *PLOS ONE, 10,* e0140771.

Iniesta, R., Hodgson, K., Stahl, D., Malki, K., Maier, W., Rietschel, M., et al. (2018). Antidepressant drug-specific prediction of depression treatment outcomes from genetic and clinical variables. *Scientific Reports, 8,* Article No. 5530.

Iniesta, R., Malki, K., Maier, W., Rietschel, M., Mors, O., Hauser, J., et al. (2016). Combining clinical variables to optimize prediction of antidepressant treatment outcomes. *Journal of Psychiatric Research, 78,* 94–102.

Iniesta, R., Stahl, D., & McGuffin, P. (2016). Machine learning, statistical learning and the future of biological research in psychiatry. *Psychological Medicine, 46,* 2455–2465.

Janes, H., Pepe, M. S., Bossuyt, P. M., & Barlow, W. E. (2011). Measuring the performance of markers for guiding treatment decisions. *Annals of Internal Medicine, 154*(4), 253–259.

Jollans, L., & Whelan, R. (2016). The clinical added value of imaging: A perspective from outcome prediction. *Biological Psychiatry: Cognitive Neuroscience and Neuroimaging, 1,* 423–432.

Katsnelson, A. (2013). Momentum grows to make "personalized" medicine more "precise." *Nature Medicine, 19,* 249.

Keefe, J. R., Wiltsey-Stirman, S., Cohen, Z. D., DeRubeis, R. J., Smith, B. N., & Resick, P. (2018). In rape-trauma PTSD, patient characteristics indicate which trauma-focused treatment they are most likely to complete. *Depression and Anxiety, 35,* 330–338.

Kessler, R. C. (2018). The potential of predictive analytics to provide clinical decision support in depression treatment planning. *Current Opinion in Psychiatry, 31,* 32–39.

Kessler, R. C., Chiu, W. T., Demler, O., & Walters, E. E. (2005). Prevalence, severity, and comorbidity of 12-month DSM-IV disorders in the National Comorbidity Survey Replication. *Archives of General Psychiatry, 62,* 617–627.

Kessler, R. C., van Loo, H. M., Wardenaar, K. J., Bossarte, R. M., Brenner, L. A., Ebert, D. D., et al. (2017). Using patient self-reports to study heterogeneity of treatment effects in major depressive disorder. *Epidemiology and Psychiatric Sciences, 26,* 22–36.

Khan, A., Leventhal, R. M., Khan, S. R., & Brown, W. A. (2002). Severity of depression and response to antidepressants and placebo: An analysis of the Food and Drug Administration database. *Journal of Clinical Psychopharmacology, 22,* 40–45.

Kircanski, K., LeMoult, J., Ordaz, S., & Gotlib, I. H. (2017). Investigating the nature of co-occurring depression and anxiety: Comparing diagnostic and dimensional research approaches. *Journal of Affective Disorders, 216,* 123–135.

Kirsch, I., Deacon, B. J., Huedo-Medina, T. B., Scoboria, A., Moore, T. J., & Johnson, B. T. (2008). Initial severity and antidepressant benefits: A meta-analysis of data submitted to the Food and Drug Administration. *PLoS Medicine, 5,* e45.

Kocsis, J. H., Leon, A. C., Markowitz, J. C., Manber, R., Arnow, B., Klein, D. N., et al. (2009). Patient preference as a moderator of outcome for chronic forms of major depressive disorder treated with nefazodone, cognitive behavioral analysis system of psychotherapy, or their combination. *Journal of Clinical Psychiatry, 70,* 354–361.

Koutsouleris, N., Kahn, R. S., Chekroud, A. M., Leucht, S., Falkai, P, Wobrock, T., et al. (2016). Multisite prediction of 4-week and 52-week treatment outcomes in patients with first-episode psychosis: A machine learning approach. *Lancet Psychiatry, 3,* 935–946.

Kraemer, H. C. (2013). Discovering, comparing, and combining moderators of treatment on outcome after randomized clinical trials: A parametric approach. *Statistics in Medicine, 32,* 1964–1973.

Kraemer, H. C., & Frank, E. (2010). Evaluation of comparative treatment trials: Assessing clinical benefits and risks for patients, rather than statistical effects on measures. *Journal of the American Medical Association, 304,* 683–684.

Kraemer, H. C., Frank, E., & Kupfer, D. J. (2011). How to assess the clinical impact of treatments on patients, rather than the statistical impact of treatments on measures. *International Journal of Methods in Psychiatric Research, 20,* 63–72.

Lam, R. W., Milev, R., Rotzinger, S., Andreazza, A. C., Blier, P., Brenner, C., et al. (2016). Discovering biomarkers for antidepressant response: Protocol from the Canadian biomarker integration network in depression (CAN-BIND) and clinical characteristics of the first patient cohort. *BMC Psychiatry, 16,* 105.

Layard, R., Clark, D., Knapp, M., & Mayraz, G. (2007). Cost–benefit analysis of psychological therapy. *National Institute Economic Review, 202,* 90–98.

Leykin, Y., Amsterdam, J. D., DeRubeis, R. J., Gallop, R., Shelton, R. C., & Hollon, S. D. (2007). Progressive resistance to a selective serotonin reuptake inhibitor but not to cognitive therapy in the treatment of major depression. *Journal of Consulting and Clinical Psychology, 75,* 267–276.

Leykin, Y., DeRubeis, R. J., Gallop, R., Amsterdam, J. D., Shelton, R. C., & Hollon, S. D. (2007). The relation of patients' treatment preferences to outcome in a randomized clinical trial. *Behavior Therapy, 38,* 209–217.

Lilienfeld, S. O., Ammirati, R., & David, M. (2012). Distinguishing science from pseudoscience in school psychology: Science and scientific thinking as safeguards against human error. *Journal of School Psychology, 50,* 7–36.

Lilienfeld, S. O., Ammirati, R., & Landfield, K. (2009). Giving debiasing away: Can psychological research on correcting cognitive errors promote human welfare? *Perspectives on Psychological Science, 4,* 390–398.

Linardon, J., Wade, T. D., de la Piedad Garcia, X., & Brennan, L. (2017). The efficacy of cognitive-behavioral therapy for eating disorders: A systematic review and meta-analysis. *Journal of Consulting and Clinical Psychology, 85,* 1080–1094.

Lo, A., Chernoff, H., Zheng, T., & Lo, S.-H. (2015). Why significant variables aren't automatically good predictors. *Proceedings of the National Academy of Sciences of the USA, 112,* 13892–13897.

Lorenzo-Luaces, L., DeRubeis, R. J., & Bennett, I. M. (2015). Primary care physicians' selection of low-intensity treatments for patients with depression. *Family Medicine, 47,* 511–516.

Lorenzo-Luaces, L., DeRubeis, R. J., van Straten, A., & Tiemens, B. (2017). A prognostic index (PI) as a moderator of outcomes in the treatment of depression: A proof of concept combining multiple variables to inform risk-stratified stepped care models. *Journal of Affective Disorders, 213,* 78–85.

Luty, S. E., Carter, J. D., McKenzie, J. M., Rae, A. M., Frampton, C. M., Mulder, R. T., et al. (2007). Randomised controlled trial of interpersonal psychotherapy and cognitive-behavioural therapy for depression. *British Journal of Psychiatry, 190,* 496–502.

Lutz, W., Hofmann, S. G., Rubel, J., Boswell J. F., Shear, M. K., Gorman, J. M., et al. (2014). Patterns of early change and their relationship to outcome and early treatment termination in patients with panic disorder. *Journal of Consulting and Clinical Psychology, 82,* 287–297.

Lutz, W., Saunders, S. M., Leon, S. C., Martinovich, Z., Kosfelder, J., Schulte, D., et al. (2006). Empirically and clinically useful decision making in psychotherapy: Differential predictions with treatment response models. *Psychological Assessment, 18,* 133–141.

Mayberg, H. S., Lozano, A. M., Voon, V., McNeely, H. E., Seminowicz, D., Hamani, C., et al. (2005). Deep brain stimulation for treatment-resistant depression. *Neuron, 45,* 651–660.

McCullough, J. P., Jr. (2003). *Treatment for chronic depression: Cognitive behavioral analysis system of psychotherapy (CBASP).* New York: Guilford Press.

McGirr, A., Berlim, M., Bond, D., Fleck, M., Yatham, L., & Lam, R. (2015). A systematic review and meta-analysis of randomized, double-blind, placebo-controlled trials of ketamine in the rapid treatment of major depressive episodes. *Psychological Medicine, 45,* 693–704.

McGrath, C. L., Kelley, M. E., Holtzheimer, P. E., Dunlop, B. W., Craighead, W. E., Franco, A. R., et al. (2013). Toward a neuroimaging treatment selection biomarker for major depressive disorder. *JAMA Psychiatry, 70,* 821–829.

McHugh, R. K., Whitton, S. W., Peckham, A. D., Welge, J. A., & Otto, M. W. (2013). Patient preference for psychological vs pharmacologic treatment of psychiatric disorders: A meta-analytic review. *Journal of Clinical Psychiatry, 74,* 595–602.

Meehl, P. E. (1954). *Clinical versus statistical prediction: A theoretical analysis and a review of the evidence.* Minneapolis: University of Minnesota Press.

Meehl, P. E. (1978). Theoretical risks and tabular asterisks: Sir Karl, Sir Ronald, and the slow progress of soft psychology. *Journal of Consulting and Clinical Psychology, 46,* 806–834.

Mergl, R., Henkel, V., Allgaier, A. K., Kramer, D., Hautzinger, M., Kohnen, R., et al. (2011). Are treatment preferences relevant in response to serotonergic antidepressants and cognitive-behavioral therapy in depressed primary care patients?: Results from a randomized controlled trial including a patients' choice arm. *Psychotherapy and Psychosomatics, 80,* 39–47.

Mickey, R. M., & Greenland, S. (1989). The impact of confounder selection criteria on effect estimation. *American Journal of Epidemiology, 129,* 125–137.

National Health Service. (2016). *Psychological therapies, annual report on the use of IAPT services—England 2015–16.* London: Health and Social Care information Centre.

National Institute for Health and Clinical Excellence. (2009). *Depression: Treatment and management of depression in adults.* London: Author.

National Research Council. (2011). *Toward precision medicine: Building a knowledge network for biomedical research and a new taxonomy of disease.* Washington, DC: National Academies Press.

Nemeroff, C. B., Heim, C. M., Thase, M. E., Klein, D. N., Rush, A. J., Schatzberg, A. F., et al. (2003). Differential responses to psychotherapy versus pharmacotherapy in patients with chronic forms of major depression and childhood trauma. *Proceedings of the National Academy of Sciences of the USA, 100,* 14293–14296.

Niles, A. N., Loerinc, A. G., Krull, J. L., Roy-Byrne, P., Sullivan, G., Sherbourne, C. D., et al. (2017). Advancing personalized medicine: Application of a novel statistical method to identify treatment moderators in the coordinated anxiety learning and management study. *Behavior Therapy, 48,* 490–500.

Niles, A. N., Wolitzky-Taylor, K. B., Arch, J. J., & Craske, M. G. (2017). Applying a novel statistical method to advance the personalized treatment of anxiety disorders: A composite moderator of comparative drop-out from CBT and ACT. *Behaviour Research and Therapy, 91,* 13–23.

Nuzzo, R. (2014). Statistical errors. *Nature, 506,* 150–152.

Osei-Bonsu, P. E., Bolton, R. E., Stirman, S. W., Eisen, S. V., Herz, L., & Pellowe, M. E. (2017). Mental health providers' decision-making around the implementation of evidence-based treatment for PTSD. *Journal of Behavioral Health Services and Research, 44,* 213–223.

Paez, J. G., Jänne, P. A., Lee, J. C., Tracy, S., Greulich, H., Gabriel, S., et al. (2004). EGFR mutations in lung cancer: Correlation with clinical response to gefitinib therapy. *Science, 304,* 1497–1500.

Papakostas, G. I., & Fava, M. (2010). *Pharmacotherapy for depression and treatment-resistant depression.* Singapore: World Scientific.

Passos, I. C., Mwangi, B., & Kapczinski, F. (2016). Big data analytics and machine learning: 2015 and beyond. *Lancet Psychiatry, 3,* 13–15.

Pauker, S. G., & Kassirer, J. P. (1980). The threshold approach to clinical decision making. *New England Journal of Medicine, 302,* 1109–1117.

Paul, G. L. (1967). Strategy of outcome research in psychotherapy. *Journal of Consulting Psychology, 31,* 109–118.

Perlis, R. H. (2013). A clinical risk stratification tool for predicting treatment resistance in major depressive disorder. *Biological Psychiatry, 74,* 7–14.

Perlis, R. H. (2016). Abandoning personalization to get to precision in the pharmacotherapy of depression. *World Psychiatry, 15,* 228–235.

Perlis, R. H., Fijal, B., Dharia, S., Heinloth, A. N., & Houston, J. P. (2010). Failure to replicate genetic associations with antidepressant treatment response in duloxetine-treated patients. *Biological Psychiatry, 67,* 1110–1113.

Perlis, R., Iosifescu, D., Castro, V., Murphy, S., Gainer, V., Minnier, J., et al. (2012). Using electronic medical records to enable large-scale studies in psychiatry: Treatment resistant depression as a model. *Psychological Medicine, 42,* 41–50.

Perlis, R. H., Patrick, A., Smoller, J. W., & Wang, P. S. (2009). When is pharmacogenetic testing for antidepressant response ready for the clinic?: A cost-effectiveness analysis based on data from the STAR* D study. *Neuropsychopharmacology, 34,* 2227–2236.

Pizzagalli, D. A. (2011). Frontocingulate dysfunction in depression: Toward biomarkers of treatment response. *Neuropsychopharmacology, 36,* 183–206.

Pizzagalli, D. A., Webb, C. A., Dillon, D. G., Tenke, C. E., Kayser, J., Goer, F., et al. (2018). Pretreatment rostral anterior cingulate cortex theta activity in relation to symptom improvement in depression: A randomized clinical trial. *JAMA Psychiatry, 75,* 547–554.

Preference Collaborative Review Group. (2008). Patients' preferences within randomised trials: Systematic review and patient level meta-analysis. *British Medical Journal, 337,* a1864.

Raza, G. T., & Holohan, D. R. (2015). Clinical treatment selection for posttraumatic stress disorder: Suggestions for researchers and clinical trainers. *Psychological Trauma: Theory, Research, and Practice, 7,* 547–554.

Renjilian, D. A., Perri, M. G., Nezu, A. M., McKelvey, W. F., Shermer, R. L., & Anton, S. D. (2001). Individual versus group therapy for obesity: Effects of matching participants to their treatment preferences. *Journal of Consulting and Clinical Psychology, 69,* 717–721.

Rosell, R., Carcereny, E., Gervais, R., Vergnenegre, A., Massuti, B., Felip, E., et al. (2012). Erlotinib versus standard chemotherapy as first-line treatment for European patients with advanced EGFR mutation-positive non-small-cell lung cancer (EURTAC): A multicentre, open-label, randomised phase 3 trial. *Lancet Oncology, 13,* 239–246.

Rosen, C. S., Matthieu, M., Stirman, S. W., Cook, J., Landes, S., Bernardy, N. C., et al. (2016). A review of studies on the system-wide implementation of evidence-based psychotherapies for posttraumatic stress disorder in the Veterans Health Administration. *Administration and Policy in Mental Health and Mental Health Services Research, 43,* 957–977.

Rosnow, R. L., & Rosenthal, R. (1989). Statistical procedures and the justification of knowledge in psychological science. *American Psychologist, 44,* 1276–1284.

Saunders, R., Cape, J., Fearon, P., & Pilling, S. (2016). Predicting treatment outcome in psychological treatment services by identifying latent profiles of patients. *Journal of Affective Disorders, 197,* 107–115.

Schleidgen, S., Klingler, C., Bertram, T., Rogowski, W. H., & Marckmann, G. (2013). What is personalized medicine: Sharpening a vague term based on a systematic literature review. *BMC Medical Ethics, 14,* 55.

Schweizer, S., Cohen, Z., Hayes, R., DeRubeis, R., Crane, C., Kuyken, W., et al. (2019). *Relapse prevention for antidepressant medication (ADM) responders with recurrent depression: Deciding between maintenance ADM and mindfulness-based cognitive therapy.* Manuscript submitted for publication.

Simon, G. E., Johnson, E., Lawrence, J. M., Rossom, R. C., Ahmedani, B., Lynch, F. L., et al. (2018). Predicting suicide attempts and suicide deaths following outpatient visits using electronic health records. *American Journal of Psychiatry, 175,* 951–960.

Simon, G. E., & Perlis, R. H. (2010). Personalized medicine for depression: Can we match patients with treatments? *American Journal of Psychiatry, 167,* 1445–1455.

Smagula, S. F., Wallace, M. L., Anderson, S. J., Karp, J. F., Lenze, E. J., Mulsant, B. H., et al. (2016). Combining moderators to identify clinical profiles of patients who will, and will not, benefit from aripiprazole augmentation for treatment resistant late-life major depressive disorder. *Journal of Psychiatric Research, 81,* 112–118.

Spengler, P. M., White, M. J., Ægisdóttir, S., Maugherman, A. S., Anderson, L. A., Cook, R. S., et al. (2009). The meta-analysis of clinical judgment project: Effects of experience on judgment accuracy. *Counseling Psychologist, 37,* 350–399.

Stephan, K. E., Schlagenhauf, F., Huys, Q. J., Raman, S., Aponte, E. A., Brodersen, K. H., et al. (2017). Computational neuroimaging strategies for single patient predictions. *NeuroImage, 145,* 180–199.

Swift, J. K., & Callahan, J. L. (2009). The impact of client treatment preferences on outcome: A meta-analysis. *Journal of Clinical Psychology, 65,* 368–381.

Swift, J. K., Callahan, J. L., & Vollmer, B. M. (2011). Preferences. *Journal of Clinical Psychology, 67,* 155–165.

Trivedi, M. H., McGrath, P. J., Fava, M., Parsey, R. V., Kurian, B. T., Phillips, M. L., et al. (2016). Establishing moderators and biosignatures of antidepressant response in clinical care (EMBARC): Rationale and design. *Journal of Psychiatric Research, 78,* 11–23.

Tversky, A., & Kahneman, D. (1974). Judgment under uncertainty: Heuristics and biases. *Science, 185,* 1124–1131.

Tversky, A., & Kahneman, D. (1983). Extensional versus intuitive reasoning: The conjunction fallacy in probability judgment. *Psychological Review, 90,* 293–315.

Uher, R., Huezo-Diaz, P., Perroud, N., Smith, R., Rietschel, M., Mors, O., et al. (2009). Genetic predictors of response to antidepressants in the GENDEP project. *Pharmacogenomics Journal, 9,* 225–233.

Uher, R,, Perlis, R., Henigsberg, N., Zobel, A., Rietschel, M., Mors, O., et al. (2012). Depression symptom dimensions as predictors of antidepressant treatment outcome: Replicable evidence for interest-activity symptoms. *Psychological Medicine, 42,* 967–980.

Uher, R., Tansey, K. E., Dew, T., Maier, W., Mors, O., Hauser, J., et al. (2014). An inflammatory biomarker as a differential predictor of outcome of depression treatment with escitalopram and nortriptyline. *American Journal of Psychiatry, 171,* 1278–1286.

van Straten, A., Tiemens, B., Hakkaart, L., Nolen, W., & Donker, M. (2006). Stepped care vs. matched care for mood and anxiety disorders: A randomized trial in routine practice. *Acta Psychiatrica Scandinavica, 113,* 468–476.

Vittengl, J. R., Clark, L. A., Thase, M. E., & Jarrett, R. B. (2017). Initial Steps to inform selection of continuation cognitive therapy or fluoxetine for higher risk responders to cognitive therapy for recurrent major depressive disorder. *Psychiatry Research, 253,* 174–181.

Vittengl, J. R., Jarrett, R. B., Weitz, E., Hollon, S. D., Twisk, J., Cristea, I., et al. (2016). Divergent outcomes in cognitive-behavioral therapy and pharmacotherapy for adult depression. *American Journal of Psychiatry, 173,* 481–490.

Walfish, S., McAlister, B., O'Donnell, P., & Lambert, M. J. (2012). An investigation of self-assessment bias in mental health providers. *Psychological Reports, 110,* 639–644.

Wallace, M. L., Frank, E., & Kraemer, H. C. (2013). A novel approach for developing and interpreting treatment moderator profiles in randomized clinical trials. *JAMA Psychiatry, 70,* 1241–1247.

Ward, J., Graham, N., Strawbridge, R., Ferguson, A., Jenkins, G., Chen, W., et al. (2018). Polygenic risk scores for major depressive disorder and neuroticism as predictors of antidepressant response: Meta-analysis of three treatment cohorts. *PLOS ONE, 13*(9), e0203896.

Wasserstein, R. L., & Lazar, N. A. (2016). The ASA's statement on *p*-values: Context, process, and purpose. *The American Statistician, 70,* 129–133.

Webb, C. A., Trivedi, M. H., Cohen, Z. D., Dillon, D. G., Fournier, J. C., Goer, F., et al. (2018). Personalized prediction of antidepressant v. placebo response: Evidence from the EMBARC study. *Psychological Medicine.* [Epub ahead of print]

Weitz, E. S., Hollon, S. D., Twisk, J., van Straten, A., Huibers, M. J., David, D., et al. (2015). Baseline depression severity as moderator of depression outcomes between cognitive behavioral therapy vs pharmacotherapy: An individual patient data meta-analysis. *JAMA Psychiatry, 72,* 1102–1109.

Westover, A. N., Kashner, T. M., Winhusen, T. M., Golden, R. M., Nakonezny, P. A., Adinoff, B., et al. (2015). A systematic approach to subgroup analyses in a smoking cessation trial. *American Journal of Drug and Alcohol Abuse, 41,* 498–507.

Williams, L. M. (2017). Getting personalized: Brain scan biomarkers for guiding depression interventions. *American Journal of Psychiatry, 174,* 503–505.

Wiltsey Stirman, S., Cohen, Z., Lunney, C., DeRubeis, R., Wiley, J., & Schnurr, P. (2019). *A prognostic index to inform selection of a trauma-focused or non-trauma-focused treatment for PTSD.* Manuscript submitted for publication.

Winter, S. E., & Barber, J. P. (2013). Should treatment for depression be based more on patient preference? *Patient Preference and Adherence, 7,* 1047–1057.

Woo, C.-W., Chang, L. J., Lindquist, M. A., & Wager, T. D. (2017). Building better biomarkers: Brain models in translational neuroimaging. *Nature Neuroscience, 20,* 365–377.

World Health Organization. (2017). *Depression and other common mental disorders: Global health estimates.* Geneva: Author.

Zilcha-Mano, S., Keefe, J. R., Chui, H., Rubin, A., Barrett, M. S., & Barber, J. P. (2016). Reducing dropout in treatment for depression: Translating dropout predictors into individualized treatment recommendations. *Journal of Clinical Psychiatry, 77,* e1584–e1590.

CHAPTER 8

The Role of Culture in Evidence-Based Practice

MANUEL BARRERA, JR.
FELIPE GONZÁLEZ CASTRO

Prominent discussions of evidence-based practice (EBP) explicate a framework in which clinical decisions about treatment are made by synthesizing knowledge from three important domains: (1) *client characteristics,* (2) *therapist attributes,* and (3) *research* findings, particularly research findings on psychotherapy mechanisms and efficacy (American Psychological Association Presidential Task Force on Evidence-Based Practice, 2006; Spring, 2007; Whaley & Davis, 2007). Within each of these general EBP domains, there are more specialized topics concerning the multifaceted concept of culture. Specifically, in this chapter we focus on considerations of (1) clients' cultural backgrounds, (2) therapists' cultural competencies, and (3) research findings on the cultural adaptation of psychotherapies. The very definition of EBP proposed by the American Psychological Association Presidential Task Force draws attention to a client's cultural background: "*Evidence-based practice in psychology* is the integration of the best available research with clinical expertise in the context of patient characteristics, culture, and preferences" (2006, p. 273). Furthermore, therapists' cultural competence exerts its influence in assessment, in the therapeutic relationship, and in the complex judgments that therapists make when they apply their understanding of clients' cultures to treatment planning and implementation. A major cultural consideration in research integration involves the utilization of both qualitative and quantitative forms of research, including mixed-methods methodologies, to better inform the cultural adaptation of evidence-based interventions (EBIs).

Thus, our purpose in this chapter is to discuss cultural considerations for each of the specific EBP domains: client cultural background, therapist cultural competence, and research findings on cultural adaptations to improve the cultural fit of interventions. Particular emphasis is given to this last topic, which includes an overview of meta-analytic research on cultural adaptation outcome studies. These reviews are resources for practitioners in their deliberations on evidence supporting the effectiveness of adaptations. We provide examples of culturally adapted interventions to illustrate how cultural perspectives were integrated into practice. This chapter concludes with recommendations for the practitioner who strives to enhance his or her own cultural competence by improving the cultural fit of interventions for his or her diverse clientele.

Definitions and Conceptualizations of Culture

Culture has been defined broadly as "a set of attitudes, behaviors, and symbols shared by a large group of people and usually communicated from one generation to the next" (Shiraev & Levy, 2010, p. 3). Culture serves an important function in sustaining human existence and well-being. Recently, the Office of Behavioral and Social Science Research (OBSSR; 2014) released a monograph titled *The Cultural Framework for Health: An Integrative Approach for Research and Program Design and Evaluation.* Written by a consensus panel, this monograph asserted that culture "is a human schema that assures survival and well-being . . . [enabling] humans to interpret the world." The panel added that cultural knowledge allows members of a group to "make sense of their world and to find meaning in and for life" (p. 12). Also, the American Psychological Association (2003) in its guidelines for multicultural practice defined *culture* as "the embodiment of a world view through learned and transmitted beliefs, values, practices, including religious and spiritual traditions. It also encompasses a way of living informed by the historical, economic, ecological, and political forces on a group" (p. 380). This definition indicates that culture includes race, ethnicity, and nationality but goes beyond those characteristics to include others, such as religion, socioeconomic status, and geographic region (also see Cohen, 2009).

An important implication of culture for EBP is that psychotherapy and other forms of sanctioned healer–sufferer relationships constitute cultural phenomena (Frank & Frank, 1993). Because culture shapes the way people make sense of the world, we can expect cultural variation in symptom displays, explanations for the causes of suffering, and the perceptions of acceptable strategies for restoring health (Benish, Quintana, & Wampold, 2011). For example, studies conducted with Chinese participants found evidence that they were more likely to express distress through somatic symptoms compared with distress expressions from those of Western cultures (Parker, Gladstone, & Chee, 2001; Ryder et al., 2008). Furthermore, somatic symptoms give rise to somatic explanations and help seeking from those who can treat bodily ailments (Ryder et al., 2008). Hispanic Americans also are thought to somaticize psychological distress (Angel & Guarnaccia, 1989). Clients enter therapy with beliefs, attitudes, conflicts, and problems shaped by their cultural roots and present-day realities (Substance Abuse and Mental Health Services Administration [SAMHSA], 2014).

Thus, the initial client–therapist engagement involves certain tasks in which the therapist explores the client's perceived causes of his or her presenting problem, and the client's perceived solutions for possibly resolving that problem. This initial engagement requires the therapist's culturally responsive analysis and understanding of the client's cultural schema regarding his or her presenting problem.

The Role of Clients' Cultural Characteristics in EBP: Relating Group-Level Cultural Characteristics to the Individual Client

An observation by Kluckhohn and Murray (1948) has been paraphrased often over the years: Every person is like all other people, some other people, and no other person. *Culture* refers to what a person shares with "some other people." Obviously, within any group, variation exists due to the uniqueness of individuals. In EBP, understanding client characteristics entails the shift from a common knowledge of the client as being "like some other people" to an individualized knowledge of the client as being "like no other person."

For example, although it is useful to know that 57% of Hispanics are Catholic, a therapist clearly needs to assess a client's religious affiliations and, more specifically, how that particular client's spiritual beliefs and practices might (or might not) be relevant in tailoring approaches for individualized treatment. Similarly, although about one-third of Mexican-heritage residents of the United States are foreign-born, the immigration stories of Mexican-heritage residents vary along dimensions such as trauma, hardship, predictability, opportunity, and resource accessibility. It is at the level of client characteristics that the complexities of acculturation and membership in multiple cultural groups are identified, clarified, and negotiated.

After showing respect for the various cultural identities that a client might have, an approach to understanding the confluence of cultural influences is to assess a client's perceptions of problems, their causes, and potential solutions. One framework for conducting such an assessment is the Cultural Formulation Interview contained in DSM-5 (American Psychiatric Association, 2013). It consists of 16 specific interview probes for evaluating clients' conceptualization of their problems, origins of problems, perceived stressors and supports, cultural identity and its possible relation to presenting problems, and cultural factors that might influence help seeking.

Complexities arise when a client's cultural views conflict, such as when an immigrant's values formed in the country of origin are incompatible with those of the host country. This issue provides a segue into the following section on *therapist cultural competence,* a capacity that confers agency to therapists in collaborating with clients on issues of culture and adjustment.

The Role of Therapists' Cultural Competence in EBP

What Is Cultural Competence?

Cultural competence refers to the capacity of a service provider to work effectively with clients from various cultural groups (Castro, 1998). This includes understanding a diverse clientele by working as much as possible with individuals in terms consistent with their own language, race, ethnicity, religious affiliation, nationality and other core aspects of their cultural identity (Sue & Sue, 1999). *Cultural competence* has also been defined as "a set of academic and interpersonal skills that allow individuals to increase their understanding and appreciation of cultural differences and similarities within, among, and between groups" (Orlandi, Weston, & Epstein, 1992, p. vi).

Components of Cultural Competence

A general model of therapists' cultural competence has identified four fundamental components of cultural competence: (1) *cultural awareness*—of own beliefs, values, attitudes, even prejudices about self and their clients; (2) *cultural knowledge*—an investment in increasing knowledge and understanding of own and of their clients' cultural worldviews; (3) *cultural knowledge of behavioral health*—an understanding of how culture interacts with health beliefs, health behavior, and other behavioral health issues to better help their clients; and (4) *cultural competence skills*—a positive attitude toward cultural learning and ongoing efforts at personal growth to enhance one's own cultural skills for working effectively with diverse clients (SAMHSA, 2014). Self-report and external-observer measures of cultural competence have been developed to assess these components (Ponterotto, Rieger, Barrett, & Sparks, 1994).

Stanley Sue wrote cogent conceptual analyses of cultural competence in which he identified components that differed slightly from those described by SAMHSA (Sue, 1998, 2006). In one framework, he proposed that there are three central attributes of cultural competence: scientific mindedness, dynamic sizing, and culture-specific skills (Sue, 2006). *Scientific mindedness* means that therapists avoid prejudging their clients' cultural influences. Instead, therapists should formulate hypotheses that can be tested over the course of therapy. *Dynamic sizing* refers to the judgments therapists make in determining to what extent generalizations about a client's ethnic background are valid. As Sue (2006, p. 239) noted, dynamic sizing is "important because one of the major dilemmas facing individuals is how to appreciate culture without stereotyping." In addition to the general components of scientific mindedness and dynamic sizing, Sue argued that knowledge and skills specific to the culture of the client (*culture-specific skills*) are an important aspect of cultural competence. Culture-specific skills include, for example, assessing and understanding the history of a client's experience of discrimination or assessing the need for pretreatment orientation that might comfort clients who are unfamiliar with therapy procedures. The ability to speak a client's native language also is an aspect of culture-specific skills. Consistent with EBP principles, the extent to which native languages are used in the provision of services should be based on the joint considerations of client preferences and the capacities of accessible service providers.

The Cultural Capacity Continuum

The capacity to work effectively with various ethnic/racial populations has been described as a continuum (Cross, Bazron, Dennis, & Isaacs, 1989) that ranges from the most negative and discriminatory attitudes toward people of different cultures to the most positive attitudes. Near the midpoint on this continuum is *cultural blindness,* which espouses that "all people are alike"; thus, all people should be "treated equally"—a "one-size-fits-all" approach. This "culturally blind" perspective ignores cultural variations in need, such that espousing "same treatment" discounts the presence of real and important differences and needs.

Advancing into the positive domain is the stage of *cultural sensitivity,* an accepting attitude toward working with issues of culture and diversity. While positive, this early stage of cultural capacity may still include simplistic or stereotypical perceptions about race, ethnicity, and other cultural issues. A more advanced stage is *cultural competence,* the capacity for an in-depth understanding of cultural issues and their nuances. Finally, the highest and most advanced stage of cultural capacity is *cultural proficiency,* which involves the capacity to conduct a "deep structure" analysis of complex cultural issues (Resnicow, Soler, Braithwait, Ahluwalia, & Butler, 2000). Cultural proficiency includes an understanding of cultural nuances, more subtle shades of meaning, as involved in attaining a more complete understanding of a client's life situation. This understanding is coupled with a more complete systems-level understanding of familial, social, cultural, and other contextual aspects of that life situation (Castro, 1998).

Cultural Adaptation of Interventions

In addition to clients' cultural backgrounds and therapists' cultural competence, the *cultural fit* of interventions with the needs and characteristics of clients is a third subdomain of EBP. To improve the fit of EBIs, particularly those that were neither created nor tested with ethnocultural groups, intervention developers sometimes culturally adapt EBIs. The *cultural adaptation of an EBI* (CA-EBI) can be defined as a purposeful modification to an EBI that "considers language, culture, and context in such a way that it is compatible with the client's cultural patterns, meanings, and values" (Bernal, Jiménez-Chafey, & Domenech Rodríguez, 2009, p. 362). Like original EBIs, CA-EBIs can be delivered in the form of standardized, manualized therapies. Because their foundation is grounded in preexisting efficacy research, CA-EBIs can be differentiated from another valid form of culturally sensitive therapies, de novo interventions, which are not adaptations of preexisting therapies; they are innovations derived from cultural theory, clinical experience, or programmatic generative research to identify cultural factors that can be leveraged in interventions. Cardemil (2010a) designated cuento therapy (Costantino, Malgady, & Rogler, 1986) and bicultural effectiveness therapy (Szapoc-

znik et al., 1986) as examples of de novo treatments developed specifically for Latino clients.

From a historical perspective, several observers (Bernal & Scharrón-del-Río, 2001; Cardemil, 2010b; La Roche & Christopher, 2009) noted that few racial and ethnic/minority clients participated in research that supported the initial listings of empirically validated/supported treatments when they first appeared in the mid-1990s (Chambless & Ollendick, 2001). They argued that assertions that these interventions are certified to be "empirically validated" or "empirically supported" were premature without more substantial demonstrations of external validity of these interventions with respect to race and ethnicity. In other words, prior research trials had not explicitly demonstrated that these interventions work as intended with certain special populations, such as Latinos or African Americans. Furthermore, to engage (e.g., recruit, retain) culturally diverse participants, some advocated modifications to EBIs to make them culturally relevant for these populations, thereby providing a better fit to participants' languages, values, and cultural preferences (Bernal & Scharrón-del-Río, 2001).

Cultural adaptations have been conducted with varying levels of sophistication. Some begin with EBIs that are supported by substantial research, then undergo systematic processes of modifications that are informed by data-driven indications that original interventions provide inadequate engagement and/or a lower level of effectiveness when applied with ethnocultural group clients (Lau, 2006). Such adaptations often result in minimal disruptions to core intervention mechanisms. For example, Hwang (2012) described the lengthy, programmatic steps taken to culturally adapt a cognitive-behavioral therapy (CBT) depression intervention for clients of Chinese heritage. But not all cultural adaptation efforts involve extensive activities that result in manualized, revised interventions. Some efforts described as cultural adaptations focus primarily on ethnic/racial matching of therapists with clients or on language used in conducting sessions. Chowdhary and colleagues (2014) observed that several studies made references to conducting "cultural adaptations," yet did not provide detailed descriptions of those modifications.

Cultural adaptations might also differ in timing. Some are made well in advance of widespread implementation (proactive), whereas others are made during implementation, including *in situ* adaptations that therapists make during sessions, perhaps because of perceived mismatches between the standard intervention and the cultural features of the person participating in therapy (reactive). Those *in situ* adaptations that are congruent with the intervention's theory are similar to therapists' tailoring of therapy methods to fit specific clients, or what Kendall and his colleagues have discussed extensively as "flexibility within fidelity" (e.g., Kendall & Beidas, 2007; Kendall, Chu, Gifford, Hayes, & Nauta, 1999).

Cultural adaptations vary in the content of what is changed and in the process that is used to identify changes. Domenech Rodríguez and Bernal (2012) reviewed the many frameworks that have been proposed for conducting systematic cultural adaptations. In broad terms, the various frameworks provide a structure for intervention developers and implementers to consider which aspects of interventions might be adapted and the steps that might be followed to determine how to make modifications. For instance, in their formulation of the ecological validity framework, Bernal, Bonilla, and Bellido (1995) identified intervention features that might be modified to improve cultural fit, features such as the languages used in sessions and treatment materials, metaphors marshaled to illustrate concepts, and intervention content.

In addition to the content of cultural adaptations, there has been attention to the process of identifying the intervention features that merit cultural adaptations (Barrera, Castro, Strycker, & Toobert, 2013). Hwang (2012) proposed a "psychotherapy adaptation and modification framework" (a top-down method emphasizing theory) and a "formative method for adapting psychotherapy" (a bottom-up method emphasizing knowledge gained from clients, therapists, and key community informants), which were integrated into the cultural adaptation of a cognitive-behavioral approach to the treatment of depressed clients of Chinese heritage. These two approaches defined strategies for specifying the *content* of cultural adaptations, as well as *strategies* for determining the steps intervention developers might follow to identify adaptations designed to improve cultural fit. The process described in the formative method for adapting psychotherapy has much in common with other stage models of cultural adaptation (Barrera & Castro, 2006; Castro, Barrera, & Holleran Steiker, 2010; Domenech Rodríguez & Bernal, 2012).

How Effective Are Cultural Adaptations?

Thus far, there have been 12 meta-analyses concerned at least in part with the efficacy of culturally adapted therapies. The most recent review was also the most comprehensive by including all of the relevant studies covered in the previous 11 meta-analyses, in addition to new studies not included in previous reviews (Hall, Ibaraki, Huang, Marti, & Stice, 2017). All of these reviews presented evidence of at least moderate effect sizes when cultural adaptations were compared to control conditions. Hall and colleagues examined several factors that might moderate the efficacy of culturally adapted therapies. One hypothesized moderator, client–therapist ethnic matching, did not show a significant effect. Culturally adapted therapies had moderate effect sizes with and without client–therapist ethnic matching. Practitioners serving children and families will find the meta-analysis by Huey and Polo (2008) particularly informative because it contains a table showing the interventions, ethnic/racial group participants, and target disorders for interventions classified as "probably efficacious" and "possibly efficacious" (p. 284).

Of the many excellent meta-analytic reviews, the one by Benish and colleagues (2011) distinguished itself with its rare, theory-inspired test of a viable mechanism underlying the effectiveness of culturally adapted therapies. They proposed that an active mechanism is the intervention's ability to change clients' *schemas,* that is, their explanatory models of illness ("illness myths"). Such models are rooted in culture and used by clients to comprehend problems they experience, the perceived etiology of these problems, and the related plausibility of proposed interventions for relieving suffering. Frank and Frank's (1993) well-known articulation of the four essential features of therapeutic practice include (1) the provision of a model that explains illness and its remedy, (2) a meaningful relationship with a culturally sanctioned healer, (3) a specialized setting that contains cultural symbols of healing, and (4) a set of procedures (healing practices) for overcoming illness. Therapeutic change occurs when ineffective explanatory models are replaced by others that mobilize hope, healthful thinking, and behavioral manifestations of agency. Benish and colleagues' analyses indicated that cultural adaptations had impressive effect sizes when compared to heterogeneous control conditions ($d = 0.41$) and other active therapies ($d = 0.32$). Furthermore, studies containing cultural adaptations that addressed clients' explanatory models appeared to account for the beneficial effects of culturally adapted psychotherapies. The meta-analysis used Barts Explanatory Model Inventory to determine if culturally adapted therapies attended to explanatory models (Rudell, Bhui, & Priebe, 2009). That assessment framework included the five aspects of explanatory models: types of symptoms expressed (e.g., somatic, mental, behavioral), perceptions of illness causes, predictions of illness course (acute, chronic, episodic), expected illness consequences, and perceptions of appropriate treatment. The authors discussed the important implications of their findings, which we summarize near the end of this chapter.

To summarize, all of these meta-analyses revealed that culturally adapted therapies were superior to control conditions. Furthermore, Benish and colleagues (2011) found that culturally adapted therapies were significantly more effective than bona fide unadapted therapies. That finding differs from the results of the review by Huey and Polo (2008), who found significant and comparable effects for culturally adapted and unadapted therapies for ethnic/minority children and adolescents. Huey and Polo cautioned that most of the studies they reviewed had low statistical power and did not include the participation of unacculturated youth. Other reviews indicated that the benefits of culturally adapted therapies were more apparent for adults and those low in acculturation than they were for children and those who were relatively acculturated (Griner & Smith, 2006; Smith, Rodriguez, & Bernal, 2011). Those findings support the prime motivation for culturally adapting psychotherapies; The adaptations appear to benefit those who are most closely affiliated with the culture for which the original psychotherapies were modified.

Examples of Culturally Adapted Interventions for EBP

La Roche, Batista, and D'Angelo (2011) observed that many have called for the inclusion of cultural characteristics in psychotherapies as a means to increase treatment engagement and effectiveness. However, studies rarely determine whether culturally adapted therapies change the hypothesized cultural variables, and whether those changes explain therapy outcomes. The research by La Roche and colleagues is noteworthy because it included the assessment of a cultural variable and evaluated its relation to anxiety treatment engagement and outcome. *Allocentrism,* the tendency to define oneself in relationship to others, was hypothesized to be an element of Latino cultures that could be incorporated in a relaxation intervention to improve its cultural fit. Specifically, guided imagery scripts that ordinarily involve individual scenes (e.g., imagining oneself sitting alone on a peaceful beach) were replaced by scripts that emphasized relatedness (e.g., imagining oneself surrounded by loved ones) (La Roche et al., 2011). In their uncontrolled, pre- and posttreatment follow-up study of 44 Latina/o adult clients who reported high levels of anxiety symptoms, allocentrism was endorsed three times more than *idiocentrism* (the tendency to define oneself in isolation of others). That finding was consistent with the investigators' hypothesis that for Latinos, allocentrism is a more prominent orientation than idiocentrism. Over 8 weeks of anxiety treatment, which included homework assignments to practice imagery-guided relaxation, Latina/o clients used allocentric imagery exercises significantly more often than idiocentric imagery exercises. Furthermore, there was a significant relation between the number of allocentric exercises performed and anxiety reduction. In summary, when a culturally compatible treatment exercise (allocentric imagery) was made available to Latina/o clients, they used it, and that use was related to anxiety reduction.

Another example illustrated how an empirically supported treatment for posttraumatic stress disorder, cognitive processing therapy, was adapted to provide a better cultural fit for refugees from the civil war in Bosnia and Herzegovina who relocated to the United States (Schulz, Huber, & Resick, 2006). The article's authors explained how critical it is for therapists to become knowledgeable about the multiple and intense traumas that challenge refugees, the somewhat unique symptom features (e.g., choking sensations), and the attitudes among some clients with low formal education, including negative views about needing to receive professional mental health services. They made specific recommendations about incorporating translators into sessions, such as the admonition to speak directly to the client (rather than to the translator) and to train translators to fully report clients' utterances (rather than censoring material they think might be embarrassing or inaccurate). The authors provided an abbreviated session transcript that illustrated concrete methods employed by the therapist to show respect for the client's explanatory model, such as when the therapist did not insist that the client reject her belief in black magic. Unlike some cultural adaptation multistep frameworks that make use of qualitative and quantitative research, the adaptation method demonstrated by Schulz and colleagues (2006) could be implemented with individual clients by culturally competent practitioners who had experience with a particular subcultural group.

The edited volume by Bernal and Domenech Rodríguez (2012) contains many chapters that illustrate cultural adaptations of psychotherapies with a variety of ethnocultural client groups. That volume is a valuable resource for practitioners who want to learn from examples of integrating culture into EBP.

Implications for EBP

The meta-analysis by Benish and colleagues (2011) included several recommendations that followed from their conclusion that understanding and then adjusting clients' explanatory models in psychotherapy might account for the salutary effects of cultural adaptations. From those recommendations, therapists should start by understanding and showing respect for clients' initial explanatory models before attempting to change them. This may be accomplished by conducting initial interviews guided by the DSM-5 Cultural Formulation Interview (American Psychiatric Association, 2013). Benish and colleagues suggested that through client–therapist collaboration or "co-creation," new explanatory models could be negotiated to better position clients for change and improvement. This focus on explanatory models, one of the four general features of therapeutic practices (Frank & Frank, 1993), differs from other cultural adaptation approaches that are directed at individual components ("ingredients") of interventions (e.g., the content of guided imagery scripts). Clearly, this is not an "either–or" proposition. Therapists can implement a general method such as explanatory model exploration, as well as adapt more specific components of a treatment regimen.

Client Variables

Thus far, research on client variables has identified two that appear to moderate the effects of culturally adapted interventions—acculturation and age of client. Adults and those who are relatively unacculturated might have a special need for culturally adapted therapies and might benefit from them the most. In the absence of data from a large number of studies, it is difficult to specify which client cultural features influence treatment engagement and outcome. Nevertheless, the study by La Roche and colleagues (2011) demonstrated how knowledge of the literature and of culture led to the identification of a client cultural variable (allocentrism) and to treatment adaptations that were correlated with engagement and symptom reduction. When practitioners work with clients of different cultural subgroups, they too can turn to the literature to learn of potentially relevant cultural variables (Castro & Hernández Alarcón, 2002), determine whether they are applicable to specific cases, and consider how they might be incorporated into treatment procedures.

Therapist Cultural Competence

In addition to culture-specific skills, Sue's (1998, 2006) analyses of cultural competence identified two general orientations, scientific mindedness and dynamic sizing, that are extensions of fundamentally sound clinical practices to issues of culture. Well-trained practitioners are familiar with the dangers of unfounded assumptions and the value of understanding the meaning and relevance of concepts for each client. Competent therapists avoid rudimentary understanding of clients' cultural backgrounds, which can promote stereotypical conceptualizations of client thinking and behavior. Culture-specific skills can be acquired. As illustrated in the example provided by Schulz and colleagues (2006), therapists can be well informed about the life experiences of clients from different cultures and the specialized circumstances impinging on their lives (e.g., civil war), particularly when there are focused efforts to provide them with programmatic clinical services. It is impossible for practitioners to be proficient in culture-specific skills for every imaginable subcultural group, but it is possible to attain such skills for some groups through study, clinical experience, and consultation with experts.

Culturally Adapted Interventions

The results of meta-analytic reviews should bring comfort to those who are considering cultural adaptations to therapies or adaptations made by others. Obviously, the meta-analyses are valuable because they provide references to studies that evaluated the efficacy of adapted versions. Even though some articles do not give adequate descriptions of adaptations to inform clinical practice, many do. As noted previously, the review by Huey and Polo (2008) has special value to child and family practitioners because it contains a table showing the interventions, ethnic/racial group participants, and target disorders for interventions classified as "probably efficacious" and "possibly efficacious."

Cultural adaptations can be done that still preserve interventions' core components. Kendall and Beidas (2007) demonstrated how "flexibility within fidelity" could be achieved with some manualized therapies, suggesting that flexibility to accommodate cultural adaptations is certainly possible. It is important to recognize that therapies vary in flexibility. For example, behavioral activation approaches that use activity schedules can incorporate salsa dancing, as well as ballroom dancing, eating Chinese food as readily as Cajun dishes. Well-known problem-solving therapies could include solution strategies grounded in any number of cultural group practices. Flexible EBIs bring the best of both worlds to EBP with subcultural group clients: the replicability of rigorously tested intervention methods with the capacity to be adapted to fit the diversity of client characteristics.

Cultural Considerations in the EBP Process

It is premature to propose a user's guide to the cultural adaptation literature similar to the consensus users' guides for incorporating research literature into medical practice. Some of the medical evidence-based user guides have specified a "hierarchy of strength of evidence for treatment decisions" for medical practitioners (e.g., Guyatt et al., 2000). For instance, the hierarchy described by Guyatt and members of the Evidence-Based Medicine Working Group placed N-of-1 randomized trials at the very top of the hierarchy followed by systematic reviews of randomized trials, single randomized trial, systematic review of observational studies addressing patient-important outcomes,

single observational study addressing patient-important outcomes, physiological studies, and unsystematic clinical observations. Because the research literature on culturally adapted treatment is still evolving, it is most appropriate to urge therapists to follow the general steps in the EBP process, a principled approach that is not rigidly prescriptive (Rubin & Bellamy, 2012). Rubin and Bellamy's *Practitioner's Guide to Using Research for Evidence-Based Practice* (2012), an excellent resource for novice and experienced practitioners, contains lucid explanations of the general EBP process, as well as concrete information about finding and evaluating research literature that can be translated into practice. Several points deserve consideration in EBP decision making about using culturally adapted psychotherapies with clients.

Recall that the defining feature of EBP is "the integration of the best available research with clinical expertise in the context of patient characteristics, culture, and preferences" (American Psychological Association Presidential Task Force on Evidence-Based Practice, 2006, p. 273). As noted previously, it is advantageous to start the integration with a thorough understanding of clients' backgrounds and their explanatory models for presenting problems (Benish et al., 2011). DSM-5's Cultural Formulation Interview (American Psychiatric Association, 2013) is a good method for assessing relevant information. One client characteristic that should be assessed is acculturation, a variable that appears to moderate the effectiveness of culturally adapted therapies (Griner & Smith, 2006; Smith et al., 2011). In the later steps of the EBP process, a practitioner might use information about a client's acculturation to favor the use of a culturally adapted intervention for an unacculturated client or use the unadapted original version for a highly acculturated client.

A practitioner's determination of a treatment, including a culturally adapted treatment, to offer a particular client can be guided by a five-step EBP process (Rubin & Bellamy, 2012). The first step is the formulation of EBP question, which might be something like "Which depression treatments have been effective for Puerto Rican adults who live in U.S. urban regions?" Questions can be tailored to fit a particular client, then expanded or contracted depending on the literature that is found in the second step—the search for evidence. The use of search engines, literature reviews, and other resources is described in detail by Rubin and Bellamy (2012). In the case of culturally adapted therapies, 12 meta-analyses are available for both identifying individual studies and accessing conclusions based on cumulative evidence. The third step is to critically evaluate the evidence found. There is no simple way to formalize the critical thinking involved in this step that depends so heavily on the breadth and quality of the pertinent knowledge. In appraising the literature, practitioners are urged to exercise caution when encountering broad terms such as *Hispanic* or *Asian* that lack meaningful specificity of nationality, regional distinctions, and urban–rural differences. Adaptations developed and evaluated with one sample (e.g., rural adults of Mexican heritage living in the Southwest) might have questionable applicability in another sample (e.g., urban Puerto Rican adults living in the Northeast). Also, practitioners might have to decide between a cultural adaptation that was evaluated in a single randomized controlled trial (RCT) and an unadapted generic therapy that was evaluated in numerous studies. Fortunately, culturally adapted therapies often retain the core components of original therapies.

As a fourth step, practitioners implement the intervention that was selected with client's input. A client's preferences not only reflect the joint influences of multiple identities that are not limited to race and ethnicity but also include the unique blend of family history, education, socioeconomic status, sexual orientation, and other client characteristics. Practicing collaboration with clients relieves therapists of the tenuous position of unilaterally judging how to incorporate all aspects of culture into interventions. A fifth step is monitoring client progress, which is a product of the intervention, the therapist's ability to implement the intervention's specific factors and to establish nonspecific therapy conditions, and client characteristics. The EBP process need not end with a client's unsuccessful experience with the initial phases of the first intervention that was selected. The fifth step might lead to a reconsideration of the other intervention approaches that were found and evaluated in earlier steps in the EBP process.

References

American Psychiatric Association. (2013). *Diagnostic and statistical manual of mental disorders* (5th ed.). Arlington, VA: Author.

American Psychological Association. (2003). Guidelines on multicultural education, training, research, practice and organizational change for psychologists. *American Psychologist, 58,* 377–402.

American Psychological Association Presidential Task Force on Evidence-Based Practice. (2006). Evidence-based practice in psychology. *American Psychologist, 61*(4), 271–285.

Angel, R., & Guarnaccia, P. J. (1989). Mind, body, and culture: Somatization among Hispanics. *Social Science and Medicine, 28*(12), 1229–1238.

Barrera, M., Jr., & Castro, F. G. (2006). A heuristic framework for the cultural adaptation of interventions. *Clinical Psychology: Science and Practice, 13,* 311–316.

Barrera, M., Jr., Castro, F. G., Strycker, L. A., & Toobert, D. J. (2013). Cultural adaptation of behavioral health interventions: A progress report. *Journal of Consulting and Clinical Psychology, 81,* 196–205.

Benish, S. G., Quintana, W., & Wampold, B. (2011). Culturally adapted psychotherapy and the legitimacy of myth: A direct comparison meta-analysis. *Journal of Counseling Psychology, 58,* 279–289.

Bernal, G., Bonilla, J., & Bellido, C. (1995). Ecological validity and cultural sensitivity for outcome research: Issues for cultural adaptation and development of psychosocial treatments with Hispanics. *Journal of Abnormal Child Psychology, 23,* 67–82.

Bernal, G. E., & Domenech Rodríguez, M. M. (Eds.). (2012). *Cultural adaptations: Tools for evidence-based practice with diverse populations.* Washington, DC: American Psychological Association.

Bernal, G., Jiménez-Chafey, M. I., & Domenech Rodríquez, M. M. (2009). Cultural adaptation of treatments: A resource for considering culture in evidence-based practice. *Professional Psychology: Research and Practice, 40,* 361–368.

Bernal, G., & Scharrón-del-Río, M. R. (2001). Are empirically supported treatments valid for ethnic minorities?: Toward an alternative approach for treatment research. *Cultural Diversity and Ethnic Minority Psychology, 7,* 328–342.

Cardemil, E. V. (2010a). The complexity of culture: Do we embrace the challenge or avoid it? *Scientific Review of Mental Health Practice, 7*(2), 41–47.

Cardemil, E. V. (2010b). Cultural adaptations to empirically supported treatments: A research agenda. *Scientific Review of Mental Health Practice, 7*(2), 8–21.

Castro, F. G. (1998). Cultural competence training in clinical psychology. Assessment, clinical intervention, and research. In A. S. Bellack & M. Hersen (Eds.), *Comprehensive clinical psychology: Sociocultural and individual differences* (Vol. 10, pp. 127–140). Oxford, UK: Pergamon.

Castro, F. G., Barrera, M., Jr., & Holleran Steiker, L. K. (2010). Issues and challenges in the design of culturally adapted evidence-based interventions. *Annual Review of Clinical Psychology, 6,* 213–239.

Castro, F. G., & Hernández Alarcón, E. (2002). Integrating cultural factors into drug abuse prevention and treatment with racial/ethnic minorities. *Journal of Drug Issues, 32,* 783–810.

Castro, F. G., & Nieri, T. (2010). Cultural factors in drug

use etiology: Concepts, methods, and recent findings. In L. M. Scheier (Ed.), *Handbook of drug use etiology: Theory, methods, and empirical findings* (pp. 305–324). Washington, DC: American Psychological Association.

Chambless, D. L., & Ollendick, T. H. (2001). Empirically supported psychological interventions: Controversies and evidence. *Annual Review of Psychology, 52*(1), 685–716.

Chowdhary, N., Jotheeswaran, A. T., Nadkarni, A., Hollon, S. D., King, M., Jordans, M. J. D., et al. (2014). The methods and outcomes of cultural adaptations of psychological treatments for depressive disorders: A systematic review. *Psychological Medicine, 44*(6), 1131–1146.

Cohen, A. B. (2009). Many forms of culture. *American Psychologist, 64*(3), 194–204.

Costantino, G., Malgady, R. G., & Rogler, L. H. (1986). Cuento therapy: A culturally sensitive modality for Puerto Rican children. *Journal of Consulting and Clinical Psychology, 54,* 639–645.

Cross, T. L., Bazron, K. W., Dennis, K. W., & Isaacs, M. R. (1989). *The cultural competence continuum: Towards a culturally competent system of care.* Washington, DC: Georgetown University.

Domenech Rodríguez, M. M., & Bernal, G. (2012). Frameworks, models, and guidelines for cultural adaptation. In G. Bernal & M. M. Domenech Rodríguez (Eds.), *Cultural adaptations: Tools for evidence-based practice with diverse populations.* (pp. 23–44). Washington, DC: American Psychological Association.

Frank, J. D., & Frank, J. B. (1993). *Persuasion and healing: A comparative study of psychotherapy.* Baltimore: Johns Hopkins University Press.

Griner, D., & Smith, T. B. (2006). Culturally adapted mental health intervention: A meta-analytic review. *Psychotherapy, 43,* 531–548.

Guyatt, G. H., Haynes, R. B., Jaeschke, R. Z., Cook, D. J., Green, L., Naylor, C. D., et al. (2000). Users' guides to the medical literature: XXV. Evidence-based medicine: Principles for applying the users' guides to patient care. *Journal of the American Medical Association, 284*(10), 1290–1296.

Hall, G. C., Ibaraki, A. Y., Huang, E. R., Marti, C. N., & Stice, E. (2017). A meta-analysis of cultural adaptations of psychological interventions. *Behavior Therapy, 47*(6), 993–1014.

Huey, S. J., Jr., & Polo, A. J. (2008). Evidence-based psychosocial treatments for ethnic minority youth. *Journal of Clinical Child and Adolescent Psychology, 37,* 262–301.

Hwang, W. C. (2012). Integrating top-down and bottom-up approaches to culturally adapting psychotherapy: Application to Chinese-Americans. In G. Bernal & M. M. Domenech Rodríguez (Eds.), *Cultural adaptations: Tools for evidence-based practice with diverse populations* (pp. 179–198). Washington, DC: American Psychological Association.

Kendall, P. C., & Beidas, R. S. (2007). Smoothing the

trail for dissemination of evidence-based practices for youth: Flexibility within fidelity. *Professional Psychology: Research and Practice, 38*(1), 13–20.

Kendall, P. C., Chu, B., Gifford, A., Hayes, C., & Nauta, M. (1999). Breathing life into a manual: Flexibility and creativity with manual-based treatments. *Cognitive and Behavioral Practice, 5*(2), 177–198.

Kluckhohn, C. E., & Murray, H. A. (1948). *Personality in nature, society, and culture.* New York: Knopf.

La Roche, M. J., Batista, C., & D'Angelo, E. (2011). A culturally competent relaxation intervention for Latino/as: Assessing a culturally specific match model. *American Journal of Orthopsychiatry, 81*(4), 535–542.

La Roche, M. J., & Christopher, M. S. (2009). Changing paradigms from empirically supported treatment to evidence-based practice: A cultural perspective. *Professional Psychology: Research and Practice, 40*(4), 396–402.

Lau, A. S. (2006). Making a case for selective and directed cultural adaptations of evidence-based treatments: Examples from parent training. *Clinical Psychology: Science and Practice, 13,* 295–310.

Office of Behavioral and Social Science Research. (2014). The cultural framework for health: An integration approach for research and program design and evaluation. Retrieved March 13, 2016, from *https://obssr-archive.od.nih.gov/pdf/cultural_framework_for_health.pdf.*

Orlandi, M. A., Weston, R., & Epstein, L. G. (1992). *Cultural competence for evaluators.* Rockville, MD: Office of Substance Abuse Prevention.

Parker, G., Gladstone, G., & Chee, K. T. (2001). Depression in the planet's largest ethnic group: The Chinese. *American Journal of Psychiatry, 158,* 857–864.

Ponterotto, J. G., Rieger, B. P., Barrett, A., & Sparks, R. (1994). Assessing multicultural counseling competence: A review of instrumentation. *Journal of Counseling and Development, 72*(3), 316–322.

Resnicow, K., Soler, R., Braithwait, R. L., Ahluwalia, J. S., & Butler, J. (2000). Cultural sensitivity in substance abuse prevention. *Journal of Community Psychology, 28,* 271–290.

Rubin, A., & Bellamy, J. (2012). *Practitioner's guide to using research for evidence-based practice.* Hoboken, NJ: Wiley.

Rudell, K., Bhui, K., & Priebe, S. (2009). Concept, development and application of a new mixed method assessment of cultural variations in illness perceptions: Barts Explanatory Model Inventory. *Journal of Health Psychology, 14,* 336–347.

Ryder, A. G., Yang, J., Zhu, X., Yao, S., Yi, J., Heine, S. J., et al. (2008). The cultural shaping of depression: Somatic symptoms in China, psychological symptoms in North America? *Journal of Abnormal Psychology, 117,* 300–313.

Schulz, P. M., Huber, L. C., & Resick, P. A. (2006). Practical adaptations of cognitive processing therapy with Bosnian refugees: Implications for adapting practice to a multicultural clientele. *Cognitive and Behavioral Practice, 13*(4), 310–321.

Shiraev, E. B., & Levy, D. A. (2010). *Cross-cultural psychology: Critical thinking and contemporary applications* (4th ed.). Boston: Allyn & Bacon.

Smith, T. B., Rodriguez, M. D., & Bernal, G. (2011). Culture. *Journal of Clinical Psychology, 67,* 166–175.

Spring, B. (2007). Evidence-based practice in clinical psychology: What it is, why it matters; what you need to know. *Journal of Clinical Psychology, 63,* 611–631.

Substance Abuse and Mental Health Services Administration. (2014). *Improving cultural competence* (Treatment Improvement Protocol [TIP] Series No. 59; HHS Publication No. SMA 14-4849). Rockville, MD: Author.

Sue, D. W., & Sue, D. (1999). *Counseling the culturally different: Theory and practice* (3rd ed.). New York: Wiley.

Sue, S. (1998). In search of cultural competence in psychotherapy and counseling. *American Psychologist, 53,* 440–448.

Sue, S. (2006). Cultural competency: From philosophy to research and practice. *Journal of Community Psychology, 34*(2), 237–245.

Szapocznik, J., Rio, A., Perez-Vidal, A., Kurtines, W., Hervis, O., & Santisteban, D. (1986). Bieultural effectiveness training (BET): An experimental test of an intervention modality for families experiencing intergenerational/intercultural conflict. *Hispanic Journal of Behavioral Sciences, 8,* 303–330.

Whaley, A. L., & Davis, K. E. (2007). Cultural competence and evidence-based practice in mental health services: A complementary perspective. *American Psychologist, 62*(6), 563–574.

CHAPTER 9

Reaching the Unreached

The Importance of Context in Evidence-Based Practice in Low-Resource Settings

SYED USMAN HAMDANI
ATIF RAHMAN

Mental, neurological, and substance use (MNS) disorders are chronic, disabling conditions. Fourteen percent of the global burden of disease is attributed to neuropsychiatric conditions (Whiteford, Ferrari, Degenhardt, Feigin, & Vos, 2015). Although absence of curative and preventative interventions contribute to huge burden of MNS disorders, evidence-based therapies, where present, are unavailable to those in need. This treatment gap is particularly huge in low- and middle-income countries (LMICs). LMICs, classified according to World Bank criteria, comprise 85% of the world's population (World Bank, 2015). Four out of five people in LMICs in need of MNS disorders services do not get them (Murray et al., 2011). Even when the services are available, they are neither evidence based nor of high quality.

Availability of mental health services in LMICs lag far behind the availability of other health-related services (Prince et al., 2007; Saxena, Thornicroft, Knapp, & Whiteford, 2007). This disparity in availability of services for MNS disorders is attributable to a number of factors both inside and outside the health sector, including but not limited to very low financing for mental health services, the stigma associated with mental illness, lack of awareness about mental health problems, the huge burden of MNS disorders, and lack of trained human resource and integration of mental health services in the primary health care systems (Kohn, Saxena, Levav, & Saraceno, 2004). The failure to prevent, treat, and protect this vulnerable population affected by MNS disorders due to nonavailability of mental health services results is a situation that has been described very accurately as the "failure of humanity" (Kleinman, 2009).

A balance between hospital- and community-based health services has been shown to be most effective in the provision of mental health services (Thornicroft & Tansella, 2004). However this has only been achieved in a few high-income countries, with adequate financial resources matched by the political will. Primary health care (PHC) systems remain the mainstay for "at scale" delivery of evidence-based mental health services in LMICs. However, lack of financial and trained human resources, inequitable distribution of scarce financial and human resources allocated for mental health services, lack of community-based mental health care, and lack of integration of community mental health services with primary health care systems have been identified as the key barriers in the scale up of evidence-based mental health services (Eaton et al., 2011; Saxena et al., 2007; Yamey, 2012).

The World Health Organization Mental Health Gap Program

To bridge the treatment gap for MNS disorders, particularly in LMICs, the World Health Organization (WHO; 2010) launched the Mental Health Gap Action Program (mhGAP), whose aim is to implement and scale up evidence-based services for priority MNS disorders. The priority of disorders is based on the burden of disease, mortality, morbidity, high economic costs, and violations of human rights associated with those disorders. The priority conditions included are depression, psychosis, bipolar disorders, epilepsy, developmental and behavioral disorders in children and adolescents, dementia, alcohol use disorders, drug use disorders, and self-harm/suicide.

A key hallmark of the WHO mhGAP is the selection of evidence-based interventions for priority mental health conditions (Dua et al., 2011). To achieve this, the WHO established a Guideline Development Group (GDG) in 2008 to create evidence-based recommendations that adhered to the Grading of Recommendations Assessment, Development and Evaluation (GRADE) principles for developing transparent, evidence-based WHO guidelines (Dua et al., 2011). Using this methodology, the group systematically synthesized and appraised the evidence base for interventions to treat priority mental health conditions in PHC settings, leading to the publication of the Mental Health Gap Intervention Guide (mhGAP-IG). While the mhGAP-IG provides guidelines for *what* to do, it does not specify *how* to do it. This becomes particularly relevant given that the settings in which mhGAP interventions are supposed to be implemented have neither the means nor the resources to implement such programs.

Task Shifting in Mental Health

There is evidence to support the idea that scale up of evidence-based mental health services is possible in LMICs if community-based models are developed and implemented to support the primary care staff in early identification and treatment of mental disorders under supervision of specialists (Murray et al., 2011; Rahman, Malik, Sikander, Roberts, & Creed, 2008). In the absence of human and financial resources for at-scale and sustainable delivery of evidence-based mental health services in low-resource settings, task shifting has been proposed as an implementation strategy to scale up mental health services (Kakuma et al., 2011; Padmanathan & De Silva, 2013). *Task shifting* involves the provision of mental health services by nonspecialists with no or little prior experience in mental health service delivery. The evidence for the effectiveness of the task-shifting strategy has been established through randomized controlled trials of evidence-based psychosocial therapies delivered by nonspecialists in low-income and fragile settings of Uganda, Pakistan, and India (Bolton et al., 2003; Patel et al., 2010; Rahman et al., 2008).

This chapter provides an account of not only the challenges but also the opportunities in implementation of evidence-based interventions by lay health workers in the low-resource settings of Pakistan. We examine one successful example in which this was attempted. The case study describes the implementation of a WHO psychological therapy program for perinatal depression, the Thinking Healthy Program (THP), delivered by nonspecialist community health workers in rural Pakistan.

As this example reflects work in Pakistan, we must begin by sharing some of the basics of the context in that country and the regions in which we work. Pakistan is the sixth most populous country of the world, with a population of more than 180 million; 70% of the population lives in rural areas. About 41 million people in Pakistan live on less than 1.25 USD purchasing power parity (PPP) per day. The rate of malnutrition in children under age 5 is over 35% (World Bank, 2013). Public spending on health is just over 1% of the gross domestic product (GDP), of which less than 5% is allocated to mental health (World Health Organization, 2009).

In rural Pakistan, Primary Health Care (PHC) is delivered through a network of Basic Health Units, each of which provides care to about 15,000–20,000 people. Each unit is staffed by a doctor, a midwife, a vaccinator, and 15–20 village-based community health workers called Lady Health Workers (LHWs). These women have completed secondary school and are trained to provide mainly preventive maternal and child health care, and education in the community. Each LHW is responsible for about 100 households in her village. About 96,000 health workers in the LHW program provide coverage to more than 80% of Pakistan's rural population (some inaccessible areas, including some of the tribal areas, are not covered). Supervision of health workers takes the form of monthly supervision meetings that take place in the respective Basic Health Units (Hafeez, Mohamud, Shiekh, Shah, & Jooma, 2011).

We share this case study from Pakistan as an illustration of the ways in which the context of delivery is essential in determining the "how" for implementing mhGAP guidelines. In so doing, we offer our work on the global mental health stage as a powerful model for evidence-based practice (EBP) generally by highlighting the importance of thinking critically and creatively about context if we are to live up to the ethical principles that undergird EBP.

Cognitive-Behavioral Therapy for Perinatal Depression Delivered by Community Health Workers: The THP

Among the chronic noncommunicable diseases, depression is the fourth leading cause of disease burden. Depression accounts for almost 12% of years lived with disability worldwide (Whiteford et al., 2013). Perinatal depression (i.e., depression during or after pregnancy) has particularly long-term devastating consequences for both the mother and the newborn. It is associated with high rates of disability, infant malnutrition, increased rates of infant diarrhea, and reduced immunization rates in infants and young children (Rahman, Bunn, Lovel, & Creed, 2007; Rahman, Iqbal, Bunn, Lovel, & Harrington, 2004). Various studies from Pakistan have reported that the prevalence of perinatal depression is from 25 to 33% (Mirza & Jenkins, 2004; Rahman, Iqbal, & Harrington, 2003).

Evidence to support the effectiveness of psychotherapeutic programs such as cognitive-behavioral therapy (CBT), interpersonal therapy, or problem solving exists in both high-income countries (HICs) and LMICs (Churchill et al., 2002; Patel et al., 2007; Rojas et al., 2007). However, the key barrier to the scale up of such evidence-based therapies is the lack of mental health professionals to deliver such interventions in low-resource settings (Saxena et al., 2007). In order for these therapies to be delivered, they need to be adapted to be delivered by nonspecialists with little or no experience in the delivery of mental health and psychosocial support. Moreover, to ensure the sustainability and scalability of such programs, they need to be integrated in the existing high-priority public health programs (Prince et al., 2007).

To overcome these barriers, Rahman and colleagues (2007, 2008) conducted groundbreaking research in rural Pakistan to develop a culturally appropriate, lay-delivered, manualized intervention for perinatal depression. Based on the formative studies and a review of evidence-based therapies for depression by a panel of local mental health experts, CBT was chosen as the approach that could be adapted for use in the rural Pakistani population. The formative studies included in-depth interviews and focus group discussions with PHC staff, community health workers, and importantly, women and their families. This allowed an in-depth understanding of the local language, culture, and context through which psychological distress would manifest. It also allowed an appraisal of the local resources that could be utilized for the successful delivery of the intervention. The "here-and-now" problem-solving CBT approach was determined to meet the requirements reported by the stakeholders, and the local resources available for its delivery. Based on the findings, the intervention was simplified and fully manualized into the THP.

The program uses the CBT techniques of active listening, collaboration with the family, *guided discovery* (i.e., a style of questioning that gently probes for family members' health beliefs and stimulates alternative ideas), and homework (i.e., trying things out between sessions, putting what has been learned into practice), and applies these to health workers' routine practice of maternal and child health education. The pilot program was integrated into the existing PHC system and delivered by village-based community health workers (Rahman et al., 2008). Through our work on the THP, we have identified a set of five challenges and opportunities that are specific to this context and that, we believe, provide a helpful model to others in thinking about the role of context in EBP. These include adapting the strategies of the program to fit the needs of local providers, integrating the program into the local routine work, adapting training and supervision to fit the local context, evaluating the outcomes in the local context, and exploring expansion through peers and technology.

Adapting Strategies to Fit the Local Context

Although CBT is an established treatment for the depression, our work was unique in adapting it for effective delivered by nonspecialists in PHC settings. For this to be achieved, the principles of CBT were simplified and a three-step approach was adopted that was repeated throughout the program (Rahman, 2007). The first step involved training the Lady Health Workers in helping expectant mothers to identify unhelpful or unhealthy thinking styles and behaviors. The second step was training LHWs to help expectant mothers to replace the unhealthy thinking and behaviors with healthy thinking and behaviors. In this step, the traditional CBT approach also was adapted to suit the local context by involving significant family members in this process. The third step was to train the LHWs to help expectant mothers to develop activities to practice healthy thinking and behaviors.

The same three steps were applied to all domains of mother and child health during the pregnancy and after the birth, including mother–infant interaction, play, nutrition, psychosocial support, and involvement of significant family members. The content of the program was tailored to the needs of individual families. The key messages and routines of the program were reinforced by providing a "health calendar" to each mother. The health calendar used culturally appropriate illustrations to depict mother, infant, and significant family members' interactions with the LHW. By using the illustrations, the LHWs helped mothers and families to identify problems in thinking and behavior and replace them with alternative thoughts and behaviors. The illustrations helped the LHWs to effectively interact with illiterate populations and avoid direct confrontation with the families in reinforcing key messages. Table 9.1 summarizes the key components of the program that were adapted to fit the local context of delivery.

Integrating Delivery into Routine Work

Among the noncommunicable diseases, mental health services in low-income countries suffer most from the lack of dedicated human and financial resources to sustain the delivery of

---

TABLE 9.1. Essential Features of the THP

- *Theoretical basis.* Based on principles of CBT.

- *Delivering agent.* Village-based LHWs. Generally have completed high school, 6 months training in preventive maternal and child health. Intervention is simple enough to be delivered by lay counselors where LHWs do not exist.

- *Structure of intervention.* Sixteen sessions organized in five modules: 4 weekly sessions (Module 1—*Preparing for the Baby*) in the last month of pregnancy, 3 fortnightly sessions (Module 2—*The Baby's Arrival*) in the first postnatal month; 9 monthly sessions (Modules 3–5—*Early, Middle, and Late Infancy*) thereafter; each session lasts approximately 45 minutes.

- *Structure of session.* Active listening followed by three steps: Step 1: identifying unhealthy (unhelpful) thinking; Step 2: replacing unhealthy thinking with healthy thinking; Step 3: practicing healthy thinking and behaviors. Homework is given for each session.

- *Areas covered.* Each module covers three areas: mother's mood and personal health; mother–infant relationship; relationship of mother with significant other.

- *Tools.* Training manual with step-by-step instructions for conducting each session; activity workbooks for mothers; health calendar for families to monitor progress and activities; THP manual cross-referenced with LHW training manual.

- *Training.* Two-day training workshop followed by 1-day refresher after 4 months; includes training videos with actors conducting sessions; role plays and discussions.

- *Supervision.* Monthly half-day session in groups of 10; discussion of problems and "brainstorming" for solutions. Check for fidelity.

- *Additional features.* Use of pictures in addition to words for nonliterates; emphasis on being active listeners, as well as trainers; special training session on dealing with difficult situations.

effective mental health interventions at scale. Scalability and sustainability of effective mental health intervention programs can be ensured by designing the programs to suit integration into existing priority health platforms (Rahman, 2015). Most of the advanced psychosocial interventions available through the WHO mhGAP can be delivered by a range of PHC workers in low-income countries.

The implementation of the THP by LHWs in Pakistan was among the first such examples of successful task shifting. The THP was integrated into a child nutrition and early development program. The LHWs were selected as the delivery agents for task shifting based on the stakeholders' consultations and formative studies in the local settings. The LHWs are well embedded in the local communities and provide extended reach to the PHC system. The training of LHWs in specific THP skills such as behavior change, communication, motivational coaching, patient education, and self-management support were deemed critical to the effective delivery of routine mother and child health (MCH) services by the LHWs in

the PHC settings. Based on its feasibility, acceptability, and effectiveness, the THP has been adopted by the WHO as a first-line psychological intervention for perinatal depression (*www.who.int/maternal_health/maternal-child/ thinking_healthy/en*).

For integration into the MCH platform, the THP was adapted using the five-pillars approach (five-PA). The adaptation allowed the program to be a more universal intervention for MCH, increased its reach through the delivery by community health workers (CHWs), such as the LHW program in Pakistan, and provided a suitable platform for sustainable delivery at scale. Table 9.2 briefly describes the five-PA.

Training/Supervision in Context

Our attention to context also has led us to consider innovative training and supervision methods, such as cascade training/experiential learning (Murray et al., 2011). Since the THP was designed to be delivered by the nonspecialists in the PHC system, the training for the program was kept short—2 days of training

---

TABLE 9.2. The Five Pillars Approach (Five-PA) to Maternal Psychosochial Well-Being

The Five-PA is an adaptation for the THP to integerate it into a child nutrition and development programme (Zafar et al., 2014). The key feautre of the approach is that it is integerated into, and facilitates the delivery of, a community health worker (CHW)-delivered intervention for early child nutrition and development. Thus, whenever the CHW delivers a session for child nutrition or development, she uses the Five-PA approach to both strengthen the key messages as well as provide the psychosocial intervention. In practice, the approach work as follows:

- *Pillar 1. Family support.* An initial home visit emphasizes family particpation, and training manual gives specific instructions on how this can be facilitated. Family members are encouraged to be active partners for the whole duration of the program. Strategies to engage key decision makers, such as mothers-in-law and husband, are emphasized.

- *Pillar 2. Empathic listening.* Each session begins in an open-ended fashion, with the CHW allowing the woman to talk freely. She uses active listening skills to convey empathy and makes a list of problems the women faced in performing the desired behaviors that the CHW might have suggested in the previous visit.

- *Pillar 3. Guided discovery using pictures.* Each new health message related to play, stimulation, or nutrition is conveyed using this approach. Using carefully researched pictures, the CHW discusses both undesired and desired behaviors. She is trained not to impose her views but to allow the mother and family to consider each viewpoint and come to their own conclusions. The idea is that the basis of any behavior change begins at the cognitive level.

- *Pillar 4. Behavioral activation.* Once the message is received and accepted, the activities related to it have to be made manageable, so that a sense of mastery is achieved. The training manual has suggestions for how each nutrition or play-related task can be broken down and monitored with the help of family members.

- *Pillar 5. Problem solving.* The CHW spends time discussing the problem the woman faced in carring out the tasks suggested in the previous session (see Pillar 2). She discusses possible soloutions, which she can generate through discussion with the family or through her supervision.

followed by 1 day of refresher training after 4 months. However, the key ingredient of the program was monthly half-day supervision meetings of the LHWs by the trainers. Regular supervision of nonspecialist-delivered intervention programs has been cited as a critical factor for the success of such lay-delivered programs (Murray et al., 2011). Delivering mental health interventions in PHC settings can be a stressful job for nonspecialists. The supervision meetings not only allow the trainers to ensure the fidelity of the intervention program and promote peer-to-peer and experiential learning among the lay counselors but also allowed the lay workers to discuss successful and problem areas of their cases, to brainstorm culturally appropriate solutions, and to develop a supportive environment for themselves (Atif et al., 2019). In-low resource settings, the presence of such support groups to promote experiential learning and provide support is a sustainable and scalable means to ensure quality program delivery and enhancement of skills in the lay counselors.

Evaluating the Outcomes in the Local Context

Following the pilot studies to evaluate the feasibility and acceptability of the program in the local settings, the effectiveness evaluation of the THP on perinatal depression in women, and infant nutrition and other health outcomes were evaluated using a cluster randomized controlled trial design in two rural subdistricts of Pakistan (Rahman et al., 2008). The THP was delivered to the mothers by 40 specially trained LHWs. The intervention consisted of a session every week for 4 weeks in the last month of pregnancy, three sessions in the first postnatal month, and nine once-monthly sessions thereafter. Mothers in the control clusters received an equal number of visits in exactly the same way as those in the intervention group, but by routinely trained LHW. These health workers in both groups received monthly supervision and were monitored by the research team to ensure that they were attending the scheduled visits.

In a poor rural community with little access to mental health care, the intervention reduced the rate of depression by half in prenatally depressed women compared with those receiving enhanced routine care. In addition to symptomatic relief, the women receiving the intervention had less disability and better social and overall functioning, and these effects were sustained after 1 year (Maselko et al., 2015).

Extending Delivery through Peers and Technology

Despite the simplification of CBT strategies, designing the program for integration into the priority MCH platform from the outset, and robust evidence for the effectiveness of the program, the integration of THP into the LHWs daily routine has not been possible. Context, again, cannot be underestimated or ignored. The failure to integrate this program is largely attributable to the overexpanded job description of the LHWs in Pakistan (Haq & Hafeez, 2009). Hence, we identified a need to explore alternative human resources to support the LHWs in their delivery of psychosocial interventions in low-resource settings. This led to the development of "peer"-delivered version of the THP, the Thinking Healthy Program—Peer Delivery (THPP). There is a wealth of literature on the feasibility, acceptability, effectiveness, and cost-effectiveness of the peer-delivered educational and behavioral interventions. The term *peer* refers to someone who shares common sociocultural characteristics as the target population and/or uses his or her own experience of overcoming a health condition to help others (Atif et al., 2016; Singla et al., 2014).

We began our exploration of working with peers in much the same way that we did our original formative work with nonspecialists. We started with a series of formative studies in India and Pakistan with women in the community and other stakeholders to evaluate the feasibility of THPP (Singla et al., 2014). The results of the formative studies showed that the psychosocial intervention delivered by the peer volunteers in the community settings would be feasible and acceptable but dependent on a number of factors, including peer volunteers' long-term motivation for this role, their ability to develop rapport with the families and the community, and whether they were from the same community and linked with the health systems. We then adapted the THP for delivery by the peer volunteers (THPP). Evaluation of the THPP is taking place in the form of randomized controlled trials in India and Pakistan.

In addition to our expansion through engaging peers, we also have encountered the need to think carefully about context in conceptualizing at-scale training and supervision (Zafar et al., 2014). At-scale training and supervision of lay health workers, including the peer volunteers, has been cited as a major challenge in the scale up of evidence-based psychosocial interventions. This is specially a problem in the context of weak and fragile health systems, displaced populations, and populations affected by humanitarian crises. Zafar and colleagues (2016) have developed a technology-assisted training and supervision system for the THP to train the lay health workers in a postconflict area of Pakistan. The evaluation of the training program took the form of a noninferiority randomized controlled trial. In the intervention arm, a lay counselor trained the LHWs in the THP using the training videos, whereas the LHWs were trained by a trainer in the control arm. The results of the evaluation indicate that the use of technology is as effective as use of the trainer (Rahmàn et al., 2019).

Conclusion

Implementation of EBP in underresourced settings presents both challenges and opportunities. Interventions need to be carefully adapted to the culture and context of the setting. The case study in this chapter demonstrates that an intervention can be simplified without losing the core ingredients that contribute to its effectiveness. Careful study of the context provides an opportunity to appraise the local resources and strengths that can be utilized for implementation. For example, peers can be effective delivery agents for an evidence-based intervention using simplified principles of CBT. Technology-based innovations such as delivery of training and supervision through online and tablet-based platforms can aid scale up. Cascade models of training and supervision allow many interventionists to be trained and supervised by a single specialist. The case study demonstrates that even in settings in which there are no mental health specialists, persons with mental health problems can access psychological interventions in an effective, acceptable, and feasible manner.

References

Atif, N., Lovell, K., Husain, N., Sikander, S., Patel, V., & Rahman, A. (2016). Barefoot therapists: Barriers and facilitators to delivering maternal mental health care through peer volunteers in Pakistan: A qualitative study. *International Journal of Mental Health Systems, 10*(1), 24.

Atif, N., Nisar, A., Bibi, A., Khan, S., Zulfiqar, S., Ahmad, I., et al. (2019). Scaling-up psychological interventions in resource-poor settings: Training and supervising peer volunteers to deliver the "Thinking Healthy Programme" for perinatal depression in rural Pakistan. *Global Mental Health, 6*, E4.

Bolton, P., Bass, J., Neugebauer, R., Verdeli, H., Clougherty, K. F., Wickramaratne, P., et al. (2003). Group interpersonal psychotherapy for depression in rural Uganda: A randomized controlled trial. *Journal of the American Medical Association, 289*(23), 3117–3124.

Churchill, R., Hunot, V., Corney, R., Knapp, M., McGuire, H., Tylee, A., et al. (2002). A systematic review of controlled trials of the effectiveness and cost-effectiveness of brief psychological treatments for depression. *Health Technology Assessment, 5*(35), 1–173.

Dua, T., Barbui, C., Clark, N., Fleischmann, A., Poznyak, V., van Ommeren, M., et al. (2011). Evidence-based guidelines for mental, neurological, and substance use disorders in low- and middle-income countries: Summary of WHO recommendations. *PLoS Medicine, 8*(11), e1001122.

Eaton, J., McCay, L., Semrau, M., Chatterjee, S., Baingana, F., Araya, R., et al. (2011). Scale up of services for mental health in low-income and middle-income countries. *Lancet, 378,* 1592–1603.

Hafeez, A., Mohamud, B. K., Shiekh, M. R., Shah, S. A. I., & Jooma, R. (2011). Lady health workers programme in Pakistan: Challenges, achievements and the way forward. *Journal of the Pakistan Medical Association, 61*(3), 210–215.

Haq, Z., & Hafeez, A. (2009). Knowledge and communication needs assessment of community health workers in a developing country: A qualitative study. *Human Resources for Health, 7*(1), 59.

Kakuma, R., Minas, H., van Ginneken, N., Dal Poz, M. R., Desiraju, K., Morris, J. E., et al. (2011). Human resources for mental health care: Current situation and strategies for action. *Lancet, 378,* 1654–1663.

Kleinman, A. (2009). Global mental health: A failure of humanity. *Lancet, 374,* 603–604.

Kohn, R., Saxena, S., Levav, I., & Saraceno, B. (2004). The treatment gap in mental health care. *Bulletin of the World Health Organization, 82*(11), 858–866.

Maselko, J., Sikander, S., Bhalotra, S., Bangash, O., Ganga, N., Mukherjee, S., et al. (2015). Effect of an early perinatal depression intervention on long-term child development outcomes: Follow-up of the Thinking Healthy Programme randomised controlled trial. *Lancet Psychiatry, 2*(7), 609–617.

Mirza, I., & Jenkins, R. (2004). Risk factors, prevalence, and treatment of anxiety and depressive disorders in Pakistan: Systematic review. *British Medical Journal, 328,* 794.

Murray, L. K., Dorsey, S., Bolton, P., Jordans, M. J., Rahman, A., Bass, J., et al. (2011). Building capacity in mental health interventions in low resource countries: An apprenticeship model for training local providers. *International Journal of Mental Health Systems, 5*(1), 30.

Padmanathan, P., & De Silva, M. J. (2013). The acceptability and feasibility of task-sharing for mental healthcare in low and middle income countries: A systematic review. *Social Science and Medicine, 97,* 82–86.

Patel, V., Araya, R., Chatterjee, S., Chisholm, D., Cohen, A., De Silva, M., et al. (2007). Treatment and prevention of mental disorders in low-income and middle-income countries. *Lancet, 370,* 991–1005.

Patel, V., Weiss, H. A., Chowdhary, N., Naik, S., Pednekar, S., Chatterjee, S., et al. (2010). Effectiveness of an intervention led by lay health counsellors for depressive and anxiety disorders in primary care in Goa, India (MANAS): A cluster randomised controlled trial. *Lancet, 376,* 2086–2095.

Prince, M., Patel, V., Saxena, S., Maj, M., Maselko, J., Phillips, M. R., et al. (2007). No health without mental health. *Lancet, 370,* 859–877.

Rahman, A. (2007). Challenges and opportunities in developing a psychological intervention for perinatal depression in rural Pakistan—a multi-method study. *Archives of women's mental health, 10*(5), 211–219.

Rahman, A. (2015). Integration of mental health into priority health service delivery platforms: Maternal and child health services. *Eastern Mediterranean Health Journal, 21*(7), 493–497.

Rahman, A., Akhtar, P., Hamdani, S., Atif, N., Nazir, H., Uddin, I., et al. (2019). Using technology to scale-up training and supervision of community health workers in the psychosocial management of perinatal depression: A non-inferiority, randomized controlled trial. *Global Mental Health, 6,* E8.

Rahman, A., Bunn, J., Lovel, H., & Creed, F. (2007). Maternal depression increases infant risk of diarrhoeal illness:—a cohort study. *Archives of Disease in Childhood, 92*(1), 24–28.

Rahman, A., Iqbal, Z., Bunn, J., Lovel, H., & Harrington, R. (2004). Impact of maternal depression on infant nutritional status and illness: A cohort study. *Archives of General Psychiatry, 61*(9), 946–952.

Rahman, A., Iqbal, Z., & Harrington, R. (2003). Life events, social support and depression in childbirth: Perspectives from a rural community in the developing world. *Psychological Medicine, 33*(7), 1161–1167.

Rahman, A., Malik, A., Sikander, S., Roberts, C., & Creed, F. (2008). Cognitive behaviour therapy-based intervention by community health workers for mothers with depression and their infants in rural Pakistan: A cluster-randomised controlled trial. *Lancet, 372,* 902–909.

Rojas, G., Fritsch, R., Solis, J., Jadresic, E., Castillo, C., González, M., et al. (2007). Treatment of postnatal depression in low-income mothers in primary-care clinics in Santiago, Chile: A randomised controlled trial. *Lancet, 370,* 1629–1637.

Saxena, S., Thornicroft, G., Knapp, M., & Whiteford, H. (2007). Resources for mental health: Scarcity, inequity, and inefficiency. *Lancet, 370,* 878–889.

Singla, D., Lazarus, A., Atif, N., Sikander, S., Bhatia, U., Ahmad, I., et al. (2014). "Someone like us": Delivering maternal mental health through peers in two South Asian contexts. *Journal of Affective Disorders, 168,* 452–458.

Thornicroft, G., & Tansella, M. (2004). Components of a modern mental health service: A pragmatic balance of community and hospital care. *British Journal of Psychiatry, 185*(4), 283–290.

Whiteford, H. A., Degenhardt, L., Rehm, J., Baxter, A. J., Ferrari, A. J., Erskine, H. E., et al. (2013). Global burden of disease attributable to mental and substance use disorders: Findings from the Global Burden of Disease Study 2010. *Lancet, 382,* 1575–1586.

Whiteford, H. A., Ferrari, A. J., Degenhardt, L., Feigin, V., & Vos, T. (2015). The global burden of mental, neurological and substance use disorders: An analysis from the Global Burden of Disease Study 2010. *PLOS ONE, 10*(2), e0116820.

World Bank. (2013). Human development indicators. Retrieved from *http://hdr.undp.org/en/countries/profiles/pak.*

World Bank. (2015). World Bank open data. Retrieved from *http://data.worldbank.org.*

World Health Organization. (2009). WHO-AIMS report on mental health system in Pakistan. Retrieved from *www.mindbank.info/item/1305.*

World Health Organization. (2010). *Mental Health Gap Action Programme (mhGAP) intervention guide for mental, neurological and substance use disorders in non-specialized health settings.* Geneva: Author.

Yamey, G. (2012). What are the barriers to scaling up health interventions in low and middle income countries?: A qualitative study of academic leaders in implementation science. *Globalization and Health, 8*(1), 11.

Zafar, S., Sikander, S., Hamdani, S. U., Atif, N., Akhtar, P., Nazir, H., et al. (2016). The effectiveness of technology-assisted cascade training and supervision of community health workers in delivering the Thinking Healthy Program for perinatal depression in a post-conflict area of Pakistan–study protocol for a randomized controlled trial. *Trials, 17*(1), 188.

Zafar, S., Sikander, S., Haq, Z., Hill, Z., Lingam, R., Skordis-Worrall, J., et al. (2014). Integrating maternal psychosocial well-being into a child-development intervention: The five-pillars approach. *Annals of the New York Academy of Sciences, 1308*(1), 107–117.

CHAPTER 10

Clinical Expertise

A Critical Issue in the Age of Evidence-Based Practice

BRUCE E. WAMPOLD
JAMES W. LICHTENBERG
RODNEY K. GOODYEAR
TERENCE J. G. TRACEY

It is probably safe to say that every psychotherapist wants to be an expert. We become therapists because we desire to assist people in distress, and we want to do it as well as we can. Yet achieving clinical expertise in psychotherapy is not at all easy. In fact, Tracey, Wampold, Lichtenberg, and Goodyear (2014) argue that there is little support for the presence of expertise within the profession of psychotherapy. Moreover, *expertise* is not even easy to define. Yet we do know much about expertise in psychotherapy: about why it is so difficult to achieve, and about the characteristics and actions of expert therapists.

In this chapter, we discuss the definition of *expertise,* as well as various alternatives for assessing it. We then turn to the issue of why it is difficult to become a psychotherapy expert and examine the research related to psychotherapy. We conclude with a discussion of the characteristics and actions of effective therapists, as well as implications for developing expertise and training of therapists.

What Is Expertise?

Generally, learning theorists define *experts* as "individuals [who] gradually acquire highly specialized competencies, which are needed for achieving consistently superior levels of per-

formance within a particular domain" (Ullén, Hambrick, & Mosing, 2016, p. 427). Three aspects of this definition are neither controversial nor debatable. The first of these is that expertise is domain specific. There is no such thing as a global expert; rather, individuals are experts in a particular domain (e.g., basketball) but not in others (e.g., music performance, or even baseball, as Michael Jordan discovered).

The second aspect is that experts' performance gradually improves over time. It is not sufficient to be really good in a domain but static in terms of skills level or performance. According to the definition of *expertise* we are using, experts continually, although gradually, improve. We return to the issue of improvement in psychotherapy later in this chapter.

The third aspect is that expertise is a designation assigned to an individual rather than to a particular performance. A baseball player with a mediocre batting average often will have more hits in a given game than a star hitter (i.e., an "expert"), as there are many factors other than the skill of the hitter that determine whether a player gets a hit at a given time at bat (Lewis, 2004).

The fourth and fifth aspects of this definition of *expertise* are more problematic when applied to psychotherapy. The definition of *expertise* mentions competencies, but as we shall see, what is meant by *competence* in psychotherapy is often not clear and may mislead us in our pursuit of expertise. The fifth aspect refers to superior levels of performance and raises the question "How do we identify those therapists who are superior performers?" We now turn to these two problematic issues, putting them in a historical context.

Competence in Psychotherapy

Often the terms *expertise* and *competence* are used synonymously. Indeed, the American Psychological Association's policy on evidence-based practice (EBP) in psychology states, "*Clinical expertise* refers to competence attained by psychologists through education, training, and experience that results in effective practice; the term is not meant to refer to extraordinary performance that might characterize an elite group (e.g., the top 2%) of clinicians" (American Psychological Association Presidential Task Force on Evidence-Based Practice, 2006, p. 274ff; original emphasis). The expertise literature, on the other hand, makes a distinction between steady growth leading to extraordinary performance as expertise, which is different than simply performing at expected levels of performance, which is competence. Nevertheless, the concept of competence in psychotherapy has arisen in many, seemingly independent discussions of psychotherapy practice. As we will see, what is discussed as competence is quite varied. And whereas the definition of *expertise* we are using speaks of competencies, simply to achieve competence by any of these understandings alone is not sufficient to achieve expertise.

Around the turn of the 21st century, educators and trainers in professional psychology, as well as other professions, including medicine, social work, and nursing, redirected their training programs toward a focus on competency-based graduate education, in response to a general movement in education to assess the knowledge and skills of students rather than assuming that achievement is a matter of matriculation toward a degree. Beginning with an initial articulation of the notion of core competencies in psychology (Peterson et al., 1992), and followed closely by the American Psychological Association's Committee on Accreditation (2002) publication of new guidelines and principles for the accreditation of graduate programs, internships, and postdoctoral residencies, a focus was placed on training for professional competence. Without

specifying what those competencies would include, competencies in professional psychology became a prominent movement in psychotherapy (Roberts, Borden, Christiansen, & Lopez, 2005; Rubin, et al., 2007). Various tasks forces, conferences, and training councils have worked to define and identify competence in professional psychology (Fouad et al., 2009; Kaslow, 2004; Kaslow et al., 2004; Rubin et al., 2007). Fouad and colleagues (2009, p. S6) provided the following definition, making a distinction between *competence* and *competencies*:

> Competence has been defined by Epstein and Hundert (2002) as the "habitual and judicious use of communication, knowledge, technical skills, clinical reasoning, emotions, values, and reflection in daily practice for the benefit of the individual and community being served" (p. 226). Competence also implies performance at an acceptable level, and presumes integration of multiple competencies. Competencies, then, are conceptualized as elements or components of competence, and consist of discrete knowledge, skills, and attitudes (Kaslow et al., 2004).

This definition has three particular difficulties relative to understanding competence as it relates to expertise. First, it is clear that competence is conceived of as a *sufficient* level of skill to perform *competently,* which is quite different than the idea of expertise as a *superior level* of performance. Of course, competence varies by level of training, and models have been proposed for stipulating and assessing competence at various levels, including doctoral education, internship, postdoctoral supervised service delivery, residency/fellowship, and professional practice levels (Fouad et al., 2009; Rodolfa et al., 2005). That is to say, what constitutes a sufficient and appropriate level of skill or professional competence is understood to differ by level of training and experience. Second, the descriptions of the competencies are quite general, and attempts to be more specific and to specify how such competencies would be assessed have not provided much clarification (e.g., Kaslow et al., 2007). A third, and related point, is that it is not clear that the competencies refer to those skills that are necessary for therapists to perform at a superior level, or even at a proficient level. For example, one of the competencies for practice is that the therapist "maintains satisfactory interpersonal relations with clients, peers, faculty, allied professionals, and the public" (Fouad et al., 2009, p. S12), although there is no evidence that good relationships with allied professionals is required to perform effectively as a therapist. Indeed, some therapists may have disrespect for other mental health professionals and still be effective therapists. Others are ambiguous, such as the behavior "Regularly uses knowledge of self to monitor and improve effectiveness as a professional" (Fouad et al., 2009, p. S13). For the most part, the competencies were developed either by borrowing from other professions, such as medicine, or through consensus among members of various tasks forces or conferences (Kaslow et al., 2004; Rubin et al., 2007), rather than being based on evidence about how psychotherapy produces benefits.

Another conceptualization of competence comes from the clinical trial literature. To adequately test the efficacy of a particular treatment, it is expected that therapists in the trial adhere to the treatment protocol competently. In their discussion of treatment integrity in clinical trials, which involves both adherence and competence, Waltz, Addis, Koerner, and Jacobson (1993) defined *competence* as "the level of skill shown by the therapist in delivering the treatment" (p. 620). Waltz and colleagues emphasized that competence is specific to the treatment being delivered, as treatments contain different ingredients, and these ingredients must be delivered skillfully. Thus, in their view, there is no such thing as general therapy competence. In terms of the learning theory definition of *expertise*, the domain is narrowed from psychotherapy generally to expertise in providing a particular treatment. Therefore, rather than the notion that there are expert therapists, there is an assumption that there are experts in delivering cognitive-behavioral therapy (CBT), experts in delivering psychodynamic therapy, and so on. In clinical trials, competence is typically measured by ratings on a treatment-specific competence measure, completed by "experts" in the treatment being delivered based on observing actual therapy. Competence conceived in this way is very different than competence discussed previously and is very much closer to the manner in which the concept in used in the definition of *expertise* in learning theory. However, as we discuss later in this chapter, competence ratings for particular treatments are problematic for a variety of reasons.

The historical context of competence in psychotherapy is highly relevant to our focus on expertise and the central issue of this volume— *evidence-based practice in psychology* (EBPP).

Across all mental health disciplines, expertise is a core component of EBP.

For example, according to the American Psychological Association Presidential Task Force on Evidence-Based Practice (2006, p. 273), EBPP "is the integration of the best available research with clinical expertise in the context of patient characteristics, culture, and preferences," forming a "three-legged stool" (i.e., evidence, clinical expertise, and patient preferences) modeled after EBP in medicine and adopted by most human service professions, including social work, nursing and education, as well as psychology. Although it would seem that the *clinical expertise* leg of the stool would comport with the learning theory definition of *expertise, clinical expertise,* as defined in the EBP statements of various professions generally and psychology particularly, is closer to the way in which competence was defined, as mentioned previously. EBPP is referring to basic competencies needed by all clinicians to be reasonably effective and is not referring to *expert performance,* as it has been defined in the expertise literature and the way we are using the term.

How Do We Identify Superior Performers?

Superior performance is a critical component of expertise. In this discussion, it is important to recall that expertise is a characteristic of therapists, as distinct from a particular instance of therapy; that is, to identify expert therapists, we need to identify therapists who consistently, but not necessarily constantly, exhibit superior performance, using whatever treatment they choose to deliver. Similar to baseball stars who may go hitless in a particular game, expert therapists will have patients who do not experience significant benefit, even though in the long run these therapists have superior performance compared to other therapists. But how should we identify therapists with superior performance? The four most frequently used strategies have been to rely on therapists' (1) degrees, credentials, or experience; (2) reputation; (3) performance; and (4) patient outcomes (Tracey et al., 2014).

The first strategy to identify psychotherapy experts is to examine their education and training, licensure in a particular jurisdiction or membership in the National Register of Health Service Providers, and advanced recognition, such as board certification by the American Board of Professional Psychology (ABPP) or awards related to practice or service to the profession. The logic of this strategy is that therapists learn from experience (e.g., by seeing more patients) and that at each stage of professional development, a greater skills level is expected and acquired. The aim of the competency movement we discussed earlier was that therapists or therapist trainees must demonstrate certain competencies before advancing, suggesting that therapists become better over time as they progress through stages of professional development. Within psychology, to become board certified by ABPP, a therapist must present a work sample and be examined by other board members, who presumably are experts. The problem with this strategy is that degrees, honors, licensure, awards, and the like, have at best a tenuous relationship to performance as a therapist (Wampold, Baldwin, Holtforth, & Imel, 2017). With the exception of the training context and the examination for board certification, for the most part, what therapists actually do in the therapy room is done outside the view of observers, so the link between these indicators of expertise and performance is most likely weak.

The second strategy involves having informants identify who are experts. In many ways, expertise in the arts and culinary pursuits is determined by art and restaurant critics, but unlike psychotherapy, these critics view the art and taste the food. In psychotherapy, nominations for expertise usually come from other therapists. Many of us are asked for referrals to therapists in our communities and we usually are agreeable to providing such referrals, although typically we make those referrals based on reputation or on interactions we have had with the therapist, but not by observing the therapist's performance in therapy or by outcomes achieved by that therapist. Major treatises on expertise and professional development are often based on experts so identified (e.g., Skovholt & Jennings, 2004). Another problem for this strategy is determining who should be the informants who identify the experts—do the informants themselves need to be experts?

The third strategy involves assessing performance in therapy, which is much closer to the phenomenon of interest (i.e., psychotherapy) than either of the two previously discussed strategies (i.e., degrees/credentials/experience and reputation). According to this strategy, *experts* are those whose performance at doing therapy is best (Hill, Spiegel, Hoffman, Kivlighan, & Gelso, 2017; Shanteau & Weiss, 2014). But what is the standard by which we judge the performance? This is a particularly difficult question for psychotherapy because we have many treatment models and debates about which models should be used (Wampold & Imel, 2015)—that is, what exactly is expert performance in psychotherapy? One possibility is to allow experts in a particular treatment decide what desired performance is. The major issue here, as we discuss more fully in the next section, is that ratings of competence are not consistently related to outcomes (Boswell et al., 2013; Webb, DeRubeis, & Barber, 2010). Thus, we might be rating aspects of the psychotherapy activity that are unimportant for the benefit of the patient.

The fourth way to identify superior performance is to focus on patient outcomes. Simply said, according to this view, superior performance is reflected by the benefits experienced by patients, and accordingly, expert therapists are those whose patients have the best outcomes. The analogy might be chess: Magnus Carlsen, the reigning World Chess Champion, is an expert because he wins games and defeats his opponents, as he did recently in the World Chess Championship against Fabiano Caruana, and not because his strategies are aesthetic or appreciated, or because he has been nominated by his peers to be an expert. In psychotherapy, according to this perspective, experts are those who help their patients to a greater extent than do other therapists. As we discuss later, it is well established that some therapists consistently achieve better outcomes than do other therapists (Baldwin & Imel, 2013; Johns, Barkham, Kellett, & Saxon, 2019). Although outcomes are thought to be the most important metric for psychotherapy success and therefore are the preferred method for identifying psychotherapy experts (Tracey et al., 2014), others have noted problems with this approach (Hill et al., 2017; Shanteau & Weiss, 2014). The problems include concerns about the validity of the outcome measures (i.e., the measures may not assess outcomes that are important to the client) and the fact that much of the variation in outcomes is due to patients (Bohart & Wade, 2013; Wampold & Imel, 2015) and other factors beyond the control of the therapist (e.g., sudden unemployment or partnership separation; Lambert & Ogles, 2004). Despite the problems, in this chapter, we argue that patient outcomes should be the primary criterion for superior performance in psychotherapy because what is important to patients is their improvement as a result of therapy.

Impediments to Expertise in Psychotherapy

Regardless of how expertise is defined or assessed, it appears that achieving expert status in psychotherapy is difficult, as Shanteau (1992) noted over a quarter of a century ago. Tracey and colleagues (2014) observed that there several impediments to achieving expertise in psychotherapy. Therapy, by its nature, is an ambiguous task, with a great deal of complexity. Even when delivering a particular treatment designed for a given disorder, there are many uncertainties, some of which involve comorbidities, patient characteristics, including racial/ethnic/cultural background, financial stability, employment status, personality, readiness for change, and context, among others. Moreover, typically, therapists do not receive reliable feedback regarding outcomes. It is rare that therapists obtain general outcome information and even rarer that they learn of outcomes beyond termination. Obtaining information about one's outcomes relative to other therapists is even rarer still. Similarly, we rarely obtain information about patient progress in therapy, and when such information is provided, it is general (e.g., "patient is not making expected progress") and fails to pinpoint what needs to change for the patient to improve. After licensure, therapists in the United States typically do not receive supervision, which further limits their learning opportunities. It also appears that most therapists do not think that supervision or consultation are career-sustaining activities (Stevanovic & Rupert, 2004). Moreover, there are concerns about whether required continuation education for licensed or credentialed counselors, social workers, psychologists, and other clinicians leads to improved performance because such activities typically are information-based rather than skills-based (Taylor & Neimeyer, 2017). Given these conditions, and as discussed at length by Lilienfeld, Ritschel, Lynn, and Latzman (Chapter 3, this volume), it is not surprising that therapists overestimate their effectiveness (Walfish, McAlister, O'Donnell, & Lambert, 2012) and fail to recognize deteriorating cases (Hannan et al., 2005; Hatfield, McCullough, Frantz, & Krieger, 2010). In addition, therapists rarely have the opportunity to practice their skills and refine their abilities outside of therapy.

Many professions, including all of those related to psychotherapy, have emphasized EBP. However, these professions have emphasized evidence related to treatments in the quest to identify the most effective treatment (Laska, Gurman, & Wampold, 2014; Wampold & Imel, 2015). Less attention has been devoted to studying therapists (Baldwin & Imel, 2013; Wampold & Imel, 2015), even though the therapist delivering a particular treatment is critical to the success of treatment (see below). Even less attention has been devoted to studying therapist expertise. We now turn to what evidence there is on the topic of expertise in psychotherapy.

Evidence Related to Therapist Expertise

There is research evidence about several aspects of therapist expertise, including (1) therapist effects, (2) gradual improvement as a function of experience, (3) characteristics and actions of effective therapists, and (4) seemingly irrelevant characteristics and actions of effective therapists.

Therapist Effects

One of the requirements for a domain to have experts is that some practitioners in the domain must be superior to others. Applied to psychotherapy, some therapists must achieve better outcomes than other therapists if they are to be experts; that is, if patients of Therapist A benefit more from psychotherapy than patients of Therapist B, and if the difference is not due to chance or differences in the patients, then Therapist A is said to be more effective than Therapist B. Whether in randomized clinical trials or naturalistic settings, patients are nested within therapists—that is, multiple patients are being treated by each therapist. Accordingly, differences among therapists typically are indexed as an intraclass correlation coefficient (ICC), which provides an estimate of the proportion of variability in outcomes that is due to the therapist within this nested structure (Baldwin & Imel, 2013; Crits-Christoph & Mintz, 1991; Johns et al., 2019; Wampold & Serlin, 2000). A significant ICC says that in terms of outcomes, the patients of the same therapist are more alike than the patients of different therapists; that is, the patients of the more effective Therapist A will have outcomes that are more similar (i.e., better outcomes generally) than will patients of a different therapist (Therapist *B*'s patients will generally be different—that is, do more poorly—than the patients of Therapist *A*).

It may seem surprising to many that therapist effects have not been a central concern of psychotherapy researchers. Yet history shows that providers of services typically have been ignored as being important sources of variation in outcome in a variety of areas. This has been true, for example, in education (teachers), agriculture (farmers), and medicine (physicians) (see Wampold, 2001; Wampold & Imel, 2015). In 1966, Kiesler identified several assumptions that were myths in psychotherapy, including the therapist uniformity assumption: "Patients are assigned to . . . psychotherapy with different therapists as if therapist differences were irrelevant" (p. 112). This pattern, with some exceptions, has been the rule (Beutler et al., 2004; Wampold & Imel, 2015).

The research evidence for therapist effects are found in two different contexts: randomized clinical trials (RCTs) and naturalistic settings. In traditional RCTs, the conditions are quite artificial, in that typically pure treatments are delivered according to manuals in controlled conditions; hence, one might expect there to be less therapist variability than in naturalistic settings, where therapists typically are free to deliver whatever treatment they desire (or, for that matter, no particular treatment at all) (Crits-Christoph & Mintz, 1991). In RCTs, therapists are carefully selected and given special training and supervision, which yields more homogeneity than would be the case in naturalistic settings. Fortunately, in the last few decades, a sufficient number of studies (46) have investigated therapist effects to warrant a meta-analysis (Baldwin & Imel, 2013; see also Johns et al., 2019), although it should be noted that the number of investigations of therapist effects pales in comparison to the number of treatment outcome trials (by 2013, over 12,000 such trials; Wampold & Imel, 2015). Baldwin and Imel (2013) found that approximately 3% and 17% of the variability in outcomes in RCTs and naturalistic settings, respectively, were accounted for by therapists. Even when therapists are well trained and supervised to provide an evidence-based treatment in specialty care, it appears that some therapists are consistently better than others (Laska, Smith, Wislocki, Minami, & Wampold, 2013). Therapists' effects seem to exist across different treatment approaches as well (Wampold & Imel, 2015).

These percentages of variability due to therapists may seem small, but they are not. First, effects due to therapists are statistically significant—in clinical trials, and more so in naturalistic settings: Some therapists consistently achieve better outcomes than others, and this is not due to chance or patient characteristics (patients are randomly assigned in RCTs, and patient characteristics are often taken into account in naturalistic settings; see, e.g., Kraus et al., 2016). Second, therapist effects are much larger than many other effects, such as differences between treatments (at most, 2% of the variability in outcomes), the effects of specific components of treatments examined in dismantling studies (effects due to specific ingredients are generally not different from zero, but they account for less than 1% of the variability in outcome when estimated liberally), and the effects due to adherence to treatment protocols (percentage of variability in outcomes close to zero) and competence with which protocols are administered (about one-half of 1% of variability in outcome) (see Laska et al., 2014; Wampold & Imel, 2015). The evidence supports the notion that the therapist giving the treatment is a more important factor than what treatment is being provided. Third, and most important, therapist effects have real-life implications. If patients of the poorer performing therapists were randomly assigned to other therapists, dramatically more patients would recover (Imel, Sheng, Baldwin, & Atkins, 2015; Kraus et al., 2016; Saxon & Barkham, 2012; Wampold & Brown, 2005). In naturalistic settings, the top quartile of therapists, defined by their outcomes, achieves effects that are twice as large as effects of those in the bottom quartile (Wampold & Brown, 2005); assigning the patients of underperforming therapists (e.g., the bottom 10%) to any other therapists dramatically increases the number of patients who would recover (Saxon & Barkham, 2012). However, it remains important to understand that much of the variability in outcomes is due to the patient (Baldwin & Imel, 2013; Bohart & Wade, 2013). Some patients, regardless of their therapist, have good outcomes because they are motivated, their comorbidity is uncomplicated, they have sufficient social support, they are ready to change, and they have enough financial resources or insurance to ensure continuous care, whereas other patients have factors that mitigate their outcomes, such as complicating personality structures, little social support, or financial problems (Bohart & Wade, 2013).

One of the hallmarks of expertise has been verified. Some therapists consistently get better outcomes than other therapists, which implies that some therapists have superior performance, as measured by outcomes.

Improvement over Time

Another hallmark of expertise that we have discussed is that the expert's performance gradually improves over time. The question of whether therapists improve over the course of their careers has been a topic of interest since the earliest days of psychotherapy research (Bergin, 1971; Beutler et al., 2004; Meltzoff & Kornreich, 1970; Myers & Auld, 1955). Early reviews suggested that experience and training have a modest effect on outcomes (Stein & Lambert, 1984, 1995), but these reviews and subsequent discussion of experience have several methodological problems, including difficulty in defining experience and the cross-sectional nature of the investigations (see Goldberg, Rousmaniere, et al., 2016; Tracey et al., 2014; Wampold & Imel, 2015). In the first large longitudinal study, Goldberg, Rousmanier, and colleagues (2016) examined the outcomes of 170 therapists treating over 6,500 patients over the course of their careers ($M = 4.73$ years, with a range from 0.44 to 17.93 years) at a college counseling center. Regardless of whether experience was operationalized as years treating patients or as the number of cases seen, overall, the therapists' effectiveness (i.e., their outcomes) actually (and significantly) *decreased* with experience, although the size of the effect was small; that is, therapists got worse with experience, although there was random variation in therapist trajectories and a minority of therapists did improve over time. Owen, Wampold, Kopta, Rousmaniere, and Miller (2016) replicated this longitudinal analysis with trainees and found that over the course of their training, the outcomes of trainees increased, although, surprisingly, the effect was quite small. As well, there are also some fairly convincing data that psychology trainees achieve outcomes comparable to those of experienced professionals (see Owen et al., 2016, for a review of studies).

The evidence from the experience literature does not support the notion of expertise in psychotherapy when experience is the criterion. Therapists do not seem to improve over time, or at least, most therapists do not appear to improve. Trainees improve over time, but the size

of the improvement is small, and novice therapists are as effective, or nearly as effective, as experienced therapists. The research on experience using longitudinal methods is recent, and clearly more research is needed to make a definitive conclusion. However, a more nuanced question needs to be asked and answered: Under what circumstances do therapists improve? Before we can address this question, we need to know the characteristics and actions of effective therapists.

Characteristics and Actions of Effective Therapists

The evidence supports the contention there is variability among therapists in terms of their effectiveness. Regardless of the treatment delivered, the person giving the treatment (i.e., the therapist) is a critical component. Although the majority of therapists do not improve over time, there are clearly therapists who are consistently more effective than others. This presents a critical question: What are the characteristics and actions of effective therapists?

Before presenting the evidence about effective therapists, we take note of the difficulty of the task. The most apparent way to identify the characteristics and actions of effective therapists is to observe what these therapists do in therapy. Unfortunately, as appealing as this is, it has a fundamental flaw. Much of what transpires in therapy is determined by the patient and the complex interaction between the patient and the therapist. An interpersonally aggressive patient will be challenging to a therapist, and the therapist in this case may well seem less skillful than otherwise would be the case (see Boswell et al., 2013). Indeed, much of the variability in adherence and competence is due to the patient rather than the therapist (Boswell et al., 2013; Imel, Baer, Martino, Ball, & Carroll, 2011). Expertise is characteristic of therapists, so to establish the characteristics and actions of effective therapists, researchers must account for patients' contributions to what is observed or assessed.

Alliance

The *alliance* is defined as a pantheoretical construct that reflects collaborative and purposeful work and has three components: the bond between the patient and the therapist, agreement about the goals of therapy, and agreement about the tasks of therapy (Bordin, 1979; Hatcher & Barends, 2006; Horvath, 2006; Horvath & Luborsky, 1993). The alliance is the most researched construct in psychotherapy process research, and the nearly 200 studies that have investigated the correlation of the alliance with outcome have found meta-analytically that there is a strong association between the alliance, measured early in psychotherapy, and the final outcome (Flückiger, Del Re, Wampold, & Horvath, 2018; Flückiger, Del Re, Wampold, Symonds, & Horvath, 2012; Horvath, Del Re, Flückiger, & Symonds, 2011). As discussed earlier, it would be tempting to say, based on this research, that a characteristic of effective therapists is that they form strong alliances, but caution is needed.

As strong as the research is relative to alliance, it is not clear that it is the therapists' contribution to the alliance that is important. Some patients come to therapy with strong social support, secure attachment style, interpersonal skills, and motivation to change. Such a patient will form a relatively strong alliance with most therapists and have relatively good outcomes; thus it might well be that it is the patient's contribution to the alliance that is important. However, just the opposite has been found. Baldwin, Wampold, and Imel (2007) disentangled the therapist and patient contributions to the alliance and found that *only* the therapist's contribution to the alliance predicted outcome, a result confirmed meta-analytically (Del Re, Flückiger, Horvath, Symonds, & Wampold, 2012). It is what the therapist offers the patient in terms of forming the alliance that produces better outcomes. The conclusion from this research is unequivocal: *Effective therapists form strong alliances across a range of patients.*

Having noted that forming an alliance across a range of patients is characteristic of effective therapists, it is important to discuss briefly that the alliance is not a straightforward concept. There is evidence that the alliance may work differently in different therapies (e.g., see Ulvenes et al., 2012; Webb et al., 2011). Webb and colleagues (2011) found that in CBT for depression, agreement on goals and tasks is important, but the bond may be a consequence of prior symptom change. Ulvenes and colleagues (2012) showed that the alliance in CBT and psychodynamic therapy of personality disorder works differently: In psychodynamic therapy, avoidance of affect in therapy suppressed the influence of the alliance on outcome, whereas

in CBT, avoidance of affect results in a stronger alliance and symptom reduction. The alliance also interacts with adherence to the treatment protocol, other common factors, and specific ingredients (Barber et al., 2006; Owen & Hilsenroth, 2011; Rubel, Rosenbaum, & Lutz, 2017). As well, the alliance may be more important to some types of patients; Lorenzo-Luaces, DeRubeis, and Webb (2014) found that in CBT for depression, alliance is strongly related to the alliance for patients with zero to two prior episodes of depression but not at all related to outcome for those with three or more episodes. Ackerman and Hilsenroth (2001), based a review of the literature, concluded that therapist attributes such as being rigid, uncertain, critical, distant, tense, and distracted, as well as the use of inappropriate self-disclosures, overly structured therapy, too many transference interpretations, and inappropriate silence, detract from forming a strong alliance.

Facilitative Interpersonal Skills

Anderson and colleagues (Anderson, Crowley, Himawan, Holmberg, & Uhlin, 2016; Anderson, McClintock, Himawan, Song, & Patterson, 2016; Anderson, Ogles, Patterson, Lambert, & Vermeersch, 2009) have an interesting method to identify the characteristics and actions of effective therapists. Instead of using material from therapy sessions or asking therapists to provide information, they presented a video of a challenging patient (i.e., a stimulus that was constant across therapists) and had the study participants respond as if they were the therapist at several of the instances in the video. In the 2009 study, Anderson and colleagues presented the stimuli to 25 therapists at a college counseling center. The responses were then coded for what the authors called *facilitative interpersonal skills* (FIS), which included verbal fluency, emotional expression, persuasiveness, hopefulness, warmth, empathy, alliance–bond capacity, and problem focus. In a multilevel model, FIS scores, at the therapist level, were used to predict the improvement of 1,141 patients seen by these therapists. The results showed that FIS scores, based on responses to the standard video stimulus, were a strong predictor of patient improvement in therapy, roughly equivalent to a correlation of 0.47 between FIS and outcome. This research suggests that effective therapists are verbally fluent, express emotion appropriately, are persuasive, communicate hopefulness, are warm and empathic, have the capacity to create a bond with patients, and focus on the patient's problems.

The Anderson and colleagues (2009) study was retrospective because FIS was assessed after the therapists had seen the patients. A similar study used a prospective design in which psychology trainees in their first weeks of training watched the psychotherapy video and their responses were recorded and coded for FIS (Anderson, Crowley, et al., 2016). The FIS scores before training in psychotherapy were then used to predict the outcomes of the therapists as they began to see patients later in their training, at least a year after the FIS was assessed. The results were not as strong as those in the previous study, most likely because the FIS was measured at the beginning of training, and the trainees' therapy experience was at least 1 year in the future. Nevertheless, the FIS of therapists did predict outcomes of patients who were seen for eight or fewer sessions. The importance of the FIS of trainees was also established in an RCT (Anderson, Crowley, et al., 2016).

Recently, Schöttke, Flückiger, Goldberg, Eversmann, and Lange (2017) conducted a study that produced results complementary to those of Anderson and colleagues. Postgraduate students in Germany, in a 5-year psychotherapy training course in either CBT or psychodynamic training, were assessed via a structured interview and by applicants' response in a group discussion with other applicants after viewing a provocative film. The interview was designed to assess interpersonally related competencies and personal strengths/capabilities, and trainees' responses were rated by experts (similar to how we often assess clinical skills in interviews with applicants for internship or professional positions). The trainees' responses in the group discussion following the provocative film, were rated on the following dimensions: (1) clarity of communication, (2) empathy and communicative attunement, (3) respect and warmth, (4) management of criticism, and (5) willingness to cooperate—actions that overlap with FIS to a great extent. The scores of the interview and the group interaction were used to predict the outcomes of patients seen during training. In a multilevel model with patients nested within therapists, the performance of the trainees in the group interaction based on the provocative stimulus predicted outcomes of patients, whereas the responses to the structured interview did not.

Professional Self-Doubt and Deliberate Practice

In a series of studies, Nissen-Lie and colleagues (2015; Nissen-Lie, Monsen, & Rønnestad, 2010; Nissen-Lie, Monsen, Ulleberg, & Rønnestad, 2013) studied therapists in practice in Norway (psychologists, psychiatrists, physiotherapists, and psychiatric nurses) using a variety of treatments by having them complete a comprehensive survey about their professional work and also measured patient outcomes. They found that therapists' self-reported professional self-doubt (PSD) predicted outcome—that is, therapists who had more doubt about their skill in helping patients (e.g., "lacking confidence that you might have a beneficial effect on a patient" and "unsure about how best to deal effectively with a patient") had better outcomes, particularly if they also had a positive sense of self.

Perhaps therapists who doubted their effectiveness also were motivated to improve. Chow and colleagues (2015) found that the amount of time therapists reported spending on improving targeted therapeutic skills outside of therapy predicted their outcomes with patients. This was a cross-sectional design, so it is not possible to determine whether the therapists who spent more time outside of therapy were improving over time or were simply better therapists than the others. Neverless, these behaviors meet the definition of *deliberate practice* (e.g., Ericsson & Lehmann, 1996), which we discuss further below.

Characteristics and Actions of Therapists That Are Not Related to Outcome

It is informative to understand what characteristics and actions of therapists are *not* related to outcome, as spending time and effort in those areas would not lead to improved outcomes. Generally, it has been found that the age, the gender, and the profession of the therapist (e.g., psychology, psychiatry, social work, professional counselor) do not predict outcome (Wampold et al., 2017; Wampold & Imel, 2015)—of course, none of these variables can be modified, and they do not help those who want to become experts.

Anderson and colleagues (2009), as discussed earlier, used a challenge test to assess FIS, as did Schöttke and colleagues (2017), who coded a discussion among trainees following a provocative video and found results similar to those of Anderson and colleagues. It appears that effective therapists display important skills in interpersonally challenging situations. However, in these studies, self-reported social skills (Anderson et al., 2009) and responses in a structured interview designed to assess clinical skills (Schöttke et al., 2017) did *not* predict outcomes. It seems that therapists' self-report of skills is not useful in identifying particular skills that need attention; rather, therapists must be observed in challenging interpersonal situations. Interestingly, supervision is often based on therapist self-report of therapy situations, and we often evaluate therapists for internship and professional positions based on therapists' discussion of their clinical skills.

Consistent with the more general literature on theoretical orientation (Wampold & Imel, 2015), the studies examining characteristics and actions of effective therapists have found that theoretical orientation does not predict therapist outcomes (Anderson, Ogles, et al., 2009; Chow et al., 2015; Schöttke et al., 2017). It is important to note that therapist adherence to treatment protocols also does not predict outcome (Boswell et al., 2013; Webb et al., 2010), which is to say, those therapists who more closely follow a treatment protocol do not achieve better outcomes. Given this result and the general lack of differences among therapies in terms of outcome (Wampold & Imel, 2015), it is possible that how a treatment is delivered is more important than the particular treatment that is offered to the patient. There is some evidence that flexibility in terms of adherence is important (Owen & Hilsenroth, 2014); flexibility is often mentioned as a candidate for a characteristics of effective therapists, although evidence is lacking in this area. Matching the treatment to the patient's personality (Beutler, Harwood, Kimpara, Verdirame, & Blau, 2011; Beutler, Harwood, Michelson, Song, & Holman, 2011) and to the cultural beliefs of the patient (Benish, Quintana, & Wampold, 2011; Huey, Tilley, Jones, & Smith, 2014) appears to be important for optimal outcomes. There is debate about whether therapists are relatively more effective with some problem areas than others (i.e., are expert at treating a particular disorder or problem area; Kraus et al., 2016; Kraus, Castonguay, Boswell, Nordberg, & Hayes, 2011; Nissen-Lie et al., 2016).

As we have discussed, it also appears that competence in delivering a particular treatment, as rated by treatment experts in clinical trials, does not predict the outcomes of therapy (Boswell et al., 2013; Webb et al., 2010). This is a curious finding because one would think that experts' ratings of competence must be related to how well the therapist performs and the outcomes achieved. It is important to emphasize that such competence measures are sensitive to *competence in a particular therapy* and do not emphasize competence in many factors discussed in this chapter, including alliance building, empathy, verbal fluency, and so forth. Another problem with competence ratings in traditional RCTS is that often, because of selection and training, there is little variability in competence ratings among therapists. Exacerbating this problem is patients' contribution to the ratings—treating more difficult patients will result in the therapist appearing less competent (Boswell et al., 2013; Imel et al., 2011). Interestingly, training therapists to be more competent in a particular therapy does not seem to improve their outcomes (see, e.g., Branson, Shafran, & Myles, 2015).

How to Become an Expert

Pablo Casals, the renowned cellist, was asked when he was in his 80s, why he practiced 4 or 5 hours a day. He responded, "I think I am making progress" (Lee, 2016, p. 895). So, although by all accounts Casals was an expert, he sought to continually improve by practicing. But practice that is necessary to improve is not simply the everyday work to which we refer when we tell people we are "in practice" as a therapist, which is very different from what Casals meant. Casals was practicing particular skills outside of performances. Recall that, in general, therapists do not progress in terms of their outcomes over the course of their careers, unlike Casals, who practiced several hours a day throughout his life despite having attained superior performance.

Anders Ericsson has developed and studied the effects of deliberate practice, which he indicates is necessary for the attainment of expertise in any domain. Specifically, deliberate practice has four components:

1. A focused and systematic effort to improve performance, pursued over an extended period.
2. Involvement of and guidance from a coach/teacher/mentor.
3. Immediate, ongoing feedback.

4. Successive refinement and repetition via solo practice outside of performance (Ericsson & Lehmann, 1996).

These are elements of practice that therapists rarely, if ever, do, even in training. Even if therapists wanted to engage in these activities, it would be difficult to accomplish for a number of reasons.

The first element of deliberate practice involves commitment to systematically work to improve. Recall that Chow and colleagues (2015) found that therapists who spent time outside of therapy on therapy-related activities achieved better outcomes than other therapists. With regard to the second components of deliberate practice, after licensure, we rarely have the opportunity to work with a coach, mentor, or supervisor to improve. And when we do, it is typically not focused and deliberate. We may consult about difficult cases, but rarely do we use an outside consultant to develop particular skills. Even in the United Kingdom, which requires lifelong supervision, the supervision that registered psychologists receive is focused predominantly on the provision of support and minimally on fostering skills development (Nicholas & Goodyear, 2015).

Third, we rarely have feedback about our performance. There is a growing movement toward routine outcome monitoring (ROM), so that therapists have access to information about patient progress. Two special issues of journals (*Psychotherapy,* Issue 4, 2015; *Psychotherapy Research,* Issue 6, 2015) were devoted to research and practice with ROM. It appears that ROM improves the quality of services (Lambert & Shimokawa, 2011; Shimokawa, Lambert, & Smart, 2010); unfortunately, it does not appear that ROM helps therapist improve over time (Goldberg, Rousmaniere, et al., 2016). ROM provides general feedback, but it does not identify skills that must be practiced and improved (Tracey et al., 2014; Wampold, 2015).

Finally, to improve, therapists need to practice particular therapy skills, ones that are important for the outcome of therapy. We have discussed several characteristics and actions of effective therapists, and it makes sense that it is these skills that should be assessed and practiced. Recall that Goldberg, Rousmaniere, and colleagues (2016) found that therapists tend to become slightly less effective over time. However, the opposite was found in an agency that emphasized deliberate practice and continual professional development and, as well, monitored outcomes to ensure that, indeed, therapists were improving—in this agency, therapists gradually improved over time (Goldberg, Babins-Wagner, et al., 2016).

Learning theorists have questioned the importance of deliberate practice in the development of expertise (see Ullén et al., 2016). They point to the fact that certain genotypes are necessary (e.g., height in basketball), and that early experiences and personality factors are necessary in addition to deliberate practice. Recall that trainees with relatively high FIS at the beginning of their training were the best therapists in future years, regardless of the effect of training, so it appears that in therapy, a certain substrate of interpersonal skills is necessary to be an expert therapist. Nevertheless, deliberate practice provides added value—it provides a way to improve, regardless of other limitation or strengths.

Conclusions

The goal of EBP is to improve the quality of mental health services. Much of the effort has been focused on identifying the most effective treatment for particular disorders (Laska et al., 2014). However, evidence from an array of perspectives is needed for the field to progress. In this chapter, we have discussed evidence related to therapists, particularly how therapists can develop expertise. The evidence we have presented is intriguing, although perhaps tenuous at this point in time. Clearly, additional research in this area is needed. Nevertheless, there are implications for selection, training, and practice that should be considered, some of which would dramatically change our current practices.

Therapist training programs, particularly those based in academic departments in research universities, typically rely on indicators of academic success to make admission decisions. These indicators, including grade point average, Graduate Record Examination scores, letters of recommendation, personal statements, and performance in interviews, have unknown but probably weak association with performance as a therapist. In two studies, trainees' interpersonal skills displayed in challenging interpersonal situations early in their training were associated with therapy outcomes several years in the future (Anderson, McClintock, et al., 2016; Schöttke et al., 2017). These observations suggest that applicants to programs that train therapists should include a protocol such as that used by Anderson and colleagues to assess interpersonal skills in challenging situations as part of the admission criteria. While selection based on interpersonal skills could increase the competence of graduates of psychotherapy training programs, attainment of expertise involves improving effectiveness over the course of the professional career. Selection based on interpersonal skills could thus serve to better ensure competence of therapists, which could then serve as a foundation for potential development of expertise.

The evidence reviewed also suggests modification of training of therapists. Practice of therapeutic skills identified to characterize effective therapists should be central to the curriculum. Stimuli, such as those used in the Anderson and colleagues (2009) study, could be used to elicit responses from trainees; these responses could be evaluated with regard to the FIS, then the trainee could repeat the response given the feedback. As well, the outcomes of trainees should be assessed so that programs can ensure that the patients of trainees are benefiting from therapy and that the trainee is improving over time. It is important to recognize that deliberate practice of particular therapeutic skills is not incompatible with teaching and learning treatment approaches; in fact, they complement each other (Wampold & Imel, 2015). The objective is to provide particular treatments skillfully. Moreover, it should be recognized that trainees whose selection is based on a relatively sophisticated set of interpersonal skills will benefit from training and will need to continue to improve to achieve expertise.

As we discussed, it is very difficult for therapists to improve after they finish their training. Most of practice involves seeing patients, with little opportunity for supervision or consultation. In cases in which supervision is used in clinical practice, it typically serves a supportive role rather than a skills building one. We have presented some preliminary evidence that therapists do not improve over their careers and may even deteriorate. However, there is also evidence that at an agency that promotes deliberate practice, the opposite result was obtained—therapists actually improved over time. However, adjusting the environment to accommodate and encourage deliberate practice is not easily accomplished (Rousmaniere, Goodyear, Miller, & Wampold, 2017) and is not particularly desired by therapists (Stevanovic & Rupert, 2004). Additionally, there is not yet sufficient evidence that such strategies would be cost-effective. However, it certainly provides an alternative to the dissemination of treatments, which is costly and may not improve the quality of mental health service (Laska et al., 2014). It is not lost on managers of care or payers that there is variation in the outcomes due to therapists. Ignoring therapist effects is a lost opportunity, as the underperforming therapists results in more unsuccessful cases. Deliberate practice is a potential means to address this issue.

Tracey and colleagues (2014) have argued for the merits of deliberate practice that is based on high-quality outcome feedback (progress within the patient over time and across different patients, long-term outcomes and across different therapists) involves careful scientific evaluation and minimizes the use of performance-inhibiting heuristics. We do not see the lack of expertise as inherent to the profession, but we think that acquisition of expertise requires explicit attention, via deliberate practice, to remedy this situation. In that sense, we see this chapter as a hopeful one, in that it suggests a means by which individual therapists can develop expertise.

References

Ackerman, S. J., & Hilsenroth, M. J. (2001). A review of therapist characteristics and techniques negatively impacting the therapeutic alliance. *Psychotherapy: Theory, Research, Practice, Training, 38*(2), 171–185.

American Psychological Association Committee on Accreditation. (2002). *Guidelines and principles for accreditation of programs in professional psychology.* Washington, DC: Author.

American Psychological Association Presidential Task Force on Evidence-Based Practice. (2006). Evidence-based practice in psychology. *American Psychologist, 61,* 271–285.

Anderson, T., Crowley, M. J., Himawan, L., Holmberg, J. K., & Uhlin, B. D. (2016). Therapist facilitative interpersonal skills and trainee status: A randomized clinical trial on alliance and outcome. *Psychotherapy Research, 26,* 511–529.

Anderson, T., McClintock, A. S., Himawan, L., Song, X., & Patterson, C. L. (2016). A prospective study of therapist facilitative interpersonal skills as a predictor of treatment outcome. *Journal of Consulting and Clinical Psychology, 84,* 57–66.

Anderson, T., Ogles, B. M., Patterson, C. L., Lambert, M. J., & Vermeersch, D. A. (2009). Therapist effects: Facilitative interpersonal skills as a predictor of therapist success. *Journal of Clinical Psychology, 65*(7), 755–768.

Baldwin, S. A., & Imel, Z. E. (2013). Therapist effects:

Finding and methods. In M. J. Lambert (Ed.), *Bergin and Garfield's handbook of psychotherapy and behavior change* (6th ed., pp. 258–297). Hoboken, NJ: Wiley.

Baldwin, S. A., Wampold, B. E., & Imel, Z. E. (2007). Untangling the alliance–outcome correlation: Exploring the relative importance of therapist and patient variability in the alliance. *Journal of Consulting and Clinical Psychology, 75,* 842–852.

Barber, J. P., Gallop, R., Crits-Christoph, P., Frank, A., Thase, M. E., Weiss, R. D., et al. (2006). The role of therapist adherence, therapist competence, and alliance in predicting outcome of individual drug counseling: Results from the National Institute Drug Abuse Collaborative Cocaine Treatment Study. *Psychotherapy Research, 16,* 229–240.

Benish, S. G., Quintana, S., & Wampold, B. E. (2011). Culturally adapted psychotherapy and the legitimacy of myth: A direct-comparison meta-analysis. *Journal of Counseling Psychology, 58*(3), 279–289.

Bergin, A. E. (1971). The evaluation of therapeutic outcomes. In A. E. Bergin & S. L. Garfield (Eds.), *Handbook of psychotherapy and behavior change* (pp. 217–270). New York: Wiley.

Beutler, L. E., Harwood, T. M., Kimpara, S., Verdirame, D., & Blau, K. (2011). Coping style. *Journal of Clinical Psychology, 67*(2), 176–183.

Beutler, L. E., Harwood, T. M., Michelson, A., Song, X., & Holman, J. (2011). Resistance/reactance level. *Journal of Clinical Psychology, 67*(2), 133–142.

Beutler, L. E., Malik, M., Alimohamed, S., Harwood, T. M., Talebi, H., Noble, S., et al. (2004). Therapist variables. In M. J. Lambert (Ed.), *Bergin and Garfield's handbook of psychotherapy and behavior change* (5th ed., pp. 227–306). Hoboken, NJ: Wiley.

Bohart, A. C., & Wade, A. G. (2013). The client in psychotherapy. In M. J. Lambert (Ed.), *Bergin and Garfield's handbook of pyschotherapy and behavior change* (6th ed., pp. 219–257). Hoboken, NJ: Wiley.

Bordin, E. S. (1979). The generalizability of the psychoanalytic concept of the working alliance. *Psychotherapy: Theory, Research, and Practice, 16*(3), 252–260.

Boswell, J. F., Gallagher, M. W., Sauer-Zavala, S. E., Bullis, J., Gorman, J. M., Shear, M. K., et al. (2013). Patient characteristics and variability in adherence and competence in cognitive-behavioral therapy for panic disorder. *Journal of Consulting and Clinical Psychology, 81*(3), 443–454.

Branson, A., Shafran, R., & Myles, P. (2015). Investigating the relationship between competence and patient outcome with CBT. *Behaviour Research and Therapy, 68,* 19–26.

Chow, D. L., Miller, S. D., Seidel, J. A., Kane, R. T., Thornton, J. A., & Andrews, W. P. (2015). The role of deliberate practice in the development of highly effective psychotherapists. *Psychotherapy, 52*(3), 337–345.

Crits-Christoph, P., & Mintz, J. (1991). Implications of therapist effects for the design and analysis of comparative studies of psychotherapies. *Journal of Consulting and Clinical Psychology, 59,* 20–26.

Del Re, A. C., Flückiger, C., Horvath, A. O., Symonds, D., & Wampold, B. E. (2012). Therapist effects in the therapeutic alliance–outcome relationship: A restricted-maximum likelihood meta-analysis. *Clinical Psychology Review, 32*(7), 642–649.

Ericsson, K. A., & Lehmann, A. C. (1996). Expert and exceptional performance: Evidence of maximal adaptation to task constraints. *Annual Review of Psychology, 47,* 273–305.

Flückiger, C., Del Re, A. C., Wampold, B. E., & Horvath, A. O. (2018). The alliance in adult psychotherapy: A meta-analytic synthesis. *Psychotherapy, 55*(4), 316–340.

Flückiger, C., Del Re, A. C., Wampold, B. E., Symonds, D., & Horvath, A. O. (2012). How central is the alliance in psychotherapy?: A multilevel longitudinal meta-analysis. *Journal of Counseling Psychology, 59*(1), 10–17.

Fouad, N. A., Grus, C. L., Hatcher, R. L., Kaslow, N. J., Hutchings, P. S., Madson, M. B., et al. (2009). Competency benchmarks: A model for understanding and measuring competence in professional psychology across training levels. *Training and Education in Professional Psychology, 3*(4, Suppl.), S5–S26.

Goldberg, S. B., Babkins-Wagner, R., Rousmaniere, T., Berzins, S., Hoyt, W. T., Whipple, J. L., et al. (2016). Creating a climate for therapist improvement: A case study of an agency focused on outcomes and deliberate practice. *Psychotherapy, 53*(3), 367–375.

Goldberg, S. B., Rousmaniere, T., Miller, S. D., Whipple, J., Nielsen, S. L., Hoyt, W. T., et al. (2016). Do psychotherapists improve with time and experience?: A longitudinal analysis of outcomes in a clinical setting. *Journal of Counseling Psychology, 63*(1), 1–11.

Hannan, C., Lambert, M. J., Harmon, C., Nielsen, S. L., Smart, D. W., Shimokawa, K., et al. (2005). A lab test and algorithms for identifying clients at risk for treatment failure. *Journal of Clinical Psychology/In Session, 61,* 1–9.

Hatcher, R. L., & Barends, A. W. (2006). How a return to theory could help alliance research. *Psychotherapy: Theory, Research, Practice, Training, 43*(3), 292–299.

Hatfield, D., McCullough, L., Frantz, S. H. B., & Krieger, K. (2010). Do we know when our clients get worse?: An investigation of therapists' ability to detect negative client change. *Clinical Psychology and Psychotherapy, 17*(1), 25–32.

Hill, C. E., Spiegel, S. B., Hoffman, M. A., Kivlighan, D. M., Jr., & Gelso, C. J. (2017). Therapist expertise in psychotherapy revisited. *The Counseling Psychologist, 45*(1), 7–53.

Horvath, A. O. (2006). The alliance in context: Accomplishments, challenges, and future directions. *Psychotherapy: Theory, Research, Practice, Training, 43*(3), 258–263.

Horvath, A. O., Del Re, A. C., Flückiger, C., & Symonds, D. (2011). Alliance in individual psychotherapy. *Psychotherapy, 48*(1), 9–16.

Horvath, A. O., & Luborsky, L. (1993). The role of the therapeutic alliance in psychotherapy. *Journal of Consulting and Clinical Psychology, 61,* 561–573.

Huey, S. J., Jr., Tilley, J. L., Jones, E. O., & Smith, C. A. (2014). The contribution of cultural competence to evidence-based care for ethnically diverse populations. *Annual Review of Clinical Psychology, 10,* 305–338.

Imel, Z. E., Baer, J. S., Martino, S., Ball, S. A., & Carroll, K. M. (2011). Mutual influence in therapist competence and adherence to motivational enhancement therapy. *Drug and Alcohol Dependence, 115*(3), 229–236.

Imel, Z. E., Sheng, E., Baldwin, S. A., & Atkins, D. C. (2015). Removing very low-performing therapists: A simulation of performance-based retention in psychotherapy. *Psychotherapy, 52*(3), 329–336.

Johns, R. J., Barkham, M., Kellett, S., & Saxon, D. (2019). A systematic review of therapist effects: A critical narrative update and refinement to review. *Clinical Psychology Review, 67,* 78–93.

Kaslow, N. J. (2004). Competencies in professional psychology. *American Psychologist, 59*(8), 774–781.

Kaslow, N. J., Borden, K. A., Collins, F. L., Jr., Forrest, L., Illfelder-Kaye, J., Nelson, P. D., et al. (2004). Competencies conference: Future directions in education and credentialing in professional psychology. *Journal of Clinical Psychology, 60*(7), 699–712.

Kaslow, N. J., Rubin, N. J., Bebeau, M. J., Leigh, I. W., Lichtenberg, J. W., Nelson, P. D., et al. (2007). Guiding principles and recommendations for the assessment of competence. *Professional Psychology: Research and Practice, 38*(5), 441–451.

Kiesler, D. J. (1966). Some myths of psychotherapy research and the search for a paradigm. *Psychological Bulletin, 65*(2), 110–136.

Kraus, D. R., Bentley, J. H., Alexander, P. C., Boswell, J. F., Constantino, M. J., Baxter, E. E., et al. (2016). Predicting therapist effectiveness from their own practice-based evidence. *Journal of Consulting and Clinical Psychology, 84*(6), 473–483.

Kraus, D. R., Castonguay, L., Boswell, J. F., Nordberg, S. S., & Hayes, J. A. (2011). Therapist effectiveness: Implications for accountability and patient care. *Psychotherapy Research, 21*(3), 267–276.

Lambert, M. J., & Ogles, B. M. (2004). The efficacy and effectiveness of psychotherapy. In M. J. Lambert (Ed.), *Bergin and Garfield's handbook of psychotherapy and behavior change* (5th ed., pp. 139–193). Hoboken, NJ: Wiley.

Lambert, M. J., & Shimokawa, K. (2011). Collecting client feedback. *Psychotherapy, 48*(1), 72–79.

Laska, K. M., Gurman, A. S., & Wampold, B. E. (2014). Expanding the lens of evidence-based practice in psychotherapy: A common factors perspective. *Psychotherapy, 51*(4), 467–481.

Laska, K. M., Smith, T. L., Wislocki, A. P., Minami, T., & Wampold, B. E. (2013). Uniformity of evidence-based treatments in practice?: Therapist effects in the delivery of cognitive processing therapy for PTSD. *Journal of Counseling Psychology, 60*(1), 31–41.

Lee, M. J. (2016). On patient safety: When are we too old to operate? *Clinical Orthopaedics and Related Research, 474,* 895–898.

Lewis, M. (2004). *Moneyball: The art of winning an unfair game.* New York: Norton.

Lorenzo-Luaces, L., DeRubeis, R. J., & Webb, C. A. (2014). Client characteristics as moderators of the relation between the therapeutic alliance and outcome in cognitive therapy for depression. *Journal of Consulting and Clinical Psychology, 82*(2), 368–373.

Meltzoff, J., & Kornreich, M. (1970). *Research in psychotherapy.* New Brunswick, NJ: Aldine.

Myers, J. K., & Auld, F., Jr. (1955). Some variables related to outcome of psychotherapy *Journal of Clinical Psychology, 11,* 51–54.

Nicholas, H., & Goodyear, R. K. (2015, August). *When credentialed psychologists are supervisees: Reports from a British sample.* Poster session at the annual meeting of the American Psychological Association, Toronto, ON, Canada.

Nissen-Lie, H. A., Goldberg, S. B., Hoyt, W. T., Falkenström, F., Holmqvist, R., Nielsen, S. L., et al. (2016). Are therapists uniformly effective across patient outcome domains?: A study on therapist effectiveness in two different treatment contexts. *Journal of Counseling Psychology, 63*(4), 367–378.

Nissen-Lie, H. A., Monsen, J. T., & Rønnestad, M. H. (2010). Therapist predictors of early patient-rated working alliance: A multilevel approach. *Psychotherapy Research, 20*(6), 627–646.

Nissen-Lie, H. A., Monsen, J. T., Ulleberg, P., & Rønnestad, M. H. (2013). Psychotherapists' self-reports of their interpersonal functioning and difficulties in practice as predictors of patient outcome. *Psychotherapy Research, 23*(1), 86–104.

Nissen-Lie, H. A., Rønnestad, M. H., Høglend, P. A., Havik, O. E., Solbakken, O. A., Stiles, T. C., et al. (2017). Love yourself as a person, doubt yourself as a therapist? *Clinical Psychology and Psychotherapy, 24*(1), 48–60.

Owen, J., & Hilsenroth, M. J. (2011). Interaction between alliance and technique in predicting patient outcome during psychodynamic psychotherapy. *Journal of Nervous and Mental Disease, 199*(6), 384–389.

Owen, J., & Hilsenroth, M. J. (2014). Treatment adherence: The importance of therapist flexibility in relation to therapy outcomes. *Journal of Counseling Psychology, 61*(2), 280–288.

Owen, J., Wampold, B. E., Kopta, M., Rousmaniere, T., & Miller, S. D. (2016). As good as it gets?: Therapy outcomes of trainees over time. *Journal of Counseling Psychology, 63*(1), 12–19.

Peterson, R. L., McHolland, J., Bent, R. J., Davis-Russell, E., Edwall, G. E., Magidson, E. (1992). *The core curriculum in professional psychology.* Washington, DC: American Psychological Association and National Council of Schools of Professional Psychology.

Roberts, M. C., Borden, K. A., Christiansen, M. D., & Lopez, S. J. (2005). Fostering a culture shift: Assessment of competence in the education and careers of professional psychologists. *Professional Psychology: Research and Practice, 36,* 355–361.

Rodolfa, E. R., Bent, R. J., Eisman, E., Nelson, P. D., Rehm, L., & Ritchie, P. (2005). A cube model for competency development: Implications for psychology educators and regulators. *Professional Psychology: Research and Practice, 36,* 347–354.

Rousmaniere, T., Goodyear, R. K., Miller, S. D., & Wampold, B. E. (Eds.). (2017). *The cycle of excellence: Using deliberate practice to improve supervision and training.* Hoboken, NJ: Wiley.

Rubel, J. A., Rosenbaum, D., & Lutz, W. (2017). Patients' in-session experiences and symptom change: Session-to-session effects on a within- and between-patient level. *Behaviour Research and Therapy, 90,* 58–66.

Rubin, N. J., Bebeau, M., Leigh, I. W., Lichtenberg, J. W., Nelson, P. D., Portnoy, S., et al. (2007). The competency movement within psychology: An historical perspective. *Professional Psychology: Research and Practice, 38*(5), 452–462.

Saxon, D., & Barkham, M. (2012). Patterns of therapist variability: Therapist effects and the contribution of patient severity and risk. *Journal of Consulting and Clinical Psychology, 80*(4), 535–546.

Schöttke, H., Flückiger, C., Goldberg, S. B., Eversmann, J., & Lange, J. (2017). Predicting psychotherapy outcome based on therapist interpersonal skills: A five-year longitudinal study of a therapist assessment protocol. *Psychotherapy Research, 27*(6), 642–652.

Shanteau, J. (1992). Competence in experts: The role of task characteristics. *Organizational Behavior and Human Decision Processes, 53*(2), 252–266.

Shanteau, J., & Weiss, D. J. (2014). Individual expertise versus domain expertise. *American Psychologist, 69*(7), 711–712.

Shimokawa, K., Lambert, M. J., & Smart, D. W. (2010). Enhancing treatment outcome of patients at risk of treatment failure: Meta-analytic and mega-analytic review of a psychotherapy quality assurance system. *Journal of Consulting and Clinical Psychology, 78*(3), 298–311.

Skovholt, T. M., & Jennings, L. (2004). *Master therapist: Exploring expertise in therapy and counseling.* Needham Heights, MA: Allyn & Bacon.

Stein, D. M., & Lambert, M. J. (1984). On the relationship between therapist experience and psychotherapy outcome. *Clinical Psychology Review, 4*(2), 127–142.

Stein, D. M., & Lambert, M. J. (1995). Graduate training in psychotherapy: Are therapy outcomes enhanced? *Journal of Consulting and Clinical Psychology, 63*(2), 182–196.

Stevanovic, P., & Rupert, P. A. (2004). Career-sustaining behaviors, satisfactions, and stresses of professional psychologists. *Psychotherapy: Theory, Research, Practice, Training, 41*(3), 301–309.

Taylor, J. M., & Neimeyer, G. J. (2017). The ongoing evolution of continuing education: Past, present,

and future. In T. Rousmaniere, R. K. Goodyear, S. D. Miller, & B. E. Wamold (Eds.), *The cycle of excellence: Using deliberate practice to improve supervision and training* (pp. 219–248). Hoboken, NJ: Wiley.

Tracey, T. J. G., Wampold, B. E., Lichtenberg, J. W., & Goodyear, R. K. (2014). Expertise in psychotherapy: An elusive goal? *American Psychologist, 69,* 218–229.

Ullén, F., Hambrick, D. Z., & Mosing, M. A. (2016). Rethinking expertise: A multifactorial gene–environment interaction model of expert performance. *Psychological Bulletin, 142*(4), 427–446.

Ulvenes, P. G., Berggraf, L., Hoffart, A., Stiles, T. C., Svartberg, M., McCullough, L., et al. (2012). Different processes for different therapies: Therapist actions, therapeutic bond, and outcome. *Psychotherapy, 49*(3), 291–302.

Walfish, S., McAlister, B., O'Donnell, P., & Lambert, M. J. (2012). An investigation of self-assessment bias in mental health providers. *Psychological Reports, 110*(2), 639–644.

Waltz, J., Addis, M. E., Koerner, K., & Jacobson, N. S. (1993). Testing the integrity of a psychotherapy protocol: Assessment of adherence and competence. *Journal of Consulting and Clinical Psychology, 61,* 620–630.

Wampold, B. E. (2001). Contextualizing psychotherapy as a healing practice: Culture, history, and methods. *Applied and Preventive Psychology, 10,* 69–86.

Wampold, B. E. (2015). Routine outcome monitoring: Coming of age—With the usual developmental challenges. *Psychotherapy, 52*(4), 458–462.

Wampold, B. E., Baldwin, S. A., Holtforth, M. G., & Imel, Z. E. (2017). What characterizes effective therapists? In L. G. Castonguay & C. E. Hill (Eds.), *How and why are some therapists better than others: Understanding therapist effects* (pp. 37–53). Washington, DC: American Psychological Association.

Wampold, B. E., & Brown, G. S. (2005). Estimating therapist variability: A naturalistic study of outcomes in managed care. *Journal of Consulting and Clinical Psychology, 73,* 914–923.

Wampold, B. E., & Imel, Z. E. (2015). *The great psychotherapy debate: The research evidence for what works in psychotherapy* (2nd ed.). New York: Routledge.

Wampold, B. E., & Serlin, R. C. (2000). The consequences of ignoring a nested factor on measures of effect size in analysis of variance. *Psychological Methods, 5,* 425–433.

Webb, C. A., DeRubeis, R. J., Amsterdam, J. D., Shelton, R. C., Hollon, S. D., & Dimidjian, S. (2011). Two aspects of the therapeutic alliance: Differential relations with depressive symptom change. *Journal of Consulting and Clinical Psychology, 79*(3), 279–283.

Webb, C. A., DeRubeis, R. J., & Barber, J. P. (2010). Therapist adherence/competence and treatment outcome: A meta-analytic review. *Journal of Consulting and Clinical Psychology, 78*(2), 200–211.

CHAPTER 11

Working Smarter, Not Harder

Comparing Evidence-Based Assessment to the Conventional Routine Assessment Process

ERIC A. YOUNGSTROM
ANNA VAN METER

Assessment has been a major component of clinical psychology for almost a century, with a core set of practices and processes that have not changed much in several decades. Yet we may be reaching a tipping point with respect to adoption of change. Evidence-based assessment (EBA) offers an exciting opportunity to change from "business as usual" to an approach that is more effective, providing better information and outcomes to more clients at the same or lower cost (Norcross, Beutler, & Levant, 2006; Youngstrom, 2013). EBA provides a framework for careful consideration of client characteristics, needs, values, and preferences, and informs clinical decision making in powerful ways. The shift from the conventional routine to EBA is daunting because it requires letting go of some familiar methods and ceding some professional autonomy (Meehl, 1997; Susskind & Susskind, 2015). In the following pages, we lay out some of the advantages and challenges of a next-generation approach to EBA, seen through the eyes and actions of two protagonists: "Old School Joe" and "EBA Jane."

Joe, a successful independent practitioner, has built up a thriving group known for its work doing psychological evaluations and treatment for a variety of clinical problems. Joe is a member of his state and national professional organizations, and he skims the associated journals, but he has not kept up on the new literature, which has caused him to change the way he practices assessment. He is selective about his choice of continuing education, always keeping an eye out for something that would add luster to his professional offerings. Like many practitioners, he has tended to keep using what has worked for him in the past rather than changing his approach to incorporate new research. Jane, a freshly licensed PhD, is joining Joe's group after completing her doctorate and internship at well-regarded clinical programs. Like many newly minted PhDs, Jane eagerly wants to put her schooling into practice, and she comes armed with the latest research as her guide for the work that lies ahead. Joe and Jane met regularly for coffee or lunch while she was completing her supervised postdoctoral hours for licensure, and they have had spirited discussions about assessment. They like each other. Joe's pragmatism and skepticism mean that he doesn't chase every shiny new trend, but he is open to hearing about new ideas and

In memory of Ethan Schafer, PhD, student, colleague, and friend, whose clinical wisdom became the model for "Joe" and whose humor and commitment to evidence inspired "Jane."

willing to adopt those that would lead to better outcomes or greater efficiency. Jane's initial suspicions that Joe was a hopeless Rorschach-hugging dinosaur, and that she would have to grit her teeth through supervision, gradually changed to grudging respect and then appreciation. Their regular discussions have influenced both of them in how they choose to conduct assessments. What have they learned from each other? And, most importantly, how might their learning apply to your own approach to evidence-based practice (EBP)?

Compare and Contrast EBA to the Old Model

The differences in how Joe and Jane approached a client began even before the first office visit. Table 11.1 outlines the steps that each typically followed in evaluating a client. Jane developed a list of clinical hypotheses based on the most common issues of individuals who come to a clinic (Meehl, 1954) (Table 11.1, Step A). After Jane had joined the practice, she asked Joe over coffee one morning if he knew what the top 10 diagnoses or problems were at the practice, and he rattled several off but had trouble coming up with 10, and he realized that he did not know percentages and would not be confident in ranking all of them in order.

Back in her office, Jane started pulling numbers from a list of prevalence rates summarized in a meta-analysis of outpatient clinics (Rettew, Lynch, Achenbach, Dumenci, & Ivanova, 2009), figuring that it would be a good first approximation because it combined data from a wide variety of different clinics (Youngstrom, Choukas-Bradley, Calhoun, & Jensen-Doss, 2014) (Table 11.1, Step B). It provided a more detailed, and reliable, starting point than Joe could offer, and Jane did not know who would walk through the door as she was just starting her practice. When Joe took a look at her list, he suggested that she needed to include learning disorders, as they accounted for a big slice of the referrals to the practice, and Jane heeded his advice, comparing Joe's armchair estimate of the rate of confirmed disabilities to some benchmarks she found with a quick search in the TRIP database (*www.tripdatabase.com*), which aggregates PubMed, Cochrane, and several other sites into a single, user-friendly interface. She summarized these as the first row in her "cheat sheet," where she gathered information about the common clinical issues, corresponding assessments, and key facts to aid their interpretation (see Table 11.2). The cheat sheet informed her practice by reminding her quickly which diagnoses she is most likely to see (which is particularly helpful for differential diagnoses or assessing comorbidity) and putting the key interpretive information for EBAs in one organized format.

Jane then set to work making sure that she had assessment tools that would help identify (Table 11.1, Step C) and track progress (Table 11.1, Steps H, I, and J) with the disorders that were most common (Youngstrom & Van Meter, 2016). The clinic assessment cabinet had a lot of cognitive and achievement measures, plus the Thematic Apperception Test, the Rorschach, the Minnesota Multiphasic Personality Inventory–2 (MMPI-2) . . . the usual suspects based on surveys of training programs and practitioners (Ready & Veague, 2014). There was a copy of the Beck Depression Inventory (BDI; Beck & Steer, 1987), but not the BDI-II ("Why pay for something when a free version gives you the same information?" Joe asked).

Jane made a table of interviews and measures that covered the gaps she identified, listing the common issues at the clinic as rows in the table, and columns for each of the key roles of assessment in *predicting* diagnosis or risk status, *prescribing* different treatments, and charting *process* and progress toward outcomes (Youngstrom, 2013). She got a jump-start on filling the table by cross-referencing her list of common clinical issues with the tables of contents from recent assessment handbooks (Hunsley & Mash, 2008), then by looking for practice parameters or systematic reviews or meta-analyses to fill in gaps. She asked Joe if he would consider buying them for the practice. Joe said, "Maybe." First, he wanted to know if there was a free option available that would accomplish the same thing. Some of the clinicians in his practice had switched from the Behavior Assessment System for Children–2 (BASC-2; Reynolds & Kamphaus, 2004) to the Strengths and Difficulties Questionnaire (SDQ; Goodman, Ford, Simmons, Gatward, & Meltzer, 2003). Jane pointed out that the SDQ covered far less, and Joe smiled and said that families might appreciate having fewer questions. Jane smiled back and said, "Actually, surveys of patients have found that they prefer doing more detailed interviews and assessments, if the information helps with the diagnosis and treatment" (Bruchmuller, Margraf, Suppiger,

TABLE 11.1. Comparing the Methods of Joe's "Assessment as Usual" versus Jane's EBA Approach

Assessment step	"Old School Joe"	"EBA Jane"
A. Identify setting's most common diagnoses.	Rely on implicit habits, and some things that rise to the level of "specializations" for which the practice group is known.	Make a "short list" of most common diagnoses and clinical issues based on practice patterns.
B. Benchmark base rates.	Not done.	Compare the short list to benchmarks from other practices and published rates; identify any potential mismatches and reflect on what might be causing the discrepancy.
C. Risks and moderators.	Some of these emerge during unstructured interview, either Joe probing to confirm a hypothesis, or the client spontaneously volunteers the information.	Build a checklist of key risk factors; also list factors that might change treatment selection or moderate outcome; develop a plan for how to routinely assess them.
D. Update patient probabilities.	Look at scores from MMPI and Rorschach, and interpret constellations of scores impressionistically.	Refer to cheat sheet with diagnostic likelihood ratios and clinical significance benchmarks for assessment instruments linked to common presenting problems; actuarial approach estimates probability informs next steps (wait, test, treat).
E. Cross-informant data patterns.	Interpret score patterns impressionistically; weave a narrative using the supporting data, if therapist has gathered it.	Gather collateral information to revise case formulation; for adults, consider parent, spouse, or roommate. Compare to typical level of agreement.
F. Add narrow, incremental assessments to clarify diagnoses and severity.	Rarely done.	Have follow-up tests available; organize so that key information is easy to integrate.
G. Finalize diagnoses and formulation.	Do an unstructured interview and discussion with client.	Administer (semi)structured interview modules; add specialized assessment until treatment threshold is crossed.
H. Treatment planning and goal setting.	Explain to the client how the favored treatment package connects with themes from the presenting problem and interview.	Screen for medical conditions and medication use. Assess family functioning, personality, comorbidity, socioeconomic status, and other potential treatment moderators.
I. Process measures ("dashboards, quizzes and homework")	"So, did you do the homework?" . . . Ask global questions, not written down and tracked.	Track homework, session attendance, medication monitoring, therapy assignments, daily report cards (Weisz et al., 2011).
J. Chart progress and outcome ("midterm and final exams").	"So, how was your week? How are things going?" Again, ask global questions, responded to empathically in the moment and explored, but not written down and tracked.	Use Jacobson and Truax (1991) benchmarks from "cheat sheet."
K. Monitor maintenance.	"Call me if things start to get bumpy. Don't wait to be in crisis." Mention proactive boosters in planned termination.	Work with client to create list of key triggers, recommendations about next action if starting to worsen.
L. Client preferences.	Watch nonverbal cues to see if client is engaged, and probe signs of being closed or defensive.	Assess client concordance with treatment plan; ask about cultural factors that might affect treatment engagement.

Note. The steps do not need to follow a strict order, and "patient preferences" in particular should be woven through the process.

TABLE 11.2. EBA Jane's"Cheat Sheet" for Common Problems, Gathering Prevalence, Screening, Follow-Up, Diagnostic Confirmation, Goal-Setting, and Outcome Measurement Information in One Place

| Step | Element | Common diagnostic hypotheses (Step A) | | | | |
		ADHD	Anxiety	Alcohol misuse	Depression	Suicide
Starting probability (Step B)	Outpatient base rate	30%	25%	8%	21%	5%
Know risk factors/ moderators (Step C)	List	Male sex (but inattentive type often missing in women); family history	Family history	Family history	Female sex (after puberty)	Female sex, family history
Broad measure (Step D)	Scale	CBCL *T* Attention Problems (Achenbach & Rescorla, 2003)	CBCL *T* Internalizing Problems (Achenbach & Rescorla, 2003)	CAGE-AID self-report (Couwenbergh et al., 2009)	Parent Mood and Feelings Questionnaire (Costello & Angold, 1988)	CBCL Suicide items (items 18 and 91; Achenbach & Rescorla, 2003; Van Meter et al., unpublished data)
	Score and DLR (source)	Score 71+, DLR = 1.98; score <64, DLR = .38 (Jarrett et al., 2016)	Score 78+, DLR = 2.03; score <50, DLR = .13 (Van Meter et al., 2014)	Score 2+, DLR = 45.5; score <2, DLR = .09 (Couwenbergh et al., 2009)	Score 11+, DLR = 6.62; score <11, DLR = .16 (Thapar & McGuffin, 1998)	Score 1+, DLR = 20.25; score <0, DLR = .92 (local data)
Cross-informant option (Step E)	Scale	TRF Attention Problems (Achenbach & Rescorla, 2003)	YSR Internalizing Problems (Achenbach & Rescorla, 2003)	—	YSR Affective Problems (Achenbach & Rescorla, 2003)	YSR Suicide items (items 18 and 91; Achenbach & Rescorla, 2003; Van Meter et al., unpublished data)
	Score and DLR (source)	Score 66+, DLR = 1.69; score <59, DLR = .48 (Jarrett et al., 2016)	Score 73+, DLR=2.35; score <42, DLR = .26 (Van Meter et al., 2014)	—	Score *raw* 7+, DLR = 6.23, score <7, DLR = .22 (Aebi et al., 2009)	Score 1+, DLR = 1.97; score <0, DLR = .97 (local data)
Narrow assessment (Step F)	Scale	Continuous Performance Test	SCARED— Parent	Proceed to interview	Child Mood and Feelings Questionnaire	Proceed to interview
	Score and DLR (source)	Hit Reaction Time SE Score 74.5+, DLR = 1.96; score <58, DLR = .39 (Jarrett et al., 2016)	Score 22+, DLR = 2.71; score <21, DLR = .55 (Van Meter et al., 2018)	—	Score 8+, DLR = 2.88; score <8, DLR = .34 (Thapar & McGuffin, 1998)	—

(*continued*)

TABLE 11.2. (*continued*)

Step	Element	ADHD	Anxiety	Alcohol misuse	Depression	Suicide
		Common diagnostic hypotheses (Step A)				
Confirmation (Step G)	Interview	MINI ADHD module (Sheehan et al., 2010)	MINI module Specific Anxiety Disorder (Sheehan et al., 2015)	MINI Alcohol Use module (Sheehan et al., 2015)	MINI Depression module (Sheehan et al., 2015)	MINI Suicidality module (Sheehan et al., 2015)
Process measurement (Step I)	Session-level tracking	Youth Top Problems (Y-TOPS; Weisz et al., 2011); track medication adherence if taking	Y-TOPS; CBT homework completion	Y-TOPS; track alcohol consumption	Y-TOPS; CBT homework completion	Ask at each session
Progress measurement (Step J)[a]	Scale 90% RCI: A: B: C:	CBCL *T* Attention 8 points <50 <66 <58	CBCL *T* Internalizing 8 points <39 <70 <56	—	CBCL *T* Internalizing 8 points <39 <70 <56	—
Maintenance monitoring (Step K)	Plan	Monitor schoolwork completion and grades	Be aware of anxiety-provoking situations; practice coping skills	Attend to situations that might increase likelihood of drinking; monitor changes in drinking	Make a list of possible mood episode triggers; track mood or energy symptoms	Monitor morbid and/or suicidal ideation and depressive symptoms

Note. RCI, Reliable Change Index, but these are scaled in the test units, not *z*-scores, so that the clinician need not convert them; 90% is the number of points required for 90% (two-tailed) or 95% (one-tailed) confidence that the construct level has changed; A, away from the clinical; B, back in the nonclinical; C, closer to the nonclinical than clinical range.

[a]Adaptation of the Jacobson clinical significance model.

& Schneider, 2011; Suppiger et al., 2009). Joe thought about it and said, "OK, let's treat it like a grant proposal. You describe the need, briefly review what's available, and show the data that a measure that costs money would significantly improve diagnosis or outcome, and *then* I'll buy it for the clinic. . . . Oh, and another thing—it needs to help with one of the common issues, like you were just saying." Anything that was available in the public domain, Jane was free to add; anything that Jane wanted to buy on her own, she could. Anything that she could make the case would significantly improve practice at the clinic, Joe would cover.

Approaching the Initial Assessment: Before the First Session

Differences also pervaded their approaches to the first session or interview. Joe used two different styles, depending on whether the person was coming for therapy or an assessment report. For therapy, Joe glanced at the note about the presenting problem before the appointment (he used to jot them on index cards; now he looked at the scheduling note on his calendar). He immediately started sizing things up, watching nonverbal behavior to form impressions of mental status and functioning, while asking the client to repeat the presenting problem and elaborate (Morrison, 2014). Joe listened for key details, probing and exploring them until he had a clear hypothesis and enough information to confirm it, and then he switched to thinking about the treatment plan and how to engage the client with it (Croskerry, 2003).

Assessments were a different story. When evaluating a young client, Joe mailed out a packet of questionnaires and checklists for the caregiver, the youth (if old enough), and a teacher to complete, and he had a developmental history packet that he asked the caregiver to complete. Adult clients skipped the developmental history and questionnaires. He used the first 15–30 minutes of the session to talk with the client and develop a sense of the hypotheses, and he had everyone do a core battery: Youth (or college students or adults doing an attention-deficit/hyperactivity disorder/learning disorder [ADHD/LD] evaluation) completed the Wechslers for ability (Wechsler, 2014), the Woodcock–Johnson Tests of Achievement (Woodcock, McGrew, & Mather, 2005), a continuous performance test (Conners, Epstein, Angold, & Klaric, 2003), and the Rorschach; adults got the Rorschach and the MMPI-2. Depending on what he found during the interview and looking at the results, Joe might supplement the battery with other specific tests in another session; but often, he thought that was enough to address the referral question (Finn & Tonsager, 1997).

Jane used a consistent approach whether the person was coming for assessment or treatment. She would send a set of checklists for the family to complete ahead of time (Table 11.1, Step D), including the caregiver, youth, and teacher ratings (Table 11.1, Step E), as well as a developmental history. She used checklists with adult clients as well (though usually limited to self-report) (e.g., Achenbach & Rescorla, 2003; Gadow, Sprafkin, & Weiss, 2004). For each clinical issue that was common or serious, Jane wanted to have a scale in the battery that would give her information about whether to explore the topic further with the client. She approached this process by looking for measures that had shown diagnostic or discriminative validity (i.e., the ability to tell apart cases with a particular diagnosis from others coming to the clinic), ideally using methods such as logistic regression or receiver operating characteristic analysis and then reporting diagnostic sensitivity or specificity, or multilevel likelihood ratios (Youngstrom & Van Meter, 2016).

Jane had developed knowledge of a set of scales that covered the most common issues that addressed the needs of more than 80% of the clients with whom she worked (Brighton, 2011; Youngstrom & Van Meter, 2016). Occasionally, she added to this core set more specialized measures relevant to new clinical settings, or when she found a particularly helpful tool that she thought might be useful in case another client had a similar concern. Jane also periodically reviewed her list to "retire" any that were no longer recommended. For example, one measure initially looked promising but then got supplanted by other measures that outperformed it in a meta-analysis; the parent-reported Young Mania Rating Scale showed statistical validity in all the papers she found (e.g., Gracious, Youngstrom, Findling, & Calabrese, 2002), but three other scales performed significantly better at teasing apart bipolar disorder from other mood or disruptive behavior disorders (Youngstrom, Genzlinger, Egerton, & Van Meter, 2015).

Jane had her "cheat sheet" that summarized this information (see Table 11.2). She had started it during her internship by printing out a copy of a table of score ranges and associated likelihood ratios from a review article, then adding the scores and diagnostic likelihood ratios (DLRs) for any new measure that she found helpful in her work over time (Youngstrom et al., 2014). Joe had never heard of DLRs. Jane explained that a DLR is an effect size, comparing how often a score would be observed among cases that truly had the disorder to the rate among those who did not have the disorder (Straus, Glasziou, Richardson, & Haynes, 2011). If an article or manual reported the sensitivity and specificity, then she could calculate the DLRs. The DLR+, attached to a high-risk score, was the ratio of the sensitivity to the "false-alarm rate" (the opposite of specificity). The DLR– divided the "false-negative rate" (the opposite of sensitivity) by the specificity. Joe did not see the point, especially since the DLRs looked more difficult to interpret. They could range from 0 to 1, and then 1 to infinity. Frankly, they looked weird.

Jane explained that the DLR was a measure of the shift in odds of having a diagnosis (Step D in the EBA model; see Table 11.2 for examples). For example, if an ADHD scale had a sensitivity of .90 and a specificity of .80, then the DLR+ would be 4.5 (Straus et al., 2011). That meant that scores above threshold were 4.5 times more likely to occur among cases with ADHD compared to cases without ADHD. The odds that an individual scoring in that range might have ADHD increase by a factor of 4.5. Conversely, a low score on the same scale would have a DLR– of .125.

Jane used the DLR to adjust the starting probability of ADHD. Using the prevalence estimate from the Rettew and colleagues (2009) meta-analysis until she got her bearings (and data) at the practice, the starting probability of an ADHD diagnosis was 38%. Joe interrupted her, "That obviously can't work: 4.5 times 38% is more than 100% probability!" Jane smiled and said, "You're right—it is 4.5 times the *odds,*

not the *probability*." The probability needs to get transformed to odds before the multiplication; the new odds could then be converted back to a revised probability.

"Sounds like a lot of work. Are people really going to do that?" Joe mused. Jane agreed—if people had to do it by hand. She showed him a probability nomogram (Figure 11.1) that used geometry to accomplish the transformations, "Like an old-fashioned slide rule! Did you ever use one of those?" Jane gently teased. There also are online calculators, apps for smartphones ("Do a Google search for 'probability calculator,' and you will find a bunch of options. . . . "). "For it to be helpful, it needs to be easy for clini-

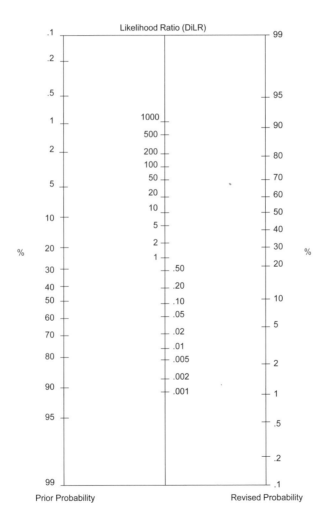

FIGURE 11.1. Probability nomogram used to combine prior probability with likelihood ratios to estimate revised posterior probability. Straus et al. (2011) provide the rationale and medical examples; Frazier and Youngstrom (2006) illustrate applying the nomogram to a client with possible ADHD.

cians to do in real time; all the evidence-based medicine gurus agree with you, Joe" (Norcross, Hogan, & Koocher, 2008; Straus et al., 2011).

Joe looked thoughtful, but not fully persuaded. "It is definitely worth it," Jane pushed. Research has shown that when clinicians have the opportunity to form their own impressions of assessment data, instead of using an algorithm to interpret the information, the algorithm consistently ties or beats clinical judgment (Ægisdóttir et al., 2006; Grove, Zald, Lebow, Snitz, & Nelson, 2000). Using the nomogram approach showed large improvements in the accuracy, and also consistency (i.e., clinicians reaching similar conclusions from the same information) of estimates and clinical decisions (Jenkins, Youngstrom, Washburn, & Youngstrom, 2011). So long as Jane had looked up (or calculated) the DLRs in advance, using the nomogram added little or no time to her work with the clients, yet it yielded big gains in consistency and accuracy. Her cheat sheet kept the key information close at hand for the tools she used routinely.

Reflecting on discussions with Jane during the early months of her tenure at his clinic, Joe made a few changes to his approach. He realized that he was probably falling into a trap of confirmation bias. Most clinicians form an initial hypothesis based on the first minutes of description about the presenting problem, then seek confirming evidence. They tend not to look for disconfirming data, and they fail to systematically consider alternative hypotheses (Croskerry, 2003). When Jane showed Joe that just jotting down a short list of contending hypotheses produced large improvements in the accuracy of diagnosis and agreement about next clinical action (Jenkins & Youngstrom, 2016)— swiftly inoculating against confirmation bias— Joe decided that there was no good reason not to make that list when meeting each client. Joe contemplated adding rating scales for his adult clients, and the discussions with Jane got him musing about why he was not gathering collateral perspectives with more of his adult clients when he found it helpful with the youth.

The First Session

Joe began the first session with a firm handshake and began to watch and listen as the client explained his take on the presenting problem. After Jane got him thinking on the limitations of his approach, he had taken to glancing down the list of contending hypotheses, perhaps adding one or crossing one off, and using it for cues about what to explore. Previously, Joe had just been listening for a few minutes, then exploring and confirming his initial hypothesis (Croskerry, 2003). For therapy cases, he was trying to settle on a sufficient diagnosis for billing; for example, if "other specified mood and related disorder" was enough, then he was not as worried about the nuances of whether a case met strict criteria for cyclothymia, pervasive depressive disorder, or a lingering adjustment disorder. After making up his mind about the billing diagnosis and the case formulation, he used the rest of the session to lay out a treatment plan (usually cognitive-behavioral therapy with a layering of insight—Joe insisted this was a coherent hybrid and not sloppy eclecticism; Stricker & Gold, 1996). He briefly described the treatment model and rationale, and connected it with his formulation of the presenting problem. Joe asked whether the person had been in therapy before, and if so, he compared and contrasted what the person had experienced in the past with the way that he typically ran sessions. He negotiated a therapeutic contract, asking the person to commit to a certain number of sessions and to doing "homework" or reflection in between sessions. Joe closed with a bit of motivational interviewing to help identify the source of pain that the client wanted to address, and connected that with the plan for change.

For assessment cases, Joe actively listened with two goals in mind: He was deciding whether he needed to augment the battery with any more specialized tests, and he wanted to be able to explain the connections between the components of the battery and the questions that the client wanted answered. For adults, he administered the Rorschach and the MMPI-2. Joe had read some of Finn's work, and he was sold on the combination of the two approaches as a way of getting detailed information about the person's style of thinking and interacting with the world (Finn, 2007; Finn & Tonsager, 1997). Finishing those two usually consumed the rest of the session, and he would schedule a follow-up debriefing session after he had the scoring done and a report drafted. Sometimes Joe would take the person on for therapy, but that occurred less than half the time. He focused on maximizing insight from the evaluation, and he believed that a good evaluation could be a fairly strong intervention in its own right (Poston & Hanson, 2010). For youth LD and psychoeducational evaluations, Joe kept the Rorschach and MMPI for Adolescents (MMPI-A) because he believed it was helpful and distinguished his reports from a typical school evaluation.

Jane aimed to start the first meeting with the checklists and measures already scored. This did not happen on every occasion, but one of her goals was to do as much of the scoring electronically as possible and to be able to drop the scores into the probability calculator or nomogram. Doing so gave her an updated set of probabilities for the common conditions (Table 11.1, Steps D and E).

The nomogram or calculator combined the initial estimate of the probability of the condition—usually the base rate at the clinic or a similar setting—with the DLR attached to the most relevant scale score to update the probability estimate. That estimate has many different aliases in the literature, including the *positive predictive value, positive predictive power, posterior probability,* and others. Evidence-based medicine suggests comparing that probability to two thresholds, the Wait–Test and the Test–Treat threshold (Straus et al., 2011). The key concept was to use the updated probability to guide the next clinical action. If the probability was below the Wait–Test threshold, then the chance of the client having that particular issue—based on the data at hand—was low enough to consider it functionally "ruled out." If the probability were above the Test–Treat threshold, then the chance was high enough to consider the condition "ruled in," and it would become a target for the treatment plan. In between the two thresholds was the "Assessment Zone," where the next clinical actions would concentrate on adding more powerful assessment strategies to resolve the ambiguity (Youngstrom, 2013) (Table 11.2, Step F). These assessments often were lengthier and more expensive, but in this instance, the investment was clearly warranted because the other data indicated too high a probability to ignore, yet not high enough to diagnose and treat.

Jane knew from experience what others had found in multiple studies: The first-wave tests were not strong enough to establish a diagnosis on their own (e.g., Van Meter et al., 2014; You, Youngstrom, Feeny, Youngstrom, & Findling, 2015). Put another way, the low base rate of most conditions, combined with the moderate-size DLR+ for checklists and screeners (typically in the 3–7 range, and rarely above 10 in studies with a clinically meaningful comparison group; Youngstrom et al., 2015) meant that the

initial evaluation would put cases in the Assessment Zone, not the Treatment Zone, based on high-risk scores. A good first assessment tool, like the Parent Mood and Feelings Questionnaire (MFQ; Costello & Angold, 1988), could move the probability of depression—a common problem in teens—from a baseline probability of ~21% to under 4% or over 64% (see the Table 11.2 "cheat sheet" for DLRs). Low scores might be enough to rule out depression if there were no other concerning signs or findings. High scores were not enough to start treatment, but they definitely signaled the need for further assessment.

This pattern is the nemesis of most screening efforts: When the condition is rare, most cases that test positive on even a good screener do not prove to have the condition (i.e., the positive predictive values is under 50%; Pepe, 2003). On the other hand, the DLR– was enough to push the base rate down into the Wait Zone for every condition on her list. This meant that Jane could use the initial results to trim her list of hypotheses, customizing it to focus only on the plausible suspects based on the presenting problem and initial results. Of course, if new information emerged that changed the probability, it could push the estimate back into the Assessment Zone. Jane also would use her clinical judgment to override the probability estimate if she learned game-changing information (Meehl, 1954), but she also knew that the literature was replete with examples of clinicians overcorrecting and performing worse than relatively simple algorithms (Ægisdóttir et al., 2006; Grove et al., 2000), so she was deliberately conservative about making changes to the formulation.

With all of this information in front of her, Jane would explain the leading hypotheses to the family, and what assessment she was going to ask them to do next to help clarify the formulation. If the family asked about something that was low probability, such as when a parent suspected that his or her child had obsessive–compulsive disorder (OCD) or bipolar disorder, then Jane would explain how the checklist scores weighed against that being likely. She also reassured them that if other data increased the risk of the diagnosis, it would be right back on the table for further evaluation. Jane and her clients liked how transparent this made the process (Harter & Simon, 2011).

The choice of the next assessment strategy depended on the specific hypothesis. Sometimes there were more specialized rating scales that could be helpful (Table 11.2, Step F). The best mania checklists, for example, could be quick additions that would tip the scale decisively toward unipolar depression or attention-deficit/hyperactivity disorder (ADHD) in many ambiguous cases (Youngstrom et al., 2015). They were not specific enough to compensate for the low base rate of bipolar disorder in most settings, but they added valuable clarification when cases were already in the "Assessment Zone." That validity profile made them inappropriate for universal screening but helpful as an intermediate measure. Similarly, continuous performance tests and some other neurocognitive measures were not specific enough to be decisive by themselves in evaluating ADHD (Pelham, Fabiano, & Massetti, 2005), but they could add useful incremental data (Frazier & Youngstrom, 2006; Jarrett, Van Meter, Youngstrom, Hilton, & Ollendick, 2016).

Jane usually followed up with a semistructured interview to rapidly confirm or disconfirm diagnoses at this point (Table 11.2, Step G). The structured aspect ensured that she was systematic in inquiring about symptoms, duration, and other key elements to make certain that she was consistent in applying the formal criteria. That would increase the reproducibility of the diagnoses (Garb, 1998). The "semi" part referred to the fact that Jane was comfortable using her own words to probe symptoms, and to rephrase things in language that was developmentally or culturally appropriate, versus sticking to a script.

Joe asked Jane why she did not just start with a structured interview for everyone. He smiled and nodded along as she pointed out that no interview covers all the possible disorders—there are more than 360 in the current DSM (American Psychiatric Association, 2013), and usually interviews concentrate on two dozen or so. Using the first wave of assessment also helps her pick which interview modules (and which optimal structured approaches) fit best for the client and presenting problem. Some have well-developed anxiety or autism modules, and others omit mania or pervasive developmental disorders completely. The semistructured aspect makes the interview more conversational, too, and helps explore which features carry particular meaning for the family. Over time, Jane had moved toward a hybrid approach, in which she picked modules from different interviews based on which topics were in the Assessment Zone at this stage. The structure helped to make sure

that she remembered all the nuances, even more so now that DSM-5 had changed the criteria for several disorders. With a bit of practice, the sets of checklists became rapid, and a seamless part of her routine: She was operating with a surgeon's precision or like a pilot preparing for takeoff (Gawande, 2010), covering the necessary elements, but able to attend to the situation and recognize when it required a different response.

After the semistructured interview, Jane still was not quite finished with the assessment. By this stage, she usually had one or more diagnoses well established. The semistructured component usually covered the differential diagnoses and explanations to be considered (e.g., make sure that the symptoms are not due to a general medical condition). There were three other things that Jane wanted to accomplish before settling on the treatment plan.

First, Jane wanted to assess whether there were any moderators that might change response to treatment (Table 11.1, Step H). For example, if the family was Hispanic, and particularly if family relationships seemed salient in the case conceptualization, then she considered whether to use an interpersonal psychotherapy (IPT) or family therapy approach instead of CBT (Mufson, Dorta, Olfson, Weissman, & Hoagwood, 2004). If there was evidence of clinically worrisome substance use, then Jane tried to explore whether it warranted simultaneous intervention (Hodge, Jackson, & Vaughn, 2012). If the child was younger or had lower verbal ability, then she shifted her treatment plans to be more behavioral and less cognitive. Comorbidity often also could influence treatment selection, as anxiety might complicate response to treatment focused on depression (Nilsen, Eisemann, & Kvernmo, 2013) and comorbid ADHD might reduce the effectiveness of interventions focused on reducing externalizing behaviors (Shelleby & Kolko, 2015). If the caregiver was depressed, then that could undermine the child's treatment, if not addressed (Shelleby & Kolko, 2015). Jane also had a checklist for reminding to ask the client about other medical conditions, any medications they were taking (including birth control), and an open-ended question about whether there was anything else of importance to the client that she had forgotten to ask.

The second consideration was patient preferences (Table 11.1, Step L). The potential cultural moderators Jane knew about were based on group data, but families differed in terms of assimilation and cultural identity, as well as other attitudes. Clients also hold different assumptions and beliefs about causes of mental illness and stances toward treatment, which are vital to know up front (Yeh et al., 2005). A medication could have a large effect size and few risks, but it would still deliver no benefit if the client was adamantly opposed to medication. Similarly, other modalities might be nonstarters for myriad reasons. Jane would rather have a quick, candid discussion rather than pitch a plan that sounded great to her and have the family not show up for the second appointment.

The third facet was to have a baseline measure of severity (Table 11.1, Step H, again). Jane wanted to be able to gauge whether treatment was helping, so she used checklists as a starting point. Often the scores from the intake checklists fit the role. If the main diagnosis was oppositional defiant disorder, then the CBCL Externalizing score would be a good touchstone for assessments spaced a couple months apart. For other diagnoses, Jane might ask the family to complete a different checklist that provided better coverage of core features and had shown good sensitivity to treatment effects. The ADHD Rating Scale or Conners included more items and potentially better sensitivity to change than the Attention Problems scale on the SDQ, for example (Lambert & Lambert, 1999). Jane's ideal measure for this role was long enough to be reasonably precise and provide good content coverage, but short enough that people would tolerate repeating it a few times over the course of treatment to evaluate progress, or even deterioration, which could serve as a strong cue to revisit the treatment plan (Lambert, Hansen, & Finch, 2001; Lambert, Harmon, Slade, Whipple, & Hawkins, 2005).

Assessing Progress, Process, and Outcomes

After the first session or two, Joe was largely done with formal assessment. He had negotiated goals with the client, and if he was using elements of CBT in his approach, he made sure that the goals were concrete and potentially measurable, as well as things that could shift incrementally ("No black-or-white thinking!"). Joe liked the scaling question from a solution-focused therapy Continuing Education (CE) workshop he had once attended: "What's the smallest change you could see, and still be sure that treatment was helping?" Each session,

he would check in with a global "So, how are things?" Sometimes he would have the person scale his or her well-being from 0 to 10, or sometimes 0 to 100. Occasionally he would try a worksheet from a manual or a scale that he found online. Joe paid attention to whether the client was doing work during the session and in between sessions. He treated client disengagement as a cue to explore rapport and whether the client was in accord with his interpretation of the goals. Joe made a point of following up any no-shows or cancellations with at least a brief exploration about alliance. A lot of the process felt intuitive to him; if the session felt "off," that was a cue to check alliance and goals.

Joe was reassured that Jane did not keep her nose buried in a manual or a stack of rating scales during session, though he was struck by how much assessment she wove through the rest of therapy. Her "cheat sheet" (Table 11.2) had four benchmarks for each scale that she used to measure baseline severity. One was the Reliable Change Index (RCI), expressed in the regular scale metric (not z-scores: "Extra work, and they do not mean anything to clients," Jane explained). They showed how much the score would need to drop in order to be 90 or 95% confident that treatment really was producing change (Jacobson & Truax, 1991). Jane walked her clients through a metaphor: "Think about a bathroom scale. We don't weigh exactly the same every time we step on it. Some days we had a big dinner; other days we are wearing different clothes. So if we are trying a diet, we shouldn't panic if we go up half a pound on Day 2, and we wouldn't celebrate if we lost half a pound, either. These numbers are how much we would need to see on this mood scale, or ADHD scale, to be sure that our treatment was working, and not just showing the usual ups and downs of life."

The other three numbers were normative benchmarks, which Jacobson called "ABC." Jane used a mnemonic to remember them (Youngstrom, 2013): A was the benchmark for moving *Away* from the clinical distribution. Jacobson suggested two standard deviations below the clinical mean (Jacobson & Truax, 1991). Jane framed it to clients by showing them a curve: "Imagine that this is 100 people with depression. Here's the average score for people with depression. If we get your score below here, then 97 out of 100 people with depression would be scoring higher. We would have gotten your level of depression away from what is typical when people are depressed." *B* stood for *Back* into the normal range. Jane drew a second curve, representing 100 people without depression. "Not having depression doesn't mean that you have zero stress, irritation, or hassles in life. Here's the average score for people who aren't depressed. Sometimes we have bad weeks, or extra stress at school or work, and that pushes scores up even though we still aren't depressed. The *Back* benchmark shows the high end of what would be typical scores without having depression. Getting your score below here means that your symptoms are back within the normal range." The third threshold, *C,* was the weighted mean combining the clinical and nonclinical benchmarks; passing it meant that the client's score was *Closer* to the nonclinical than to the clinical distribution. Jane looked at the baseline score, then picked the closest of the ABC benchmarks as a target, along with the RCI. "If treatment helps, then after six or so sessions, we should see definite improvement (aiming for more than the RCI), and we should be able to reach this first benchmark." Jane was setting expectations about the rate of change, negotiating a measurable goal, and scheduling a midterm evaluation. She usually picked the sixth session as the time to repeat the severity scales for the primary treatment targets. Six sessions was long enough for the treatment to have gained traction if it was working (Lambert et al., 2005), and early enough to allow course correction if not—before the client got frustrated and dropped out (Swift & Greenberg, 2012). The midterm format avoided burdening the client with lengthy rating scales every session (Table 11.1, Step J).

Jane also had weekly ratings of progress, which she wrote down and tracked diligently (Table 11.2, Step I). She borrowed heavily from the Youth Top Problems approach (Y-TOPS; Weisz et al., 2011), asking the client to pick up to three things that he or she wanted to focus on changing in therapy. They rated how bad the problem was on a 0- to 10-point scale, then updated their rating every session. Three items was fast and low burden, and because the client picked them, they reinforced the sense of engagement. If Jane was working with a youth, she asked the caregiver to pick three problems as well, and she checked regularly about them. She knew that if the caregiver did not feel engaged or see progress, the child was not going to drive him- or herself to the session. Joe asked if it was overkill to have clients do both the severity scales and the Y-TOPS. Jane pointed out that together they combined both nomothetic and idiographic approaches to assessment. The Jacobson approach was norm-referenced, comparing the level of symptoms to external benchmarks, including results from treatment studies (Weersing, 2005). The Y-TOPS was personalized, and the frequency let it detect critical incidents and put them on the table for discussion in session. It also would expose when clients got stuck on a plateau, not making headway several sessions in a row. That could be another indication to revisit the formulation or treatment approach.

The Y-TOPS approach proved to be common ground for Jane and Joe. That sort of goal setting meshed with Joe's idiographic, motivational approach, but it provided a quantitative element and regular measurement that he had been lacking. He could see how it might improve outcomes. Joe could imagine how well a diet would work if someone never stepped on a scale and just talked about whether he or she felt lighter. It also got him thinking about whether he had gotten into a rut in which he offered everyone the same default treatment, versus looking for clues that he should try a different approach or make adaptations or adjustments along the way. Jane's approach made her shift plans more often and guided her in choosing new skills to add to her toolkit. For example, she realized that substance misuse issues were a common complication with many of her adolescent and adult clients, and she needed more in her toolkit to assess and manage those issues, as well as a good list of referrals when the problems became too severe. It was more work at times, but it also kept her growing as a clinician.

Learning Client Preferences and Goals

Joe made a point of getting client input. He asked clients if they had any questions, or things that they wanted him to elaborate on. He made sure that they had a shared goal they were working toward in therapy. Joe also paid attention to whether the client completed work between sessions, though he rarely logged it. He watched for nonverbal cues about whether the client was engaged and made sure to probe signs of being closed or defensive. Joe and the client decided intuitively when treatment was winding down.

Jane used a different system to solicit client preferences for treatment (Table 11.1, Step L).

Specifically, she discussed the pros and cons of each possible treatment option with clients. She also wanted to know about alternative treatments that her clients might find of interest or prefer (e.g., fish oil, or a light box, prayer, reflexology, as well as any psychotropic medication—whatever the client added), and she helped clients track their usage, so that it was an ongoing conversation. Jane made a point of tracking homework and skills use between sessions, and periodically she and the client would graph the week-by-week history of change on the client's top problems, overlaying the homework and skills tracking. Often the client saw the connection between doing the work and reaping the progress or, conversely, not implementing the tactics and feeling stuck.

Jane's regular tracking also created opportunities to check on therapeutic alliance and adherence (Table 11.1, Step I). Talking with Joe, as well as tracking her own clients, Jane realized that client concordance about the goals was important to consider, along with adherence. When clients were concordant with goals and adherent with recommendations, things went swimmingly. It was possible to be adherent but not on board with the goals—this routinely happened when the caregiver dragged an unmotivated child to session. This scenario was a cue for Jane to attend to the alliance and to renegotiate goals that were intrinsically more motivating for the client. Nonadherence when the client was concordant with the goals was a different situation: Jane knew that her job was to help problem-solve, debugging the implementation of the skill or creating more external supports for the person to be able to follow through. She used the diet analogy—even when people understand that a diet would be good for them, it can be hard to follow through. Planning and support become key to success. If the client was discordant about the goals and not adherent, Jane knew that she had to make big changes quickly to get the client engaged, or else treatment was likely to end. The midterm and final exam repetitions of the severity measure (Table 11.1, Step J) also triggered conversation about goals, helping shift the frame to more of a big picture rather than weekly perspectives.

After the Last Session: Monitoring

If the client stuck with therapy all the way to a planned termination session, then Joe made a point of celebrating the successes, and also planting the seed that the client could call and schedule a booster session or come back at any time. Joe emphasized not waiting until there was a crisis; a quick booster session could prevent much more serious problems. "You've got my number, and my e-mail. Get in touch if you get worried. Don't wait for it to get bad."

Jane was impressed with Joe's proactive approach and liked how he built long-term relationships with the clients. She had never experienced that opportunity, in part due to all the changes in placement and moves for internship during her training. Jane incorporated Joe's strategies and went a step further in terms of writing things down: During the last sessions with the client, they worked together on a list of triggers and danger situations. They discussed low-friction assessments—such as lifestyle or health tracking apps—that were easy and helpful enough to be worth continuing. They discussed and agreed on operational definitions of warning signs that would elicit a call (e.g., 3 nights of sleeping 3 hours less than usual; starting marijuana again; daily happiness scores below 5 for 4 days in a row). Jane also made short lists of coping strategies and techniques that the client had found effective, creating a sort of "care package" that the client could unpack whenever needed (Table 11.1, Step K). She was mashing up Meehl (1973), Gawande (2010), and the coping cards from dialectical behavior therapy with smartphone apps. Joe liked her reasoned eclecticism.

Predictions: The Friendly Wager

Several weeks into supervision, Joe and Jane both started to loosen up and discuss their differences more openly. Watching Jane set up her checklists and cheat sheets, Joe shared, "I have thought about trying some of that stuff. But my clients would not go for it. It would take too long; it would ask about too many things that aren't an issue for each person (vs. me using my judgment to home in on the key themes) . . . so it would hurt rapport. I bet that people would burn out and drop out early. I'm not sure there's a point to adding all the extra assessment. If I can't read my client and tell what's going on, I'm not doing my job as a clinician."

Jane thought about it for a moment. "Joe, there are some testable predictions in there. One is that my assessments will take longer than yours. Another is that clients won't like the assessment process, or that you'll have better rapport with clients at the end. About it being pointless—I would wager that the extra assessment would lead to better outcomes on average." Joe smiled, "You'd wager . . . ?" They roughed in a plan to keep track of the next 20 consecutive cases. The easy part would be pulling the number of sessions from the record; and it was easy enough to add the length of the assessment sessions to the progress note. Measuring client satisfaction with the assessment was an extra step; they agreed to e-mail the 10 item, one-page survey from Suppiger and colleagues (2009) after finishing the intake assessment. It included a mix of questions about burden, degree of understanding gained, and first impressions about rapport. They also used the Working Alliance Inventory—Short Form (Munder, Wilmers, Leonhart, Linster, & Barth, 2010) after each session (to avoid missing data), completed by both them and the client. "Outcomes" was sticky because Joe did not have—nor did he want to have—a standard rating scale, and Jane changed her primary outcome measure depending on the client. For the purposes of settling the bet, they decided to use the clinical global improvement scale (again rated by them and the client), which rated overall improvement on a scale from 1 to 7, and also tracking planned versus premature termination. Joe teased, "After we're done with the great meal you'll be buying us, we can talk about how you can streamline your practice to be more like mine." Jane smiled, "My results are going to eat yours for lunch, and I'll still be hungry for that dinner you'll be buying."

The Data and the Dinner

Based on the data, Jane's approach wins on these points: Patients prefer it (Bruchmuller et al., 2011; Suppiger et al., 2009), diagnoses are more accurate (Jensen-Doss, Youngstrom, Youngstrom, Feeny, & Findling, 2014), treatments better match diagnoses and agreement about next clinical action is stronger (Jenkins, Youngstrom, Youngstrom, Feeny, & Findling, 2012; Jensen-Doss & Weisz, 2008), outcomes are better (Lambert et al., 2001), and treatment response is faster and retention is higher (Lambert, 2003; Lambert et al., 2005). To Joe's astonishment, the approach added little time to the first session. Most of the rating scales were

quickly completed, scored, and integrated into a summary, often before the client walked into the room. The targeted follow-up with the semi-structured interview took less time than Joe spent giving the Rorschach. The time spent on interpretation was much shorter for Jane's method, too, compared to the investment in scoring and interpreting the Rorschach or poring over the output from the MMPI scoring. Jane could not resist zinging Joe, pointing out that the time scoring was not contact hours, so not billable time for a lot of third-party payors.

Where do the data fall in Joe's favor? Joe wins decisively on clinician preference, especially established clinicians (Bruchmuller et al., 2011). It appears hard to change our ways once we are done with training. This is not limited to psychology; it is true of the professions in general (Susskind & Susskind, 2015), and of the diffusion of innovation (Rogers, 2003). So it is commonplace, but is that really "winning"? At first glance, it looked like a tie on rapport scores—both Joe's and Jane's clients agreed that rapport tended to be excellent. But after reflection, Joe gave the point to Jane, saying that she had a higher retention rate, and his clients who dropped out might not have been feeling as great about rapport. Jane did not argue the point, but said that she was impressed by his attention to rapport. She had always understood its importance, and watching Joe, she had picked up some skills to improve her ability to connect with kids. She also was struck by his deftness in building the reputation of the practice. Jane was learning from his networking with other professionals and his follow-up with clients. There were important skills that were not directly quantified in routine outcome assessment.

They decided to split the check: Joe paid for dinner, acknowledging that Jane's approach did better at the main ingredients of the meal. Jane paid for the drinks and the tip, acknowledging that Joe had reminded her of the importance of informal ways of building and tending to relationships. Also, she understood the personal interaction and flexibility required to deliver EBAs and treatments in practice, and Joe's deft touch in doing so. Their discussion led them both to a middle way: using EBA approaches could work smarter, quickly integrating a lot of information, while avoiding some common cognitive heuristics; but having it connect with the client requires a degree of reflectiveness, avoiding the trap of being an "expert" or relying only on numbers. EBA provides better technique but does not contradict the need for relationship. They are better together, and together they provide a powerful combination of rigor and relevance (Schon, 1983).

References

Achenbach, T. M., & Rescorla, L. A. (2003). *Manual for the ASEBA Adult Forms and Profiles*. Burlington: University of Vermont Press.

Aebi, M., Winkler Metzke, C., & Steinhausen, H.-C. (2009). Prediction of major affective disorders in adolescents by self-report measures. *Journal of Affective Disorders, 115,* 140–149.

Ægisdóttir, S., White, M. J., Spengler, P. M., Maugherman, A. S., Anderson, L. A., Cook, R. S., et al. (2006). The Meta-Analysis of Clinical Judgment Project: Fifty-six years of accumulated research on clinical versus statistical prediction. *The Counseling Psychologist, 34,* 341–382.

American Psychiatric Association. (2013). *Diagnostic and statistical manual of mental disorders* (5th ed.). Arlington, VA: Author.

Beck, A. T., & Steer, R. A. (1987). *Beck Depression Inventory manual*. San Antonio, TX: Psychological Corporation.

Brighton, H. (2011). The future of diagnostics: From optimizing to satisficing. In G. Gigerenzer & J. A. Muir Gray (Eds.), *Better doctors, better patients, better decisions* (pp. 281–294). Cambridge, MA: MIT Press.

Bruchmuller, K., Margraf, J., Suppiger, A., & Schneider, S. (2011). Popular or unpopular?: Therapists' use of structured interviews and their estimation of patient acceptance. *Behavior Therapy, 42,* 634–643.

Conners, C. K., Epstein, J. N., Angold, A., & Klaric, J. (2003). Continuous performance test performance in a normative epidemiological sample. *Journal of Abnormal Child Psychology, 31,* 555–562.

Costello, E. J., & Angold, A. (1988). Scales to assess child and adolescent depression: Checklists, screens, and nets. *Journal of the American Academy of Child and Adolescent Psychiatry, 27,* 726–737.

Couwenbergh, C., Van Der Gaag, R. J., Koeter, M., De Ruiter, C., & Van den Brink, W. (2009). Screening for substance abuse among adolescents validity of the CAGE-AID in youth mental health care. *Substance Use and Misuse, 44,* 823–834.

Croskerry, P. (2003). The importance of cognitive errors in diagnosis and strategies to minimize them. *Academic Medicine, 78,* 775–780.

Finn, S. E. (2007). *In our clients' shoes: Theory and techniques of therapeutic assessment*. New York: Taylor & Francis.

Finn, S. E., & Tonsager, M. E. (1997). Information-gathering and therapeutic models of assessment:

Complementary paradigms. *Psychological Assessment, 9,* 374–385.

Frazier, T. W., & Youngstrom, E. A. (2006). Evidence-based assessment of attention-deficit/hyperactivity disorder: Using multiple sources of information. *Journal of the American Academy of Child and Adolescent Psychiatry, 45,* 614–620.

Gadow, K. D., Sprafkin, J., & Weiss, M. D. (2004). *Adult Self-Report Inventory 4 manual*. Stony Brook, NY: Checkmate Plus.

Garb, H. N. (1998). *Studying the clinician: Judgment research and psychological assessment*. Washington, DC: American Psychological Association.

Gawande, A. (2010). *The checklist manifesto*. New York: Penguin.

Goodman, R., Ford, T., Simmons, H., Gatward, R., & Meltzer, H. (2003). Using the Strengths and Difficulties Questionnaire (SDQ) to screen for child psychiatric disorders in a community sample. *International Review of Psychiatry, 15,* 166–172.

Gracious, B. L., Youngstrom, E. A., Findling, R. L., & Calabrese, J. R. (2002). Discriminative validity of a parent version of the Young Mania Rating Scale. *Journal of the American Academy of Child and Adolescent Psychiatry, 41,* 1350–1359.

Grove, W. M., Zald, D. H., Lebow, B. S., Snitz, B. E., & Nelson, C. (2000). Clinical versus mechanical prediction: A meta-analysis. *Psychological Assessment, 12,* 19–30.

Harter, M., & Simon, D. (2011). Do patients want shared decision making and how is this measured? In G. Gigerenzer & J. A. Muir Gray (Eds.), *Better doctors, better patients, better decisions* (pp. 53–58). Cambridge, MA: MIT Press.

Hodge, D. R., Jackson, K. F., & Vaughn, M. G. (2012). Culturally sensitive interventions and substance use: A meta-analytic review of outcomes among minority youths. *Social Work Research, 36,* 11–19.

Hunsley, J., & Mash, E. J. (Eds.). (2008). *A guide to assessments that work*. New York: Oxford University Press.

Jacobson, N. S., & Truax, P. (1991). Clinical significance: A statistical approach to defining meaningful change in psychotherapy research. *Journal of Consulting and Clinical Psychology, 59,* 12–19.

Jarrett, M. A., Van Meter, A., Youngstrom, E. A., Hilton, D. C., & Ollendick, T. H. (2016). Evidence-based assessment of ADHD in youth using a receiver operating characteristic approach. *Journal of Clinical Child and Adolescent Psychology, 45,* 1–13.

Jenkins, M. M., & Youngstrom, E. A. (2016). A randomized controlled trial of cognitive debiasing improves assessment and treatment selection for pediatric bipolar disorder. *Journal of Consulting and Clinical Psychology, 84,* 323–333.

Jenkins, M. M., Youngstrom, E. A., Washburn, J. J., & Youngstrom, J. K. (2011). Evidence-based strategies improve assessment of pediatric bipolar disorder by community practitioners. *Professional Psychology: Research and Practice, 42,* 121–129.

Jenkins, M. M., Youngstrom, E. A., Youngstrom, J. K., Feeny, N. C., & Findling, R. L. (2012). Generalizability of evidence-based assessment recommendations for pediatric bipolar disorder. *Psychological Assessment, 24,* 269–281.

Jensen-Doss, A., & Weisz, J. R. (2008). Diagnostic agreement predicts treatment process and outcomes in youth mental health clinics. *Journal of Consulting and Clinical Psychology, 76,* 711–722.

Jensen-Doss, A., Youngstrom, E. A., Youngstrom, J. K., Feeny, N. C., & Findling, R. L. (2014). Predictors and moderators of agreement between clinical and research diagnoses for children and adolescents. *Journal of Consulting and Clinical Psychology, 82,* 1151–1162.

Lambert, M. J. (2003). Is it time for clinicians to routinely track patient outcome?: A meta-analysis. *Clinical Psychology: Science and Practice, 10,* 288–301.

Lambert, M. J., Hansen, N. B., & Finch, A. E. (2001). Patient-focused research: Using patient outcome data to enhance treatment effects. *Journal of Consulting and Clinical Psychology, 69,* 159–172.

Lambert, M. J., Harmon, C., Slade, K., Whipple, J. L., & Hawkins, E. J. (2005). Providing feedback to psychotherapists on their patients' progress: Clinical results and practice suggestions. *Journal of Clinical Psychology, 61,* 165–174.

Lambert, M. J., & Lambert, J. M. (1999). Use of psychological tests for assessing treatment outcome. In M. E. Maruish (Ed.), *The use of psychological testing for treatment planning and outcomes assessment* (2nd ed., pp. 115–151). Mahwah, NJ: Erlbaum.

Meehl, P. E. (1954). *Clinical versus statistical prediction: A theoretical analysis and a review of the evidence.* Minneapolis: University of Minnesota Press.

Meehl, P. E. (1973). Why I do not attend case conferences. In P. Meehl (Ed.), *Psychodiagnosis: Selected papers* (pp. 225–302). New York: Norton.

Meehl, P. E. (1997). Credentialed persons, credentialed knowledge. *Clinical Psychology: Science and Practice, 4,* 91–98.

Morrison, J. (2014). *Diagnosis made easier: Principles and techniques for mental health clinicians* (2nd ed.). New York: Guilford Press.

Mufson, L. H., Dorta, K. P., Olfson, M., Weissman, M. M., & Hoagwood, K. (2004). Effectiveness research: Transporting interpersonal psychotherapy for depressed adolescents (IPT-A) from the lab to school-based health clinics. *Clinical Child and Family Psychology Review, 7,* 251–261.

Munder, T., Wilmers, F., Leonhart, R., Linster, H. W., & Barth, J. (2010). Working Alliance Inventory— Short Revised (WAI-SR): Psychometric properties in outpatients and inpatients. *Clinical Psychology and Psychotherapy, 17,* 231–239.

Nilsen, T. S., Eisemann, M., & Kvernmo, S. (2013). Predictors and moderators of outcome in child and adolescent anxiety and depression: A systematic review of psychological treatment studies. *European Child and Adolescent Psychiatry, 22,* 69–87.

Norcross, J. C., Beutler, L. E., & Levant, R. F. (Eds.). (2006). *Evidence-based practices in mental health.* Washington, DC: American Psychological Association.

Norcross, J. C., Hogan, T. P., & Koocher, G. P. (2008). *Clinician's guide to evidence based practices: Mental health and the addictions.* London: Oxford University Press.

Pelham, W. E., Jr., Fabiano, G. A., & Massetti, G. M. (2005). Evidence-based assessment of attention deficit hyperactivity disorder in children and adolescents. *Journal of Clinical Child and Adolescent Psychology, 34,* 449–476.

Pepe, M. S. (2003). *The statistical evaluation of medical tests for classification and prediction.* New York: Wiley.

Poston, J. M., & Hanson, W. E. (2010). Meta-analysis of psychological assessment as a therapeutic intervention. *Psychological Assessment, 22,* 203–212.

Ready, R. E., & Veague, H. B. (2014). Training in psychological assessment: Current practices of clinical psychology programs. *Professional Psychology: Research and Practice, 45,* 278–282.

Rettew, D. C., Lynch, A. D., Achenbach, T. M., Dumenci, L., & Ivanova, M. Y. (2009). Meta-analyses of agreement between diagnoses made from clinical evaluations and standardized diagnostic interviews. *International Journal of Methods in Psychiatric Research, 18,* 169–184.

Reynolds, C. R., & Kamphaus, R. (2004). *BASC-2 Behavior Assessment System for Children.* Circle Pines, MN: American Guidance Service.

Rogers, E. M. (2003). *Diffusion of innovations.* New York: Free Press.

Saunders, J. B., Aasland, O. G., Babor, T. F., De la Fuente, J. R., & Grant, M. (1993). Development of the Alcohol Use Disorders Identification Test (AUDIT): WHO collaborative project on early detection of persons with harmful alcohol consumption—II. *Addiction, 88,* 791–804.

Schon, D. A. (1983). *The reflective practitioner: How professionals think in action.* New York: Basic Books.

Sheehan, D. V., Sheehan, K. H., Shytle, R. D., Janavs, J., Bannon, Y., Rogers, J. E., et al. (2010). Reliability and validity of the Mini International Neuropsychiatric Interview for Children and Adolescents (MINI-KID). *Journal of Clinical Psychiatry, 71*(3), 313–326.

Shelleby, E. C., & Kolko, D. J. (2015). Predictors, moderators, and treatment parameters of community and clinic-based treatment for child disruptive behavior disorders. *Journal of Child and Family Studies, 24,* 734–748.

Straus, S. E., Glasziou, P., Richardson, W. S., & Haynes, R. B. (2011). *Evidence-based medicine: How to practice and teach EBM* (4th ed.). New York: Churchill Livingstone.

Stricker, G., & Gold, J. R. (1996). Psychotherapy integration: An assimilative, psychodynamic approach. *Clinical Psychology: Science and Practice, 3,* 47–58.

Suppiger, A., In-Albon, T., Hendriksen, S., Hermann, E., Margraf, J., & Schneider, S. (2009). Acceptance of structured diagnostic interviews for mental disorders in clinical practice and research settings. *Behavior Therapy, 40,* 272–279.

Susskind, R., & Susskind, D. (2015). *The future of the professions: How technology will transform the work of human experts.* New York: Oxford University Press.

Swift, J. K., & Greenberg, R. P. (2012). Premature discontinuation in adult psychotherapy: A meta-analysis. *Journal of Consulting and Clinical Psychology, 80,* 547–559.

Thapar, A., & McGuffin, P. (1998). Validity of the shortened Mood and Feelings Questionnaire in a community sample of children and adolescents: A preliminary research note. *Psychiatry Research, 81,* 259–268.

Van Meter, A., You, D. S., Halverson, T., Youngstrom, E., Birmaher, B., Fristad, M., et al. (2017). Diagnostic efficiency of caregiver report on the SCARED for identifying youth anxiety disorders in outpatient settings. *Journal of Clinical Child and Adolescent Psychology, 46,* 1–13.

Van Meter, A., Youngstrom, E., Youngstrom, J. K., Ollendick, T., Demeter, C., & Findling, R. L. (2014). Clinical decision making about child and adolescent anxiety disorders using the Achenbach System of Empirically Based Assessment. *Journal of Clinical Child and Adolescent Psychology, 43,* 552–565.

Wechsler, D. (2014). *Wechsler Intelligence Scale for Children—5th edition.* San Antonio, TX: NCS Pearson.

Weersing, V. R. (2005). Benchmarking the effectiveness of psychotherapy: Program evaluation as a component of evidence-based practice. *Journal of the American Academy of Child and Adolescent Psychiatry, 44,* 1058–1062.

Weisz, J. R., Chorpita, B. F., Frye, A., Ng, M. Y., Lau, N., Bearman, S. K., et al. (2011). Youth Top Problems: Using idiographic, consumer-guided assessment to identify treatment needs and to track change during psychotherapy. *Journal of Consulting and Clinical Psychology, 79,* 369–380.

Woodcock, R. W., McGrew, K. S., & Mather, N. (2005). *Woodcock–Johnson Psychoeducational Battery—III NU Complete.* Rolling Meadows, IL: Riverside.

Yeh, M., Hough, R. L., Fakhry, F., McCabe, K. M., Lau, A. S., & Garland, A. F. (2005). Why bother with beliefs?: Examining relationships between race/ethnicity, parental beliefs about causes of child problems, and mental health service use. *Journal Consulting and Clinical Psychology, 73,* 800–807.

You, S. D., Youngstrom, E. A., Feeny, N. C., Youngstrom, J. K., & Findling, R. L. (2015). Comparing the diagnostic accuracy of five instruments for detecting posttraumatic stress disorder in youth. *Journal of Clinical Child and Adolescent Psychology, 44,* 1–13.

Youngstrom, E. A. (2013). Future directions in psychological assessment: Combining evidence-based medicine innovations with psychology's historical strengths to enhance utility. *Journal of Clinical Child and Adolescent Psychology, 42,* 139–159.

Youngstrom, E. A., Choukas-Bradley, S., Calhoun, C. D., & Jensen-Doss, A. (2014). Clinical guide to the evidence-based assessment approach to diagnosis and treatment. *Cognitive and Behavioral Practice, 22,* 20–35.

Youngstrom, E. A., Genzlinger, J. E., Egerton, G. A., & Van Meter, A. R. (2015). Multivariate meta-analysis of the discriminative validity of caregiver, youth, and teacher rating scales for pediatric bipolar disorder: Mother knows best about mania. *Archives of Scientific Psychology, 3,* 112–137.

Youngstrom, E. A., & Van Meter, A. (2016). Empirically supported assessment of children and adolescents. *Clinical Psychology: Science and Practice, 23,* 1–13.

PART III

ILLUSTRATIONS OF EVIDENCE-BASED PRACTICE IN ACTION

CHAPTER 12

An Idiographic Hypothesis–Testing Approach to Psychotherapy

Using Case Formulation and Progress Monitoring to Guide Treatment

JACQUELINE B. PERSONS
LISA S. TALBOT

Ann was intensely distressed when she spoke on the telephone to the therapist who was screening callers at the clinic. She reported, "I have completely lost social confidence. I'm so sick of being at home by myself, but I'm terrified to go anyplace where I have to socialize. I force myself to go to my community college classes, but that's about it." Ann answered the therapist's questions over the phone in a straightforward, very brief way, and made an appointment for an evaluation at the clinic.

When Ann appeared for her appointment, she was attractively dressed in slacks and a sweater, with neat hair and a slight build. She appeared timid and frightened. She was hunched in her chair, and she spoke so softly that the therapist had to lean in to hear her. However, Ann also demonstrated warmth, flashing occasional smiles. Her eye contact appeared natural, though less frequent than might be expected. She rarely volunteered information and spoke only in response to the therapist's inquiries, giving very little detail, so that the therapist had to frequently ask her to elaborate on her answers. Ann appeared conscientious and earnest and worked hard to answer the therapist's questions in a thoughtful way. She described her experiences during social interactions, including her high fear, sensations of fluttering heartbeat and flushing, and her common thoughts ("I'm so

boring!" or "Ugh, that was such a weird thing to say" or "He's checking out my hair—it must look bad"). Ann fidgeted with her fingers throughout the interview and repeatedly smoothed her hair with her hands. She became tearful numerous times, particularly when discussing her longstanding anxiety in social situations, her dispiriting loneliness, and her hopelessness that things could ever be different for her.

Ann reported that she had been shy since childhood. As an elementary school student, she spoke to few children in her class at school. At times she made casual friends, but her reticence mostly kept her disconnected. Ann reported that her mother had told her that her withdrawal had become more pronounced when she was 4 years old, when her parents' marriage broke up due to her father's alcoholism. Her father then moved to another state and had little contact with Ann or her mother. Ann assumed that her behavior had somehow caused his departure, and she became wary of developing relationships for fear that she'd mess up and be rejected again.

Ann suffered another huge interpersonal loss in eighth grade, when her best friend, Angela, suddenly and abruptly stopped returning her texts or calls and began avoiding Ann at school. Angela instead began spending all her time with one of the most popular girls in the school. Angela's abandonment of Ann was sudden, unexpected, and devastating. Ann felt confused about what had happened. She thought about it endlessly, listing all the ways she felt she didn't measure up to Angela's new friend and speculating about all the things she might have done to provoke Angela to leave her.

As a consequence of Angela's rejection of her, Ann became even more careful about her interactions with others. She began to expect that others were very likely to find her unacceptable in some way and reject her. She avoided social contact as much as possible. And when she did interact with others, Ann focused her attention not on the person she was talking to, but instead on how she perceived herself to be coming across to the other person, and she constantly evaluated how she felt she was doing and how the interaction was going. She tried to assess whether the person had a good impression of her (e.g., found her interesting, "normal"). For example, in one interaction, she felt that her face had a serious expression. She had the thought "I'm not being friendly enough!" and quickly forced a smile. Indeed, Ann constantly monitored her facial expression to try to ensure that it appeared interested, relaxed, and friendly. She minimized self-disclosure so as to avoid exposing features of herself that the other person might dislike.

Ann's social anxiety and disconnectedness really began to interfere with her functioning when she began college and needed to make new friends. Instead of getting to know her classmates, she avoided social contact more than ever. Ann did not join a study group to work on her class assignments, and this meant that the quality of her work suffered, and her grades began to suffer as well. Ann's social isolation and poor academic performance led to self-criticism, depressed mood, hopelessness, and other depressive symptoms. Finally, she became so miserable and desperate that she called the clinic to ask for help.

*   *   *

We describe here an idiographic hypothesis-testing approach to psychotherapy that relies on a case formulation and progress monitoring data, and we illustrate it with the example of Ann's case. An idiographic hypothesis-testing approach to psychotherapy is an elegant strategy for providing evidence-based care. Using the scientific method, the therapist develops a hypothesis (formulation) about the factors that

cause and maintain the patient's problems and interfere with the patient's accomplishing his or her goals, uses the formulation to guide treatment, and collects data as the treatment proceeds in order to evaluate the effectiveness of the treatment and test the formulation hypotheses (Persons, 2006).

The therapist using an idiographic hypothesis-testing approach also relies on several types of data and findings:

• Treatment protocols that have been shown to be effective in empirical studies, including randomized controlled trials, uncontrolled trials, and single case studies.

• Interventions and practices (cf. John Weisz's [Weisz, Ugueto, Herren, Afienko, & Rutt, 2011] distinction between ears [treatments] and kernels [interventions]) that have been shown to be effective in empirical studies. An example is the evidence-based practice (EBP) of progress monitoring (Lewis et al., 2018).

• Formulations of psychopathology that are supported by evidence, especially formulations that underpin the empirically supported treatments (ESTs), EBPs, and evidence-based interventions. An example is the evidence that safety behaviors maintain negative beliefs and symptoms of social anxiety (Wells, Clark, & Salkovskis, 1995), which supports the cognitive-behavioral formulations of social anxiety as resulting from faulty beliefs and avoidance behaviors that prevent disconfirmation of those beliefs (Clark & Wells, 1995; Rapee & Heimberg, 1997).

• Assessment tools and strategies that are supported by evidence from controlled studies (see Youngstrom & Van Meter, Chapter 11, this volume; see also Hunsley & Mash, 2018) or that have some evidence of utility in the treatment of the case at hand.

• Findings about the process of change in psychotherapy (e.g., that trajectory of change is generally nonlinear, with early rapid improvement followed typically followed by a slower rate of change [Lutz, Martinovich, & Howard, 1999] or that cognitive preparation enhances the beneficial effects of video feedback in the treatment of social phobia [Harvey, Clark, Ehlers, & Rapee, 2000]), or that exposure is more successful at treating social anxiety when even the most subtle avoidance behaviors are identified and eliminated [Wells et al., 1995]).

- Findings from basic science, such as evidence that inhibitory learning is fragile and highly context-dependent (Craske et al., 2008).

- Evidence from this patient's own history or experience. An example is that Ann connected better socially with slightly older peers than with same-age or younger peers.

We describe here our approach to providing idiographic hypothesis-testing psychotherapy based on a case formulation and progress monitoring data. Our example uses cognitive-behavior therapy (CBT), but the concepts and methods we describe are not specific to that treatment modality and can be used in any modality of psychotherapy.

We provide an overview of CBT guided by an idiographic hypothesis-testing approach and progress monitoring data, and we describe each step of the assessment and treatment process, giving special attention to the steps of developing a case formulation and using the formulation to guide treatment. We illustrate our account with examples from the treatment of Ann, described at the outset of the chapter.

Overview of an Idiographic Hypothesis-Testing Approach to CBT

In this approach to CBT (Persons, 2008), depicted in Figure 12.1, the therapist begins by collecting assessment data to obtain a diagnosis and an initial formulation (conceptualization) of the case. The *formulation* is a hypothesis about the mechanisms causing and maintaining the patient's problems. The therapist uses the formulation (and other information) to develop a *treatment plan and obtain the patient's informed consent to it.* Then *treatment* begins. The therapist uses the formulation to select treatment targets and interventions, and to guide other clinical decisions. As treatment proceeds, the patient and therapist collect assessment data to evaluate whether the patient is making progress toward accomplishing his or her treatment goals. The assessment data also help patient and therapist test the formulation and evaluate whether the patient is attending to, learning, remembering, and using the concepts and skills the therapist is teaching. Treatment ends when the patient's goals are met or the progress monitoring data indicate that the patient is not likely to improve, and the therapist makes a referral to another provider. All of these steps are carried out in the context of a *collaborative therapeutic relationship.*

Assessment to Obtain a Diagnosis and an Initial Case Formulation

The therapist begins by working with the patient to obtain a diagnosis and an initial case formu-

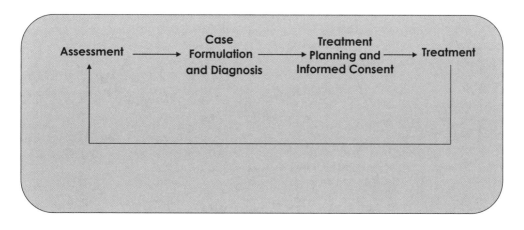

□ = the therapeutic relationship

FIGURE 12.1. Case formulation-driven CBT.

lation that guide treatment planning. Diagnosis is important for several reasons, including that much of the scientific literature, especially the treatment literature, is tied to diagnosis.

But diagnosis is not enough to guide treatment. A case formulation is also needed. A *case formulation,* unlike a diagnosis, describes and proposes relationships among the psychological mechanisms and other factors that are causing and maintaining all of a particular patient's disorders and problems. The formulation helps the therapist and patient understand how all the patient's disorders and problems are related, describes the idiographic features of these disorders and problems, and helps the therapist design and implement effective treatment.

The National Institute of Mental Health's (NIMH) Research Domain Criteria (RDoC) project proposes that the best way to address psychopathology is to focus on understanding dysfunctions that are defined and measured dimensionally *across* diagnoses rather than through categorical, symptom-defined approaches (Insel et al., 2010). This way of thinking about psychopathology aligns well with the case formulation approach to psychopathology and its treatment that we describe here.

Elements of a Case Formulation

A complete case formulation includes all of the following elements and ties them together into a coherent whole: all of the patient's *symptoms, disorders,* and *problems*; the *mechanisms* causing the symptoms, disorders, and problems; the *precipitants* of the symptoms, disorders, and problems; and the *origins* of the mechanisms. The case formulation that Ann's therapist used to guide her therapy appears in Figure 12.2. This formulation includes all of Ann's problems, as well as hypotheses about the mechanisms causing and supporting the problems, and also describes relationships among the problems, especially the way that social isolation led to problems at school and depression.

Ann's therapist also developed a detailed formulation of Ann's social anxiety using the worksheet provided at *http://psychology-tools.com/cognitive-model-of-social-anxiety. html.* As shown in Figure 12.3, Ann's therapist fleshed out this nomothetic model of social anxiety with the idiographic details of Ann's social anxiety symptoms.

Thus, Ann's therapist relied on two formulations, one of the case (Figure 12.2), which includes all the problems and symptoms and how

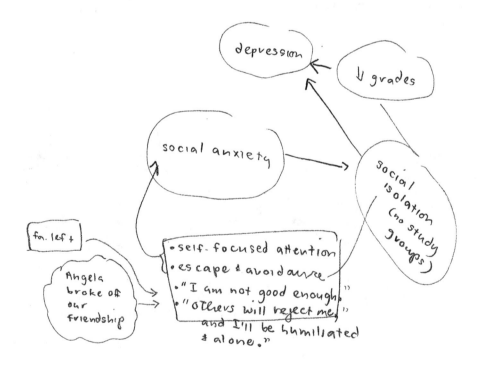

FIGURE 12.2. A diagram of the formulation of Ann's case.

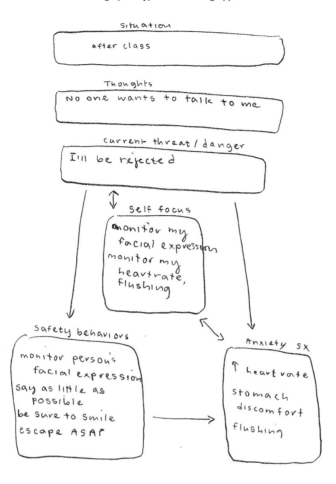

FIGURE 12.3. A diagram of the formulation of Ann's social anxiety.

they are related, and another (Figure 12.3) of Ann's social anxiety disorder. In fact, Ann's therapist relied on multiple formulations. She often used a Thought Record with Ann to examine the details of her automatic thoughts and behaviors and emotions in a particular situation, and the Thought Record itself was a formulation—a formulation of Ann's experience in a particular situation. The therapist develops all of these formulations collaboratively with the patient.

The Process of Developing an Initial Case Formulation

We describe the process of developing two of the key elements of the initial case formulation: the comprehensive Problem List, and the initial mechanism hypotheses.

Developing a Comprehensive Problem List

Why develop a comprehensive problem list? Obtaining a comprehensive list is critical for at least four reasons. First, important problems can be missed if the therapist simply focuses on the problems the patient wishes to focus on or that are in plain view. Patients frequently wish to ignore serious problems such as substance abuse, self-harming behaviors, or others that can interfere with successful treatment of the problems on which the patient *does* want to focus. Second, a comprehensive problem list often reveals common elements or themes that cut across problems. Awareness of these themes can help the therapist generate mechanism hypotheses for the formulation. Third, the presence of some problems (e.g., major medical problems that might make it difficult for the patient to keep reliable therapy appointments) can affect treatment of the others. Finally, although often the treatment focuses quite a bit on a particular disorder or disorders (as in Ann's case, in which the therapist focuses on her social anxiety disorder and her depression), a key perspective of the case formulation-driven approach to treatment is that the therapist is treating not the *disorder* or disorders, but the *patient*.

To obtain a comprehensive list of the patient's problems, the therapist assesses the patient's psychiatric and medical problems, any difficulties the patient has in obtaining and making good use of treatment for those problems (e.g., noncompliance), as well as any difficulties in the areas of interpersonal, occupational, school, financial, housing, legal, and leisure functioning.

Note that in the Problem List, the therapist begins to translate diagnostic information into terms that facilitate conceptualization and intervention from a cognitive-behavioral point of view. The Problem List does this in part by detailing the important symptoms of the patient's psychiatric disorders and psychosocial problems and by describing, whenever possible, the cognitive, behavioral, and emotional components of problems. Both of these features of the Problem List are illustrated in the formulation of Ann provided earlier.

To obtain a Problem List, the therapist collects data from multiple sources, including the clinical interview, structured diagnostic interviews, self-report scales, self-monitoring data provided by the patient, observations of the patient's behavior, and reports from the patient's family members and other treatment providers. At the Oakland Cognitive Behavior Therapy Center, we send patients to our website and ask them to download, complete, and bring to their initial consultation session an intake packet that includes an Adult Intake Questionnaire that asks questions about previous and current treatment, family and social history, previous and current substance use, trauma, and legal and other problems, as well as a self-report diagnostic screening form that we developed, and several standardized scales. Many of these are available free at *https://oaklandcbt.com*.

Standardized assessment scales that we are currently using for all our patients include the Beck Depression Inventory (Beck, Steer, & Garbin, 1988), the Beck Anxiety Inventory (Beck, Epstein, Brown, & Steer, 1988), and a standardized assessment of functioning, the Work and Social Adjustment Scale (Mundt, Marks, Shear, & Greist, 2002), which assesses functioning in the domains of work, home management, social and private leisure activities, and relationships, and a self-report diagnostic screening tool (the diagnostic screening tool was developed at the San Francisco Bay Area Center for Cognitive Therapy and is in the public domain and available at *https://oaklandcbt. com/forms-and-tools-for-clinicians*). Based on the information obtained in the initial telephone contact, the therapist may also ask the patient to complete scales to assess other symptoms and problems. Ann's therapist asked her to complete the Liebowitz Social Anxiety Scale (Liebowitz, 1987) in addition to the measures listed earlier. When the patient arrives for the initial session, the therapist asks the patient's permission to take the first five minutes of the session to review all of this information in order to be able to prioritize the topics taken up in the interview (e.g., to identify whether suicidality must be assessed), and uses it to guide the interview.

Developing a Mechanism Hypothesis

The heart of the formulation is the *mechanism hypothesis,* which describes mechanisms or processes that cause and maintain symptoms. A core part of the case formulation approach is the development of an idiographic mechanism hypothesis for each particular case. Mechanisms can include biological mechanisms (e.g., thyroid dysfunction) but we emphasize and focus here on psychological mechanisms.

Mechanisms in cognitive-behavioral formulations include such things as attentional biases, exaggerated expectations of harm and danger, perfectionism, faulty contingencies, repetitive negative thinking (e.g., worry, rumination), avoidance, and a view of the self as worthless. Note that some of these phenomena may also be considered symptoms. For example, the last three items in the list just given—repetitive negative thinking, avoidance, and the belief that the self is worthless—may be viewed either as symptoms or as mechanisms; that is, some phenomena that are problems, or symptoms, may also be viewed as mechanisms. If this is the case, in which section of the formulation does the clinician place these phenomena? In problems? Or in mechanisms? The rule of thumb that we recommend the therapist use to answer this question is to place the phenomenon in either the problem section or the mechanism section, or both, and make the decision based on which view of the phenomenon is most helpful in guiding the treatment. In the case of Ann, her self-focused negative automatic thoughts were distressing symptoms that she hoped to address in treatment. However, when her therapist laid out the cognitive model of social anxiety, Ann could see that her thoughts also served as mechanisms that contributed to her distress, and she reported that viewing them as mechanisms was helpful to her in her treatment.

To develop an idiographic mechanism hypothesis, the therapist relies, as described earlier, on any or all of the types of data described at the beginning of the chapter. A key source of data is the findings from randomized controlled trials of ESTs that treat the patient's presenting problems and disorders. Ann met criteria for social anxiety disorder and major depressive disorder, so the therapist consulted the nomothetic formulations underpinning those ESTs and used them to guide the development of the formulation of Ann's case. The formulation of Ann's case relied heavily on the formulation of social phobia developed by Clark and Wells (1995) and Rapee and Heimberg (1997) and the formulations of depression offered by Beck, Rush, Shaw, and Emery (1979) and by Martell, Addis, and Jacobson (2001).

The model developed by Rapee and Heimberg (1997) stipulates that individuals with social phobia are hyperaware of the fact that they are observed by others, whom they perceive as quite critical. When interacting with others, they focus their attention not on the person with whom they are interacting but instead on a mental comparison of how they believe they appear to that person, and the other person's standard for them; that is, they monitor for the potential threat of failing to meet the other person's standard. In addition, they experience inflated expectations of the *likelihood* and the *consequences* of failing to meet the standard. These processes frequently lead the individual to conclude that he or she failed to meet others' standards and, as a result, experience cognitive, behavioral, and physical symptoms of social anxiety.

Ann's therapist used this nomothetic model of social anxiety disorder to develop an idiographic case formulation for Ann by filling in the details of the model as they applied to her case (see Figure 12.3). Her therapist determined that Ann's monitoring for potential threat consisted especially of hypervigilant attention to the fa-

cial expression of the person to whom she was speaking in order to assess whether that person seemed interested in what Ann was saying. Her physiological symptoms of anxiety consisted primarily of increased heart rate, stomach discomfort, and blushing. Her behavioral response was to say as little as possible when she was in a social situation, and to escape and avoid social contact whenever possible.

In addition, the therapist laid out, in the case formulation (Figure 12.2), a model that accounted for all of Ann's symptoms, including her poor academic functioning and social isolation, and hypothesized that both resulted directly from Ann's avoidance of social contact. To conceptualize the depressive symptoms, the therapist used Beck's and Martell and colleagues' (2001) models to hypothesize that she had negative cognitions about herself and others ("I am not likable, others find me boring") and suffered a loss of positive reinforcers as a result of her social isolation and half-hearted participation in her schoolwork. Consequently, Ann became depressed.

A key clinical question related to the development of the mechanism hypothesis is, When more than one model can be used to formulate a case, how does the therapist choose? For example, multiple evidence-based formulations are now available for unipolar depression, including Beck's cognitive model (Beck et al., 1979), behavioral activation (Martell et al., 2001), Lewinsohn's behavioral model (Lewinsohn, Hoberman, & Hautzinger, 1985), and the problem-solving model developed by Nezu and Perri (1989). This question is a fascinating one. We list here several factors that we consider when working with Ann and other clients, which allows us to select a model on which to base a case formulation:

- The degree to which the details of the patient's case, as assessed using standardized scales or idiographic logs, match any particular formulation (Haynes, Kaholokula, & Nelson, 1999).
- The degree to which the patient's formulation of his or her own case matches a particular formulation.
- The patient's receptiveness to interventions based on a formulation, as assessed by observing the patient's receptiveness and willingness to use interventions that flow out of a formulation.
- The patient's progress (as assessed via a stan-

dardized symptom scale at every session) in treatment based on a particular formulation.

- The patient's treatment history (e.g., he or she may have failed previous treatment guided by a particular formulation).
- The therapist's training or experience, or preference.
- The formulation the therapist finds that he or she can use most easily to aid in treatment.

Another important question is: "Must the therapist choose between models or can he or she use more than one model simultaneously?" Often our cognitive-behavior models are not mutually exclusive; that is, both the cognitive (Beck et al., 1979) and the behavioral activation (Martell et al., 2001) formulations could account for a particular patient's symptoms of depression. And both can provide useful intervention ideas. For these reasons, to guide Ann's treatment, we relied both on Beck's model (to focus on the very prominent thoughts and to use the thought record to intervene to address Ann's depression), and on the behavioral activation model (to help Ann understand how her avoidance behavior left her isolated and unhappy).

Finally, we emphasize that the therapist develops the initial case formulation in the context of a collaborative relationship with the patient. Ideally, this happens gradually, as a process of mutual discovery (Kuyken, Padesky, & Dudley, 2009) rather than in a session in which the therapist authoritatively informs the patient about the details of the formulation in one fell swoop. For example, Ann worked with her therapist to track her mood and her social contact for 2 weeks to test the hypothesis that the two were related. Ann learned from this log that she repeatedly experienced a mood boost following social interactions—even when she didn't think the interactions were as positive as she had hoped—and she experienced chronic low mood when she was socially isolated. After doing this experiment, Ann understood and agreed with the therapist's formulation that her social isolation was a major cause of her depression.

We also emphasize that the formulation is a hypothesis, and one on which the therapist and patient work collaboratively to fine-tune and revise as treatment proceeds. In Ann's case, monitoring her mood after social activities led to a change in her view of her behavior in a social situation. Ann found it difficult to attend social activities, so she and the therapist made a plan to ask her friend Joan to come with her to parties

on campus. However, Ann was surprised to find that when she attended a party with Joan, she actually socialized less at the event, and she did not enjoy the event and feel the mood improvement she usually felt after she pushed herself to engage in social activities. After discussing the situation with her therapist, Ann realized that her friend Joan was so anxious and clung to her so tightly that Ann found it very easy to avoid socializing, so that when she left the party, she felt even more alone than she had beforehand. Ann learned that taking Joan with her to parties was actually a safety behavior. Ann tested this hypothesis by attending the next event on her own and pushing herself to engage with people. Although she found it difficult to do this, when she did, she enjoyed herself, and when she left the party, she noticed that her mood was quite a bit brighter than when she had attended with Joan.

Treatment Planning and Obtaining Informed Consent

Treatment Planning

The function of the formulation is to guide effective treatment (Hayes, Nelson, & Jarrett, 1987). A key way the formulation does this is by identifying the targets of treatment, which are generally the mechanisms that the formulation proposes are causing the symptoms.

The formulation also guides treatment planning by helping the therapist think about and coordinate all of the therapies the patient is receiving, not just the treatment the individual therapist is providing. For example, Ann discussed her symptoms with her primary care provider (PCP), who recommended that when Ann felt anxious in interactions, she try to slow her breathing, then check to see if her heart pounding decreased. When Ann discussed this plan with her therapist, the therapist reviewed the formulation and pointed out that self-focused attention ("Am I slowing down my breathing?") and monitoring for threat ("Is my heart beating too hard?") were actually mechanisms *contributing* to Ann's heightened physiological arousal, anxiety, and urges to escape.

Ann quickly understood this formulation and decided not to follow her PCP's recommendations. She and her therapist worked together to help Ann explain to her PCP why she had elected not to follow the recommendations. Ann was successful at asserting herself, and her PCP was receptive to her input. The key to successful collaboration of Ann's two treatment providers was the shared formulation.

Obtaining Informed Consent for Treatment

Obtaining the patient's consent to treatment before treatment begins is ethically necessary (American Psychological Association, 2002). It is also clinically helpful in numerous ways. For example, it can help prevent nonadherence by obtaining the patient's agreement to the goals and interventions of treatment before beginning it. Working with the patient to obtain a collaborative case formulation aids in the process of obtaining informed consent because most patients are not willing to go forward in treatment unless they have confidence that the therapist truly understands their difficulties and will provide treatment that addresses them. A careful process of agreeing on a treatment plan also sets the stage for revisiting the plan if progress monitoring data show that treatment is failing (Persons, Beckner, & Tompkins, 2013).

There are multiple elements of the process of obtaining informed consent. Specifically, in this process, the therapist:

- Provides an assessment, including a diagnosis and formulation, of the patient's condition.
- Recommends a treatment, describes it, provides a rationale for the recommendation, and describes any risks.
- Negotiates a treatment plan with which both therapist and patient are comfortable.
- Describes alternative treatment options.
- Obtains the patient's agreement to proceed with the agreed-upon treatment plan.

All of the elements of therapy described so far (initial assessment, diagnosis, case formulation, treatment planning, and informed consent) comprise the pretreatment phase of the therapy. This phase of therapy lasts one to four sessions, depending largely on the complexity of the case. If these elements are successfully accomplished, and patient and therapist can agree on a treatment plan, treatment begins.

Treatment

Treatment is guided by the *formulation,* which describes the mechanisms that cause and maintain the patient's symptoms, and the therapist uses this information to plan interventions that reduce symptoms by modifying the mechanisms that the formulation hypothesizes drive the symptoms. In Ann's case, the formulation led to interventions aimed to help her shift her attention away from the comparison of herself with her mental ideal to the conversation at hand, drop her avoidance behaviors, and revise her beliefs about others' expectations of her and about the consequences of failing to meet others' expectations.

To target Ann's negative comparisons with her ideal social performance, her therapist taught her to focus her attention on the content of the conversation at hand, as well as more positive (rather than threatening) aspects of her conversational partner. Ann began to attend to her conversational partner's verbal cues (positive) more than his or her facial expression (often ambiguous and perceived by Ann as threatening). Focusing on the verbal cues from the partner helped Ann attend to the conversation at hand rather than her performance, and provided more reliable, explicit feedback that her partner was interested in the conversation. If the partner continued the conversation, Ann was instructed to attend to it and consider it positive feedback.

This attentional shift also helped ease Ann's physical symptoms of anxiety, as her focus on her symptoms tended to exacerbate them. Ann and her therapist conducted several behavioral experiments in which Ann tracked her anxiety and her enjoyment of the conversation when she attended as usual to her conversational partner's expression and her own performance, and when she shifted her attention to the content of the conversation. Ann learned that when she shifted her attention to the content of the conversation, her anxiety decreased, and she actually began enjoying her some of her interactions with others.

Ann and her therapist also worked to drop her avoidance behaviors, and Ann began to stay in conversations regardless of her perceived performance. In addition, Ann worked with her therapist to set goals to help her approach her goal of joining some of the small group meetings her fellow students had established. These goals were set in a graduated fashion, to help Ann feel confident that she could achieve them (particularly important given the high level of behavioral avoidance delineated in the formulation). For example, the first week Ann only had to learn the logistics of the small group meetings (i.e., when, where). Subsequent goals included attending a small group meeting without participating, then attending and participating, and eventually volunteering to take the lead on some group tasks. And Ann and her therapist also role-played conversations in which Ann expanded her self-disclosure—another component of her behavioral avoidance—and Ann began practicing more self-disclosure outside the session.

Ann also worked with her therapist to schedule more activities, particularly pleasant and social ones. These interventions were based on the case formulation mechanism hypothesis that Ann had a lack of positive reinforcers, and in particular a lack of social interaction, which contributed to isolation and consequent depressed mood. Ann initiated a study session with another shy young woman, Susan, and over time, Susan became a regular "study buddy" and a friend.

Progress Monitoring

As treatment proceeds, patient and therapist collect data to monitor the process and outcome of therapy and, directly or indirectly, to test the formulation hypotheses (e.g., with Ann, that self-focused attention increases anxiety in social situations). The therapist collects some data formally, using written or online tools, and collects other data informally, observing the patient's behavior in the session, for example. Data collection allows patient and therapist to answer questions such as the following: Are the symptoms remitting? Is the patient achieving her goals? Does the patient accept the formulation the therapist has offered? Is the patient doing her therapy homework? Are the mechanisms described in the formulation changing as expected? Are problems in the therapeutic relationship interfering?

It is not feasible to collect formal data to evaluate all aspects of outcome and progress. However, we do recommend that the therapist monitor symptoms at every session in writing or using a software or online tool. This can be done using a standardized assessment instrument or idiographic measures. Ann's therapist used the Beck Anxiety Inventory (Beck, Epstein, et al., 1988) and the Beck Depression Inventory (Beck, Steer, et al., 1988) to track her symptoms at every session. Ann's therapist asked her to come 5 minutes early for her session and to fill out the two forms in the waiting room. Then, when Ann arrived, her therapist scored the measures, plotted the scores, and reviewed the plot with her at the start of the therapy session. The plots appear in Figure 12.4.

Ann's therapist also used self-report data to monitor the change process. For example, in several of her behavioral experiments, Ann provided ratings of predicted, peak, and postlevels of anxiety in social situations. These data helped Ann learn that her anxiety predictions

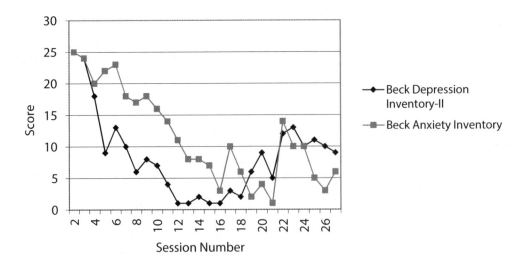

FIGURE 12.4. Ann's scores on the Beck Depression Inventory and Burns Anxiety Inventory during treatment.

were typically higher than her actual experience, and this information helped her approach feared situations more easily. The ratings also helped her therapist see that the exposures Ann was doing were having the desired effect, as Ann's peak anxiety ratings were decreasing over time.

Ann's therapist also monitored her progress by observing Ann's behavior in the session. The therapist noted that as treatment proceeded, Ann came to her session looking brighter and with a lighter step. Her hunched posture from her early sessions began to disappear, and she spontaneously volunteered information with more enthusiasm than the therapist had previously seen from her. And Ann now spoke in a normal volume, in contrast to her near whispers in the intake session. These in-session behavioral observations suggested that Ann's social anxiety was easing and her mood was improving.

The data the therapist collects are used to test the formulation hypothesis. The therapist tests the formulation indirectly by monitoring the degree to which the treatment plan based on the formulation helps the patient accomplish his or her treatment goals. To test the formulation more directly, the therapist can collect data to examine the degree to which changes in symptoms and mechanisms covary in the way the formulation predicts (e.g., see Iwata et al., 1994; Turkat & Maisto, 1985). For example, if the formulation predicts that changes to target mechanisms ought to produce changes in symptoms, but progress monitoring data show that changes in mechanisms occur but changes in symptoms do not, these data suggest that the formulation is incorrect (Persons et al., 2013). In Ann's case, her observations that attending parties with her friend Joan reduced her participation in the event and dampened her mood indicated that being with Joan was a safety behavior thus led to a revision in the formulation and in the treatment plan.

In addition to its key role in the hypothesis-testing process, progress monitoring helps the therapist identify nonadherence and setbacks early, so that they can be addressed before they undermine the therapy. Ann made excellent progress in treatment, as shown in the progress plot in Figure 12.4. However, after a period of improved social functioning and engagement, at about Session 21 (see Figure 12.4), Ann began arriving late to her therapy sessions. Her mood level dropped and she stopped pushing herself to attend social activities.

Ann's lateness to sessions and the increase in her symptoms that appeared in the progress monitoring data alerted the therapist to the fact that treatment was going off track. The therapist queried Ann about these things and learned that Ann was very upset about her interactions with her mother's partner. Ann often spent the night or weekend at her mother's house, and her relationship and comfort with her mother was a source of positive reward. But Ann felt upset by what she perceived as her mother's partner's expectations that Ann take over the role of kitchen cleanup whenever she was there and by the unpleasant jokes and sarcasm that her mother's partner directed at her. Ann's response was to stop spending time at her mother's house.

Ann's therapist reviewed the situation with Ann and helped her see that she had slipped back into her usual coping strategy of avoidance, and that it was not serving her. Ann's therapist revised the formulation to highlight the importance of asserting herself to solve interpersonal problems, and worked with Ann to teach her skills to handle interpersonal conflict. Ann was able to speak up effectively to her mother's partner, resume her positive relationship with her mother, and get back on track with her therapy and planned social activities.

Termination

Termination occurs when the goals of treatment have been met, when patient and therapist agree that treatment has failed, or when logistical or other obstacles arise and cannot be solved. Progress monitoring data often provide a good read on whether the patient has reached his or her goals. Sometimes the formulation and progress monitoring data, viewed together, can help patient and therapist decide whether termination is indicated. For example, progress monitoring data that indicate a depressed patient's symptoms remitted because she went on vacation, not because she solved the problems that are making her miserable at work, suggest that termination is premature. The fact that no change has occurred in the mechanisms (in this case, problem-solving skills deficits) that appear to cause the depressive symptoms indicates that more treatment is needed.

Often reductions in symptoms seen in the progress monitoring data, coupled with changes in the target behaviors described in the formulation, provide good evidence that the patient is ready to end her treatment. In Ann's case, after 26 sessions, her symptoms of anxiety and depression had remitted (see Figure 12.4), and she was consistently engaging in social interactions. She had developed some friends at school and was participating in study groups. Ann's grades were better, and she felt happier and more confident. After spending a session reviewing her progress and helping her identify the skills she needed to keep practicing, Ann and her therapist agreed that she was ready to bring her therapy to an end.

The Therapeutic Relationship

The therapeutic relationship supports all of the other elements of the therapy. Additionally, case formulation-driven CBT relies on a dual view of the relationship. One part of the relationship is the necessary-but-not-sufficient view. In this view, the trusting collaborative relationship is the foundation on which the technical interventions of CBT rest.

The other view of the relationship is itself an assessment (Turkat & Brantley, 1981) and intervention tool (Kohlenberg & Tsai, 1991), as illustrated in the case of Ann. In our work with her, we observed that Ann tended to describe her problems in vague, general terms, such as "It's been a nerve-wracking week," and to resist giving details of her struggles and distress. When the therapist gently pointed out to Ann how difficult it was to get detailed information from their conversations, a good discussion ensued that provided details about the mechanisms driving Ann's reluctance to provide details. Ann reported that she feared that if she provided more information about her experiences, the therapist would find her unappealing and want to stop working with her. It was this discussion that led to the discovery that minimizing self-disclosure was a key avoidance behavior that Ann used to protect herself from harm in social situations. Thus, a detailed examination of the interactions between Ann and her therapist provided important information that contributed to the case formulation and to the treatment.

Ann's therapist also used the therapeutic relationship to treat Ann's fear of self-disclosure, using ideas from functional analytic psychotherapy (Kohlenberg & Tsai, 1991). When Ann shared more personal details, the therapist took care to spontaneously, warmly, and immediately let Ann know that the therapist felt closer to Ann and experienced her as more interesting and appealing in that moment.

The case formulation-driven approach also helps the therapist establish a strong and positive relationship at the beginning of therapy because the collaborative process of building a shared formulation provides a kind of superglue that binds therapist and patient together in an important joint enterprise, and motivates the patient—and the therapist—to work hard in therapy.

Summary

We have described an idiographic hypothesis-testing approach to treatment that provides an elegant strategy for providing evidence-based psychotherapy, and we illustrated the model with an example from CBT with a client who was socially anxious and depressed. The essential elements of a hypothesis-testing approach to therapy guided by a case formulation (the hypothesis) and progress monitoring data that are used to test the hypothesis are not limited to CBT and may be employed by psychotherapists using any psychotherapy modality or orientation (e.g., see Eells, 2007).

CBT can seem to be the route to EBP because so many randomized controlled trials have shown CBT to be effective, and fewer randomized controlled trials have been conducted to examine efficacy of other modalities of psychotherapy. However, the EBP of psychotherapy and psychotherapy based on ESTs are not one and the same. In fact, sometimes, oddly enough, training in ESTs seems to impede clinicians from using an empirical hypothesis-testing approach to their work (Shiloff, 2015). Strikingly, most ESTs do not include one of the essential elements of evidence-based psychotherapy: progress monitoring. Collecting data to monitor progress and test the formulation hypothesis is, we argue, an essential element of an empirical approach to clinical work. In addition, progress monitoring is an EBP (see review by Lewis et al., 2018). As a result, psychotherapy trainees who are learning to provide evidence-based treatment by learning to adhere to EST protocols often fail to learn to use an empirical hypothesis-testing approach to their cases (Shiloff, 2015). Instead, these trainees learn to make clinical decisions by searching the treatment manual for answers to their questions.

Providing psychotherapy based on an individualized case formulation and the results of progress monitoring data is a difficult enterprise. Challenges clinicians face include lack of library access, and lack of the time and skills needed to digest voluminous, technical, and constantly changing literatures. Another impediment is the difficulty accessing inexpensive data collection tools for assessment and progress monitoring. Training in these difficult skills can also be difficult to access. We encourage the field to develop tools and mechanisms to address these challenges, so that practitioners have the support they need to provide evidence-based care to their patients. And we encourage trainees and experienced clinicians alike to utilize the idiographic hypothesis-testing approach described in this chapter as a guide to integrating the research evidence to support best practice with their clients.

References

American Psychological Association. (2002). *Ethical principles of psychologists and code of conduct.* Washington, DC: Author.

Beck, A. T., Epstein, N., Brown, G., & Steer, R. (1988). An inventory for measuring clinical anxiety: Psychometric properties. *Journal of Consulting and Clinical Psychology, 56,* 893–897.

Beck, A. T., Rush, J. A., Shaw, B. F., & Emery, G. (1979). *Cognitive therapy for depression.* New York: Guilford Press.

Beck, A. T., Steer, R. A., & Garbin, M. G. (1988). Psychometric properties of the Beck Depression Inventory: Twenty-five years of evaluation. *Clinical Psychology Review, 8,* 77–100.

Clark, D. M., & Wells, A. (1995). A cognitive model of social phobia. In R. G. Heimberg, M. R. Liebowitz, D. A. Hope, & F. R. Schneier (Eds.), *Social phobia: Diagnosis, assessment, and treatment* (pp. 69–93). New York: Guilford Press.

Craske, M. G., Kircanski, K., Zelikowsky, M., Mystkowski, J., Chowdhury, N., & Baker, A. (2008). Optimizing inhibitory learning during exposure therapy. *Behaviour Research and Therapy, 46,* 5–27.

Eells, T. D. (Ed.). (2007). *Handbook of psychotherapy case formulation* (2nd ed.). New York: Guilford Press.

Harvey, A. G., Clark, D. M., Ehlers, A., & Rapee, R. M. (2000). Social anxiety and self-impression: Cognitive preparation enhances the beneficial effects of video feedback following a stressful social task. *Behaviour Research and Therapy, 28,* 1183–1192.

Hayes, S. C., Nelson, R. O., & Jarrett, R. B. (1987). The treatment utility of assessment: A functional approach to evaluating assessment quality. *American Psychologist, 42,* 963–974.

Haynes, S. N., Kaholokula, J. K., & Nelson, K. (1999). The idiographic application of nomothetic, empirically based treatments. *Clinical Psychology: Science and Practice, 6,* 456–461.

Hunsley, J., & Mash, E. J. (Eds.). (2018). *A guide to assessments that work.* New York: Oxford University Press.

Insel, T., Cuthbert, B., Garvey, M., Heinssen, R., Pine, D. S., Quinn, K., et al. (2010). Research domain criteria (RDoC): Toward a new classification framework for research on mental disorders. *American Journal of Psychiatry, 167*(7), 748–751.

Iwata, B. A., Pace, G. M., Dorsey, M. F., Zarcone, J. R., Vollmer, T. R., & Smith, R. G. (1994). The functions of self-injurious behavior: An experimental-epidemiological analysis. *Journal of Applied Behavior Analysis, 27,* 215–240.

Kohlenberg, R. J., & Tsai, M. (1991). *Functional analytic psychotherapy: Creating intense and curative therapeutic relationships.* New York: Plenum Press.

Kuyken, W., Padesky, C. A., & Dudley, R. (2009). *Collaborative case conceptualization: Working effectively with clients in cognitive-behavioral therapy.* New York: Guilford Press.

Lewinsohn, P. M., Hoberman, T., & Hautzinger, M. (1985). An integrative theory of depression. In S. Reiss & R. Bootzin (Eds.), *Theoretical issues in behavior therapy* (pp. 331–359). New York: Academic Press.

Lewis, C. C., Boyd, M., Puspitasari, A., Navarro, E., Howard, J., Kassab, H., et al. (2018). Implementing measurement-based care in behavioral health: A review. *JAMA Psychiatry.* [Epub ahead of print]

Liebowitz, M. R. (1987). Social phobia. *Modern Problems in Pharmacopsychiatry, 22,* 141–173.

Lutz, W., Martinovich, Z., & Howard, K. I. (1999). Patient profiling: An application of random coefficient regression models to depicting the response of a patient to outpatient psychotherapy. *Journal of Consulting and Clinical Psychology, 67,* 571–577.

Martell, C. R., Addis, M. E., & Jacobson, N. S. (2001). *Depression in context: Strategies for guided action.* New York: Norton.

Mundt, J. C., Marks, I. M., Shear, M. K., & Greist, J. M. (2002). The Work and Social Adjustment Scale: A simple measure of impairment in functioning. *British Journal of Psychiatry, 180*(5), 461–464.

Nezu, A. M., & Perri, M. G. (1989). Social problem-solving therapy for unipolar depression: An initial dismantling investigation. *Journal of Consulting and Clinical Psychology, 57,* 408–413.

Persons, J. B. (2006). Case formulation-driven psychotherapy. *Clinical Psychology: Science and Practice, 13,* 167–170.

Persons, J. B. (2008). *The case formulation approach to cognitive-behavior therapy.* New York: Guilford Press.

Persons, J. B., Beckner, V. L., & Tompkins, M. A. (2013). Testing case formulation hypotheses in psychotherapy: Two case examples. *Cognitive and Behavioral Practice, 20*(4), 399–409.

Rapee, R. M., & Heimberg, R. G. (1997). A cognitive-behavioral model of anxiety in social phobia. *Behaviour Research and Therapy, 35,* 741–756.

Shiloff, N. (2015). The scientist-practitioner gap: A clinical supervisor self-discloses. *Clinical Science, 18*(3), 21–23.

Turkat, I. D., & Brantley, P. J. (1981). On the therapeutic relationship in behavior therapy. *Behavior Therapist, 4,* 16–17.

Turkat, I. D., & Maisto, S. A. (1985). Personality disorders: Application of the experimental method to the formulation and modification of personality disorders. In D. H. Barlow (Ed.), *Clinical handbook of psychological disorders: A step-by-step treatment manual* (pp. 502–570). New York: Guilford Press.

Weisz, J. R., Ugueto, A. M., Herren, J., Afienko, A. R., & Rutt, C. (2011). Kernels vs. ears and other questions for a science of treatment dissemination. *Clinical Psychology: Science and Practice, 18*(1), 41–46.

Wells, A., Clark, D. M., & Salkovskis, P. (1995). Social phobia: The role of in-situation safety behaviors in maintaining anxiety and negative beliefs. *Behavior Therapy, 26,* 153–161.

CHAPTER 13

Collaborative Case Conceptualization

A Bridge between Science and Practice

SHADI BESHAI
WILLEM KUYKEN
ROB KIDNEY

Brenda, a 34-year-old mother of two, was born in Mainland China but moved to Vancouver, Canada, with her parents and grandparents when she was only an infant. Brenda's parents became devout Christians when she was a child, so Brenda was raised in accordance with strong Christian values and traditions. In the years leading up to her adolescence, Brenda described a very close and supportive relationship with her parents and grandparents. When Brenda moved away for college, she described a resurgence of interest and pride in her cultural and religious roots.

During college, Brenda met her husband, Kelvin, and soon after graduating, they married and conceived their first child, Jon. Brenda and Kelvin separated when Brenda was 24 and pregnant with her second child, Emma. Brenda described the separation as a "difficult time" but explained that her closeness to God and her parents made the process more bearable.

At the time of her treatment, Brenda was working as a registered nurse and described a fulfilling and supportive, yet at times very stressful work environment. In the last 8 months, she had been suffering from low mood, fatigue, poor concentration, and disrupted appetite and sleep. Furthermore, Brenda described intense and recurrent thoughts of worthlessness; these feelings made it very difficult for her to resume her normal activi-

ties. For example, although Brenda had typically enjoyed an active social life, she described intense anxiety, especially in the midst of strangers. This anxiety had made it difficult for her to consider the prospect of dating, although she was open to starting a new relationship. For example, Brenda described frequent blushing and feelings of being "tongue-tied" around new romantic partners. Brenda stated that these concerns began shortly after the dissolution of a brief and recent romantic relationship. She reported that "cultural differences" between herself and her partner were the main reason for the dissolution of this relationship. Brenda's treatment goals were to increase her confidence and comfort when dating and to improve her mood.

*   *   *

The central aims of scientific psychology are to describe, explain, and predict human behavior, thought, and emotion. By extension, the aims of clinical science are to describe, explain, and predict behavior and emotional responses that create psychological disorders, and provide evidence-based psychological treatments for these disorders. Accordingly, clinical scientists have developed hundreds of theories and corresponding therapies that are believed to account for and treat various psychological disorders. However, there is a tension between attempts to explain, predict, and treat psychological disorders—and in doing so potentially reducing such disorders to theories and treatment protocols developed for populations—and missing the inescapable diversity of human experience. For example, although Brenda presented with a number of typical clinical features of depression (e.g., low mood, disruptions of sleep and appetite), she also presented with a number of unique and important factors (e.g., her religious faith and familial belonging; social anxiety symptoms). These idiosyncratic features may render standardized treatment delivery unnecessary or suboptimal.

The diversity of human experience makes clinical science not only challenging but also interesting. Researchers are now beginning to build evidence-based processes within treatment protocols to account for individual differences. As such, a one-size-fits-all approach, which may at best be unhelpful and at worst be harmful to patients, is replaced by the flexible adaptation and application of treatment protocols.

In this chapter, we define our approach to embracing the central aims of scientific psychology and the wonderful diversity of psychological problems. We define our approach—collaborative case conceptualization (CCC)—and illustrate its use to guide our description, explanation, prediction, and treatment of Brenda's presenting concerns. The conceptualization process functioned to socialize Brenda to the cognitive model, improve her engagement and buy into treatment, plan ways to dismantle negative behaviors and thoughts, and build her resilience. Treatment with Brenda spanned 17 sessions and progressed in accordance with manualized cognitive therapy for depression and anxiety; that is, the focus early in treatment was on psychoeducation and self-monitoring, and progressed to behavioral interventions, and ended with higher-order work on cognitive restructuring and challenging. Although this specific case example is fictitious, Brenda represents an amalgamation of clinical features of a number of clients we have worked with in the past. We illustrate our work with her through description, with sample transcripts from sessions and "think-aloud" sections in which we reflect on our interactions with her, and examples of completed worksheets.

What Is CCC?

Given the evidence base that supports the use of cognitive-behavioral therapy (CBT) for depression and anxiety disorders (Gloaguen, Cottraux, Cucherat, & Blackburn, 1998; Hofmann & Smits, 2008), we adopted a cognitive-behavioral approach in the treatment of Brenda's presenting issues. CBT, one of the most tested and widely adopted of all psychological treatments (Butler, Chapman, Forman, & Beck, 2006), is defined as a set of treatment approaches that emphasizes the role of cognitions (thought content, pattern, and structure) and behaviors in the onset and maintenance of abnormal responses (Beck & Haigh, 2014). For example, the "mediational" hypothesis in CBT dictates that "desired behavior change may be affected through cognitive change" (Dobson, 2010, p. 4). Accordingly, any treatment approach that devotes considerable therapeutic time to the identification and restructuring of thoughts can be conceptualized under the general CBT rubric (Blagys & Hilsenroth, 2002).

As CBT is hypothesis-driven, case conceptualization (used here interchangeably with *case formulation*) stands at the heart of this approach. Although there is some variability in the way case conceptualization is defined, most sources agree on the essential features and functions of this process in therapy. Broadly defined, *case conceptualization* is the process by which therapists "provide a clear, theoretical explanation of *what the client is like* as well as theoretical hypotheses for *why the client is like this*" (Berman, 2014, p. xi; original emphasis). Thus, case conceptualization is a hypothesis-driven process designed to describe and explain client distress. During this process, a treatment plan that maps onto these hypotheses is created in order to address current concerns and prevent reemergence of these concerns. The case conceptualization process is not unique to CBT, as many other therapeutic approaches champion the use of this process in therapy (Needleman, 1999). The case conceptualization process has been described as a core skill of CBT and other evidence-based approaches (Bieling & Kuyken, 2003; Eells, 1997).

There are a number of case conceptualization models that exist in CBT and other evidence-based treatments. However, we believe that many case conceptualization models focus disproportionately on client problems, while neglecting strengths. Moreover, case conceptualization in many models is often static, presented only once during therapy, and delivered in a top-down manner, with little to no collaborative input from the client. Our work on the CCC model seeks to address these limitations. CCC can be defined as "the process whereby therapist and client work collaboratively first to describe and then to explain the issues a client presents in therapy. Its primary function is to guide therapy in order to relieve client distress and build client resilience" (Kuyken, Padesky, & Dudley, 2009, p. 3). The developers of this unique conceptualization model argue that this clinical process is guided by three overarching principles (Kuyken at al., 2009): (1) levels of conceptualization, (2) collaborative empiricism, and (3) a strengths focus.

Within the CCC model, case conceptualization is a process rather than a milestone; that is, the term *levels of conceptualization* refers to the unfolding of the conceptualization process in correspondence with the understanding of the therapist and client. Accordingly, increasingly complex conceptualization models are discussed and created throughout treatment.

Collaborative empiricism stands at the heart of the CCC model. *Collaborative empiricism* is the process by which therapist and client collaboratively agree on client issues and goals of treatment. Collaborative empiricism also involves the collaborative efforts of therapist and client to design and implement tests of the client's beliefs (Beck, Rush, Shaw, & Emery, 1979; Kazantzis, MacEwan, & Dattilio, 2005; Tee & Kazantzis, 2011).

As a strengths focus is an important facet of the CCC model, definitional clarity about strength, as well as risk and vulnerability, is in order. Risk factors in psychopathology are any factors that are associated with the increased likelihood of experiencing or developing a condition (Masten & Garmezy, 1985; Rutter, 1987). Accordingly, risk factors do not necessarily play a causal role in the development of psychopathology (e.g., being female is a risk factor for depression, but it does not cause depression). On the other hand, vulnerability factors are associated with the mechanisms of a disorder and so are implicated causally in the development of a condition (Rutter, 1987). Rutter (1987) defined *resilience factors* as the dynamic, individual differences that are linked to coping successfully in response to risk and environmental stressors. *Protective factors,* on the other hand, are directly related to vulnerability.

Accordingly, protective factors are believed to be associated with "amelioration of the reaction to factors that would otherwise lead to a maladaptive outcome" (Rutter, 1987, p. 317). Rutter indicated that there is a constant negotiation between risk, vulnerability, resilience and protective factors, and the outcome of this negotiation can mean the difference between health and disorder. Finally, *strengths* are defined as "any psychological processes that consistently enable a person to think and act so as to yield benefits to himself or herself and society" (McCullough & Snyder, 2000, p. 3). Accordingly, resilience factors are dynamic, whereas strengths are more stable characteristics.

Within the CCC model, there is a strong emphasis on the training and skills development of therapists. Similar to conceptualization processes in treatment, training also unfolds in a graded fashion and in accordance with the skills level of the trainee. Kuyken, Padesky, and Dudley (2009) adapted Bennett-Levy's (2006; Bennett-Levy & Haarhoff, Chapter 25, this volume) three-part model in developing case conceptualization skills. This model emphasizes declarative, procedural, and reflective learning. *Declarative learning* is defined as the acquisition of knowledge of CBT theory, techniques, and treatment structure. *Procedural learning* is concerned with the application of knowledge acquired in the declarative learning stage, while *reflective learning* is defined as "standing back" from one's practice and reflecting on experiences in order to improve skills (Kuyken et al., 2009, p. 256).

What Is the Crucible of CCC?

In chemistry, a *crucible* is a vessel used to contain chemical elements when heated. A crucible is typically made of materials capable of withstanding very high temperatures. Kuyken and colleagues (2009) liken the case conceptualization process to a crucible: a vessel used to contain the necessary ingredients of change in CBT. Specifically, these necessary ingredients include client experiences, CBT theory, research, and techniques. Accordingly, the case conceptualization process represents the vessel containing the interaction of these active ingredients. Within the CCC model, the whole of the interactions between ingredients is invariably more than the sum of their parts; that is, and much like the transformational process that comes from heating chemical elements, the systematic "fusion" of client experiences with CBT theory and research is key in the process of therapeutic change (see Figure 13.1).

Consistent with the crucible metaphor, "heating" in the CCC model is achieved through collaboration between client and therapist (i.e., collaborative empiricism); that is, a unilateral approach—either top-down from therapist to client or bottom-up, from client to therapist—will be insufficient in producing enough "heat" to instill transformation. As such, the CCC model heavily emphasizes a collaborative approach, and indeed, this approach stands as one of the guiding principles in the current model. Kuyken and colleagues (2009) argued that this emphasis on collaboration during the conceptualization process is an extension of already extant emphasis within CBT as a whole (Beck et al., 1979).

Within the crucible, each of the guiding principles of CCC is active. The first guiding principle, namely, *levels of conceptualization,* emphasizes the evolving nature of conceptualization in CBT. To optimize utility and effectiveness, the conceptualization process must transform gradually to reflect level of therapist understanding and client readiness. Accordingly, the function and nature of conceptualizations evolve from description to explanation to prediction. *Collaborative empiricism,* the second guiding principle, highlights the need for therapist and client to work together to integrate client experiences with CBT theory and research. As such, over-involvement of one member of the therapeutic dyad (e.g., therapist) increases the likelihood of improper integration of important elements of change (e.g., client experiences). The third guiding principle, *incorporation of client strengths,* acknowledges that most current CBT protocols focus almost exclusively on the client's problems, which is believed to reduce client engagement in treatment. As such, a strengths focus is thought to increase client's commitment to the treatment and enhance clients' sense of agency (Kuyken et al., 2009, 2015; Kuyken, Padesky, & Dudley, 2008).

Functions of CCC in CBT

Sound clinical theories (e.g., the CCC model) are intended to be useful; that is, to serve as tools to help the clinician and client. The CCC model serves 10 important functions that, as a whole, seek to alleviate distress and cultivate resilience in practice (Kuyken et al., 2009). We illustrate each of these with examples from our work with Brenda.

1. Synthesize the unique characteristics and histories of the client with relevant CBT theory and research. In Brenda's case, research on depression and social anxiety is of particular relevance. The challenge, which is made easier through the adoption of the CCC model, would be to incorporate Brenda's unique cultural and spiritual frameworks within these existing theories.

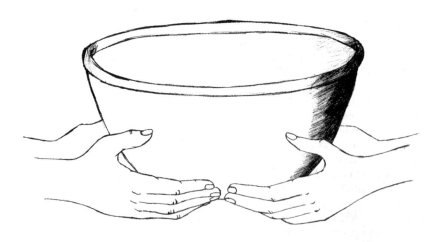

FIGURE 13.1. CCC as a crucible, with collaboration between client and therapist as "heat" source.

2. Normalize the client's presenting concerns and reduce self-stigma. Early in treatment, Brenda said, "I am afraid to tell my closest friends of what has been going on because I can't imagine anyone would understand." Accordingly, most clients are distressed about their own distress, so, in our experience, providing psychoeducation through the case conceptualization process often brings a sense of relief and empowerment.

3. Engender client engagement in treatment. Evidence suggests that engagement in CBT is a predictor of treatment success (Strunk, Brotman, & DeRubeis, 2010). As such, one of the goals of case conceptualization is to promote engagement and "buy" into the treatment. In Brenda's case, presenting a descriptive conceptualization early in treatment that closely fits her experiences (unhelpful automatic thoughts in reaction to her own emotions, which in turn generates a cascade of other negative thoughts and emotions) underscored the intuitiveness and simplicity of the cognitive model, which in turn engaged the client in the treatment.

4. Increase the manageability of the numerous and often complex presenting issues. This function serves both clients and therapists, as the process may reveal common threads that run through seemingly disconnected concerns. For example, and during the cross-sectional conceptualizations, Brenda identified her working unhelpful assumption: "If people notice my weaknesses, they will judge me." This helped Brenda and therapist to better understand the connection between most of her seemingly disconnected presenting concerns (e.g., anxiety when meeting potential romantic partners; low mood when feeling overwhelmed at work).

5. Organize, select, and order appropriate therapeutic techniques. Cognitive-behavioral therapists may feel bewildered by the dizzying array of techniques and interventions in CBT. Accordingly, the fifth function of conceptualization is to support therapists by allowing them to select techniques that map well onto agreed-upon clinical issues. As an illustration, Brenda identified that her anxiety and self-doubt around potential romantic interests was her most pressing concern. Accordingly, Brenda and her therapist selected behavioral techniques as a first therapeutic step in order to alleviate such anxiety.

6. Identify client strengths and suggest avenues for bolstering these strengths. This function is aligned with the third guiding principle of CCC and further highlights the holistic approach of the model. In the case of Brenda, her closeness with family, her Christian faith, and pride in her cultural heritage were all identified early on as potential sources of strength.

7. Maximization of cost-efficiency of treatment is now often at the forefront of academic and clinical inquiry. Case conceptualization can suggest the most cost-efficient avenue for treatment, which is prioritized more often today, as financial accountability is increasing as a function of limited resources in many settings. For Brenda, starting with behavioral techniques and ending with cognitive restructuring of faulty assumptions comprised the most cost-efficient route for treatment.

8. Anticipate and prevent problems in therapy. As dropout is a frequent problem in CBT (Shottenbauer, Glass, Arnkoff, Tendick, & Gray, 2008), we believe that the case conceptualization process should build in mechanisms to avoid this potential concern. In Brenda's case, the conceptualization models pointed to the salience of social judgment cognitions as a *modus vivendi* for the client. As such, the therapist was careful to preempt the activation of such cognitions in the context of the therapeutic relationship; that is, the therapist was careful to point out to Brenda that "setbacks" in treatment are normal and can be framed as an opportunity for further growth.

9. Anticipate and prevent treatment nonresponse. A large minority (30–45%) of patients who complete a course of CBT do not experience a significant remediation in symptoms (Whisman, 2008). As such, the case conceptualization process is designed to anticipate this potential nonresponse and suggest alternative fruitful avenues. Conducting a collaborative conceptualization with Brenda helped the therapist anticipate lack of response due to her engagement in safety behaviors in the context of the behavioral interventions. Accordingly, the model was able to preempt such lack of response and intervene to reduce safety behaviors.

10. Allow for high-quality supervision of trainees and consultation. According to Kuyken and colleagues (2009), high-quality treatment, which describes, explains client presenting concerns, and fosters resilience, is similar to the supervision process.

Painting a Portrait: Descriptive Conceptualization

It is common for clinicians to find themselves facing the often complex, intricate, and over-whelming nature of clients' presenting issues. Brenda's therapist was no exception; he was led quickly into complicated and difficult terrain shortly after starting the session.

THERAPIST: Brenda, perhaps you could tell me what brings you here today?

BRENDA: I really don't know where to start. The last few months have just been very hard.

THERAPIST: I am very sorry to hear that. You said your life in the last few months has been very hard. What exactly has been troubling you?

BRENDA: I can hardly get out of bed. I have a job that I love, but I feel like I am not doing the best that I can. I am pretty miserable all the time, which makes me feel even worse, because I know that I have a good life in comparison to a lot of people, and I know I shouldn't really feel this way.

THERAPIST: It sounds like a lot of things are on your mind and have been affecting you lately. Anything else in particular that has made the last few months hard for you?

BRENDA: Well, I really want to find someone that I can share my life with, but I feel like I am no good to anyone. Worse yet, I feel like people judge me when I am in public; like they can see all my flaws; or that I will say something that will show how stupid I am or unworthy I am.

The goal of a descriptive case conceptual-ization is to render an accurate portrait of the client's presenting issues and prioritize them to pave the way for an efficient and effective treat-ment plan. The goal also is to normalize some of these client's struggles and engage the client early in treatment. The first task is to identify and prioritize top issues, and rate their impact:

THERAPIST: You mentioned a lot of issues that have been affecting your life in the last few months. To make treatment as useful as pos-sible, let's make a list of these issues. How does that sound?

BRENDA: I guess we can do that. It might be a long list.

THERAPIST: That's OK. First, let's try and think of the issues that are impacting your life the most and then we will make our way down. Does that sound OK?

BRENDA: Yeah, that sounds good.

THERAPIST: So, what has been bothering you the most lately?

BRENDA: I suppose how sad I get sometimes. My low mood can get really overwhelming for me. When I feel that way, I keep think-ing about how people at work may notice, and then I have trouble concentrating and feel like I am doing a lot of mistakes.

THERAPIST: Let's jot that down in our list. (*Hands Brenda a structured form on which she can list issues and strengths in descend-ing order of impact/importance*)

Think-Aloud: It was important that the therapist encourage Brenda to write down simple present-ing issues and their behavioral impact on her life. For example, if Brenda had only identified "low mood" as her top presenting issue, the therapist would have prompted Brenda, in order to uncover the specific impact of low mood on her function-ing: "What things does your low mood get in the way of?"

In our experience, it is unlikely for patients to report their strengths spontaneously. Accord-ingly, it is important that the therapists ask cli-ents directly about what they view as strengths and resilience factors:

THERAPIST: We talked a lot about some of the issues that have been impacting your life of late. Let's talk about the other side of the coin: things that you do particularly well, or things that are going right for you at the mo-ment, and effective ways you've learned to deal with your stress.

BRENDA: Not sure if there is much going right for me at the moment. Everything feels like its falling apart.

THERAPIST: I know it may feel that way, but even in our short time together here, I have noticed that despite all the issues that have been impacting you lately, there seems to be a lot of things you're getting right. Our job is to bring those things to light and to-gether help strengthen them over the course of treatment. For example, one thing I no-ticed is that you seem to get a lot of pride and strength from your family and heritage, and both seem to help you deal with stressful situations in your life. Am I getting that right?

BRENDA: I suppose you're right. My parents can sometimes be a source of stress for me, but overall, they have been really supportive toward me and the kids. I am also really proud of being Chinese. Sometimes when I feel like I don't even know who I am any more, I start thinking about where I come from and feel like I am connected to something. I also have a lot of people that care about me at the church that I go to. I've called on them to support me before and they were happy to help. They always remind me that no matter how I feel about myself, God still loves me. It's a nice feeling.

Think-Aloud: Note how the therapist uses words like *our* and *together* to stress the collaborative nature of treatment. Also note how the therapist in this example uses self-disclosure: When he noticed that the client was "stuck" on presenting issues and their impact, he prompted her to think of her strengths by informing her of what he had noticed during their brief interaction.

In addition to identifying and prioritizing presenting issues, it is important that therapists contextualize these issues in the descriptive level of the conceptualization process. The five part model (Padeskey & Mooney, 1990) is a popular method of contextualizing presenting issues, and pictorial models of conveying this information are often helpful means of introducing the cognitive-behavioral framework by stressing the relationships between cognitions, behaviors, emotions, and physiological responses (see Figure 13.2). As can be seen in Brenda's five-part model, the therapist and client worked together to identify how environmental diatheses may have interacted with existing vulnerabilities to produce some of the presenting complaints.

More than the Sum of the Parts: Cross-Sectional Conceptualization

Cross-sectional conceptualization refers to the level of conceptualization that links theory with particular client experiences. This level works on a "higher level" (Kuyken et al., 2009, p. 172)

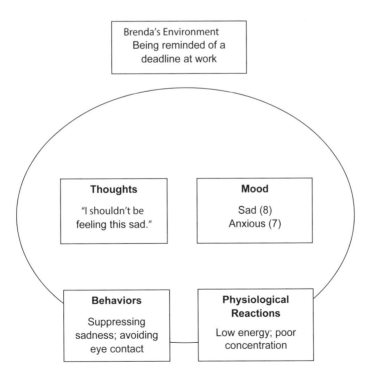

FIGURE 13.2. Brenda's five-part model.

by identifying key cognitive and behavioral mechanisms that maintain or exacerbate presenting concerns. The first goal of the cross-sectional conceptualization is to help clients identify proximal vulnerability factors unique to them and develop interventions that disrupt this cycle of vulnerability. The second goal of this level of conceptualization is identifying common threads that run across the patient's presenting issues. Kuyken and colleagues (2009) recommend a four-step process to establish a cross-sectional conceptualization, as described below. Note that although we do not discuss session details between the construction of the descriptive and cross-sectional conceptualizations, this work is foundational for appropriate progression in treatment. Important milestones after the descriptive conceptualization include appropriate self-monitoring and introduction to some early behavioral techniques (e.g., exposure; activation). The first step in this process is to gather recent examples of the patient's top concerns. In doing so, the therapist can also help the patient establish mechanisms related to the client's distress. Brenda had identified "low mood" and "poor concentration" as top priorities in her treatment. Accordingly, the therapist and Brenda worked together to uncover as many recent examples in her life as possible when these issues occurred, and to identify whether there were similarities among these seemingly unconnected occurrences.

THERAPIST: We have been talking about your mood and the fact that you notice your mood dip from time to time. You mentioned that last week you noticed that you felt sad at work. Do you remember any other instances when your mood was that low?

BRENDA: On Monday last week, I was grocery shopping, and then I started feeling sad. It felt completely out of the blue, but I almost broke down in tears in the middle of the store.

THERAPIST: That sounds really hard, Brenda. Maybe we can try to find a link between these two situations during which you felt this way. Let's look back at your five-part model that we put together a few sessions ago. I notice here that you identified the thought "I shouldn't be sad" and an associated physical reaction of being out of energy and having poor concentration. Am I getting that right?

BRENDA: Yeah, that sounds right.

THERAPIST: If you think back, what were the thoughts and the physical sensations that went along with your low mood that time when you were in the grocery store?

BRENDA: Now that I think about it, I did have a wave of fatigue that hit me. I also remember thinking, "Here it comes again. I won't even have energy to finish shopping for the kids. This is not normal and unacceptable."

Think-Aloud: Assuming Brenda was engaged with homework related to self-monitoring of thoughts, emotions, behaviors, and physical sensations, discussions such as the one we just presented work to further solidify observations made in, and hypotheses generated by, the descriptive conceptualization.

After the identification of a number of recent examples when Brenda felt low and sad, the therapist and client worked to develop a model of triggers and maintenance factors to help account for her top presenting issues:

THERAPIST: From the list of examples we wrote down, can you see a pattern that connects these different situations together?

BRENDA: I see that my mood is almost always connected with thoughts about how I shouldn't feel a certain way or that people will notice and will judge me. My low mood seems to also be connected with how tired I feel.

THERAPIST: I am seeing this, too. What do you make of all of this?

BRENDA: I am starting to see that my depression is making me question myself as a nurse and a mother. I guess the more I think that way, the more fatigued I feel and harder it is for me to concentrate on what I am doing, and less likely for me to get what I need done. It's kind of like a self-fulfilling prophecy.

THERAPIST: That seems like it fits with what has been going on. If you could, how would you connect your thoughts, feelings, behaviors, and physical sensations across these different situations, then?

BRENDA: If I had to guess, across these situations, I probably start noticing something about my depression, like my sadness or how tired I am, and then I start thinking about how I shouldn't feel this way or that people will think less of me if they know, and that makes me even more sad and tired. I always remember the thought "I have to hide this," because

I can't imagine anyone understanding what is happening to me. The thought that I have to hide it doesn't help with my concentration.

THERAPIST: It sounds like you may be on to something here, Brenda.

Think-Aloud: Here, the therapist challenges Brenda to think about her own thinking and generate her own hypotheses that function to link thoughts, behaviors, and emotions across time and situations.

As we can see, together with the therapist, Brenda was able to devise a working model of her low mood: Physical primes of her low mood and fatigue may lead to negative thoughts about her need to "hide" the symptoms, which lead to intense feelings of sadness and fatigue, which then make it less likely for her to carry out her duties (e.g., work-related deadlines) and may reinforce the original unhelpful thoughts ("This is not normal"; "I shouldn't feel this way"). In the coming sessions, Brenda and her therapist uncover a potential unhelpful underlying assumption that may work to maintain her low mood: "If people notice my moments of weakness, they will judge me." Brenda and the therapist then work together on a brief conceptualization of this hypothesized model (Figure 13.3).

In the next step of cross-sectional conceptualization, Brenda and the therapist identify targeted interventions to disrupt this hypothesized cycle of vulnerability. During this step, Brenda also identifies how her resilience and strengths, namely, the support of her parents and friends, can help break the cycle. For example, Brenda indicated that she would solicit help from her parents around the house during instances when she is feeling extremely fatigued. She also agreed to solicit help from her coworkers when she is feeling particularly sad or is need of a short break while on the job. In soliciting this kind of support, Brenda also began to modify her underlying assumption: "Even if I cannot always be strong, I know I can still get support from people around me, and they will not judge me."

In subsequent sessions, the therapist and Brenda began developing another maintenance model surrounding Brenda's social anxiety:

THERAPIST: I know that one of your other concerns was how anxious you get around others. I am curious if you think your mood and anxiety are connected somehow?

BRENDA: Now that I think back, every time I get really anxious around strangers is when

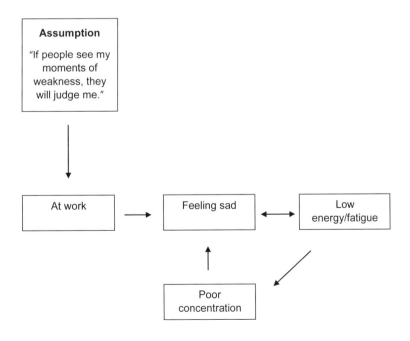

FIGURE 13.3. Cross-sectional conceptualization.

that thought pops back in my head: "People can't see me sad," "Feeling this way is not normal," or "I will be judged." As soon as I have these thoughts, I start feeling like there is something wrong with me and that people will see it and judge me.

Related to the underlying assumption that triggers and maintains her low mood, Brenda identified that she "feels judged" when she does not maintain an appearance of energy and excitement around others. Accordingly, she becomes anxious in the company of her romantic interests, which works to increase her fatigue and poor concentration, and maintain the cycle of anxiety.

During last stage of the cross-sectional level of conceptualization, the therapist and Brenda revised and expanded the original maintenance model. For instance, Brenda noticed that at times, she preempts feeling judged by others and starts acting with hostility and defensiveness around them, which makes her feel guilty later. Note that the models created in this and other levels of the conceptualization process are tentative in nature. Thus, all models are subject to revision when evidence that is unsupportive of such models arises.

From Then to Now and Beyond: Longitudinal Conceptualization

In the longitudinal level of the conceptualization process, Brenda and her therapist explore key developmental events that may have contributed to formation of unhelpful underlying assumptions and schemas. Together, they connect her life history to her present struggles. As is argued by Kuyken and colleagues (2009), a longitudinal conceptualization may not always be necessary, especially when treatment goals have been met during the cross-sectional conceptualization stage. However, if progress seems volatile and/or if more pervasive clinical issues have been identified, a longitudinal conceptualization is recommended. Accordingly, the goals of a longitudinal conceptualization are to address causes of unstable remission and to elucidate why patients may continue to experience symptoms across varying environmental circumstances. Finally, longitudinal conceptualizations are intended to predict and prevent future relapse and mobilize protective factors when vulnerability factors have been activated.

Longitudinal conceptualizations comprise two stages. In the first stage, the patient and therapist use CBT theory to establish a connection between current issues and developmental experiences. In the second stage, patient and therapist use the conceptualization to develop and select interventions that may break this association. As with other stages in the conceptualization process, movement between these two stages is driven by how well the conceptualization fits with the evidence.

The assessment phase of Brenda's treatment revealed two important developmental events. Brenda reported being ridiculed by other children for her ethnicity in middle school. She reported feeling "different," and that she worked hard to "blend in" with the other children. Also, in her late adolescence, Brenda reported developing a romantic interest in a boy at her church. She reported that her Youth Pastor became aware of this relationship and voiced his disapproval of this interest on religious grounds.

THERAPIST: Brenda, I noticed on your thought records from last week you had the thoughts "It's awful if they know what's really going on" and "I shouldn't be feeling this way." Do these sound familiar to you?

BRENDA: I guess I had similar thoughts a couple weeks ago. Now that I think about it, I had really similar thoughts a few weeks before then, too.

THERAPIST: Yeah, I noticed that, too. What do you make of this?

BRENDA: I am not sure.

THERAPIST: I remember when we were talking about your history in the first couple of sessions and you had mentioned something about your experience of being bullied in middle school.

BRENDA: That's right. Kids were awful to me just because I didn't look the same or because I showed up with a different lunch than most of them. That year didn't do my self-esteem very good.

THERAPIST: I also remember that the low mood and other issues you came to treatment with started shortly after you and your most recent boyfriend broke up because of how close you are with your parents.

BRENDA: That's right. He just didn't understand that this is how it is for me and how it will always be. He just couldn't accept that fact.

THERAPIST: Do you see a connection there?

BRENDA: Do you mean both are about my culture?

THERAPIST: Yes, there's that. But I am also curious to know how you perceived these events then and now?

BRENDA: Well, I usually feel very confident about where I come from, but in both of these instances, I guess I felt a bit of shame or that I need to be like everyone else, which is ridiculous.

Here, Brenda discovered that there may be a connection between her being bullied in middle school and the events that led to the dissolution of her most recent romantic relationship. The therapist then used Socratic questioning to bring this possible connection to light. Brenda confirmed that she experienced similar thoughts and symptoms as a reaction to both events. Later, the therapist and Brenda make another connection between her current "need" to be strong around others and her experience of intense sadness when she perceives her strength or the appearance of it as wavering (e.g., when she is unable to concentrate at work).

Subsequently, Brenda and her therapist devise a working longitudinal conceptualization connecting her developmental history with her current functioning (Figure 13.4). In addition to the conceptualization of vulnerability, Brenda and her therapist developed a "resilience" longitudinal conceptualization (Table 13.1). As we mentioned in the opening section of this chapter, there is continual negotiation between risk and resilience factors, and the relative strengths and weight of each of these factors may dictate long-term remission or relapse. As such, we believe it is important to develop a resilience model, as tapping into resilience and protective factors may help dismantle the effects of vulnerability factors, even if the latter set of factors are not dealt with in a direct manner.

The Science of Case Conceptualization: What Does the Evidence Say?

Despite the stated importance of case conceptualization and formulation in cognitive therapy (Butler, 1998), few studies to date have examined the effects of conceptualization on treatment outcome per se. Initial research efforts in this area examined the level of interrater agreement on different aspects of the conceptualization process (Dudley, Park, James, & Dodgson, 2010). This research revealed that although there was higher agreement on the descriptive aspects of conceptualization, more inferential elements produced only modest inter-clinician agreement (Kuyken, Fothergill, Musa, & Chadwick, 2005; Mumma & Smith, 2001).

Several lines of research have found that training and expertise function to improve the validity and utility of case conceptualizations in treatment. Evidence suggests that clinicians with more experience and specialized training produce more reliable conceptualizations (Kuyken et al., 2005, 2015; Persons & Bertagnolli, 1999). For example, clinicians with more experience were more likely to agree on the same patients' underlying cognitive schemas than those with less experience. Furthermore, therapists with greater expertise were found to produce higher quality (Mumma & Mooney, 2007) and more parsimonious (Bieling & Kuyken, 2003) conceptualizations. For example, experienced clinicians' schema conceptualizations were more predictive of patients' distress than those of novice clinicians (Mumma & Mooney, 2007).

Investigations that attempted to examine the effects of quality of formulation on treatment outcome are scant, and existing studies have generated mixed results (Chadwick, Williams, & Mackenzie, 2003). That said, there is emerging evidence of its importance in treatment. For example, in a recent trial, Abel, Hayes, Henley, and Kuyken (2016) found that therapists who demonstrated higher CCC competence also displayed sudden gains in CBT with clients who suffer from treatment-resistant depression. Sudden gains in this trial were associated with a more stable and long-term remission. CBT case conceptualization may function to improve outcome by enhancing other process-related variables. For example, Tee and Kazantzis (2011) found that use of a collaborative approach in treatment improved clinicians' understanding of their clients' viewpoints and enhanced the therapeutic alliance. This was replicated in a recent study by Nattrass, Kellett, Hardy, and Ricketts (2015) in a sample of patients with obsessive–compulsive disorder. Furthermore, some researchers have hypothesized that adopting a strengths and resilience approach in treatment will function to improve outcome (Padesky & Mooney, 2012; Slade, 2009); however, most of

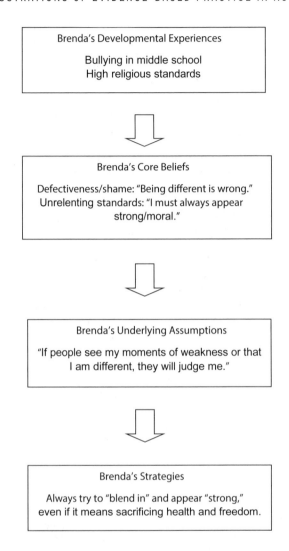

FIGURE 13.4. Brenda's top longitudinal case conceptualizations.

these hypotheses have not been empirically validated. In addition, Persons, Roberts, Zalecki, and Brechwald (2006) found that the use of case conceptualization was significantly associated with outcome in effectiveness trials. Finally, Kuyken and colleagues (2015) found that clinician scores on the Collaborative Case Conceptualization Scale (CCC-RS) were significantly and positively correlated with CBT competence in general, as assessed by the Cognitive Therapy Scale (CTS).

Considering the entirety of the evidence base, there are few studies that have directly examined the effects of case conceptualization on therapy outcome, and such early studies are supportive of the use of case conceptualization to improve outcome, especially for comorbid diagnoses or complex presentations (e.g., Persons et al., 2006); however, much work remains to be done. Our interpretation of the extant literature suggests that (1) case conceptualization may be enhanced through training; (2) case conceptualization may improve other process-related factors (e.g., therapeutic alliance), which may in turn produce favorable outcomes; and (3) some elements of the CCC model (e.g., strength focus and collaborative approach) may overall be therapeutically beneficial.

TABLE 13.1. Brenda's Resilience Model

Development	Core beliefs	Assumptions	Strategies
Strong familial connection	"I am loved."	"If I am ever in need, I can count on those around me."	Solicit help from others.
Sense of pride from Chinese heritage	"I belong."	"If I am ever lost, I can look to my culture for answers."	Use wisdom of culture in explaining everyday experiences and struggles.
Religious upbringing	"God loves me."	"Even if I am different or not always strong, I am still loved."	Use spirituality to feel accepted even in the midst of adversity or personal struggles.

Although the results of these preliminary studies are suggestive, more research is needed to support the role of conceptualizations in CBT. For example, future studies should directly examine whether the quality (e.g., reliability and validity) of case conceptualizations predicts outcomes later in treatment. Furthermore, and given the recent development of a rating scale of CCC skills in CBT (Kuyken et al., 2015), future studies should directly examine the relationship of such skills with outcomes in treatment. Finally, the utility of many elements of the CCC model specifically (e.g., the levels of conceptualization) has yet to be empirically tested; therefore, we encourage researchers to examine the incremental value of such elements in CBT.

Summary

Decades of careful clinical research have generated useful theories about the human condition and the nature of distress. Importantly, this research has revealed that these theories do not always apply, or they do not apply in the same manner to all sufferers. For this reason, a reflective, deliberate, and flexible approach to alleviating distress is necessary. The CCC approach in CBT is a blueprint for how to effectively use clinical theories built on solid evidence in a flexible manner that is respectful of human complexity and diversity; that is, both our clients and psychological science bring to therapy useful, rich theories to help describe and explain the human condition and how distress is caused and maintained. They also provide ways to describe and explain resilience.

The CCC approach in CBT provides a crucible in which these personal and psychological theories come together, with the therapist and client collaboratively building an understanding that can help the client move toward his or her treatment goals. For Brenda and her presenting issues, history, strengths, and faith are all part of the conceptualization in the service of both helping her to not only address her mood and relationship problems but also lead a happy and fulfilling life.

In using the CCC model, we hope that mental health practitioners can appreciate and embrace the richness and complexity of clinical practice. Furthermore, in writing this chapter, we also hoped to emphasize to practitioners the value of collaboration in the context of treatment; rather than a practitioner-led approach to treatment, the work is a partnership. Many therapists have said that this is a relief, as responsibility is fully shared with the client. Finally, and through use of and proficiency in the CCC model, we hope that practitioners are able to better identify and build on patients' strengths and work not just to address patients' vulnerability but very explicitly develop their resilience.

References

Abel, A., Hayes, A. M., Henley, W., & Kuyken, W. (2016). Sudden gains in cognitive-behavior therapy for treatment-resistant depression: Processes of change. *Journal of Consulting and Clinical Psychology, 84*(8), 726–737.

Beck, A. T., & Haigh, E. A. (2014). Advances in cognitive theory and therapy: The generic cognitive model. *Annual Review of Clinical Psychology, 10,* 1–24.

Beck, A. T., Rush, A. J., Shaw, B. F., & Emery, G. (1979). *Cognitive therapy of depression*. New York: Guilford Press.

Bennett-Levy, J. (2006). Therapist skills: A cognitive model of their acquisition and refinement. *Behavioural and Cognitive Psychotherapy, 34,* 57–78.

Berman, P. S. (2014). *Case conceptualization and treatment planning: Integrating theory with clinical practice.* Thousand Oaks, CA: Sage.

Bieling, P. J., & Kuyken, W. (2003). Is cognitive case formulation science or science fiction? *Clinical Psychology: Science and Practice, 10*(1), 52–69.

Blagys, M. D., & Hilsenroth, M. J. (2002). Distinctive activities of cognitive-behavioral therapy: A review of the comparative psychotherapy process literature. *Clinical Psychology Review, 22*(5), 671–706.

Butler, A. C., Chapman, J. E., Forman, E. M., & Beck, A. T. (2006). The empirical status of cognitive-behavioral therapy: A review of meta-analyses. *Clinical Psychology Review, 26*(1), 17–31.

Butler, G. (1998). Clinical formulation. In A. S. Bellack & M. Hersen, M. (Eds.), *Comprehensive clinical psychology* (pp. 1–23). Oxford, UK: Pergamon

Chadwick, P., Williams, C., & Mackenzie, J. (2003). Impact of case formulation in cognitive behaviour therapy for psychosis. *Behaviour Research and Therapy, 41*(6), 671–680.

Dobson, K. S. (2010). *Handbook of cognitive-behavioral therapies* (3rd ed.). New York: Guilford Press.

Dudley, R., Park, I., James, I., & Dodgson, G. (2010). Rate of agreement between clinicians on the content of a cognitive formulation of delusional beliefs: The effect of qualifications and experience. *Behavioural and Cognitive Psychotherapy, 38*(2), 185–200.

Eells, T. D. (1997). *Psychotherapy case formulation: History and current status.* New York: Guilford Press.

Gloaguen, V., Cottraux, J., Cucherat, M., & Blackburn, I.-M. (1998). A meta-analysis of the effects of cognitive therapy in depressed patients. *Journal of Affective Disorders, 49*(1), 59–72.

Hofmann, S. G., & Smits, J. A. (2008). Cognitive-behavioral therapy for adult anxiety disorders: A meta-analysis of randomized placebo-controlled trials. *Journal of Clinical Psychiatry, 69*(4), 621–632.

Kazantzis, N., MacEwan, J., & Dattilio, F. M. (2005). A guiding model for practice. In N. Kazantzis, F. P. Deane, K. R. Ronan, & L. L'Abate (Eds.), *Using homework assignments in cognitive behavior therapy* (pp. 359–407). New York: Routledge/Taylor & Francis Group.

Kuyken, W., Beshai, S., Dudley, R., Abel, A., Görg, N., Gower, P., et al. (2015). Assessing competence in collaborative case conceptualization: Development and preliminary psychometric properties of the Collaborative Case Conceptualization Rating Scale (CCC-RS). *Behavioural and Cognitive Psychotherapy, 44*(2), 179–192.

Kuyken, W., Fothergill, C. D., Musa, M., & Chadwick, P. (2005). The reliability and quality of cognitive case formulation. *Behaviour Research and Therapy, 43*(9), 1187–1201.

Kuyken, W., Padesky, C. A., & Dudley, R. (2008). The science and practice of case conceptualization. *Behavioural and Cognitive Psychotherapy, 36*(6), 757–768.

Kuyken, W., Padesky, C. A., & Dudley, R. (2009). *Collaborative case conceptualization: Working effectively with clients in cognitive-behavioral therapy.* New York: Guilford Press.

Masten, A. S., & Garmezy, N. (1985). Risk, vulnerability, and protective factors in developmental psychopathology. In B. B. Lahey & A. E. Kazdin (Eds), *Advances in Clinical Child Psychology* (pp. 1–52). New York: Plenum Press.

McCullough, M. E., & Snyder, C. R. (2000). Classical sources of human strength: Revisiting an old home and building a new one. *Journal of Social and Clinical Psychology, 19*(1), 1–10.

Mumma, G. H., & Mooney, S. R. (2007). Comparing the validity of alternative cognitive case formulations: A latent variable, multivariate time series approach. *Cognitive Therapy and Research, 31*(4), 451–481.

Mumma, G. H., & Smith, J. L. (2001). Cognitive-behavioral–interpersonal scenarios: Interformulator reliability and convergent validity. *Journal of Psychopathology and Behavioral Assessment, 23*(4), 203–221.

Nattrass, A., Kellett, S., Hardy, G. E., & Ricketts, T. (2015). The content, quality and impact of cognitive behavioural case formulation during treatment of obsessive compulsive disorder. *Behavioural and Cognitive Psychotherapy, 43*(5), 590–601.

Needleman, L. D. (1999). *Cognitive case conceptualization: A guidebook for practitioners.* London: Routledge.

Padesky, C. A., & Mooney, K. (1990). Clinical tip: Presenting the cognitive model to patients. *International Cognitive Therapy Newsletter, 6,* 1–2.

Padesky, C. A., & Mooney, K. A. (2012). Strengths-based cognitive-behavioural therapy: A four-step model to build resilience. *Clinical Psychology and Psychotherapy, 19*(4), 283–290.

Persons, J. B., & Bertagnolli, A. (1999). Inter-rater reliability of cognitive-behavioral case formulations of depression: A replication. *Cognitive Therapy and Research, 23*(3), 271–283.

Persons, J. B., Roberts, N. A., Zalecki, C. A., & Brechwald, W. A. (2006). Naturalistic outcome of case formulation-driven cognitive-behavior therapy for anxious depressed outpatients. *Behaviour Research and Therapy, 44*(7), 1041–1051.

Rutter, M. (1987). Psychosocial resilience and protective mechanisms. *American Journal of Orthopsychiatry, 57*(3), 316–331.

Schottenbauer, M. A., Glass, C. R., Arnkoff, D. B., Tendick, V., & Gray, S. H. (2008). Nonresponse and dropout rates in outcome studies on PTSD: Review and methodological considerations. *Psychiatry, 71*(2), 134–168.

Slade, M. (2009). *Personal recovery and mental illness: A guide for mental health professionals*. New York: Cambridge University Press.

Strunk, D. R., Brotman, M. A., & DeRubeis, R. J. (2010). The process of change in cognitive therapy for depression: Predictors of early inter-session symptom gains. *Behaviour Research and Therapy, 48*(7), 599–606.

Tee, J., & Kazantzis, N. (2011). Collaborative empiricism in cognitive therapy: A definition and theory for the relationship construct. *Clinical Psychology: Science and Practice, 18*(1), 47–61.

Whisman, M. A. (Ed.). (2008). *Adapting cognitive therapy for depression: Managing complexity and comorbidity*. New York: Guilford Press.

CHAPTER 14

Integrating Basic Research into a Phase Approach to Guide Clinical Practice

BETHANY A. TEACHMAN
RACHEL K. NARR

Paige, a 19-year-old, single, white, undergraduate female majoring in economics, was referred to our psychology department's in-house training clinic for outpatient therapy by her university psychiatrist following a marked decrease in her academic performance over the first semester of her sophomore year and clear presentation of moderate to severe depressive symptoms. Paige reported that her academic performance and depressive symptoms had been problematic for at least the past 1½ years, and likely longer (on a somewhat waxing and waning course, but with no evident periods of remission or euthymia). She had been put on academic probation after just barely passing her first-semester classes and failing the majority of her second-semester classes.

Paige reported that she "hated herself," felt unhappy most of the time, had no appetite and ate irregularly, struggled to pull herself away from the television to attend class, had disturbed sleep (varying between sleeping excessively and difficulty falling and staying asleep), and could not come up with any activities that she enjoyed. She also struggled when faced with any uncertainty and felt intense pressure to make the "most effective" decision, often leading her to avoid making any decisions or taking any actions, even when she knew what she needed to do. Paige had some friends in her hometown and at college but had not become involved in any extracurricular activities in college (despite having

volunteered at a homeless shelter and played for her school's soccer team in high school), and she rarely left her dorm room. Instead, she spent the majority of her time watching television or surfing the Internet, sometimes smoking pot with her roommate to relieve stress. She denied any active suicidal ideation, intent, or plan, and had never made an attempt, though she endorsed some occasional passive ideation. She denied all past or current homicidal ideation. She disclosed occasional binge drinking and use of marijuana, but substance abuse was not deemed to be a primary presenting problem or critical therapy-interfering behavior at intake.

Despite the obvious impairment associated with her depressive symptoms, Paige's stated goal for therapy was not to address her depression but to increase her academic motivation to pass her classes and earn her degree. Paige was reluctant to accept that her depression was linked to her low motivation and academic difficulties. She felt that to use depression to explain any part of her problems was "not taking responsibility" for what she "should be doing." She presented with a great deal of hopelessness about being less depressed or improving her quality of life, and ambivalence about whether therapy could be helpful for her, repeatedly suggesting that she was not worth the therapist's valuable time.

As evidence of her pessimism about the likelihood of therapy being helpful, Paige explained her lack of response to prior treatments. Over the summer between her first and second years of college, she initially sought therapy and medication for depression in her hometown at the suggestion of her past residential advisor. Paige said that she met with the therapist weekly during this time but did not find therapy helpful. When asked about the treatment model, Paige stated, "I'm not really sure. He didn't say it was called anything specific. He asked about my family a lot and how we got along." Furthermore, although Paige reported that she had been on multiple medications for depression over the past year, she felt ambivalence about taking medication and took medication very erratically, often skipping days or even weeks before stopping altogether. She explained that the reason for her lack of adherence was less tied to side effects than to her belief that she "should" be able to function without medication.

Understanding Paige requires consideration of her sociocultural background and family history. Paige felt tremendous shame about her academic problems and tried to hide the degree of her struggles from family and friends. She had come to the university from a small, rural town on a diversity scholarship aimed at economically disadvantaged students, and she was the first in her family to attend college. Paige believed it was critical to do well to prove that she could break the cycle of poverty that had been her model growing up. She was set on the idea of attaining an MBA after college, primarily because she believed this would demonstrate that she was able to get through a difficult, prestigious college major, and it would set her up to succeed in business after getting her degrees. Paige was an only child; growing up, she had lived with her mother, stepfather, and an older cousin, who had dropped out of high school and joined the Army a few years earlier. Her biological father had left the family shortly after her birth; Paige had not talked with him since she was in elementary school, and he had not provided financial support in over a decade. Paige's mother had moderately severe obesity- and alcohol-induced cirrhosis, which left her unable to work. The major source of income for the family came from an uncle who lived in another town. Paige described her mother as reckless and irresponsible. Paige spoke of how her mother wasted the majority of the family's income and recounted multiple occasions on which she was hospitalized due to alcohol abuse despite her cirrhosis. Paige deeply resented her mother, and much of her disappointment in herself was compounded by her fear of "ending up like her mother."

* * *

There are few experiences in life that are simultaneously as challenging and gratifying as conducting therapy. It is a privilege to play a part in someone making important changes in her life and feeling better able to reach her full potential. Yet how to facilitate these changes can also feel uncertain and at times unattainable. This is particularly true in working with clients like Paige, who begin treatment with long-standing problems and a track record of not being helped by other mental health interventions. We are thankful that there is a rich empirical literature to help guide this process, both in terms of overall treatment packages that can be delivered in personalized and innovative ways (as other chapters in this volume emphasize) and in terms of basic and applied research that clarifies the mechanisms of cognitive, emotional, behavioral, motivational, and relational change. In our work, we draw from research across numerous disciplines (clinical, of course, but also educational, health, developmental, cultural, and social psychology, among others) to guide our thinking and treatment planning. In this chapter, we illustrate our approach in the context of our ongoing work with Paige.

Our goal in sharing our work with Paige (who started treatment with Narr as a third-year doctoral student being supervised by Teachman) is to illustrate the "real" challenges that arise in clinical care and how they can be approached using an evidence-based perspective. This is not a clean case with a perfect happy ending. It is messy, and writing this chapter has brought to the fore decision points that we wish we had handled differently in hindsight. But we expect this is likely to be the norm for difficult cases. We view treatment planning as an iterative process that typically plays out across multiple phases of treatment (Woody, Detweiler-Bedell, Teachman, & O'Hearn, 2003), so we do not view our missteps as devastating errors that should be hidden from a book designed to promote best practices. Rather, we believe that foundational to an evidence-based approach is the very process of routinely asking whether the treatment may be heading down a less productive path, and trying something new if an initial plan is not successful. The first author (Teachman) has taught an adult intervention course to clinical doctoral students early in their training for well over a decade, and the most common complaint from students each year is that almost all the case studies they read are "too perfect." This gives students the false impression that therapy sessions are like sitcoms that wrap up neatly, with an epiphany and great lesson each time, which means students judge themselves as failing when their own sessions do not match this idealized view.

Thus, in this chapter, we show ourselves working on a tough problem across multiple sessions, recognizing and recovering from missteps in clinical decision making and the often nonlinear nature of change. We illustrate how a nomothetic approach (using the treatment outcome literature to establish what types of treatment are likely to be successful for a given problem area) can be integrated with an idiographic approach that uses the broader research literature (drawing from fields such as goal setting and motivation, growth mindset, reinforcement learning and behavior change, developmental theories on the growth of autonomy and relatedness, and transactional family systems) to identify and alter specific mechanisms of change. In the context of this integration, we also highlight strategies to monitor outcomes specific to the individual's unique goals and how to use this monitoring to improve care and highlight questions for future research.

Treatment Planning Using a Phase Approach

A phase approach to treatment planning is based on the idea that for complex cases, it is not generally feasible or productive to try to tackle many different problems at once (see Woody et al., 2003). One can easily end up doing many things inadequately and nothing sufficiently. Instead, by explicitly planning out treatment in different phases, one picks a manageable number of problems on which to focus at a given time, with the idea that additional problems can be addressed in subsequent phases. This helps convert an overwhelming list of problems that can seem insurmountable (to both client and therapist) to a series of well-laid-out steps that follow from a strong case conceptualization about the functional links between problems. Phases typically do not last more than a few months and typically focus on not more than two to four aims.

The selection of initial aims is based on what problem areas are most severe or pressing, the client's desired focus of treatment, where prog-

ress seems most likely, what changes are most likely to generalize to improve other problems, and what is feasible given the constraints of the practice setting (e.g., if only six sessions of care will be possible). Critical to the phase model is the idea that progress on aims will be routinely monitored and establishment of a new phase will be based on periodic review of progress. One can move to a new phase because of making good progress (e.g., ready to tackle new problem areas or terminate), or because of lack of progress (e.g., the need to consider a different approach or revisit the case conceptualization), or because of intermediate progress (e.g., some gains have been made but you want to facilitate more dramatic improvements or work on maintaining gains), or because a new problem area has become more pressing (e.g., increase in substance use or suicidality, or a crisis such as losing one's job). Regardless, fundamental to the approach is iteratively setting out a small set of aims (that contribute to larger treatment goals) and regularly evaluating progress on those aims to determine when to shift to a new phase of therapy.

The idea of a phase approach to therapy has been in the literature for many decades (e.g., Rogers, 1958) and is not unique to any one theoretical orientation (Beitman, Goldfried, & Norcross, 1989). It is central to many approaches to therapy, especially for complex cases, such as persons with personality disorders (e.g., dialectical behavior therapy for borderline personality disorder; Linehan, 1993, among many others), and is often a practical necessity given the limited availability of long-term uninterrupted care in most settings (Haas & Cummings, 1991). Importantly, there is empirical evidence consistent with the effectiveness of multiple, brief "doses" of therapy even for chronic, serious problems (see Budman & Gurman, 1988; see Woody et al., 2003). Furthermore, an analogous model from Heinssen, Levendusky, and Hunter (1995) that applied a sequence of phases across many different inpatient and outpatient settings found benefits to treatment compliance and cost-effective therapeutic outcomes using a phase approach.

Selection of Treatment Aims and Associated Strategies

Applying the phase approach to treatment planning with Paige, we elected to focus on alleviating her depressive symptoms as the primary focus of the initial phase of treatment given her symptom severity and our conceptualization that her academic difficulties were functionally tied to her depression. Planning treatment followed a two- to three-session assessment phase that began with our clinic's standard intake interview (a semistructured biopsychosocial review of major problem areas, time course and precipitants of the central problems, social/school/work/health/treatment/familial history, and current stressors and supports). This was complemented by a validated personality inventory and general quantitative measure of symptoms, role functioning, and interpersonal distress that could subsequently be used to track progress. This combination of baseline assessments is typical in our setting and is often followed by administration of specific disorder modules from a standardized diagnostic assessment (e.g., the *Structured Clinical Interview for DSM*) based on what information has arisen

during the interview. In Paige's case, given that dysthymic symptoms had likely been evident for very close to 2 years and she was currently in a depressive episode, her diagnostic presentation was understood as persistent depressive disorder of moderate severity with the DSM-5 specifier "with intermittent major depressive episodes, with current episode" (American Psychiatric Association, 2013). We thus also included a measure specific to depressive symptoms (see Table 14.1 for specific measures used). Note that the assessment stage with new clients at our clinic also involves giving feedback on the assessments we have administered to address any questions clients may have and to ensure client understanding of the material being used to form the therapist's case conceptualization. We find that giving feedback allows for both better informed consent from the client and more collaborative treatment planning, which in turn increases the client's motivation for therapy.

TABLE 14.1. Phase 1: Treatment Aims and Associated Strategies

Aim 1: Decrease self-critical, pessimistic thinking (to reduce depression symptoms).
1. Thought Records and other cognitive restructuring exercises to reevaluate cognitive distortions tied to negative self-evaluation.
2. Mindfulness to increase acceptance of thoughts.

Aim 2: Increase rewards from the environment (to reduce depression symptoms and increase motivation).
1. Schedule and complete activities that promote mastery and pleasure (e.g., getting involved in a social group, playing intramural sports).
2. Plan rewards for small successes (e.g., attending class).

Aim 3: Increase tolerance of uncertainty (to facilitate decision making).
1. Plan and carry out everyday tasks (e.g., when to begin homework) despite not knowing the "best" option.
2. Thought Records and other cognitive restructuring exercises to reevaluate cognitive distortions about need for certainty before taking action.

Aim 4: Increase motivation and perseverance in academic domains.
1. Use alarm clocks, schedules, and so forth, to provide environmental supports.
2. Break down tasks into small steps.
3. Decrease barriers to motivation (e.g., self-defeating thoughts) through cognitive restructuring.
4. Functional analysis to explore antecedents and consequences of difficulties with motivation.
5. Decisional balance exercises to evaluate pros/cons of choices.

Starting Date: November 2013   Progress Review Date: April 2014

Measures of progress

Aim 1: Outcome Questionnaire (OQ) Symptom Distress subscale; Beck Depression Inventory–II (BDI-II).

Aim 2: Weekly tracking of planned positive activity completion; OQ Symptom Distress subscale; OQ Interpersonal Relations subscale; BDI-II.

Aim 3: Intolerance of Uncertainty Scale (IUS).

Aim 4: Weekly tracking of class attendance and homework completion.

Based on our understanding of Paige's presenting problems, our aims for reducing her depression symptoms derived directly from the research on mechanisms underlying depression, including the following:

1. Reducing negative, self-critical thinking (emphasized in cognitive models of therapy for depression that have shown very good efficacy; see Beck, 2011; Leahy, 2003; Young, Rygh, Weinberger, & Beck, 2014) and obtaining some acceptance of those thoughts via mindfulness (e.g., McKay, Wood, & Brantley, 2007; Roemer & Orsillo, 2014).

2. Obtaining reinforcement from the environment to both decrease depressive symptoms (as emphasized in models of behavioral activation that have shown very positive outcomes; see Dimidjian, Martell, Herman-Dunn, & Hubley, 2014; Jacobson, Martell, & Dimidjian, 2006) and increase motivation and self-efficacy (based on basic learning principles showing the value of reinforcement to encourage behavior; see Higgins, Heil, & Lussier, 2004).

3. Dcreasing intolerance of uncertainty given recent evidence that it may be a transdiagnostic factor underlying numerous forms of psychopathology (see Mahoney & McEvoy, 2012), including depression (see Gentes & Ruscio, 2011).

The strategies employed to achieve these aims followed from both basic research and well-established therapy guides and treatment manuals, as noted earlier. However, the particular combination of aims and strategies, sequence of techniques administered across sessions, and relative emphasis does not follow from any particular source, and reflects the adaptation of these nomothetic principles to form an idiographic treatment plan. For example, our decision to spend more time on cognitive change strategies in session, relative to acceptance, was informed by our impression of Paige's difficulty identifying distortions, paired with our commitment to be responsive to her preferences and strong desire "to be logical and rational." Cognitive restructuring was a primary strategy to address distorted thoughts that seemingly led Paige to disparage herself and not engage in behaviors that would support her making desired changes. We did this by identifying and reevaluating negative automatic thoughts, then encouraging her to develop "balanced" thoughts that were more helpful and promoted more flexible thinking. In addition, we taught Paige several mindfulness techniques to help her observe her negative thoughts and feelings as they arose, without judging them as severely or attributing "ultimate truth" to them.

Finally, we included one aim directly tied to academic motivation given that this was Paige's primary concern and the research showing that outcomes are enhanced when clients have a strong therapeutic alliance (e.g., Arnow et al., 2013) and perceive that their therapist shares their goals (Bachelor, 2013). The strategies used to improve academic motivation and perseverance followed from the literature on the value of using environmental supports to facilitate behavior change (e.g., in the health literature; Rothman et al., 2015), and the value of graded task assignments and breaking down tasks to reduce feelings of being overwhelmed and provide frequent opportunities for success (see Chartier & Provencher, 2013). These strategies also align directly with core components of a behavioral treatment for depression. Furthermore, given the goal of encouraging change behaviors that required motivation, some motivational interviewing approaches were incorporated (e.g., decisional balance exercise) given the considerable evidence for the value of this approach to address ambivalence (see Miller & Rollnick, 2012).

As recommended in most cognitive and behavioral approaches to therapy (e.g., Leahy, 2003), homework assigned at the end of each session was tied to the skills that had been the focus of a given session (e.g., completing a thought record or functional analysis, or engaging in rewarding activities). This emphasis on homework was based on evidence that completing homework enhances outcomes (Kazantzis, Dattilio, Cummins, & Clayton, 2014), presumably by providing increased practice and encouraging generalization of skills outside the clinic, which can enhance self-efficacy.

In our clinic, we encourage trainees to prepare treatment plans that make their selection of aims and strategies very explicit (see Table 14.1). In addition, we require therapists to set a date for when they expect to review progress on the aims they have established for the first phase of treatment (typically about 3 months after therapy begins) and to list the measures they will use to assess progress on the aims they have laid out. Measures used for the initial assessment with Paige included the Personality Assessment Inventory (this measure was included because our training clinic requires administration of a personality assessment at intake; we used it for treatment planning but not as an outcome measure), the Outcome Questionnaire (OQ; this provides a measure of overall distress, as well as interpersonal and role functioning, and is administered approximately monthly in our clinic), the Intolerance of Uncertainty Scale (IUS; Buhr & Dugas, 2002) and the Beck Depression Inventory–II (BDI-II; Beck, Steer, & Brown, 1996). A personality assessment (either the Personality Assessment Inventory or the Minnesota Multiphasic Personality Inventory) is administered to all clients at intake in our training clinic. Similarly, the OQ is used to monitor progress for most clients at our clinic (and basically all clients supervised by Teachman), whereas selection of the other questionnaires was based on the client's specific presenting problems. We often use a mix of both questionnaire and behavioral indicators, and our clinic policy requires that progress in treatment be monitored but gives the therapist and supervisor considerable leeway in deciding which instruments will be most helpful for a given case.

Paige's scores indicated high levels of distress consistent with depression on the Personality Assessment Inventory and OQ; surprisingly, she did not have a particularly elevated score on the BDI-II; she scored 13 initially, which falls in the minimal depressive symptoms range (her subsequent score was an 8). We speculated that the relatively low BDI-II score may have occurred because the BDI-II asks about recent changes in symptoms, and for someone like Paige, who has been depressed for an extended period, responses such as "I am more critical of myself than I used to be" may not capture her long-standing symptoms accurately. Paige also scored approximately one standard deviation (SD) above the population mean on the IUS (this measure has continuous scoring and no set "cutoffs"). Specifically, she initially scored 69 on the IUS (population mean = 54; $SD = 17$) and subsequent scores were 67, then 51.

Addressing Barriers to Change

Paige understood the proposed strategies quite readily and was capable of implementing most of them, but she frequently did not complete planned therapy homework, so much of her

therapy work was limited to once-per-week, in-session practice. She could not effectively articulate what was difficult for her about doing therapy homework; however, this mirrored her lack of regular academic work and so served as a useful in-session model of a process we also hoped to address outside the therapist's office (Kiesler, 1988; Teyber & McClure, 2010). Determining the mechanisms maintaining this lack of follow-through was challenging given that Paige was otherwise quite reliable and had become relatively open to treatment (e.g., she was always on time for appointments, and therapist and client seemingly had good rapport). Furthermore, Paige appeared to find the rationale for the homework credible and have the requisite skills to complete the tasks, as evidenced by the fact that she easily remembered and processed information in therapy.

We repeatedly discussed barriers, checked understanding of the rationale for homework assignments, set up environmental supports with planning and reminders, and broke assignments into small steps, with encouragement to incorporate rewards for steps completed. Nonetheless, progress was slow with (too) much of the work happening in session. Notably, in hindsight, it seems evident that we persisted in repeatedly trying the same strategies to encourage homework completion far longer than was wise. We did not adhere to our planned progress review date, in part due to an inadequate reminder system for ourselves (e.g., Teachman usually writes a reminder about upcoming progress reviews in her daybook as a cue, but she had not done so), and in part because of a sense that we "were close" and just needed a couple more weeks to get the therapy moving forward more rapidly. Needless to say, keeping the progress review date is especially critical in these cases because this is precisely the review process that can catch these stuck points, so that "a couple more weeks" does not get repeatedly extended.

In our clinic, in addition to individual supervision, early-stage clinicians are given weekly opportunities to present cases to fellow students and our clinic director for consultation. At this stage, in response to this case presentation, a colleague referred us to protection motivation theory (Floyd, Prentice-Dunn, & Rogers, 2000). This theory is well aligned with both cognitive-behavioral therapy and motivational interviewing ideas and approaches, and suggests that changing a response pattern requires strong reasons to change the behavior (in the form of rewards for changing, costs for not changing, or both), and believing that change attempts will be efficacious and that one is capable of making changes. The concept of "protection motivation" as a driver of behavior derives from work by R. W. Rogers (1983). We sought out more information about the evidence supporting this approach. Our review identified meta-analyses suggesting that the key model components—severity of a problem, vulnerability, response efficacy, self-efficacy, and response costs—are all related to intentions and behaviors; however, self-efficacy and perceived response efficacy are the components most highly correlated with concurrent and future behavior (Floyd et al., 2000; Milne, Sheeran, & Orbell, 2000).

Using this theory to evaluate why Paige might be stuck, we hypothesized that Paige's lack of follow-through likely derived from disbelief that she could effectively make changes rather than any actual skills deficits or problematic reward contingencies. We presented this model to Paige, and she agreed that she had strong reasons to change and few reasons not to change, but a large hurdle was her belief that she would be unable to follow-through with planned changes, and feeling uncertain that the techniques we planned would work for her. Protection motivation theory offered a digestible model to which Paige could relate.

PAIGE: I *know* I need to do stuff differently. It's not that hard; I should be able to.

NARR: I'm glad you brought that up—it's something I've been thinking about a lot, and I have some thoughts about what might be going on. If you think about why people choose to do one thing and not another, there are a whole bunch of reasons, but you can often boil them down to what you get out of it, and what it costs you. Does that make sense?

PAIGE: Well, yeah, but not doing stuff is costing me a lot, and I would benefit from doing it. It's stupid.

NARR: Yes, it does cost a lot. It's not stupid, though, because here's the thing. You know there are costs to not doing your work, and you know there are benefits to doing it. *But* there are also costs to *doing* your work, and benefits to *not* doing it. You don't enjoy doing your schoolwork; that's a cost. If you don't do it, you can spend more time watching TV or hanging out with friends. And, something

else that I think might be relevant for you, a big part of what determines what decisions people make isn't only weighing the costs and benefits of both possible actions—it's if you feel like you'll be able to follow through on the choice that might take more effort.

PAIGE: What do you mean? I just don't have any motivation.

NARR: It's hard to be motivated if you don't believe you can do something. For a lot of people, it's easier to not try and not risk failure than it is to put yourself on the line that way. Then you can say you failed because you didn't try, not because you *couldn't* do it.

PAIGE: I guess that is less awful. I hate failing. I don't want to fail. I wish I knew for sure if I'm actually as smart as I always thought. My grades don't show it, but, yeah . . . I'm not really trying. I guess I am worried about if I'd be able to do it even if I did try.

Bolstering the therapeutic alliance by working with Paige as a more fully engaged treatment planning partner, and helping Paige to see that her difficulties could be explained (and directly targeted), increased Paige's self-efficacy and openness to collaborative problem solving. She was then better able to generate and actually implement specific strategies, such as blocking her Internet access for periods of time to increase her engagement in therapy homework and schoolwork. We also spent time discussing different situations in Paige's life in which she tolerated uncertainty on a daily basis, and practiced taking small chances to test the outcome rather than giving up before trying.

With this progress, Paige passed her spring semester classes, and slightly increased her willingness to recognize when she had successfully implemented a change strategy rather than discounting it. In addition, her small successes resulting from treatment helped her to better tolerate uncertainty in other parts of her life and take occasional risks without being sure of the outcome (e.g., going on a date with someone new). However, her general tendency to engage in negative rigid thinking persisted, and while her OQ showed some mild decreases in distress, the score was not markedly different from when she began treatment.

Following the end of spring semester, Paige then spent over a month in her hometown (during which time we were not in contact) before returning to start summer session classes, which provided a natural transition to shift to a new phase of treatment. When she returned, she reported overall better mood and lower distress. Although interactions with her mother had at times been stressful at home, Paige had mostly "steered clear" of her and had been able to reconnect with some old friends at home and very much enjoyed the break from feeling like she was failing at school. This was obviously a positive shift in her mood, but we felt this improvement was difficult to trust given that her distress was so clearly tied to academic concerns and she was currently between classes. Notwithstanding, given her improved mood, we shifted our focus more fully to her low motivation and academic self-handicapping behaviors to further support her school performance, which remained her primary goal for treatment (see Table 14.2).

This phase of treatment lasted from the middle of Paige's summer break through roughly the middle of the fall semester. We continued using the OQ to measure progress given that it assesses distress and multiple aspects of role functioning. We also kept the IUS given its tie to Paige's self-handicapping behaviors, such as avoidance of making basic decisions due to fears that she might not be making the "right" decision (e.g., what subject to study first on a given night). And we added Paige's own weekly reports of her class attendance, (academic) homework completion, and mood check-ins during our sessions. We opted to stop

administering the BDI-II given that it had not shown good sensitivity to Paige's depression symptoms, and we were using other measures that seemed more useful. This choice to include both a standardized outcome measure (i.e., the OQ) along with more idiographic assessments unique to the client's goals (e.g., report of class homework assignments completed) is common in our clinic. Our intent is to obtain the benefits of relying on measures with good psychometric properties and established treatment sensitivity, while also including measures that most directly address the individual's priorities (but which do not have known psychometric properties). It is worth noting that we often use behavioral indicators, such as classes attended, in addition to questionnaires.

Increasing Paige's low motivation and removing (typically self-imposed) barriers to change were prioritized during this phase of treatment based on a review of our case conceptualization for Paige (e.g., the functional relationships between her different problem areas) and her uneven progress (e.g., evident grasp of, but lack of application of, the skills). Much of the work in therapy to that point had been oriented toward cognitive-behavioral therapy, which had been partly effective but had assumed Paige had a more consistent motivation to change than was perhaps warranted. Thus, in this phase of therapy, we placed greater emphasis on a motivational interviewing framework (Miller & Rollnick, 2012) given empirical evidence that it can be ef-

---

TABLE 14.2. Phase 2: Treatment Aims and Associated Strategies

Aim 1: Increase academic motivation, complete assignments, and attend class.

1. Motivational interviewing around academic goals.
2. Provision of scientific articles on growth mindset, motivation, and achievement.
3. Reminder e-mails sent by therapist daily for 2 weeks.

Aim 2: Decrease self-handicapping cognitions/behaviors that get Paige "stuck."

1. Discussion of pros–cons of changing versus not changing self-handicapping behaviors.
2. Exposures to making plans and decisions, as well as "experimenting" with new techniques to improve homework completion.
3. Cognitive restructuring to address the idea that she "shouldn't" feel negative emotions, stress about school, and so forth.

Starting Date: July 2014   Progress Review Date: November 2014

Measures of progress

Aim 1: Weekly tracking of planned academic goal completion; Outcome Questionnaire (OQ) Symptom Distress subscale.

Aim 2: OQ Symptom Distress subscale.

ficacious for many different problem areas and patient characteristics (see Lundahl et al., 2013). We also drew from the closely aligned transtheoretical stages-of-change model (see the application in Prochaska, Norcross, & DiClemente, 2013), which suggests that prior to taking action, people typically first pass through earlier stages of nonreadiness (precontemplation), getting ready (contemplation), and being ready (preparation), before actually taking action. Critically, different interventions are thought to be effective at each stage of readiness. Applying this model to Paige, we suspected that we had been attempting to work on "action" strategies with Paige before she was ready, and we wondered whether Paige would have benefited from an earlier phase of treatment focused on reducing her mixed feelings and beliefs about her ability to benefit from treatment before shifting to the action-focused strategies. We thus stepped back and focused on "contemplation" work: helping Paige to resolve her ambivalence about making changes. We spent a great deal of time discussing her Desire, Ability, Reasons, and Need for change (this preparatory change talk is referred to as DARN within motivational interviewing), with a goal of increasing her ratio of change talk to sustain talk. As this approach led to increased change talk, we then added in decisional balance exercises and discussions of her barriers to change. We also paired this with discussions about her intolerance of uncertainty given that this was one major roadblock for Paige with regard to her perception of her ability for change. We continued our earlier discussions and experiments to find places in Paige's life where she already made "uncertain" decisions without negative repercussions and regularly planned small exercises to encourage her to take steps without certainty (e.g., reading 10 pages in a textbook despite being unsure whether that was "enough").

In an effort to keep Paige as an active collaborator in planning her treatment, and because she expressed interest in psychological research, we gave her accessible journal articles (e.g., Dweck, 1986) on a "growth mindset" (the idea that abilities are not fixed and can be improved through effort and learning), and handouts designed for clients on the stages-of-change framework (Prochaska & DiClemente, 1984; Whalley, 2008). These resources allowed Paige to better understand the rationale for our treatment, normalized her experiences (which helped to reduce her self-blame), and increased her sense of agency that she could both understand and change her behaviors. Notably, even though we do not typically give clients basic psychology research articles to read (as we opted to do for Paige), we regularly use the basic research on learning principles, goal setting, motivation, and numerous other basic psychology principles to guide treatment planning. The standard treatment outcome literature (e.g., randomized controlled trials on a given treatment package for a given disorder) is enormously helpful, but it is also limited, so we routinely turn to the basic literature in healthy samples and to the psychopathology literature (e.g., research on mechanisms guiding extinction learning, emotion regulation, and other research on evidence-based principles of change; Craske, Treanor, Conway, Zbozinek, & Vervliet, 2014; Mennin, Ellard, Fresco, & Gross, 2013; Payne, Ellard, Farchione, Fairholme, & Barlow, 2014).

Maintaining an Evidence-Based Approach When Treatment Priorities Shift

Paige passed her summer classes and was increasingly willing to accept new ideas without requiring certainty (or at least to test out propositions before dismissing them), but it was clear that she was beginning to "lose steam," and she continued to struggle with motivation. The beginning of the next semester brought numerous, serious challenges for Paige: She began taking a full class load again (which meant a dramatic increase in school stress); she was no longer able to obtain financial aid because of her history of academic probation; she sustained shin splints after attempting to go running (which was especially upsetting to her because she had committed to exercising for the emotion regulation benefits; see Powers, Asmundson, & Smits, 2015); she was unable to get a physical therapy appointment for several weeks and eventually developed a stress fracture; and her mother was hospitalized for the fifth time in 2 years. Critically, the lack of financial aid contributed to Paige being unable to afford to eat properly (though part of her poor eating also concerned not prioritizing activities such as purchasing groceries or preparing food), and she began to lose weight. As one would expect, the insufficient eating increased Paige's daily fatigue and diminished her motivation. She turned more and more to television as a distraction and once again found it difficult to recognize any successes she had. Each of these stressors would have been difficult to manage on its own; together, they were devastating.

At this stage, we were alarmed by Paige's health, and therapy shifted to supporting her self-care (see Table 14.3). We did also continue to spend some time on academic issues because of their continued central importance to Paige (it is common in a phase approach to therapy for some aims to change across phases, while others remain the same), but we focus here on the self-care issues that dominated this phase of care. Also, in retrospect, we wonder whether we should have focused more on challenging Paige's idea that her self-worth was inevitably tied to her academic performance earlier in therapy, but it is difficult to know whether such a focus would have led to Paige leaving therapy altogether given concerns that the therapist and client did not share the same goals (see Rector, Zuroff, & Segal, 1999).

During this phase of treatment, we continued administering the OQ, and also administered the Hamilton Depression Rating Scale to monitor depression symptoms (and we routinely checked for increases in suicidality). As noted, we had stopped using the BDI-II for this case but felt the wording of the Hamilton items might fit Paige's presentation better. We also stopped administering the IUS given that Paige had made gains in this area and was scoring just below the population average (final score = 51). More than the questionnaires, our primary measures of progress during this phase were Paige's tracking of her self-care goals (e.g., we asked her to track number of meals she ate each day, and whether she had taken medication, gotten dressed, and attended class). We completed these goal charts retrospectively in session when Paige missed recording the information on a daily basis, so while the records were almost certainly not fully accurate, they provided a reasonable indication of Paige's progress.

A major focus in this phase of treatment was breaking larger goals, such as eating regularly, down into smaller, more manageable subgoals. This form of goal setting has been found to be helpful in treating many different problems, such as addictions, including behavioral addictions such as the excessive use of television and Internet surfing that was an element of Paige's presentation (Dau, Hoffman, & Banger, 2015).

TABLE 14.3. Phase 3: Treatment Aims and Associated Strategies

Aim 1: Increase academic motivation and goal completion (see Phase 2).

Aim 2: Increase self-care tied to physical and emotional health (stabilize eating, medication, injury management, and social support).

1. Continue motivational interviewing strategies.
2. Continue cognitive restructuring to address Paige's belief that she isn't worth caring for.
3. Problem solving and scaffolding to obtain necessary institutional supports (e.g., talk with residential advisor, financial aid office, local food banks, medical doctors).
4. Midweek phone check-ins with therapist to encourage between-session focus on goals.
5. Problem solving to support flexible implementation of self-care activities based around Paige's schedule (e.g., exercising or fixing meals during commercial breaks; working out ways to get to the grocery store).
6. Closer consultation with psychiatrist about lack of medication adherence.
7. Activity scheduling with focus on activities that could provide pleasure and social support (vs. mastery-focused activities).
8. Continued efforts to use environmental control strategies to limit television and other unhealthy "escape" behaviors that interfered with Paige's self-care.

Starting Date: November 2014   Progress Review Date: February 2015

Measures of progress

Aim 1: Weekly tracking of planned academic goal completion; Outcome Questionnaire (OQ) Symptom Distress subscale.

Aim 2: Weekly tracking of caloric intake and other self-care goals (e.g., showering, medication adherence); weekly tracking of hours of television watched; weekly tracking of planned pleasant activity completion; Hamilton Depression Rating Scale.

Moreover, repeatedly setting small goals paired with self-monitoring is central to behavioral activation treatment for depression as individuals try numerous activities that can increase opportunities for reinforcement from the environment. Having Paige record her completion of small, routine subgoals, such as eating breakfast or getting dressed rather than staying in pajamas, allowed Paige to immediately and frequently "check off" her successes. The tracking was designed to serve as both an assessment and an intervention because frequently noting small accomplishments can enhance self-efficacy and enable recognition of gradual change over time. Critically, this feeling of self-efficacy in effecting change increases the likelihood of sustaining behavioral changes over time (DiClemente, Prochaska, & Gibertini, 1985; Miller & Rollnick, 2012).

We began implementing a midweek phone check-in after a session during which Paige expressed that she often remained motivated for a few days after therapy, then would begin to forget or ignore what she had intended to do. We first spent some time in supervision considering whether adding this check-in would be helpful. Our ultimate goals were to empower Paige and increase her self-efficacy and ability to independently follow through on her goals, so we worried that we might inadvertently increase dependence on the therapist and reduce Paige's sense of personal responsibility (and accomplishment). However, given Paige's prior difficulty with follow-through (e.g., even setting daily electronic reminders did not prove helpful), seriousness of her self-care difficulties, and her strong connection to the therapist, we decided that temporarily providing a lot of structure and "active helping" was likely warranted in this case. Also, the provision of between-session coaching is common in behavioral interventions for severe or complex cases when encountering challenges in independent skill application is typical (e.g., it is a common component of dialectical behavior therapy for borderline personality disorder, and is not unusual for challenging cases of exposure and response prevention for obsessive–compulsive disorder), and we felt some of the same needs also applied in this case. Requiring Paige to plan for only 3 or 4 days at a time rather than 7 fits with research suggesting that people experiencing depression perceive time as passing more slowly than do nondepressed individuals (Gil & Droit-Volet, 2009), so typical breaks between sessions may feel very extended. This midweek check-in and assistance with problem solving seemed to improve Paige's ability to maintain change behaviors.

We also applied this more active helping model to help facilitate Paige's communication with other members of the community who could help address Paige's problems. Although we typically focus our efforts on encouraging the client to work directly with other providers and social services, rather than directly engaging ourselves (beyond standard consultations for treatment planning with psychiatrists, etc.), we complemented this encouragement with a more directly involved role in this case, with Paige's permission. This included speaking with Paige's residential advisor (who had also reached out to us) and talking to Paige's psychiatrist about nonmedication options for Paige given her lack of adherence to any medication regimen over the course of multiple years, despite numerous providers' attempts to encourage more consistent use of antidepressant medication. While Paige and her psychiatrist did not pursue these alternative options, our minor intervention ensured that Paige's psychiatrist was better informed about Paige's ambivalence about taking medication, which we hoped would open better lines of communication between them moving forward.

Although Paige had provided permission for us to speak with the residential advisor and psychiatrist, this nonetheless (understandably) created some discomfort for Paige about "what had been said" about her. In retrospect, we see now that it likely would have been more effective to have Paige present during those conversations, especially given research showing that promoting autonomy involves providing empowering supports for people to succeed at a task versus being directive or doing the task for them (Martin, Liao, & Campbell, 2013; see Boud, 2012). After playing "phone tag" with the residential advisor and psychiatrist, it had simply been convenient to talk with them directly when we were able to connect, but waiting to find a time when Paige could have joined in and helped lead the calls would likely have been wiser. Fortunately, this threat to rapport was fairly readily remedied, but it provided a good lesson to us not to let expedience guide decision making in treatment.

Ultimately, Paige improved multiple aspects of her self-care, including obtaining some additional financial support, reducing time spent watching television and surfing the Internet, receiving medical attention for her injury, and stabilizing her eating (though not her medication use). Thus, the primary aim of this phase was mostly achieved. However, Paige continued to struggle academically, and a month into our revised treatment plan, Paige withdrew from her classes for the semester to avoid receiving failing grades and being unable to return to the university. Despite the obvious severity of this decision, unlike prior times when she had to take a leave from school, Paige did not catastrophize the break in the same way. For the first time, she was able to say that taking time to work on her depression would likely help improve her academic motivation and school performance. She used the time off to reengage with her social supports (and actually be more open with them about her struggles) and to practice some emotion regulation skills we had worked on early in her therapy, including mindfulness and cognitive restructuring.

The Importance of Readiness for Change and Consideration of Sociocultural Context

This brings us to Paige's current phase of care. Since her return to school and to therapy, we have seen a number of positive changes in Paige's evident motivation and flexibility. Paige's readiness for change, by and large, has progressed from contemplation to preparation and, at times, action. She has been significantly more willing to make and implement her own action plans and struggle through more independent problem solving. Her reduction in intolerance of uncertainty and rigid self-critical thinking about what she "must" accomplish has helped her be more willing to take steps without guarantees that they will be successful, and to persist even when she is not feeling motivated. This has been paired with greater acceptance of both her negative emotions and her (still precarious) academic situation. She decided to change from majoring in economics to minoring in it, and instead major in political science. This option, she feels, allows her to still earn a degree in economics as she desires, but it puts her less at risk of failing given that she typically finds political science classes a little easier and the assignments less intimidating. She recognizes that although this is not her ideal situation, it is likely a good option at this time. Thus, we are cautiously optimistic that Paige (and the

therapist) are now at a more advanced stage of readiness for Paige to meet her initial goal of increasing her academic motivation and follow-through, while also maintaining her gains in self-care and managing her reduced, but not remitted, depressive symptoms.

When Paige returned to school, it provided us an opportunity to reflect together on her initial assessment information and course of treatment. Doing so highlighted the critical role of Paige's background and current sociocultural context. Paige continues to face many challenges, including serious financial pressures and lack of familial support. It is impossible to understand Paige's challenges at school and in therapy without considering these factors. Paige often felt she did not "fit in" at this prestigious university that has many wealthy students, and we have little doubt this made it harder for her to maintain her academic motivation and use available resources (e.g., joining study groups with other students or going to professors' office hours). There is considerable research on the impact of not "belonging" and how it can hurt academic achievement, especially for minority students (see Walton, Cohen, Cwir, & Spencer, 2012). Although Paige is not a racial or ethnic/minority student, she is an underrepresented student, being the first in her family to attend college. She also comes from a family with a history of abrupt life disruptions due to mental health and substance use problems. While these issues were discussed on occasion in the therapy, stepping away from our weekly work with Paige to reflect on her care broadly made us aware that it may be important to consider the impact of these challenges more fully in therapy going forward. At times, the therapist and supervisor did not adequately consider how Paige's lack of stable family support growing up meant that she had missed key developmental experiences, such as the development of appropriate autonomy during adolescence, which is tied to the development of self-esteem, intrinsic motivation, and self-efficacy (Hare, Szwedo, Schad, & Allen, 2014).

Her challenging home life also meant that Paige grew up observing ineffective ways of solving problems, which likely contributed to her initial difficulty employing active coping strategies at school. For instance, while Paige's substance use, which we assessed fairly regularly, did not increase to such a level that it needed to become a primary focus of treatment, her tendency to spend many hours a day watching television as a way to temporarily avoid her negative affect and ignore her problems likely reflected a similar (maladaptive) reinforcement pattern. Thus, while she was not "turning into her mother" (one of her biggest fears), she did have a tendency to use an analogous unhealthy, avoidant coping style.

Conclusion

Working with Paige has been both challenging and rewarding. Clearly, her progress has not been linear, and the complexities of her case meant it was not sufficient to apply a brief, disorder-driven, empirically supported protocol in its standard form. In fact, responding to the complexity and unpredictable course of events in working with Paige and clients like her makes replying on the empirical literature even more important. We have illustrated how we used treatment elements that have clear empirical support in the nomothetic literature (e.g., cognitive restructuring, activity scheduling, goal setting, problem solving, motivational interviewing, mindfulness) and applied these approaches in an idiographic, phase-specific manner. Using our case conceptualization as a starting point, the phase approach to therapy was followed with new phases determined in large part by our monitoring of the client's progress on a given set of aims. In this way, it is a sequenced approach that iteratively asks how the research evidence can guide targeting the specific aims for that phase of care, and draws from both treatment outcome research and basic research on mechanisms of change in healthy and clinical samples.

We have shared openly our "mistakes" in therapy and how it is possible to recover from such missteps. There were certainly periods when the client felt hopeless and the therapist and supervisor felt frustrated as the case seemed "stuck" or even to grow worse. The use of a phase approach, which assumes that treatment planning will be a dynamic process and that it is not a failure to need to "switch course," was helpful in this regard. Our "mistakes" are valuable also in highlighting potential avenues for future research, and our work with clients like Paige helps to identify gaps in the empirical literature.

For instance, more research on how to help change a rigid self-concept when it is not shifting in line with behavior changes would be helpful (e.g., even when Paige made positive steps, we spent months with her still believing she could not improve and was a "failure" who was "not worth the therapist's time"; this negative self-view was very demotivating and interfered with further progress). There are many models in the social cognition and health literature examining how behavior and attitude change can be discordant (e.g., when a person values exercise but has trouble actually going to the gym), but these often focus on attitude change not resulting in behavioral follow-through. While Paige certainly routinely experienced this exact type of difficulty, she also experienced a challenge in the other direction when she made positive behavioral changes, such as attending classes, but her self-concept (especially regarding her low self-efficacy) stayed rigidly negative. More research on how to promote identity shifts among clients who have had a disorder for a very long time would be valuable.

We are regularly reminded of how difficult it is to know for sure whether what we are doing is "working" given how challenging it is to determine the source of a client's changes (see Lilienfeld, Ritschel, Lynn, Cautin, & Latzman, 2014), even when monitoring outcomes in a collaborative way. But we feel very privileged to be a part of this process and hope that our joy in doing therapy—even for hard cases—has come through. Conducting therapy provides a unique blend of intellectual and emotional challenge; it provides an amazing opportunity to try to understand at a deep level the functional relationships between a person's thoughts, feelings, behaviors, relationships, and their environment. The brainstorming and "puzzle solving" that occurs in therapy and in supervision, and the bidirectional "on the ground" link between research and practice make it endlessly fascinating, and the opportunity to (we hope) be part of someone's change process makes it endlessly rewarding.

References

American Psychiatric Association. (2013). *Diagnostic and statistical manual of mental disorders* (5th ed.). Arlington, VA: Author.

Arnow, B. A., Steidtmann, D., Blasey, C., Manber, R., Constantino, M. J., Klein, D. N., et al. (2013). The relationship between the therapeutic alliance and treatment outcome in two distinct psychotherapies for chronic depression. *Journal of Consulting and Clinical Psychology, 81*(4), 627–638.

Bachelor, A. (2013). Clients' and therapists' views of the

therapeutic alliance: Similarities, differences and relationship to therapy outcome. *Clinical Psychology and Psychotherapy, 20*(2), 118–135.

Beck, A. T., Steer, R. A., & Brown, G. K. (1996). *Manual for the Beck Depression Inventory–II.* San Antonio, TX: Psychological Corporation.

Beck, J. S. (2011). *Cognitive behavior therapy: Basics and beyond* (2nd ed.). New York: Guilford Press.

Beitman, B. D., Goldfried, M. R., & Norcross, J. C. (1989). The movement toward integrating the psychotherapies: An overview. *American Journal of Psychiatry, 146,* 138–147.

Boud, D. (Ed.). (2012). *Developing student autonomy in learning.* New York: Routledge.

Budman, S. H., & Gurman, A. S. (1988). *Theory and practice of brief psychotherapy.* New York: Guilford Press.

Buhr, K., & Dugas, M. J. (2002). The intolerance of uncertainty scale: Psychometric properties of the English version. *Behaviour Research and Therapy, 40*(8), 931–945.

Chartier, I. S., & Provencher, M. D. (2013). Behavioural activation for depression: Efficacy, effectiveness and dissemination. *Journal of Affective Disorders, 145*(3), 292–299.

Craske, M. G., Treanor, M., Conway, C. C., Zbozinek, T., & Vervliet, B. (2014). Maximizing exposure therapy: An inhibitory learning approach. *Behaviour Research and Therapy, 58,* 10–23.

Dau, W., Hoffman, J. D. G., & Banger, M. (2015). Therapeutic interventions in the treatment of problematic internet use—Experiences from Germany. In C. Montag & M. Reuter (Eds.), *Internet addiction: Neuroscientific approaches and therapeutical interventions* (pp. 183–217). Cham, Switzerland: Springer International.

DiClemente, C. C., Prochaska, J. O., & Gibertini, M. (1985). Self-efficacy and the stages of self-change of smoking. *Cognitive Therapy and Research, 9*(2), 181–200.

Dimidjian, S., Martell, C. R., Herman-Dunn, R., & Hubley, S. (2014). Behavioral activation for depression. In D. H. Barlow (Ed.), *Clinical handbook of psychological disorders: A step-by-step treatment manual* (5th ed., pp. 353–393). New York: Guilford Press.

Dweck, C. S. (1986). Motivational processes affecting learning. *American Psychologist, 41*(10), 1040–1048.

Floyd, D. L., Prentice-Dunn, S., & Rogers, R. W. (2000). A meta-analysis of research on protection motivation theory. *Journal of Applied Social Psychology, 30*(2), 407–429.

Gentes, E. L., & Ruscio, A. M. (2011). A meta-analysis of the relation of intolerance of uncertainty to symptoms of generalized anxiety disorder, major depressive disorder, and obsessive–compulsive disorder. *Clinical Psychology Review, 31*(6), 923–933.

Gil, S., & Droit-Volet, S. (2009). Time perception, depression, and sadness. *Behavioural Processes, 80*(2), 169–176.

Haas, L. J., & Cummings, N. A. (1991). Managed outpatient mental health plans: Clinical, ethical, and practical guidelines for participation. *Professional Psychology, 22,* 45–51.

Hare, A. L., Szwedo, D. E., Schad, M. M., & Allen, J. P. (2014). Undermining adolescent autonomy with parents and peers: The enduring implications of psychologically controlling parenting. *Journal of Research on Adolescence, 25*(4), 739–752.

Heinssen, R. K., Levendusky, P. G., & Hunter, R. H. (1995). Client as colleague: Therapeutic contracting with the seriously mentally ill. *American Psychologist, 50,* 522–532.

Higgins, S. T., Heil, S. H., & Lussier, J. P. (2004). Clinical implications of reinforcement as a determinant of substance use disorders. *Annual Review of Psychology, 55,* 431–461.

Jacobson, N. S., Martell, C. R., & Dimidjian, S. (2006). Behavioral activation treatment for depression: Returning to contextual roots. *Clinical Psychology: Science and Practice, 8*(3), 255–270.

Kazantzis, N., Dattilio, F. M., Cummins, A., & Clayton, X. (2014). Homework assignments and self-monitoring. In S. G. Hofmann (Ed.), *The Wiley handbook of cognitive behavioral therapy* (Vol. 1, pp. 311–330). Hoboken, NJ: Wiley.

Kiesler, D. J. (1988). *Therapeutic metacommunication: Therapist impact disclosure as feedback in psychotherapy.* Palo Alto, CA: Consulting Psychologists Press.

Leahy, R. (2003). *Cognitive therapy techniques: A practitioner's guide.* New York: Guilford Press.

Lilienfeld, S. O., Ritschel, L. A., Lynn, S. J., Cautin, R. L., & Latzman, R. D. (2014). Why ineffective psychotherapies appear to work: A taxonomy of causes of spurious therapeutic effectiveness. *Perspectives on Psychological Science, 9*(4), 355–387.

Linehan, M. M. (1993). *Cognitive-behavioral treatment of borderline personality disorder.* New York: Guilford Press.

Lundahl, B., Moleni, T., Burke, B. L., Butters, R., Tollefson, D., Butler, C., et al. (2013). Motivational interviewing in medical care settings: A systematic review and meta-analysis of randomized controlled trials. *Patient Education and Counseling, 93*(2), 157–168.

Mahoney, A. E., & McEvoy, P. M. (2012). A transdiagnostic examination of intolerance of uncertainty across anxiety and depressive disorders. *Cognitive Behaviour Therapy, 41*(3), 212–222.

Martin, S. L., Liao, H., & Campbell, E. M. (2013). Directive versus empowering leadership: A field experiment comparing impacts on task proficiency and proactivity. *Academy of Management Journal, 56*(5), 1372–1395.

McKay, M., Wood, J. C., & Brantley, J. (2007). *Dialectical behavior therapy skills workbook: Practical DBT exercises for learning mindfulness, interpersonal effectiveness, emotion regulation, and distress tolerance.* Oakland, CA: New Harbinger.

Mennin, D. S., Ellard, K. K., Fresco, D. M., & Gross, J. J. (2013). United we stand: Emphasizing commonalities across cognitive-behavioral therapies. *Behavior Therapy, 44*(2), 234–248.

Miller, W. R., & Rollnick, S. (2012). *Motivational interviewing: Helping patients change behavior* (3rd ed.). New York: Guilford Press.

Milne, S., Sheeran, P., & Orbell, S. (2000). Prediction and intervention in health-related behavior: A meta-analytic review of protection motivation theory. *Journal of Applied Social Psychology, 30,* 106–143.

Payne, L. A., Ellard, K. K., Farchione, T. J., Fairholme, C. P., & Barlow, D. H. (2014). Emotional disorders: A unified transdiagnostic protocol. In D. H. Barlow (Ed.), *Clinical handbook of psychological disorders: A step-by-step treatment manual* (5th ed., pp. 237–274). New York: Guilford Press.

Powers, M. B., Asmundson, G. J., & Smits, J. A. (2015). Exercise for mood and anxiety disorders: The state-of-the science. *Cognitive Behaviour Therapy, 44*(4), 237–239.

Prochaska, J. O., & DiClemente, C. C. (1984). *The transtheoretical approach: Crossing traditional boundaries of therapy.* Homewood, IL: Dow/Jones Irwin.

Prochaska, J. O., Norcross, J. C., & DiClemente, C. C. (2013). Applying the stages of change. *Psychotherapy in Australia, 19*(2), 10–15.

Rector, N. A., Zuroff, D. C., & Segal, Z. V. (1999). Cognitive change and the therapeutic alliance: The role of technical and nontechnical factors in cognitive therapy. *Psychotherapy: Theory, Research, Practice, Training, 36*(4), 320–328.

Roemer, L., & Orsillo, S. M. (2014). An acceptance-based behavioral therapy for generalized anxiety disorder. In D. H. Barlow (Ed.), *Clinical handbook of psychological disorders: A step-by-step treatment manual* (5th ed., pp. 206–236). New York: Guilford Press.

Rogers, C. R. (1958). A process conception of psychotherapy. *American Psychologist, 13,* 142–149.

Rogers, R. W. (1983). Cognitive and physiological processes in fear appeals and attitude change: A revised theory of protection motivation. In J. T. Cacioppo & R. E. Petty (Eds.), *Social psychophysiology* (pp. 153–176). New York: Guilford Press.

Rothman, A. J., Gollwitzer, P. M., Grant, A. M., Neal, D. T., Sheeran, P., & Wood, W. (2015). Hale and hearty policies: How psychological science can create and maintain healthy habits. *Perspectives on Psychological Science, 10*(6), 701–705.

Teyber, E., & McClure, F. H. (2010). *Interpersonal process in therapy: An integrative model* (6th ed.). Belmont, CA: Brooks/Cole.

Walton, G. M., Cohen, G. L., Cwir, D., & Spencer, S. J. (2012). Mere belonging: The power of social connections. *Journal of Personality and Social Psychology, 102*(3), 513–532.

Whalley, M. (2008). Stages of change [worksheet]. Retrieved from *http://psychology.tools/stages-of-change.html.*

Woody, S. R., Detweiler-Bedell, J., Teachman, B. A., & O'Hearn, T. (2003). *Treatment planning in psychotherapy: Taking the guesswork out of clinical care.* New York: Guilford Press.

Young, J. E., Rygh, J. L., Weinberger, A. D., & Beck, A. T. (2014). Cognitive therapy for depression. In D. H. Barlow (Ed.), *Clinical handbook of psychological disorders: A step-by-step treatment manual* (5th ed., pp. 275–331). New York: Guilford Press.

CHAPTER 15

The Practice of Dialectical Behavior Therapy with Multidiagnostic and Suicidal Patients

CHELSEY R. WILKS
MARSHA M. LINEHAN

Jay had recently attempted suicide and wanted to get help. Two weeks earlier, he had been drinking a lot of vodka and had jumped off a pier into water, with the intent to drown himself. When he hit the cold water, he no longer wanted to die and swam to shore. Since then, he has been trying to cut down on his drinking and thinking about getting help. He was referred to our clinic by a family friend who had visited the clinic's website. He called to inquire about available services, and asked to be seen for therapy. We set up an assessment appointment for later that week.

When Jay arrived for the assessment, he reported that he had been having difficulties for years but had never sought help. He explained that he and his family moved permanently to the United States in 2005, following the death of his father. His mother, who was born and raised in Mongolia, had met his father while attending college in the United States. Jay's father worked for an international organization in a position that required constant travel and, as such, the family had lived in many different locations around the globe. Jay had a 16-year-old sister, also born in Mongolia, with whom he was very close given unique and mutual life experiences. When Jay was 13, the family was living in the Middle East, and his father was violently assassinated. According to Jay's recollection, his mother brought him to the room where his father's body lay and then instructed him to fold down the sheet from his deceased father's face and to give his father a kiss on the forehead. According to Jay, following this event, he experienced several "blackouts" in which he would replay images of his father lying on the table and seeing his father's wounded face. After his father's death, Jay recounted that his mother decided to bring their family to the United States to be closer to his father's immediate family. Jay's sister was living at home and attending a public high school, and Jay's mother had recently remarried. Jay and his sister, being half-American and moving to the United States as young adolescents, were more acculturated to the "American way of life" than their mother. However, Jay was very proud of his cultural heritage, and he actively participated in cultural activities at home, which was a considerable source of strength.

At the time Jay called to request treatment, he had stopped attending college in order to focus solely on "getting better." He was living with five of his closest friends near a college campus and was drinking heavily. He reported consuming, on average, 10 standard alcoholic beverages a day, which was the norm among his roommates and strongly reinforced in his living environment. Jay kept his departure from school a secret from his mother. He reported that his mother highly valued education and that his decision to stop school would be heavily punished. He also kept from his mother his drinking, his suicide attempt, and seeking help from a therapist. In fact, Jay would text his mother daily about how his "classes" were going and would fabricate his well-being to give the impression that he was doing well and everything was fine.

In truth, things were far from fine. Including his most recent suicide attempt, Jay reported attempting suicide three times in his lifetime in response to the Suicide Attempt and Self-Injury Interview (SASII; Linehan, Comtois, Brown, Heard, & Wagner, 2006). He attempted suicide for the first time when he was 16 years old by consuming "a large amount of alcohol" and overdosing on over-the-counter pain medication. Jay reported that his mother found him unconscious in his room, and he was immediately transported to the hospital. According to Jay, when he thought his heart had stopped, he experienced himself as "finally at peace." The other time he attempted suicide was 2 months prior to his referral. Jay reported that one of his roommates found him trying to stab himself in the heart with a kitchen knife, although according to Jay, he was highly intoxicated and the knife only superficially punctured his skin.

We conducted the Structured Clinical Interview for Axis I and Axis II DSM-IV Disorders (First, Spitzer, Gibbon, & Williams, 1995; First, Spitzer, Gibbon, Williams, & Benjamin, 1996). Jay was threshold for six of the nine criteria for borderline personality disorder (BPD), including interpersonal instability, unstable sense of self, impulsivity, suicidality, anger, and affect instability. Jay also met criteria for major depressive disorder, alcohol dependence, and post-traumatic stress disorder (PTSD). Jay reported severe problems with regulating emotions, scoring a 152 out of a possible 180 on the Difficulties of Emotion Regulation Scale (DERS; Gratz & Roemer, 2004), which is two standard deviations higher than normative scores, and scoring 37 on the State–Trait Anger Expression Inventory Anger Expression subscale (STAXI; Lievaart, Franken, & Hovens, 2016; Spielberger, 1999), which is almost four standard deviations higher than normative levels.

*   *   *

BPD is a chronic disorder characterized by instability in affect, behavior, identity, and relationships (American Psychiatric Association, 2013). As a result, BPD is quite debilitating; although only up to 5% of U.S. adults meet criteria for BPD, in primary care settings, the prevalence of BPD is approximately four times higher than that in the general population, indicating

that individuals with BPD tend to be high users of services (see Leichsenring, Leibing, Kruse, New, & Leweke, 2011). Furthermore, individuals with BPD often meet criteria for multiple other diagnoses. Specifically, among clinical samples, approximately 50% of individuals with BPD have a co-occurring diagnosis of PTSD (Harned, Jackson, Comtois, & Linehan, 2010) and 57% have an alcohol use disorder (AUD; Grant et al., 2008). Risk for suicide increases precipitously among those with BPD and co-occurring PTSD (Pagura et al., 2010) or AUD (Preuss et al., 2006). Given this, we believed Jay would be very high risk and could very likely attempt or even die by suicide while in treatment.

Dialectical behavior therapy (DBT; Linehan, 1993, 2014) is an empirically supported treatment for highly suicidal, complex, and multidiagnostic clients (see Kliem, Kröger, & Kosfelder, 2010). DBT is a comprehensive modular treatment consisting of individual therapy, group skills training, telephone coaching, and a therapist consultation team. Underlying DBT is the biosocial theory, which states that BPD is a disorder of pervasive emotion dysregulation; DBT therapists operate under the assumption that behaviors involving BPD criteria function to regulate emotions or are consequences of emotion dysregulation (Linehan, 1993).

DBT is conceptualized as a stage-based treatment; in other words, treatment is organized to prioritize target behavior based on severity. Given the frequent co-occurrence of BPD with other disorders, within stages, DBT is guided by a hierarchical framework in which specific behaviors are targeted by severity. At Stage 1, treatment is broken down into the following behavioral targets: (1) decrease life-interfering behavior (e.g., suicide attempts) because treatment does not work if the client is dead; (2) decrease therapy interfering behavior (e.g., missing treatment) because treatment does not work if the client does not do treatment; (3) decrease quality-of-life-interfering behavior (e.g., homelessness, addictive behavior); and (4) increase skillful behavior to replace dysfunctional behavior (Linehan, 1993).

Given the high comorbidity, specifically, between BPD and PSTD, a protocol for DBT plus prolonged exposure (PE) has been developed specifically for suicidal individuals meeting criteria for both disorders (Harned, Korslund, & Linehan, 2014). Within this framework, PTSD is treated once clients enter "Stage 2" of treatment, or when clients' behavioral dyscontrol is stabilized but emotional suffering is not. In order to determine one's readiness to begin PE in the context of DBT, clients have to establish that they (1) are no longer at high risk for suicide, (2) are capable of experiencing intense emotions without escaping or avoiding, (3) want to treat their PTSD, and (4) are not engaging in significant therapy-interfering behaviors, which may include missing sessions or homework noncompliance (Harned, Korslund, Foa, & Linehan, 2012). While Jay's frequent binge-drinking behavior was a concern on the onset of treatment, the DBT plus PE treatment protocol does not require abstinence from alcohol, but rather no drinking during exposure homework and 2 hours after exposure homework. Therefore, Jay needed to be armed with a set of distress tolerance strategies that he could access during and after exposure tasks.

In this chapter, we describe use of the DBT and PE protocol with Jay. We determined that the integrated DBT and PE protocol was the best of available options because (1) PE has the most empirical support for targeting trauma; (2) PE is highly compatible with DBT because of its focus on tolerating intense emotions without avoiding or escaping; (3) DBT plus PE has been empirically evaluated and shown to be safe, effective, and acceptable; and (4) Linehan (1993) recommended exposure in her initial publication of the DBT treatment manual. Beyond the theoretical and empirical justification for implementing the DBT plus PE protocol, Jay wanted to try exposure. Throughout his life, Jay had never directly addressed what had happened to him, and he was initially very willing (albeit timid) to implement an exposure-based treatment. Finally, Jay (and his mother) had a strong devotion toward science, evidence, and research and were enthusiastic about the empirical and theoretical justification for this treatment.

Jay stated that he entered treatment because he wanted to live, to find freedom from suffering related to his trauma history, and to cope better with life's stressors.

Course of Treatment

Orientation and Commitment (Sessions 1–4)

Given Jay's recent suicide attempt and hospitalization, we classified him as "high risk"; thus, we immediately focused on obtaining Jay's commitment to stay alive for the duration of treatment. Another complicating factor was the

"double life" that Jay was living. Specifically, he was keeping several secrets from his family, for example, (1) that he was no longer in school and (2) that he was in psychotherapy. As a result, he requested that we keep his secret, and we initially obliged.

The orientation of DBT is conducted by first obtaining from Jay his goals for therapy and asking him to commit to staying alive while in therapy and to work toward his wise mind goals. Jay's treatment goals were to develop stronger interpersonal relationships and to go back to school. Finally, Jay indicated that the thing he wanted most in the world was to be a stay-at-home dad. In DBT, we use a commitment technique called "Devil's advocate," in which we have the client argue for why he wants to live and engage in treatment. This is how it went with Jay:

THERAPIST: I am confident that we can get you to your goals, but here's the deal. This treatment doesn't work if you're dead—so you have to stay alive for the duration of our treatment. That means suicide is off the table. Can you commit to that?

JAY: Umm, I don't know. Suicide has always been my escape button, and I'm nervous about giving that up.

THERAPIST: Yeah (*pause*) and this is going to require a huge leap of faith from you to trust me that we can develop new skills you can turn to when urges to die are high. I'm asking you to take a leap of faith and give up suicide as your escape button.

JAY: (*pause*) OK, that makes sense. I am committed to giving it up.

THERAPIST: You're committed?

JAY: Yes!

THERAPIST: Let me ask you this. You just said that suicide has been your "go to" strategy. Why would you agree to participate in a treatment that is asking you to give that up?

JAY: Well, there's lots of things I want from life, and I don't want to give up. I want to get better.

THERAPIST: But, wouldn't you prefer to be in a treatment that isn't requiring this level of commitment from you?

JAY: I don't want to be in a treatment that's OK with me killing myself.

This commitment session proved immensely valuable for Jay, as it instilled in him a sense of hope that things could get better. It was also during these first four sessions that we assessed what prompted Jay's previous suicide attempts to better understand what factors set off Jay's suicidal behavior. We had Jay begin to fill out a daily diary card in order to track behaviors of interest. We tracked specific emotions (e.g., anger, sadness, shame, and joy), as well as urges to die, and quantity of alcoholic beverages. The diary card informed our assessment (and guided treatment as we continued its use each week to set the agenda based on highest priority treatment targets).

Based on our discussions and the diary card over the first four sessions, Jay appeared to be particularly sensitive to experiencing invalidation from his friends and family, and he struggled to tolerate emotions that occurred in the presence of invalidation. Jay reported that he was a "sensitive kid," and that his mother would punish him for displaying any amount of negative emotions (i.e., "You've cried enough! Stop it!"). Jay learned to avoid displaying and experiencing emotions as much as possible. After the death of his father, his negative emotions were intolerable; thus, he eventually turned to binge drinking as his primary method of emotion regulation. Jay would also fantasize about suicide in order to escape painful emotions or memories. These behaviors were maintained by the immediate relief from negative emotions. Jay was fearful that if he allowed himself to feel sad or grieve the death of his father, then he would never recover, and because he never allowed himself to feel any emotions other than anger, it appeared that he never learned that his emotional responses would eventually decrease. Jay also experienced numerous negative consequences as a result of his avoidance behaviors, including dropping out of school, interpersonal problems (exacerbated by alcohol use), and stopping hobbies that he previously enjoyed (e.g., drawing, basketball). It also became clear that Jay's high impulsivity and proclivity for consuming large amounts of alcohol to the point of blacking out were major risk factors. We had to arm Jay with strategies to regulate emotions and tolerate distress in order to weather crises without turning to suicide (Linehan, 2014).

Decreasing Life- and Quality-of-Life-Interfering Behaviors and Increasing Skills Use (Sessions 5–16)

As we have mentioned, DBT is a principles-based intervention that hierarchically organizes treatment based on severity. To accomplish this, DBT therapists rely heavily on the diary card to guide therapy from week to week. As clients enter the therapy office and sit down, often the first words out of the therapist's mouth are "Do you have your diary card?" The therapist then looks it over to see whether the client engaged in any life-threatening behaviors (e.g., nonsuicidal self-injury [NSSI], suicide attempt, increase in urges to die by suicide) or had significant increases in suicidal urges over the past week. If the diary card shows no indication of life-interfering behaviors, then the therapist evaluates the presence of therapy-interfering behaviors, which might include (1) not going to skills group, (2) not having his or her diary card, (3) not doing the assigned homework, and/or (4) not attending the session. If there are no life- or therapy-interfering behaviors, the therapist moves on to evaluate significant quality-of-life-interfering behaviors. If and when a target behavior shows up on the diary card (or if there is not a diary card), therapist and client work together to figure out "How in the world did that happen?"

In this way, DBT is an iterative therapy that ebbs and flows week to week. DBT therapists are forced to continually assess and monitor suicidal behaviors, but they are also guided by the client's case conceptualization. In other words, while DBT therapists consistently monitor, assess, and attempt to reduce dysfunctional behaviors, therapist and client work together to understand how the client's behavior fits in with broader behavioral patterns, in order to solve the "core problem." Nonetheless, overarching treatment targets also become moving targets as client and therapist unravel the client's life history, behavioral repertoire, and expectations.

Prioritizing Suicidal Behavior

At the beginning of treatment, Jay indicated that he frequently thought of suicide; thus, early treatment targeted methods to reduce frequency and intensity of suicidal ideation. Our assessment indicated that his suicidal ideation functioned to help him escape painful memories and/or emotions. We targeted suicidal ideation in several ways. First we tracked it using the diary card so that Jay could become more mindful of the frequency and intensity of his suicidal thoughts. Whenever Jay endorsed an elevated urge to die (defined as a 3-point increase from the previous week on a 6-point Likert scale), we were prompted to fill out a Linehan Risk Assessment and Management Protocol (LRAMP; Linehan, Comtois, & Ward-Ciesielski, 2012). The LRAMP includes several risk and protective factors, and allows clinicians to document their crisis plans. Second, we taught Jay the DBT skill of "mindfulness of current thoughts," in which the suicidal thought is treated as "just a thought," in order to reduce the saliency of the thought. Third, as Jay's suicidal thoughts functioned to reduce acute distress, we collaboratively brainstormed ways in which Jay could distract himself with other thoughts that were more in line with his long-term goals. At the fifth week of treatment, Jay reported that he no longer had the thought to go to suicide as an escape or a fantasy. These thoughts ultimately stopped after he reported having a candid conversation with his sister while he was visiting his mother, in which his sister conveyed that his suicide would destroy her. Ultimately, Jay's conversation with his sister gave him another reason for living, and he was more motivated to use skillful means to reduce suicidal thoughts.

After our 11th session, we received a phone call from an attending psychiatrist who reported that Jay was in the hospital after a suicide attempt. The psychiatrist reported that Jay was transported to the hospital after ingesting a large quantity of pain pills. Additional testing at the hospital indicated that Jay had a life-threatening level of alcohol intoxication. The psychiatrist reported that Jay was stable and would likely be discharged in 1 day. Jay's suicide attempt and subsequent hospitalization resulted in his mother acknowledging his current mental health status and his departure from college. Subsequently, Jay moved in with his mother and stepfather.

When Jay returned to our next sessions, we discussed the fact that because he had engaged in suicidal behavior, the clock to administer PE for his trauma was reset to eight more weeks to establish that he was not imminently suicidal (Harned et al., 2012). We also prioritized conducting the chain of events that led to the attempt. Jay reported that the thought of suicide entered his mind as soon as he saw the bottle of pain medication; furthermore, his reported urge to die was a 3 out of 5 on the LRAMP. According to Simon and colleagues (2002), impulsive suicide attempts constitute approximately one-fourth of attempts. Specifically, in a sizable proportion of suicide attempters, the thought to die by suicide and the act occur less than 5 minutes apart. We recognized that despite the motivation elicited by Jay's connection with his sister, those reasons for living were not strong enough to counteract the risk created by alcohol use. At this point, we were very clear that treatment needed to shift to making a stronger effort to reduce Jay's drinking.

Reducing Alcohol Consumption

Jay entered treatment reportedly drinking 10–12 standard drinks a day for over a year. As a result, he had developed physical and psychological dependence on alcohol. As alcohol was a large contributing factor for Jay's suicidal behavior as well as a facilitator of his avoidance of emotions, it was important to target drinking. Furthermore, Jay indicated that he feared "becoming an alcoholic," and he entered treatment with the goal of reducing his drinking. Initially, we assessed what he liked and did not like about drinking, ultimately identifying ways in which drinking interfered with his long-term treatment goals and how reducing his drinking would stimulate positive change.

In the beginning of treatment, Jay decided that he wanted to reduce the frequency and quantity of his drinking, as well as engage in safer drinking practices. We adapted a harm reduction module (Larimer et al., 1998) for Jay. This treatment approach differed slightly from the DBT addiction skills (Linehan, 2014), which emphasize abstinence as an ultimate behavioral goal. Initially, Jay was hesitant about choosing abstinence as a drinking goal because his roommates (who were all drinkers) were huge social supports, and he believed that he would have to cut them out of his life in order to stop drinking. We also learned through the alcohol literature about the importance of having clients establish a drinking goal for themselves versus a forced choice (e.g., Adamson & Sellman, 2001).

Almost immediately, Jay reduced his drinking from about 60 standard drinks a week to an average of 20 standard drinks a week (see Figure 15.1). Jay attributed his success to switching his drink of choice from vodka to beer and opting not to drink on weekdays. Jay was also diligent about filling out his diary card (which included tracking his drinking), and he found that as he tracked his alcohol consumption, he organically reduced his drinking. Given the severity of Jay's alcohol use, we closely monitored his alcohol reduction and subsequent withdrawal symptoms; we also consulted with a psychiatrist when Jay reported significant distress associated with alcohol withdrawal. After Jay moved in with his mother and stepfather (Week 11), his alcohol consumption dropped from an average of 15 standard drinks a week to less than two. The sudden reduction in alcohol consumption resulted in an increase alcohol withdrawal symptoms that included sleeping difficulty, profuse sweating, and agitation; fortunately, these symptoms did not require medical attention.

Increasing Emotion Regulation Capabilities

As we were taking away Jay's two major coping strategies (e.g., drinking and suicidal ideation), we needed to replace those behaviors with some skills that would serve the same function (i.e., reduce distress) but be in accordance with his treatment goals (e.g., going to school, being a dad).

Throughout treatment, it became clear that Jay was incapable of sitting with negative emotions. If an emotional topic came up (e.g., the death of his father), he would laugh it off, change the subject, or shut down. He had learned from an early age to avoid expressing his emotions. Subsequently, Jay indicated that he was very uncomfortable with the emotion of sadness and would often become angry at himself for feeling sad. This was particularly troublesome because Jay had a habit of drinking alcohol more quickly and in greater quantities when he was angry. In addition, he would be at high risk of attempting suicide whenever he was highly intoxicated and angry. So, in order to increase Jay's ability to tolerate negative emotions (which could ultimately keep him alive), we started by informally exposing him to negative affect in session.

JAY: I wish my dad was alive because my life would be a lot better.

THERAPIST: OK, let's pause right here at this moment. What emotion are you feeling?

JAY: Sadness . . . I don't like it.

THERAPIST: Describe to me where you feel this emotion in your body.

JAY: Heavy in my chest (*pause*) my throat is tight (*pause*) tenseness in my stomach.

THERAPIST: I want you to sit with the sadness right now. On a scale from 1, low, to 10, high, how sad are you at this moment?

JAY: 7.

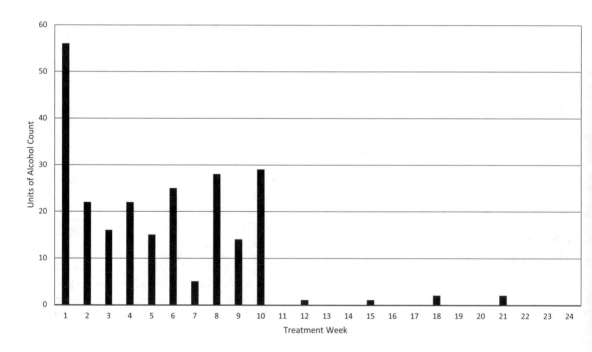

FIGURE 15.1. Units of alcohol consumption over the course of treatment.

THERAPIST: Good. (*after 1 minute*) Same scale, how sad are you now?

JAY: 9.

THERAPIST: (*after 1 minute*) And now?

JAY: (*shaking his head*) OK, I'm done, 1.

THERAPIST: How was that for you to sit with that emotion?

JAY: Annoying.

THERAPIST: You did it, and that's really impressive! It's completely reasonable to avoid things we don't like (*pause*) and sometimes avoidance can interfere with our long-term goals. How has avoiding feeling sad affected you?

JAY: I don't like to think about my dad because it makes me sad, and I want to be able to think about him.

THERAPIST: That makes sense.

Jay had never learned that emotions ebb and flow; as a result, it took several iterations of this informal exposure for Jay to learn that he could sit with and ride the emotion wave without escaping or avoiding it. Initially, we only conducted informal exposure in session,

so that he could build mastery in a safe environment. For between-session homework, Jay was instructed to practice "mindfulness of emotions," in which he observed his emotions rise and fall while listening to music, viewing artwork, and watching television. Eventually, Jay reported experiencing emotions without suppressing them as they naturally occurred in his environment (e.g., watching a movie or talking to a friend). In the beginning of treatment, Jay rolled his eyes during and after informal exposure to emotions. Thus, it was important to continuously link the rationale for this treatment strategy to his long-term goals and values (i.e., reengaging in school, treating PTSD). He also experienced natural positive outcomes of not suppressing his emotions (e.g., not engaging in target behavior). By the end of treatment, Jay's level of emotion dysregulation was still above the normative range for men (e.g., 80.6; Gratz & Roemer, 2004); however, his score had decreased by almost three standard deviations since the start of treatment (see Figure 15.2). In addition, Jay's anger was reduced substantially from the beginning of treatment. As can be seen in Figure 15.3, Jay scored below normative levels on the STAXI

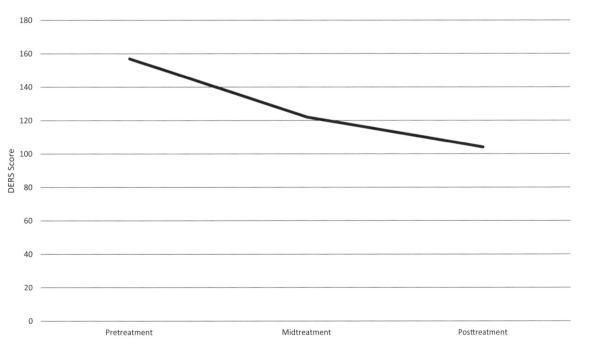

FIGURE 15.2. DERS total score over the course of treatment.

by the end of treatment (Lievaart et al., 2016; Spielberger, 1999).

Trauma Treatment (Sessions 17–23)

Jay entered into treatment highly motivated to reduce his PTSD symptoms. Following the DBT plus PE protocol outlined by Harned and colleagues (2012), we collaboratively determined that trauma treatment would begin once we believed that Jay was engaging in effective coping strategies when distressed. Specifically, because Jay was no longer at imminent risk of suicide, attended sessions regularly, and no longer relied on alcohol use as a form of emotion regulation, we were confident in our decision to embark on trauma-focused work.

Because Jay was living back at home, we decided to invite Jay's mother and stepfather into the session to describe PTSD, PE, and common reactions to trauma. Initially, Jay's mother communicated suspicion of Jay's clinical diagnoses due to a lack of observed symptomatic distress from Jay. She requested that we spend more time working to get Jay back into school rather than "solving Jay's made up problems." Indeed, Jay exhibited a tremendous amount of inhib-

ited grieving, as well as apparent competence. Specifically, Jay avoided experiencing negative emotions (*inhibited grieving*) and would present as though he was doing well (*apparent competence*); the net result of this behavioral presentation was a tendency for his family and friends to inadvertently invalidate his emotions (Linehan, 1993). Thus, it was reasonable for his mother to believe that he did not have PTSD. As a result, we spent more time thoroughly describing the symptoms of PTSD and which ones affected Jay's ability to reattend school (e.g., avoidance and reexperiencing). Jay's mother eventually acknowledged that treating his PTSD would facilitate his (and his mother's) larger goals about school. Finally, Jay's mother valued the strong scientific evidence in support of PE, as well as the theoretical rational behind exposure, and was supportive of Jay's treatment decision.

The PE component of the DBT plus PE protocol is very similar to standard PE. That being said, in order to make room for PE, clients either come in for an extra 1-hour session a week or complete one 90-minute session. During the PE portion of DBT, treatment is focused on (1) understanding the nature of the trauma(s) (Session 1 of PE), (2) providing a rational for PE (Ses-

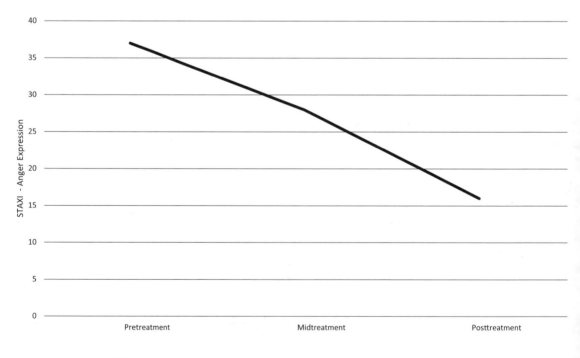

FIGURE 15.3. STAXI anger expression score over the course of treatment.

sion 1 of PE), (3) completing an *in vivo* exposure hierarchy (Session 2), and (4) conducting imaginal exposure (Session 3+ of PE). For Jay, we developed an exposure hierarchy for Jay's *in vivo* practice outside of session, which included watching war-related movies, going to hospitals, and being in crowds. We also discussed a postexposure skills plan for Jay to use to prevent ineffective coping (e.g., binge drinking, physical fights). This included DBT skills such as "mindfulness of current emotions," "distraction," and "self-soothing." Specifically, during the exposure practice, he would notice his emotions rise and fall. Jay would also describe where he experienced his emotions in his body. If he experienced intense urges to engage in dysfunctional behavior (i.e., binge drinking), he would actively distract himself from the emotion by watching TV, playing basketball, or talking to friends.

In Session 19, we began imaginal exposure for the entire traumatic event, followed by emotional processing. At this time, Jay endorsed high levels of distress, guilt, and anger; however, he displayed flat affect during both the imaginal and processing portion of the session. We conceptualized Jay as being *underengaged,* or as having a difficult time accessing the emotional components of the trauma memory (Foa, Hembree, & Rothbaum, 2007). In addition, while Jay completed his homework for imaginal exposure, which was listening to the in-session recording and completing an exposure recording form, he reported flat affect and increased anger. Jay's underengagement was consistent with his learning history (i.e., punishment for displaying affect and fear of losing emotional control). Furthermore, given Jay's relative comfort with the emotion of anger, and aversion to experiencing fear or sadness, his anger and frustration with the treatment made sense.

In order for the treatment to work, we needed Jay to fully experience his emotional reaction in response to imaginal exposure. Jay had shielded himself from the memory of seeing his dead father, and every time the memory entered his mind, he pushed it away as quickly as possible—through drinking and experiencing emotions that would temporarily alleviate his suffering but extend his misery in the long term. In fact, as Jay recognized, the more he fought to avoid remembering his trauma, the more frequent and stronger the memories were. PE works because it enables the client to purposely confront the memory and the emotions that naturally occur as a result of revisiting the memory. Eventually, the individual with PTSD acknowledges the memory as just a memory rather than something to fear. That being said, we needed Jay to acknowledge his memory, and the natural emotions and behaviors in response to his memory. Therefore, we followed suggestions from Foa and colleagues (2007); specifically, we reintroduced the rationale for exposure and asked brief, probing questions related to sensory information (e.g., "How does it smell?"; "What are you thinking?"). As Jay was immensely committed to treatment, he took the rationale very seriously and was visually more emotional at the subsequent sessions of imaginal exposure. Specifically, Jay teared up and spoke more slowly during his story. Furthermore, because we had been practicing mindfulness of current emotions during previous sessions (i.e., having Jay observe the sensations in his body), Jay recognized the benefits of experiencing his emotions, particularly in session. The imaginal component of PE lasted for several more sessions, until we decided to focus on "hot spots," or aspects of the memory that were particularly distressing and salient. For Jay, his hot spot was the moment in which he pulled the sheet from his father's body and kissed his father on the forehead.

Ultimately, the goal for imaginal exposure is not to forget what happened but to accept what happened. During the processing component of imaginal exposure, which lasts roughly 20–30 minutes after retelling the story, Jay found that he was coming more to terms with what happened in his life. Prior to entering treatment, Jay had yet to accept the death of his father, and he feared that if he allowed himself to think about that day, he would never recover from the overwhelming sadness that his father was no longer alive. By purposely attending to that day in his life, he recognized that he did eventually recover from his sadness, and he had the secondary outcome of allowing himself to remember positive moments about his father. As the course of PE was completed, Jay still felt sad when the memory of his father entered his mind; however, he no longer experienced a frantic effort to avoid the memory—or anything that could remind him of his father. Finally, results from the PTSD Checklist (PCL; Blanchard, Jones-Alexander, Buckley, & Forneris, 1996) indicated large reductions in Jay's PTSD symptoms.

Concluding Treatment

In Session 22, Jay had significant improvements in emotion dysregulation—specifically with anger, reductions in drinking, and reduced distress associated with PTSD. Following the insistent urging of his mother to stop therapy (according to her, he did not need it), Jay decided that he would like to conclude treatment. Based on his treatment measures at this point (see Figures 15.1–15.4), it was clear that Jay had made substantial gains and, most importantly, he was no longer suicidal, he no longer met criteria for an AUD, and he was no longer traumatized by PTSD. Furthermore, at this point, his sessions included far fewer agenda items because Jay at this point could successfully manage both minor and major challenges on his own.

At Week 23, we scheduled a termination session to review progress, answer questions, provide treatment referrals if needed in the future, and say good-bye. Jay reported that being in DBT enabled him to experience a "paradigm shift" in his perception of the world; specifically, Jay indicated that he "now holds a nonjudgmental stance" toward himself and others. Finally, while good-byes in DBT can be difficult, we invited Jay to stay in touch with us as his "ex-therapist," meaning that we would remain in his life as advocates and cheerleaders.

Summary of Outcomes

When Jay entered treatment, he was diagnosed with BPD, PTSD, and a severe AUD. He had high emotion dysregulation (as indicated on the DERS), and consumed, on average, 10 standard alcoholic drinks a day. By the end of treatment, he no longer met criteria for BPD and was only considered subthreshold for the BPD criteria "uncontrollable anger" and "affect instability." While Jay was still in the "clinical range" on the DERS at the end of treatment, he reduced his DERS score by roughly three standard deviations. Another indicator of emotion dysregulation is uncontrollable anger. At the end of treatment, Jay's scores on the STAXI Anger Expression subscale was reduced from a score of nearly 40 (nearly the highest possible score) to roughly 15, indicating a significant reduction in anger expression. At the end of treatment, we also conducted the PTSD Symptom Interview Scale—Interview (PSS-I; Powers, Gillihan, Rosenfield, Jerud, & Foa, 2012), which indicated that Jay no longer met criteria for PTSD. Finally, Jay was only drinking about one to four

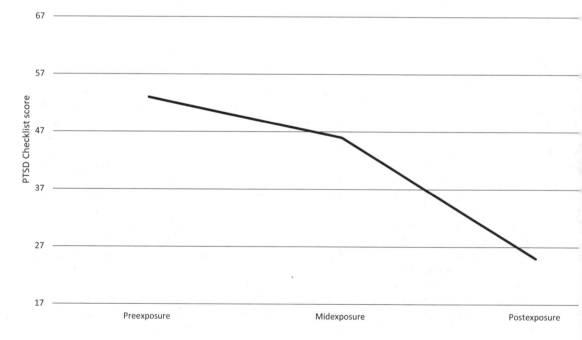

FIGURE 15.4. PCL score during the course of PE.

standard drinks a week, which was a considerable reduction from where he started when he entered treatment.

Lessons Learned: Cultural Considerations

Of the approximately 0–5% of U.S. adults with a BPD diagnosis (Leichsenring et al., 2011), men, Asians, and particularly Asian men, have significantly lower prevalence rates (Grant et al., 2008; Skodol & Bender, 2003; Tomko, Trull, Wood, & Sher, 2014). Jay was both a first-generation Mongolian and an American male; thus, he belonged to a small demographic/cultural group that has been noticeably underrepresented in DBT treatment research. Given Jay's minority status, we had to consider several issues when conceptualizing and implementing his treatment.

DBT was originally developed specifically to treat women presenting with chronic problems with self-harm and/or suicidal behaviors, and the majority of studies done on the clinical applications of DBT has remained within this trajectory. While promising results have been obtained, academic attention and research on male samples have been mostly restricted to correctional or forensic settings, and have tended to focus on small subgroups of men exhibiting specific types of overtly problematic and socially detrimental behavioral presentations (e.g., violent tendencies; Evershed et al., 2003; Shelton, Sampl, Kesten, Zhang, & Trestman, 2009). Moreover, DBT treatment outcome research on ethnic minorities also remains an underresearched area. To our knowledge, only one study to date has examined the effectiveness of DBT treatment for racial/ethnic minorities (e.g., American Indian/Alaskan Natives; Beckstead, Lambert, DuBose, & Linehan, 2015).

Ultimately, we had to turn to the literature in order to develop a better treatment plan for Jay. One important consideration stemmed from evidence suggesting that Easterners and Westerners tend to exhibit different styles of reasoning (Masuda & Nisbett, 2001; Peng & Nisbett, 1999). For instance, Peng and Nisbett (1999) found that Chinese students favor the dialectical approach to resolving contradictions by accepting and integrating opposing propositions ("both–and"), while American students favored the "either–or" approach in which one proposition is logically ruled out for the other ("either–or"). As such, thought-challenging approaches used in standard cognitive therapy may be less effective for Asian Americans, particularly as they relate to resolving apparent contradictions using formal logic. Fortunately, DBT is inherently dialectical—it is *dialectical* behavior therapy after all. Simply put, dialectics mean that two seemingly opposite concepts, actions, and/or thoughts can be true at the same time (e.g., Linehan, 1993). Moreover, DBT also emphasizes behavioral change over cognitive change because cognitive modification can be perceived as invalidating (i.e., "You're thinking is wrong"). As such, because DBT shares theoretical roots with the dialectical mode of thinking found to be dominant in collectivist and Asian cultures, third-wave acceptance-based psychotherapies that incorporate mindfulness (e.g., DBT), may show greater promise for application with Asian American clients. In agreement with this, we did observe Jay to be strongly on board with the underlying theoretical rationale of DBT.

In addition, we also frequently used a consultation team when we were confronted with case conceptualization and treatment planning challenges rooted in culture. Whenever client or therapist complications arose, team members identified other solutions (or problems) that we could use to refine treatment. This was particularly important when working with a racial and cultural minority, as team members were able to provide new perspectives to such clients' families; ultimately, this engendered greater compassion toward Jay and his mother. Team members also helped us to radically accept Jay's decision to discontinue treatment.

In summary, cultural considerations bear important treatment implications, as they inform and shape worldviews, values, and the ways in which oneself, others, and relationships are perceived and conceptualized in rather profound ways. The recognition and integration of culture cannot be overlooked when considering treatment plans and approaches for clients whose cultural background has been underrepresented in the body of research evidence on which empirically supported treatment models are founded.

Acknowledgments

Marsha M. Linehan receives royalties from The Guilford Press for books she has written on dialectical behavior therapy (DBT) and from Behavior Tech,

LLC, for DBT training materials. She also owns Behavioral Tech Research, Inc., a company that develops online learning and clinical applications that include products for DBT. Both authors are compensated for providing DBT training and consultation.

References

Adamson, S. J., & Sellman, J. D. (2001). Drinking goal selection and treatment outcome in out-patients with mild–moderate alcohol dependence. *Drug and Alcohol Review, 20*(4), 351–359.

American Psychiatric Association. (2013). *Diagnostic and statistical manual of mental disorders* (5th ed.). Arlington, VA: Author.

Beckstead, D. J., Lambert, M. J., DuBose, A. P., & Linehan, M. (2015). Dialectical behavior therapy with American Indian/Alaska Native adolescents diagnosed with substance use disorders: Combining an evidence based treatment with cultural, traditional, and spiritual beliefs. *Addictive Behaviors, 51,* 84–87.

Blanchard, E. B., Jones-Alexander, J., Buckley, T. C., & Forneris, C. A. (1996). Psychometric properties of the PTSD Checklist (PCL). *Behaviour Research and Therapy, 34*(8), 669–673.

Evershed, S., Tennant, A., Boomer, D., Rees, A., Barkham, M., & Watson, A. (2003). Practice-based outcomes of dialectical behaviour therapy (DBT) targeting anger and violence, with male forensic patients: A pragmatic and non-contemporaneous comparison. *Criminal Behaviour and Mental Health, 13*(3), 198–213.

First, M. B., Spitzer, R. L., Gibbon, M., & Williams, J. B. W. (1995). *Structured Clinical Interview for Axis I DSM-IV Disorders—Patient edition (SCID-I/P)*. New York: Biometrics Research Department, New York State Psychiatric Institute.

First, M. B., Spitzer, R. L., Gibbon, M., Williams, J. B. W., & Benjamin, L. (1996). *User's guide for the Structured Clinical Interview for for DSM-IV Axis II Personality Disorders (SCID-II)*. New York: Biometrics Research Department, New York State Psychiatric Institute.

Foa, E. B., Hembree, E. A., & Rothbaum, B. O. (2007). *Prolonged exposure therapy for PTSD*. New York: Oxford University Press.

Grant, B. F., Chou, S. P., Goldstein, R. B., Huang, B., Stinson, F. S., Saha, T. D., et al. (2008). Prevalence, correlates, disability, and comorbidity of DSM-IV borderline personality disorder: Results from the Wave 2 National Epidemiologic Survey on Alcohol and Related Conditions. *Journal of Clinical Psychiatry, 69*(4), 533–545.

Gratz, K. L., & Roemer, L. (2004). Multidimensional assessment of emotion regulation and dysregulation: Development, factor structure, and initial validation of the difficulties in emotion regulation scale. *Journal of Psychopathology and Behavioral Assessment, 26*(1), 41–54.

Harned, M. S., Jackson, S. C., Comtois, K. A., & Linehan, M. M. (2010). Dialectical behavior therapy as a precursor to PTSD treatment for suicidal and/or self-injuring women with borderline personality disorder. *Journal of Traumatic Stress, 23*(4), 421–429.

Harned, M. S., Korslund, K. E., Foa, E. B., & Linehan, M. M. (2012). Treating PTSD in suicidal and self-injuring women with borderline personality disorder: Development and preliminary evaluation of a dialectical behavior therapy prolonged exposure protocol. *Behaviour Research and Therapy, 50*(6), 381–386.

Harned, M. S., Korslund, K. E., & Linehan, M. M. (2014). A pilot randomized controlled trial of dialectical behavior therapy with and without the dialectical behavior therapy prolonged exposure protocol for suicidal and self-injuring women with borderline personality disorder and PTSD. *Behaviour Research and Therapy, 55,* 7–17.

Kliem, S., Kröger, C., & Kosfelder, J. (2010). Dialectical behavior therapy for borderline personality disorder: A meta-analysis using mixed-effects modeling. *Journal of Consulting and Clinical Psychology, 78*(6), 936–951.

Larimer, M., Marlatt, G. A., Baer, J., Quigley, L., Blume, A., & Hawkins, E. (1998). Harm reduction for alcohol problems. In G. A. Marlatt (Ed.), *Harm reduction: Pragmatic strategies for managing high-risk behaviors* (pp. 69–108). New York: Guilford Press.

Leichsenring, F., Leibing, E., Kruse, J., New, A. S., & Leweke, F. (2011). Borderline personality disorder. *The Lancet, 377,* 74–84.

Lievaart, M., Franken, I. H., & Hovens, J. E. (2016). Anger assessment in clinical and nonclinical populations: Further validation of the State–Trait Anger Expression Inventory–2. *Journal of Clinical Psychology, 72*(3), 263–278.

Linehan, M. M. (1993). *Cognitive-behavioral treatment of borderline personality disorder*. New York: Guilford Press.

Linehan, M. M. (2014). *DBT® skills training manual* (2nd ed.). New York: Guilford Press.

Linehan, M. M., Comtois, K. A., Brown, M. Z., Heard, H. L., & Wagner, A. (2006). Suicide Attempt Self-Injury Interview (SASII): Development, reliability, and validity of a scale to assess suicide attempts and intentional self-injury. *Psychological Assessment, 18*(3), 303–312.

Linehan, M. M., Comtois, K. A., & Ward-Ciesielski, E. F. (2012). Assessing and managing risk with suicidal individuals. *Cognitive and Behavioral Practice, 19*(2), 218–232.

Masuda, T., & Nisbett, R. E. (2001). Attending holistically versus analytically: Comparing the context sensitivity of Japanese and Americans. *Journal of Personality and Social Psychology, 81*(5), 922–934.

Pagura, J., Stein, M. B., Bolton, J. M., Cox, B. J., Grant, B., & Sareen, J. (2010). Comorbidity of borderline personality disorder and posttraumatic stress disorder in the US population. *Journal of Psychiatric Research, 44*(16), 1190–1198.

Peng, K., & Nisbett, R. E. (1999). Culture, dialectics, and reasoning about contradiction. *American Psychologist, 54*(9), 741–754.

Powers, M. B., Gillihan, S. J., Rosenfield, D., Jerud, A. B., & Foa, E. B. (2012). Reliability and validity of the PDS and PSS-I among participants with PTSD and alcohol dependence. *Journal of Anxiety Disorders, 26*(5), 617–623.

Preuss, U. W., Koller, G., Barnow, S., Eikmeier, M., & Soyka, M. (2006). Suicidal behavior in alcohol-dependent subjects: The role of personality disorders. *Alcoholism: Clinical and Experimental Research, 30*(5), 866–877.

Shelton, D., Sampl, S., Kesten, K. L., Zhang, W., & Trestman, R. L. (2009). Treatment of impulsive aggression in correctional settings. *Behavioral Sciences and the Law, 27*(5), 787–800.

Simon, T. R., Swann, A. C., Powell, K. E., Potter, L. B., Kresnow, M. J., & O'Carroll, P. W. (2002). Characteristics of impulsive suicide attempts and attempters. *Suicide and Life-Threatening Behavior, 32*(1, Suppl.), 49–59.

Skodol, A. E., & Bender, D. S. (2003). Why are women diagnosed borderline more than men? *Psychiatric Quarterly, 74*(4), 349–360.

Spielberger, C. D. (1999). *State–Trait Anger Expression Inventory–2 (STAXI-2) Professional manual.* Tampa, FL: Psychological Assessment Resources

Tomko, R. L., Trull, T. J., Wood, P. K., & Sher, K. J. (2014). Characteristics of borderline personality disorder in a community sample: Comorbidity, treatment utilization, and general functioning. *Journal of Personality Disorders, 28*(5), 734–750.

CHAPTER 16

Implementing Cognitive–Behavioral Therapy to Treat a Fear of Morphing in Obsessive–Compulsive Disorder

ROZ SHAFRAN
EVA ZYSK
TIM WILLIAMS

Joanne, in her late 30s, had suffered from symptoms of obsessive–compulsive disorder (OCD) since childhood. She recalled reading a biology textbook at about the age of 7 and having the sensation that she had not fully understood the passage. This sensation made her extremely anxious and she reread the passage until she was sure she fully understood it. Joanne's parents were not particularly academic, but Joanne had excelled at school. She had won prizes for both achievement and effort, and these had been valued by her parents, who had praised her for them. Joanne considered that they were extremely proud of her, and she felt she had let them down by failing to study at Oxford or Cambridge due to a poor exam grade. She had gone on to teacher training college and become a teacher, but she had a strong sense that she had not lived up to her potential. Although she was functioning at work, she was working excessive hours, was exhausted due to lack of sleep, and was constantly worried that she would make a mistake.

Joanne had been receiving therapy involving exposure and response prevention for OCD in a community setting but had not responded well to the intervention. She was referred to our program for expert treatment of OCD and had a specific interest in targeting some of her primary OCD symptoms. In our first meeting with Joanne, she expressed concerns that she might lose her intelligence and become immoral. She feared that if she stood near someone undesirable, then she could become like them through a negative atmosphere. She feared that she would become like them in terms of key aspects of herself (i.e., her intellect, morality, values, and emotional well-being) and that she could become physically diminished in terms of both her height and attractiveness. She believed she had to take every possible opportunity to maximize her potential and ensure a full understanding of whatever situation or conversation in which she participated. Joanne also had fears about a "reverse" process through which she could infect other people with her mood and thoughts, and others could take away her positive traits. She reported a strong belief in her thoughts but had insight that they were irrational, and they were not held with delusional intensity. Joanne also reported that she experienced a range of other co-occurring difficulties, including perfectionism (particularly focused on work), low mood, and generalized anxiety. She was markedly disorganized and had irregular patterns of sleeping and eating that impacted her performance at work.

Joanne shared that her first experience of treatment in adolescence comprised a lengthy period of psychological treatment based on exposure and response prevention (ERP). Given that many patients report having received ERP but in fact have not received the key aspects of ERP or an adequate dose (Stobie, Taylor, Quigley, Ewing, & Salkovskis, 2007) or it has not been delivered optimally (Gillihan, Williams, Malcoun, Yadin, & Foa, 2012), we asked Joanne detailed questions about her previous therapy. Her previous ERP had involved exposure hierarchies based solely on reducing repeated checking and washing. From her report, the treatment appeared to have been delivered well and in accordance with the key principles. Additional past therapies received on two occasions had included face-to-face counseling support based on reducing perfectionism and anxiety about work, telephone support, and fluoxetine for depression and anxiety. Joanne described all of these interventions as "very unhelpful." However, she clearly wanted help.

* * *

Many people consider cognitive-behavioral therapy (CBT) to be impersonal, stylized and unable to be tailored to an individual. One of us was horrified recently to hear a clinician say (rather proudly) that he had never had a client he could "make fit into those CBT boxes." However, a major aspect of CBT is being able to listen to what the client says and work together to see how one's knowledge base from theory and clinical practice can be married to the client's personal experience and viewpoint. With OCD, there are multiple challenges and rewards because it is such a heterogeneous disorder. One of its many forms that has been the focus of recent, growing clinical interest is known as mental contamination (Rachman, 2006; Rachman, Coughtrey, Shafran & Radomsky, 2015).

Mental contamination is the experience of feeling dirty and polluted despite the absence of physical contact with a contaminant. Unlike the traditional concept of *contact contamination,* in which contamination fears are evoked by direct physical contact with an item or place associated with disease, dirt, or harm, mental contamination evokes predominantly internal feelings of dirtiness and pollution; it often appears elusive, obscure, and intangible. Mental contamination and contact contamination regularly co-occur due to a number of overlapping features. In both forms clients report feelings of discomfort and dread that generate strong urges to wash, clean, and avoid recontamination. However, the key distinguishing feature is that mental contamination arises without physical contact with a contaminant. The primary

source of mental contamination is human rather than an object or substance, and clients feel they are uniquely vulnerable to the polluting effects of the contaminant.

There are different forms of mental contamination described in the literature, one of which is known as *morphing fear* (Rachman, 2006; Zysk, Shafran, Williams, & Melli, 2015). This form of mental contamination has also been referred to as *transformation obsessions* (Monzani et al., 2015; Volz & Heyman, 2007). It involves the worry that the person can be contaminated by or acquire unwanted mental, physical, or social characteristics from others. In extreme cases, patients even fear being changed into this "undesirable" person (Rachman, 2006). The impact of ERP on mental contamination in general, and on morphing fears in particular, has yet to be established. Joanne's previous treatment using ERP had, understandably, focused on reducing the compulsions and avoidance associated with morphing fears. However, they had not directly addressed the fear of morphing, and Joanne had not engaged well with ERP, which led us to think a more cognitive intervention might be helpful.

Joanne's primary symptoms of OCD, her co-occurring problems with low mood and perfectionism, and the lack of benefit associated with prior ERP created a clinical challenge, but one that was familiar to us. We were committed to doing evidence-based practice (EBP), but there was no clear evidence to guide our practice. A particular challenge was whether to focus on the low mood, the perfectionism, or the mental contamination. Joanne was clear that she wished to address the contamination and felt that was the cause of her low mood, anxiety, and perfectionism. We conducted our work with Joanne as part of a broader program of research at our University that was specifically aimed at (1) developing a measure to assess the fear of morphing and (2) evaluating CBT for the fear of morphing. Treatment with Joanne was provided by the first author (Shafran), an experienced clinical psychologist and cognitive therapist. Each session was audiotaped. Therapy was conducted around a large high table to facilitate shared reviewing of documents, without the typical uncomfortable crouching around a low coffee table. In this chapter, we describe our work with Joanne to illustrate the ways in which we implement EBP, specifically using the five steps as articulated by Spring, Marchese, and Steglitz (Chapter 1, this volume). More details about the case and treatment can be found elsewhere (Zysk, Shafran & Williams, 2018).[1]

The Five Steps of EBP in Action with Joanne

Step 1: Asking Clinically Informative Questions

Assessment comprised standard clinical interview questions about the reasons for referral, current difficulties, development of the difficulties, current functioning, past history of treatment, family situations and responses, and treatment goals. Given Joanne's low mood, a risk assessment was also conducted, in which she expressed occasional suicidal ideation but no plans to harm herself and an optimism that treatment would help her difficulties. In addition, a broad assessment of mental contamination was conducted. The assessment of mental contamination in a clinical interview seeks to elicit information about the extent to which the contamination arises in the absence of contact and is persistent, and seeks to establish the nature by which contamination is acquired and spread (Coughtrey, Shafran, & Bennett, 2017). Unlike contact contamination, the source of mental contamination is typically human, and that there is some aspect of "unique vulnerability" in which the patient feels that he or she would become polluted/infected in the presence of the contaminant but that others would not be affected. For example, standing near a "stupid" person made Joanne fear that she would be vulnerable to losing her intellect, but if the therapist was standing near the same person, his or her intellect would be unaffected. Mental contamination is also often associated with moral violations, which are discussed in the assessment (Rachman, 2006). Given the nature of mental contamination and previous treatment protocols that outline key differences between standard CBT and CBT for mental contamination (cf. Coughtrey, Shafran, Lee, & Rachman, 2013), the following areas were assessed:

1. *Understanding the current problem and its impact in detail.* Joanne was asked for a specific and recent example of her morphing fear to elicit thoughts, feelings, and counterproductive behaviors (e.g., "What do you do when you are near someone that you consider has the potential to make you a weak or inferior person?"). Joanne gave the recent example of being in a

_____
[1] The case in that paper is referred to as "James."

nightclub and standing near some women who were scantily and provocatively dressed. She said she felt that they were immoral, and that she had become immoral by being in the same nightclub as such people. This indicated to the therapist that Joanne found it difficult to distinguish between her fear of becoming immoral and her belief that she was immoral or had already become immoral by being near particular people.

2. *The source(s) of contamination,* in particular human sources and hypervigilance to these sources. This included asking questions about how her vulnerability to morphing would operate. When Joanne described taking on the undesirable characteristics of others, she was asked, "How would that happen?" Some of the responses sounded reasonably rational on the surface (e.g., "If I am in a negative mood, then that brings everyone down"), but had a large amount of magical thinking (e.g., "It is like their characteristics permeate my skin"). When asked by the therapist, "What would happen if *I* were in conflict and contact with someone who was morally questionable?", Joanne replied, "Nothing," but when the question was directed at herself, Joanne replied, "I could become like them." When asked to explain this discrepancy, she responded, "You don't believe it could happen, so it couldn't, but because I believe it, then it makes it able to be so." This was a clear illustration of Joanne's sense of unique vulnerability.

3. *History.* A detailed history of the development of the problem, such as time and speed of onset, and the client's understanding of the issue is common in psychological treatment, but it is particularly important for mental contamination. Specifically, Joanne was asked, "How do you make sense of the problem?"; "If that had happened to someone else, do you think they would become contaminated?"; "What was happening in your life when the problem first started?"; and "What do you fear would be the worst outcome?" Trying to understand the relationship between Joanne's checking behavior, contamination fears, and fear of morphing was difficult, but we hypothesized that Joanne was checking to ensure that she did not become another person, that she retained her morality, and that her intellect was fully intact.

4. *Psychological violations and betrayals.* Rachman (2010) has identified previous or cur-

rent physical and psychological violations and betrayals as critical in the development of contamination fears. We began by asking Joanne, "Can you tell me about anyone who has been particularly helpful to you? What were their characteristics?" before moving on to questions such as "Can you tell me about anyone who has been particularly unhelpful to you? You don't have to identify them if you don't wish to. What were their characteristics?" In Joanne's case, the therapist sought to understand the association between any betrayal and the current presenting issues around becoming a negative person. Joanne's responses revealed her perception that her parents were highly critical with regard her failure to achieve high standards and, even more importantly, failing to live up to her potential.

5. *Spread of contamination.* As is standard, Joanne was asked about the nature of the spread of mental contamination. She was asked, "Do new items/persons/places ever become contaminated? How do they become contaminated?" Her responses painted a picture of places becoming contaminated if she had had a conflict there, or if immoral or underachieving people had been present in that place. She subsequently avoided those places.

6. *Mental imagery.* Joanne was asked, "Are there any pictures that cause you to feel contaminated?" This also included questions about protective images—"Are there any pictures in your mind that you use to protect yourself?" In response to these questions, Joanne revealed that she often ruminated after a perceived conflict or after being near someone who was immoral or had failed to live up to his or her potential. Such rumination was mostly verbal and not in the form of pictures in her head, and Joanne would subsequently feel the need to engage in action (typically walking for hours at a time) in order to clear her head and ensure she had not lost any of her intellectual capacity. She did not have any protective imagery.

7. *Avoidance.* Joanne was asked questions about her avoidance of people, places, and situations, along with questions about cognitive avoidance (e.g., "Is there anything that you avoid thinking about?"). For Joanne, a lack of contemplation of current affairs and deep philosophical questions such as the meaning of life and what happens when you die would indicate that she had lost her intellectual capacity. She

therefore actively engaged in thinking about these issues, although, paradoxically, they triggered questions about her intellectual capacity and whether she had lived up to her potential, thereby causing her further distress. Establishing the range of people, places, and situations she avoided behaviorally was straightforward.

8. *Compulsive washing and checking, and other behavioral responses.* Joanne was asked about the nature, frequency, and intensity of her washing and checking behavior in detail. As is typical with washing behavior in mental contamination, any relief from washing was transient; Joanne still felt dirty after conflict, and she was articulate in describing how the washing of her skin did not alleviate the "dirtiness from my mind." Her repetitive checking of her height and appearance in the mirror to establish whether she had physically changed was assessed in depth. She was asked, "How often do you look in the mirror?"; "Where are the mirrors in your house?"; "What sizes are the mirrors?"; "Can you see all of yourself in the mirror?"; "What parts of yourself do you look at when you look in the mirror?"; "How long do you spend looking in the mirror?"; and "How do you feel when you look in the mirror?" At first, the question of whether Joanne had comorbid body dysmorphic disorder (BDD) was raised in the therapist's mind, but despite a resemblance to some features of BDD, the difficulties were considered to be better explained as related to her OCD, in part because they were not held with delusional intensity. Joanne was also asked about her walking behavior, as she had described solitary walking "to clear her head." She walked for 3–4 hours a night, usually after midnight, which was considered both risky to her safety and unhelpful to her daily routine and general well-being. This late-night walking resulted in her feeling chronically tired and impacted her work; she would often miss work due to tiredness and sleep throughout the day.

9. *Other difficulties.* Joanne described difficulties with the following areas: perfectionism, chronic worry, depression, and anxiety in social situations.

To enhance the clinical interview component of our assessment process, we used a range of standardized measures. In selecting what measures to use, we were guided by the following principles and priorities.

1. *Morphing Fear Questionnaire* (MFQ; Zysk et al., 2015). This measure assesses the presence and severity of morphing fears. Joanne's score of 29 indicated high morphing fear. Her responses to this measure also were consistent with responses of patients with OCD, more so than patients with anxiety or depression only.

2. *Vancouver Obsessional Compulsive Inventory—Mental Contamination* Scale (VOCI-MC; Rachman, 2006). Joanne's score on this 20-item measure was 59, and she scored high on items such as "Certain people or places that make me feel dirty or contaminated leave everyone else completely unaffected." Her scores were higher than the mean of patients with general contamination fears (Radomsky, Rachman, Shafran, Coughtrey, & Barber, 2014).

3. *Obsessive–Compulsive Inventory—Revised* (OCI-R; Foa et al., 2002). Joanne scored 52 before treatment, which indicated high levels of general OCD symptoms, including those relating to checking and washing compulsions (e.g., "I wash my hands more often and longer than necessary").

4. *Beck Anxiety Inventory* (BAI; Beck & Steer, 1990). Joanne's score of 24 was similar to the clinical mean of 25 in those with a primary anxiety disorder (Beck, Epstein, Brown, & Steer, 1988) and higher than nonclinical norms (Creamer, Foran, & Bell, 1995; Gillis, Haaga, & Ford, 1995).

5. *Beck Depression Inventory–II* (BDI-II; Beck, Steer, & Brown, 1996). Joanne was significantly depressed, with a mean score of 42—approximately twice as high as the clinical mean for those with depression, which is 21.9 (Beck et al., 1996).

6. *Yale–Brown Obsessive Compulsive Scale* (Y–BOCS; Goodman, Price, Rasmussen, Mazure, Delgado, et al., 1989; Goodman, Price, Rasmussen, Mazure, Fleischmann, et al., 1989). Joanne's score of 31 using this "gold standard" assessment measure indicated that she had significant OCD (Tolin, Abramowitz, & Diefenbach, 2005).

7. *Visual Analogue Scales* (VAS). We constructed a series of 10-cm VAS to measure self-report ratings of anxiety, feelings of general contamination, feelings of internal contamination, and washing and neutralizing urges/behaviors, ranging from *Not at all* to *Extremely.*

The VAS comprised eight scales, four of which ask the patient to rate current symptoms, and four of which ask about symptoms over the previous week. VAS are sensitive to clinical change (cf. McCormack, Horne, & Sheather, 1988), and data collected using VAS have been shown to be reliable and valid (Reips & Funke, 2008). These VAS were used each session due to the importance of monitoring treatment progress and improving outcome (Egan & Hine, 2008; Lambert et al., 2001).

Step 2: Acquiring the Best Available Research Evidence

The National Institute for Health and Care Excellence (NICE; *www.nice.org*) is a U.K. government body that provides evidence-based guidance for a range of health and social care issues. Its website additionally provides a range of evidence-based services, including a search for evidence and access to journals and databases. While we would like to think that it is the first port of call for the majority of practicing clinicians in the United Kingdom, our own research indicates that research evidence is not the primary source of information when it comes to decision making (Gyani, Shafran, Myles, & Rose, 2014) and NICE guidelines for the treatment of OCD are largely ignored in primary care (Gyani, Shafran, & Rose, 2012).

Nevertheless, the guidelines produced for the treatment of OCD (Clinical Guideline 31, published in 2005 [*www.nice.org.uk/guidance/cg31*] and updated in 2015) state that adults such as Joanne, who have moderate functional impairment and have not responded to less intensive (fewer than 10 therapist sessions) CBT (including ERP), should be offered the choice of either a course of an selective serotonin reuptake inhibitor (SSRI) or more intensive CBT (including ERP) because these treatments appear to be comparably efficacious.

These guidelines are clear; however, our dilemma was that an adequate dose of both of these treatments had been tried previously without success. Furthermore, we questioned the extent to which the clinical trials on which the research evidence was based were designed to inform the care of people like Joanne with mental contamination. Thus, while Joanne clearly met criteria for OCD, it was unclear to what extent the evidence generalizes to this particular type of OCD, let alone to morphing fears.

We decided to consult the primary literature

by searching journals using search terms such as transformation obsessions, morphing, mental contamination, and *treatment-refractory OCD*. We also searched using U.S. terms such as *empirically supported treatments for OCD*. We used Google Scholar for these searches rather than Science Direct or any journals that require a University subscription/pass. The reasons we used Google Scholar first were (1) ease of searching, (2) ease of obtaining the paper, and (3) ease of communicating with our clinical colleagues. We then also searched PubMed and Science Direct. Given the rarity of the problem, we also looked at U.K. Charity websites for OCD such as *OCD-UK* and *Obsessive Action*. The reason for this is that we felt there may be people with similar issues who were sharing their personal stories of treatment. It was from that search that the term *emotional obsessions* was identified as being used in the same way as morphing fears or transformation obsessions (Hevia, 2009). We therefore reran our literature searches, adding this new term. Although we did not discover much more than we had identified previously, it was helpful to understand the different ways in which the same construct was being labeled and identified.

As a final additional step, we contacted our colleagues working in this field (there are not many of us!) to seek additional advice and information as to other sources of evidence, including their personal experience of treating such cases. The conversation took the form of an informal supervision in which we presented the problem and the clinical dilemmas, then asked for guidance about how to conduct an evidence-informed intervention. This was a helpful process in that it necessitated synthesizing and summarizing a complex case and to formulate a clear question to guide treatment. After receiving useful advice and formulating a treatment plan, we then stopped our thorough search.

Step 3: Appraising the Evidence Critically

It is hard to objectively and critically appraise the evidence after having worked in the field for so long and being so close to the topic. It is also challenging to objectively reconcile the presenting issues with the research literature. For this reason, the first and second authors, Shafran and Zysk, first discussed the treatment plan and approach based on the available literature, then in supervision with Williams, the third author. This may by some be labeled as reassurance seeking but perhaps it can be considered best clinical practice (!). Williams was able to bring in a different angle from the viewpoint of a practitioner who treated younger people with OCD and magical thinking/thought–action fusion, providing a developmental perspective to treatment. Such a perspective draws attention to the both the strengths and weaknesses of the existing literature.

We reviewed the main large clinical trials to establish whether it was likely that they included or excluded people with morphing fears but were left unsure. It is possible that someone with Joanne's difficulties of mental contamination and morphing could have been misunderstood as having delusions (in particular, the belief that she could physically change in stature) and therefore be excluded from the majority of trials. Certainly, there was no mention of Joanne's problem in the large randomized controlled trials (RCTs), and even if people like her were included, we had no information about the extent to which the treatments were helpful, specifically, in addressing the nature of her concerns.

The literature that appeared most relevant was the description of treatment from Rachman (2006), existing case series with younger people on transformation obsessions (Volz & Heyman, 2007), our own case series on mental contamination (Coughtrey et al., 2013) and the case study of Hevia (2009). These sources emphasized that there is much about standard unadapted CBT that could and should be used to treat Joanne, but that some specific additional interventions might be warranted if Joanne failed to respond to the existing interventions.

It was not a difficult decision to decide to use CBT including some ERP based on the literature. What *was* difficult was planning how best to use the exposure tasks. Their traditional use involves creating a graded hierarchy based the view that patients' anxiety habituates with repeated exposure and therefore decreases over time. We were not inclined to use this model because it had been unsuccessful with Joanne previously and did not capture the nature of her presenting issues. Moreover, the habituation model is based on an outdated learning model rather than an empirically based one of inhibitory learning (Craske, Treanor, Conway, Zbozinek, & Vervliet, 2014), which provides multiple ways of optimizing exposure (e.g., by focusing on expectancy violation). Thus, in considering the cognitive nature of the presenting problem, the lack of cognitive input into previous treatments, the clinical guidance from NICE, the case series emphasizing behavioral experiments in the treatment of mental contamination (Coughtrey et al., 2013), and the literature showing equivalence between CBT and ERP (for a review, see Öst, Havnen, Hansen, & Kvale, 2015), we decided to offer a cognitively focused CBT with an emphasis on behavioral experiments incorporating some exposure to test beliefs. Our treatment manual served as a starting point and overall guide (Rachman et al., 2015).

Our use of CBT with an emphasis on behavioral experiments would specifically address Joanne's fear of morphing. However, Joanne was also experiencing a wide range of related co-occurring difficulties, including low mood, perfectionism, and disorganization/lack of structure, all of which were impacting her work and daily functioning. We faced what is perhaps the most common clinical dilemma in practice—how to address comorbidity. It is truly baffling (and scandalous) that psychological treatments, trials, and guidance historically focus on one specific diagnosis, yet estimates indicate that 45% of those with mental health problems have multiple disorders (Kessler, Chiu, Demler, & Walters, 2005), and this figure rises to 62% among people with OCD (Torres et al., 2006).

The comorbidity of mental disorders and the lack of literature on how to address them presents a critical dilemma about implementing evidence-based treatment. It is the problem of comorbidity that is partially responsible for the surge of interest in "transdiagnostic" treatments for anxiety disorders, such as those developed by David Barlow (Farchione et al., 2012) and Peter Norton (McEvoy, Nathan, & Norton, 2009). However, this research is in its relative infancy. Two alternatives to the transdiagnostic approach are to sequence interventions or to apply multiple different evidence-based protocols simultaneously. There is little literature to guide such clinical decision making, and nothing existed that was specifically relevant to Joanne's case.

We expanded our search to consider relevant studies that addressed anxiety problems broadly. Two studies related to the treatment of comorbidity seemed to be potentially informative for Joanne's treatment plan. The first indicated that remaining focused on CBT for

panic disorder may be more beneficial for both principal and comorbid diagnoses than combining CBT for panic disorder with "straying" to CBT for comorbid disorders (Craske et al., 2007). The second was a subanalysis from an RCT on depression, which found that more time and effort spent addressing anxiety in session predicted less improvement in both depression and anxiety over the course of treatment (Gibbons & DeRubeis, 2008). Taken together, we concluded from this research that it is better to focus on one problem than to become distracted by providing multiple interventions or drifting from the main focus of therapy, and our own subsequent work in the United Kingdom supports that decision (Shafran, Wroe, Nagra, Pissaridou, & Coughtrey, 2018).

In summary, it was clear that there was a need to synthesize the key information in the literature with the realities of Joanne's experience. Joanne had not responded to ERP or psychopharmacology previously. She had an unusual form of OCD that had not been well researched, and it was unclear whether this form had been included in trials. Furthermore, there was a great deal of comorbidity on which the literature failed to provide adequate guidance in the treatment of such a case. It was also notable that the Joanne's current behavior was exhausting her; not only was such exhaustion leading to practical problems with regard to her work, but we also recognized that it could be an issue for implementing treatment strategies. A final consideration was the need to balance the potential benefit and harm of the intervention and, as with our other patients, we considered it essential to keep a record of any potential adverse events resulting from therapy. After consideration of the available evidence with regard to the treatment of OCD in general, mental contamination, nonresponsiveness to interventions, addressing comorbidity, and the urgent need to help Joanne improve her functioning at work for both psychological and practical reasons, we opted to do the following:

1. Focus on addressing morphing fears rather than adopting a transdiagnostic approach, but briefly and regularly monitor other concerns (in particular, mood, perfectionism, and worry).
2. Use CBT with a heavily cognitive focus, in which Joanne's key maladaptive cognitions would be challenged, alongside behavioral experiments incorporating exposure to help

challenge fears, as with other cases of mental contamination.

3. Use session-by-session measurement to evaluate specific, measurable goals such as reduction of compulsive acts and having a better routine to help reduce number of days off work.

Step 4: Applying the Evidence

We met with Joanne twice weekly for the first 2 weeks in order to maximize momentum, then moved to a weekly then fortnightly schedule for the majority of treatment and toward the end as part of relapse prevention work. Fifteen sessions were provided in total over a 24-week period. The sessions did not start with setting an agenda as is often the case; instead we began by reviewing homework before setting the agenda, as has been done in the treatment of eating disorders for many years (Wilson, Fairburn, & Agras, 1997). This is a personal choice, but is used so that items arising from the homework can be easily incorporated into the agenda, and the homework is the very first thing asked about in treatment, which helps convey its importance. Below, we describe the major treatment strategies we used with Joanne. Some interventions took place in a single session (e.g., formulation), whereas others, particularly behavioral experiments, were conducted across multiple sessions.

Formulation

A devised individualized formulation of the maintenance of Joanne's problem was based on the theory of mental contamination (Rachman, 2006) and an appraisal-based cognitive-behavioral model of OCD. The formulation focused on triggers of mental contamination, beliefs relating to contamination, and maintaining behaviors (e.g., compulsive washing and avoidance). A historical formulation was also constructed to help Joanne make sense of the problem (Beck, 1976). This historical formulation focused on her early experiences, any critical incidents, and beliefs that arose from those. Joanne reiterated that the key memory of failing to understand a biology textbook at age 7 was a pivotal moment in the development of her difficulties, and that her early experiences revolved around schoolwork and performance at school. She said she had "always" considered her self-worth to be contingent on academic achievement and that doing well was "who I am." Joanne's

maintenance formulation is shown in Figure 16.1. This initial formulation evolved over time.

Psychoeducation

Psychoeducation was provided in the first session about mental contamination in general and morphing fears in particular, for example, about the stability of characteristics and the possibility of transference of qualities. The distinction between mental and contact contamination was made, with particular emphasis on the human source of contamination and personal vulnerability. An illustration of the psychoeducation is as follows:

"Most work has been done on understanding and treating the feelings of dirtiness that come from touching something that is considered contaminated or dirty—for example, touching dog mess. Everyone would agree that if anyone touches dog mess, then it is important to wash one's hands to stop it from spreading and get rid of any germs there may be. Mental contamination has only recently been identified as a type of OCD in which the same feelings of dirtiness are experienced, not from touching something that is considered dirty but instead from one's own thoughts, from being near particular types of people, or even from seeing something, similar to the symptoms you report. In mental contamination, the source of the dirtiness is often a person rather than a particular object/thing. Also, in mental contamination, people often feel that they alone can become contaminated from the thoughts or being near certain types of people, or seeing things, and that other people are unaffected. People with OCD who have mental contamination very often have contact contamination, too—there is a lot of overlap between the two forms."

Some psychoeducation was provided about the mislabeling of mood states (i.e., feeling "dirty" or "diminished" rather than "anxious"); differentiating among thoughts, feelings and facts; the connection between mood and visual perception, based on work in eating disorders; and biases such as thought–action fusion and ex-consequentia reasoning. The role of hypervigilance and selective attention was also discussed with regard to seeking internal evidence of retention of intellect. More general psychoeducation about the importance of sleep and the

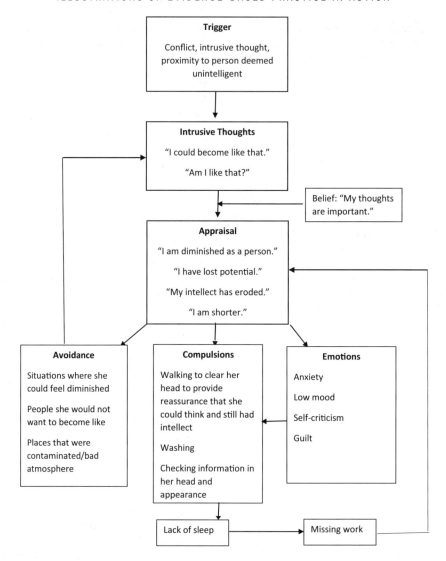

FIGURE 16.1. A formulation of the maintenance of Joanne's difficulties.

relationship between sleep, mood, and intrusions was provided.

Monitoring

Joanne was asked to keep a record in real time of her triggers, intrusions, appraisals, and behavior, and to reflect on these at the end of each day. An example is on next page.

Behavioral Experiments

A range of behavioral experiments were conducted to test Joanne's beliefs that she "lost in-

tellect" or became shorter as a result of being near, or in conflict with, people she perceived to be immoral. Joanne was asked to take a photograph of herself next to a height chart before and after such interactions. Together, in session, we showed these photos to colleagues and asked them to "spot the difference" in terms of her physical appearance, with Joanne predicting that people would see her as shorter and less intelligent in the "after" picture. This was not the case. We did behavioral experiments to see what would happen if Joanne had a relaxing bath instead of walking after fearing that she had lost her intellect. We operationalized "los-

Situation	Trigger	Intrusion	Appraisal	Behavior	Reflection
With a friend	Argument	Need to drop the argument	Need to understand where the argument went wrong to ensure I understand	Needing to bridge the argument in head and recall sentences; otherwise, I will be diminished	Angry at myself, as I knew it wouldn't make a difference

ing intellect" and "losing potential" by using time to complete a crossword as a proxy for intellectual performance.

Addressing the Meaning of Morphing

We addressed the meaning of morphing into an "unintelligent" person who, for example, could not produce a coherent argument based on logic, by discussing the relationship among diminished intellect, reduced stature, and quality of life. Joanne was asked to construct a pie chart of the multifaceted nature of her personality to help broaden her sense of self-identity (based on Fairburn's [1995] self-evaluation pie chart for treatment of eating disorders). The role of self-perceptions is of increasing interest and relevance to contamination fears (Doron, Sar-El, & Mikulincer, 2012), and addressing these fears via information gathering and consideration of self-identify can be helpful; such interventions are not considered "reassurance seeking," as they are not providing repeated assurances but rather are about exploring the construct of self-identity. The permanent nature of Joanne's personality in terms of a dislike for Marmite (a type of sandwich spread made from yeast extract) and country music was reviewed to help strengthen her identity, and we asked people close to her who have known her many years, such as her parents, to list her immutable characteristics. Asking her parents to help with treatment also assisted in decreasing Joanne's secrecy and encouraged her to confide in others. She had been reluctant to confide in her parents for fear that they would be critical and confirm her view that she was less successful than her siblings. In fact, her parents revealed they had suspected Joanne was struggling for many years but did not know what the struggle was about or how to help her. They assured her that her job was worthwhile, and that they were proud of her for being a teacher.

Imagery

Imagery was a not a significant issue for Joanne and was not a central focus on treatment.

Relapse Prevention

In the final two sessions, with the aid of the therapist, Joanne devised a relapse prevention plan reviewing what was done in treatment, what she found to be useful, how to distinguishing between a lapse and relapse, and how to spot the early signs of a relapse. She was asked to consider the main message of therapy and to summarize this in a format akin to a "tweet." Joanne's tweet was "Not everything you do is a statement," which was not exactly what the therapist had in mind (!) but, on talking it through, Joanne explained it meant that she needed to remember that she could just be herself. Given the broad emphasis of the intervention that had included work on depression and perfectionism in the latter stages of treatment, Joanne's explanation and tweet made sense. The impact of reducing the compulsive walking on her exhaustion and increasing her attendance at work was a key aspect of the relapse prevention work.

Step 5: Analyzing the Effects and Adjusting Practice

We measured the effects of our interventions throughout our work with Joanne. Her outcome using standardized measures (Table 16.1) and her session-by-session VAS (Figure 16.2) indicated that the intervention had been highly successful at addressing her fear of morphing and scores on the other measures, including depression and anxiety, had significantly reduced. However, she was still experiencing some symptoms of mental contamination, OCD, and fluctuating anxiety more broadly.

TABLE 16.1. Outcomes of Standardized Measures Collected over Five Assessments

Week no.	Treatment stage	ADIS-IV diagnoses	Y-BOCS	MFQ	VOCI-MC	OCI-R	BAI	BDI-II
0	Assessment	OCD, depression, mild social phobia, mild GAD	31	29	59	52	24	42
9	Start of treatment	OCD, depression, mild social phobia, GAD	27	28	56	37	12	43
20	Midtreatment (Session 10)	OCD, depression, mild social phobia, GAD	27	10	N/A	N/A	N/A	N/A
28	Midtreatment (Session 13)	Mild OCD, mild social phobia, mild GAD	20	3	13	12	4	18
36	End of treatment (Session 15)	Mild OCD, mild GAD	14	1	37	15	4	2

Note. GAD, generalized anxiety disorder; OCD, obsessive–compulsive disorder.

Reflecting on our work with Joanne and her progress over time highlights some intriguing questions about the intervention process. It might have been helpful to have given the Obsessive Beliefs Questionnaire (Obsessive Compulsive Cognitions Working Group, 2003) to assess perfectionist beliefs within the context of OCD. Understanding perfectionism would have helped guide the treatment intervention. It might have been helpful to incorporate some of the burgeoning work on self-identify in OCD (Doron et al., 2012) and possibly self-compassion (Gilbert, 2009). However, even as we are thinking of that, we know that our enthusiasm for such methods should not go too far ahead of the empirical support for these interventions (both generally and in the context of mental contamination). We also want to keep an eye on the great risk of therapist drift (Waller, 2009). By trying to do too much, it is possible that we would have risked achieving very little. We believe that the behavioral experiments were essential ingredients of Joanne's care, allowing us to address the cognitive and behavioral components of Joanne's difficulties, without getting caught up in prolonged and ultimately futile philosophical debates with her. It is also striking how more mundane aspects of work, such as ensuring that Joanne got sleep, are so often neglected in case presentations and research outcomes. Without such fundamentals, it is hard to see how therapy can get off the ground.

Summary

One of the joys (and challenges) of working with OCD is the heterogeneity of the disorder. It requires drawing on wide-ranging expertise and information. We had a head start in working previously with patients with fear of morphing and with OCD generally; also, some of our previous expertise on the treatment of eating disorders and mirror checking proved particularly helpful for Joanne. At the same time, having knowledge of the treatment of perfectionism made it tempting to "drift" from the focus on morphing and try to address multiple problems simultaneously—even though there is no empirical support for doing this, and some data even indicate that it may be unhelpful.

The reality of clinical practice is that time is very pressured, and clinicians are required to make decisions about how to proceed in the face of great complexity and partial evidence. There often is a lack of time to gather the research evidence and reflect on one's clinical practice, then incorporate patient values and preferences, and revise the plan. It is challenging to create time to for deliberation and reflection. Without this, however, CBT can become impersonal, rote, and rigid. Also, even when one has made sound decisions in collaboration with the client and is guided by the literature, it is easy to get off track. Recognizing this chal-

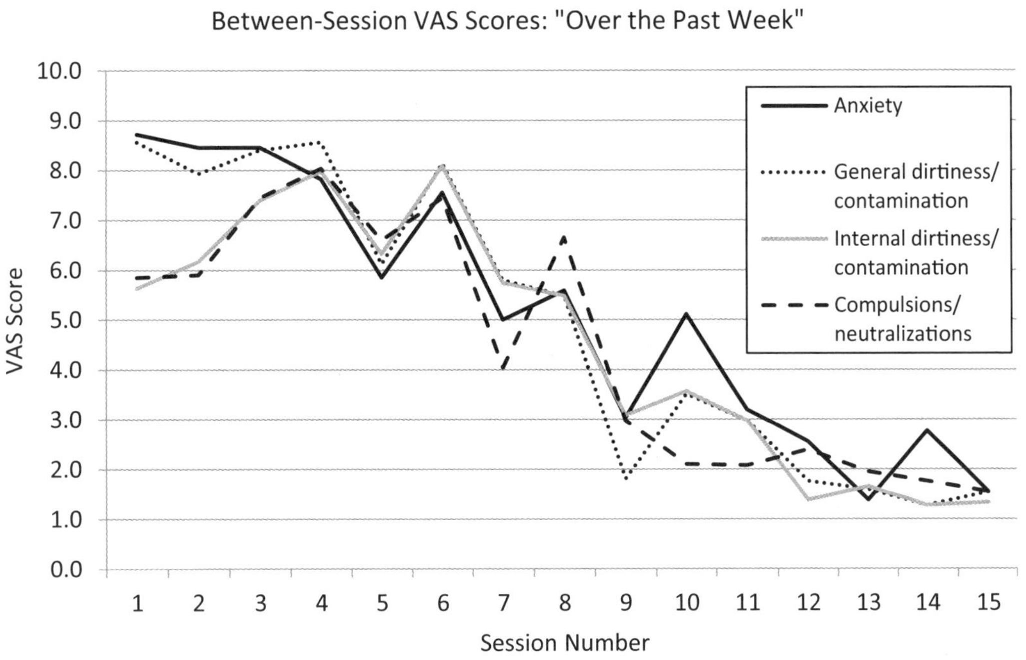

Between-Session VAS Scores: "Over the Past Week"

FIGURE 16.2. Session-by-session VAS measures for treatment targets.

lenging context, we offer the following key pieces of advice:

1. Balance "flexibility" with "fidelity." Kendall's description of how to apply evidence-based treatment flexibly but with fidelity to a protocol is unsurpassed (e.g., Kendall & Beidas, 2007). Take these principles with you and enjoy the creativity that such an approach gives within the safety of an empirically supported approach.

2. Keep it simple. Maintain your focus on the main presenting problem, but monitor symptoms that are not the immediate focus of the intervention.

3. If you are recording your sessions, take a couple of minutes at the end to reflect on the session and plan for the next one. It really is worth it. Play that small section back at the beginning of your next session. Chris Fairburn taught us this, and it has been an invaluable tool. We used it in each session of our work with Joanne.

4. Use supervision well. Prepare for it properly by scheduling preparation time in your diary, keeping meaningful notes about the is-

sues arising from supervision and thinking through your chosen supervision question. Discuss the research literature with one another, particularly when the supervisor has a different perspective. Doing this was also key in our work with Joanne.

5. Collaboration and curiosity are essential. Humor helps if it is used appropriately, and genuine curiosity about the client's experience is a must. If you think you are losing that curiosity, it is time to step back and reflect on reasons why.

There will never be an evidence base for each individual variant of OCD, so knowing how to acquire and extrapolate from the existing data are essential skills, as we have illustrated in this chapter. Also, knowing how to apply interventions in flexible and personalized ways is critical. In fact, in our view, the most pressing research priority is providing an evidence base on how to address multiple co-occurring difficulties. Given the high proportion of comorbidities between disorders, the lack of data is truly appalling. Such information would be of benefit to the large proportion of clients who currently do not receive evidence-based treatments (Lilienfeld et al., 2013) or who fail to respond to existing interventions (e.g., Loerinc et al., 2015).

References

Beck, A. T. (1976). *Cognitive therapy and the emotional disorders.* New York: International Universities Press.

Beck, A. T., Epstein, N., Brown, G., & Steer, R. A. (1988). An inventory for measuring clinical anxiety: Psychometric properties. *Journal of Consulting and Clinical Psychology, 56,* 893–897.

Beck, A. T., & Steer, R. A. (1990). *Beck Anxiety Inventory manual.* San Antonio, TX: Psychological Corporation.

Beck, A. T., Steer, R. A., & Brown, G. K. (1996). *Manual for the Beck Depression Inventory–II.* San Antonio, TX: Psychological Corporation.

Coughtrey, A., Shafran, R., & Bennett, S. (2017). Mental contamination. In J. Abramowitz, D. McKay, & E. Storch (Eds.), *The Wiley handbook of obsessive-compulsive disorders* (Vol. 1, pp. 457–473). Hoboken, NJ: Wiley Blackwell.

Coughtrey, A. E., Shafran, R., Lee, M., & Rachman, S. J. (2013). The treatment of mental contamination: A case series. *Cognitive and Behavioral Practice, 20*(2), 221–231.

Craske, M. G., Farchione, T. J., Allen, L. B., Barrios, V., Stoyanova, M., & Rose, R. (2007). Cognitive behavioral therapy for panic disorder and comorbidity: More of the same or less of more? *Behaviour Research and Therapy, 45*(6), 1095–1109.

Craske, M. G., Treanor, M., Conway, C. C., Zbozinek, T., & Vervliet, B. (2014). Maximizing exposure therapy: An inhibitory learning approach. *Behaviour Reseach and Therapy, 58,* 10–23.

Creamer, M., Foran, J., & Bell, R. (1995). The Beck Anxiety Inventory in a non-clinical sample. *Behaviour Research and Therapy, 33,* 477–485.

Doron, G., Sar-El, D., & Mikulincer, M. (2012). Threats to moral self-perceptions trigger obsessive compulsive contamination-related behavioral tendencies. *Journal of Behavior Therapy and Experimental Psychiatry, 43,* 884–890.

Egan, S. J., & Hine, P. (2008). Cognitive behavioural treatment of perfectionism: A single case experimental design series. *Behaviour Change, 25*(4), 245–258.

Fairburn, C. G. (1995). *Overcoming binge eating.* New York: Guilford Press.

Farchione, T. J., Fairholme, C. P., Ellard, K. K., Boisseau, C. L., Thompson-Hollands, J., Carl, J. R., et al. (2012). The unified protocol for the transdiagnostic treatment of emotional disorders: A randomized controlled trial. *Behavior Therapy, 3,* 666–678.

Foa, E. B., Huppert, J. D., Leiberg, S., Langner, R., Kichic, R., Hajcak, G., et al. (2002). The Obsessive-Compulsive Inventory: Development and validation of a short version. *Psychological Assessment, 14*(4), 485–496.

Gibbons, C. J., & DeRubeis, R. J. (2008). Anxiety symptom focus in sessions of cognitive therapy for depression. *Behavior Therapy, 39,* 117–125.

Gilbert, P. (2009). Introducing compassion-focused therapy. *Advances in Psychiatric Treatment, 15*(3), 199–208.

Gillihan, S. J., Williams, M. T., Malcoun, E., Yadin, E., & Foa, E. B. (2012). Common pitfalls in exposure and response prevention (EX/RP) for OCD. *Journal of Obsessive–Compulsive and Related Disorders, 1*(4), 251–257.

Gillis, M. M., Haaga, D. A. F., & Ford, G. T. (1995). Normative values for the Beck Anxiety Inventory, Fear Questionnaire, Penn State Worry Questionnaire, and Social Phobia Anxiety Inventory. *Psychological Assessment, 7,* 450–455.

Goodman, W. K., Price, L. H., Rasmussen, S. A., Mazure, C., Delgado, P., Heninger, G. R., & Charney, D. S. (1989). The Yale–Brown Obsessive Compulsive Scale: II. Validity. *Archives of General Psychiatry, 46,* 1012–1016.

Goodman, W. K., Price, L. H., Rasmussen, S. A., Mazure, C., Fleischmann, R. L., Hill, C. L., et al. (1989). The Yale–Brown Obsessive Compulsive Scale: I. Development, use, and reliability. *Archives of General Psychiatry, 46,* 1006–1011.

Gyani, A., Shafran, R., Myles, P., & Rose, S. (2014). The gap between science and practice: How therapists make their clinical decisions. *Behavior Therapy, 45*(2), 199–211.

Gyani, A., Shafran, R., & Rose, S. (2012). Are the NICE guidelines for OCD being used in primary care? *Primary Health Care Research and Development, 13,* 92–97.

Hevia, C. (2009). Emotional contamination: A lesser known subtype of OCD. *OCD Newsletter, 23*(4), 10–12.

Kendall, P. C., & Beidas, R. S. (2007). Smoothing the trail for dissemination of evidence-based practices for youth: Flexibility within fidelity. *Professional Psychology: Research and Practice, 38,* 13–19.

Kessler, R. C., Chiu, W. T., Demler, O., & Walters, E. E. (2005). Prevalence, severity, and comorbidity of 12-month DSM-IV disorders in the National Comorbidity Survey Replication. *Archives of General Psychiatry, 62,* 617–627.

Lambert, M. J., Whipple, J. L., Smart, D. W., Vermeersch, D. A., Nielsen, S. L., & Hawkins, E. J. (2001). The effects of providing therapists with feedback on patient progress during psychotherapy: Are outcomes enhanced? *Psychotherapy Research, 11,* 49–68.

Lilienfeld, S. O., Ritschel, L. A., Lynn, S. J., Cautin, R. L., & Latzman, R. D. (2013). Why many clinical psychologists are resistant to evidence-based practice: Root causes and constructive remedies. *Clinical Psychology Review, 33*(7), 883–900.

Loerinc, A. G., Meuret, A. E., Twohig, M. P., Rosenfield, D., Bluett, E. J., & Craske, M. G. (2015). Response rates for CBT for anxiety disorders: Need for standardized criteria. *Clinical Psychology Review, 42,* 72–82.

McCormack, H. M., Horne, D. J. D., & Sheather, S. (1988). Clinical applications of visual analogue scales: A critical review. *Psychological Medicine, 18,* 1007–1019.

McEvoy, P. M., Nathan, P., & Norton, P. J. (2009). Efficacy of transdiagnostic treatments: A review of published outcome studies and future research directions. *Journal of Cognitive Psychotherapy, 23,* 27–40.

Monzani, B., Jassi, A., Heyman, I., Turner, C., Volz, C., & Krebs, G. (2015). Transformation obsessions in paediatric obsessive–compulsive disorder: Clinical characteristics and treatment response to cognitive behaviour therapy. *Journal of Behavior Therapy and Experimental Psychiatry, 48,* 75–81.

Obsessive Compulsive Cognitions Working Group. (2003). Psychometric validation of the Obsessive Beliefs Questionnaire and the interpretation of intrusions inventory: Part 1. *Behaviour Research and Therapy, 41,* 863–878.

Öst, L. G., Havnen, A., Hansen, B., & Kvale, G. (2015). Cognitive behavioral treatments of obsessive–compulsive disorder: A systematic review and meta-analysis of studies published 1993–2014. *Clinical Psychology Review, 40,* 156–169.

Rachman, S. J. (2006). *The fear of contamination: Assessment and treatment.* Oxford, UK: Oxford University Press.

Rachman, S. J. (2010). Betrayal: A psychological analysis. *Behaviour Research and Therapy, 48,* 304–311.

Rachman, S. J., Coughtrey, A. E., Shafran, R., & Radomsky, A. S. (2015). *The Oxford guide to the treatment of mental contamination.* New York: Oxford University Press.

Radomsky, A. S., Rachman, S. J., Shafran, R., Coughtrey, A. E., & Barber, K. C. (2014). The nature and assessment of mental contamination: A psychometric analysis. *Journal of Obsessive–Compulsive and Related Disorders, 3,* 181–187.

Reips, U. D., & Funke, F. (2008). Interval-level measurement with visual analogue scales in Internet-based research: VAS Generator. *Behavior Research Methods, 40*(3), 699–704.

Shafran, R., Wroe, A., Nagra, S., Pissaridou, E., & Coughtrey, A. (2018). Cognitive behaviour treatment of co-occurring depression and generalised anxiety in routine clinical practice. *PLOS ONE, 13*(7), e0201226.

Stobie, B., Taylor, T., Quigley, A., Ewing, S., & Salkovskis, P. M. (2007). "Contents may vary": A pilot study of treatment histories of OCD patients. *Behavioural and Cognitive Psychotherapy, 35*(3), 273–282.

Tolin, D. F., Abramowitz, J. S., & Diefenbach, G. J. (2005). Defining response in clinical trials for obsessive–compulsive disorder: A signal detection analysis of the Yale–Brown Obsessive Compulsive Scale. *Journal of Clinical Psychiatry, 66*(12), 1549–1557.

Torres, A. R., Prince, M. J., Bebbington, P. E., Bhugra, D., Brugha, T. S., Farrell, M., et al. (2006). Obsessive–compulsive disorder: Prevalence, comorbidity, impact, and help-seeking in the British National Psychiatric Morbidity Survey of 2000. *American Journal of Psychiatry, 163,* 1978–1985.

Volz, C., & Heyman, I. (2007). Case series: Transformation obsession in young people with obsessive–compulsive disorder (OCD). *Journal of the American Academy of Child and Adolescent Psychiatry, 46*(6), 766–772.

Waller, G. (2009). Evidence-based treatment and therapist drift. *Behavioural Research and Therapy, 47*(2), 119–127.

Wilson, G. T., Fairburn, C. G., & Agras, S. W. (1997). Cognitive-behavioral therapy for bulimia nervosa. In D. M. Garner & P. E. Garfinkel (Eds.), *Handbook of treatment for eating disorders* (2nd ed., pp. 67–93). New York: Guilford Press.

Zysk, E., Shafran, R., & Williams, T. I. (2018). A single-subject evaluation of the treatment of morphing fear. *Cognitive and Behavioral Practice, 25*(1), 168–181.

Zysk, E., Shafran, R., Williams, T., & Melli, G. (2016). Development and validation of the Morphing Fear Questionnaire (MFQ). *Clinical Psychology and Psychotherapy, 23*(6), 533–542.

CHAPTER 17

Using an Experimental Therapeutics Approach to Target Psychopathy

EMILY KEMP
ARIELLE BASKIN-SOMMERS

Mr. A was often bored growing up. School made him restless and challenged him too little. His hyperactive behavior made him hard to control, and he was unable to get along with his teachers. From an early age, he began to initiate verbal and physical fights, ignore the rules made by his parents, and consistently skip school. He casually recounted "the incident" that led to a string of 50+ school suspensions and expulsions. This "incident" included "whooping" his teacher and breaking her finger. He was 8 years old at the time. It was this same year that he earned his first arrest for stealing dirt bikes, which Mr. A claimed never to regret doing, as the days of dirt bike racing were the "happiest of [his] life."

Since adolescence, Mr. A moved around a lot, running away from home for months at a time and "shacking up" with his many sexual partners. From the age of 14, he lived with at least 11 different women, many of whom were much older. They provided for him financially. He bragged that he had always been a "ladies' man" and explained that none of these relationships were "real." He stated that he used his manicured charms and simply feigned emotions of love and caring to beguile and manipulate his supposed romantic partners into providing free housing, money, and sex. While taking advantage of these women, Mr. A often committed sexual infidelities. When asked about this, he laughed, coolly described being caught in the act, and proclaimed that he "never thought much of it."

Mr. A's unusual interpersonal style extended beyond that of sexual relationships. He had no close friendships and felt little interest in securing them. He explained that he often feels "detached" from others, as he "laughs when people cry" and thinks it weak to show true emotions. Furthermore, he admitted to lying often and claimed that he can "talk [his] way out of anything." He felt no sympathy for those he fooled and added "those who get conned are naive."

While in prison, Mr. A tended to keep to himself. He looked down on the other inmates, described his intelligence as far superior to theirs, and asserted that "they have no common sense, nothing intellectual to offer." He avoided having "anything to do with them," except to gain something from them, such as money or commissary goods. When he was motivated to cozy up to another inmate, he was often successful and boasted that they would "live like kings," while he profited from the relationship. As soon as the profits ran dry, however, Mr. A never hesitated to move on to the next opportunity.

Mr. A rarely found it necessary or even interesting to contemplate his past. When confronted about his crimes, including theft, assault, drugs, and murder, he replied that he "often feels indifferent about what happened" and "didn't think about a victim ever in [his] life." He elaborated that he felt no sympathy for the man he murdered because he (the victim) had stolen from him, and "it was a matter of respect." He did feel strongly, however, that many others were to blame for his incarceration, including the individual who "ratted" on him, his "horrible" defense attorney, who was a "poor planner," and the "rigged" trial. When asked about his future, Mr. A was confident and nonchalant as he listed goals, which included "owning stuff," like his own business, and "having no problems." He felt little concern that his criminal past would present an obstacle to these goals, as he boasted, "I've had felonies since 8 and always got a job."

At the time of this interview, Mr. A was an inmate in a state correctional facility, serving time for drug possession. He consented to participating in our study of personality and decision-making factors that influence people's problems with the law. In reviewing his case file, we noted that Mr. A had been in correctional custody 15 times and that he had participated in a number of prison-based treatment programs (at least four documented), none of which seemed to result in any positive behavioral change. Our assessment of Mr. A revealed that he met criteria for a class of individuals typically referred to as psychopathic. Psychopathy has captured the attention of the media, lay public, legal authorities, and scholars. Most people are familiar with the names of "famous" psychopathic individuals, such as Jeffrey Dahmer, Ted Bundy, and John Wayne Gacy. That said, it is important to note that not all psychopathic individuals commit crimes as extreme as these individuals, and not all psychopathic individuals are the same in terms of the types of characteristics they display. So what are the core personality characteristics of psychopathic individuals?

Psychopathic individuals exhibit a chronic and flagrant disregard for moral, social, and oftentimes, legal norms. They display an inability to form genuine relationships with parents, teachers, friends, or lovers; limited and superficial affective processing, especially with respect to anticipatory anxiety and remorse; and an impulsive behavioral style, including a general failure to evaluate anticipated actions and inhibit inappropriate ones. Many, especially those like Mr. A, demonstrate a chronic antisocial lifestyle starting early in life, which entails great costs to society and to the affected individual (e.g., incarceration) (Hare, 2006; Skeem & Cooke, 2010). Both Mr. A's life history narrative and his presentation of self during our interview showed him to be simultane-

ously charming and callous, deliberate and impulsive, and criminally repetitive, as well as versatile. And similar to other psychopathic individuals, his temperament interfered with normal socialization throughout life and later, with therapeutic intervention.

* * *

Although their numbers in the general population are small (approximately 1%), psychopathic individuals commit two to three times more violent and nonviolent crimes and recidivate at a much higher rate than nonpsychopathic individuals (Hare, 2006; Hare & Neumann, 2009). This persistent antisocial behavior is responsible for a disproportionate share of the estimated $2.34 trillion in annual costs associated with crime in the United States (Anderson, 1999; Kiehl & Hoffman, 2011). Furthermore, psychopathic individuals account for between 15 and 25% of the prison population (Hare, 1996). Nonetheless, a clear understanding of the complexity of their behavior remains somewhat elusive, and many clinicians, like those who determined the fate of Mr. A, believe that there is little possibility that psychopathic individuals are at all amenable to treatment.

Is it the case that psychopathic individuals are destined to fail all treatments? Or is it possible that a new approach to translating scientific knowledge about psychopathic behavior into treatment interventions may provide cause for greater optimism? In this chapter, we explain that the failure of traditional therapies may be rooted in the lack of attention to the relatively unique cognitive–affective dysfunctions associated with psychopathy. Using the case of Mr. A, we suggest that if progress in treatment is to be made, interventions must specifically target the cognitive–affective problems evident among psychopathic individuals.

How Problematic are Treatments for Psychopathic Individuals?

Historically, the prognosis for psychopathy has been poor. Research consistently suggests that psychopathic individuals are resistant to various treatment approaches. Compared to nonpsychopathic individuals, they demonstrate poor program adjustment and higher attrition (Berger, Rotermund, Vieth, & Hohnhorst, 2012; Ogloff, Wong, & Greenwood, 1990; Olver & Wong,

2009, 2011), and achieve lower levels of therapeutic gain (Chakhssi, de Ruiter, & Bernstein, 2010; Hughes, Hogue, Hollin, & Champion, 1997; Roche, Shoss, Pincus, & Ménard, 2011). Furthermore, in some studies, treatment appears to be associated with heightened rates of recidivism for psychopathic individuals (Hare, Clark, Grann, & Thornton, 2000; Rice, Harris, & Cormier, 1992). This was true in the case of Mr. A, who received prison-based treatment during each of his incarcerations, and whose self-reports and official records confirm high rates of repeat offending following these treatments.

To what types of treatment are most prison inmates exposed? Typically, the vast majority revolves around some form of cognitive-behavioral therapy (CBT). Evaluations of the efficacy of CBT within prison populations, in general, are equivocal. However, and importantly, studies have clearly shown CBT, individual or group, to be ineffective for psychopathic individuals. Hitchcock (1994) compared the effects of CBT in psychopathic and nonpsychopathic inmates and found that this form of treatment had little effect in either sample. Other studies evaluating the efficacy of CBT reported that (1) psychopathy correlated negatively with clinical improvements in forensic patients (Hughes et al., 1997), (2) offenders with elevated levels of psychopathy were more likely to reoffend despite showing improvements due to treatment (Olver, Lewis, & Wong, 2013; Seto & Barbaree, 1999), (3) sexual offenders with high levels of psychopathy were more likely to quit the program and to recidivate (Olver & Wong, 2009), and (4) the interpersonal–affective characteristics (e.g., glibness/charm, callousness, shallow affect) of psychopathy, especially the affective characteristics, were a strong positive predictor of violent recidivism, despite participation in CBT treatment (Olver et al., 2013). Thus, the pattern of findings in studies using CBT in offender populations suggest no or very limited treatment efficacy. This lack in efficacy is especially true with higher levels of psychopathy.

CBT also has been integrated into other types of interventions. For instance, it has been incorporated into milieu therapy, which uses therapeutic communities to effect behavior change. Though there are differences across milieu therapy settings, this combined approach generally implements techniques that support self-examination, the development of accountability, and the enhancement of effective interpersonal engagement through CBT strategies. Similar to individual therapy, this integrated approach has not been effective in psychopathic individuals. Rice and colleagues (1992) evaluated a therapeutic community program that targeted the development of empathy and responsibility, which was believed to be a good approach for treating psychopathy. A follow-up evaluation, conducted approximately 10.5 years after treatment ended, showed that participants with psychopathy, compared to those without psychopathy, had a higher rate of violent recidivism. In contrast, offenders without psychopathy who followed the treatment had a lower rate of reoffending. These findings led Hare (2006) to suggest that "some of the most popular prison treatment and socialization programs may actually make psychopaths worse than they were before. . . . Group therapy and insight oriented programs help psychopaths develop better ways of manipulating, deceiving and using people but do little to help them understand themselves" (p. 717).

Another study of incarcerated offenders found that those with psychopathy tended to invest less time in the program and were less motivated to change their behavior, while nonpsychopathic offenders did benefit from the treatment (Ogloff et al., 1990). Hobson, Scott, and Rubia (2011) reported similar results. They demonstrated that the interpersonal–affective traits of psychopathy, such as shallow affect and charm, were strongly associated with disruptive behaviors in the therapeutic community and on the ward. Thus, research indicates that therapeutic communities may be useful for treating offenders in general but not psychopathic offenders in particular.

Overall, there is little evidence that traditional psychological interventions are effective for psychopathic individuals. Most consistently, psychopathic individuals are found to be unresponsive to individual, group, and community CBT. It should be noted, though, that most of the psychopathy-related treatment studies have been plagued by issues such as flawed design, relatively small sample size, inaccurate characterization of target populations, and use of outcome measures that some have deemed inappropriate (D'Silva, Duggan, & McCarthy, 2004; Harris & Rice, 2006). In light of these shortcomings, some have argued that it is premature to draw the general conclusion that treatment does not work in populations with high levels of psychopathy (D'Silva et al., 2004;

Salekin, Worley, & Grimes, 2010). That said, it is clear that current treatment options for psychopathy fall short. The question remains: Are these individuals untreatable, or are they just not receiving the correct treatment? We believe that in order to address the psychopathic individual's abject failure to adhere to social norms, it is essential to develop treatment programs that capitalize on an understanding of the specific processes underlying this form of psychopathology.

What Are the Core Deficits of Psychopathic Individuals?

Over the past several decades, discoveries in neurobiology, cognitive neuroscience, and other disciplines have led to significant revisions in our understanding of the underlying cognitive–affective mechanisms contributing to psychopathy. The behavior of psychopathic individuals has most often been understood in the context of the low-fear model (Lykken, 1957). However, this traditional view tends to undervalue the role that cognitive–affective and cortical–subcortical brain interactions have in modulating the behavior of psychopathic individuals. Thus, more recent theoretical and empirical models of psychopathy attempt to integrate cognitive and affective patterns, and their influence on prototypical psychopathic behavior. In this section, we review briefly the evidence supporting different etiological models of psychopathy.

Many of the most prominent models of psychopathy attribute the behavior of psychopathic individuals to core deficits in experience of emotion, which prevents them from generating negative affect responses to aversive stimuli and limits their capacity for empathic experience sharing with others (Lykken, 1995; Patrick, 2007). Consistent with this suggestion, psychopathic individuals show deficits in viewing (e.g., processing facial emotions; Marsh & Blair, 2008), responding to (e.g., startle reflex while viewing emotional pictures; Levenston, Patrick, Bradley, & Lang, 2000; Patrick, 1994), and utilizing (e.g., attributing mental states to onself and others; Shamay-Tsoory, Harari, Aharon-Peretz, & Levkovitz, 2010) emotion information. Additionally, psychopathic individuals show widespread structural and functional neural abnormalities (Baskin-Sommers, Neumann, Cope, & Kiehl, 2016; Koenigs, Baskin-Sommers, Zeier, & Newman, 2011), particularly in

brain regions important for emotion processing. For example, psychopathic individuals show reduced recruitment of amygdala and medial orbitofrontal cortex (mOFC) during tasks that ask about moral dilemmas (Decety, Chen, Harenski, & Kiehl, 2013; Glenn, Iyer, Graham, Koleva, & Haidt, 2009), blunted amygdala responsiveness during tasks that ask participants to take the emotional perspective of others (Decety, Chen, et al., 2013; Marsh et al., 2013), and weaker mOFC engagement in response to tasks related to empathic processing (Decety, Skelly, & Kiehl, 2013) and emotional faces (Hyde, Byrd, Votruba-Drzal, Hariri, & Manuck, 2014). Finally, psychopathic individuals demonstrate reduced structural and functional connectivity between the amygdala and mOFC (Craig et al., 2009; Motzkin, Newman, Kiehl, & Koenigs, 2011), which indicates that psychopathic individuals have poorer tissue health connecting these regions and improper recruitment of cognitive functions to regulate emotions. These emotion deficits are clear in the case of Mr. A, who reported feeling "detached" from others, inappropriate affect in response to emotional or risky situations, indifference about hurting others, and little concern for his victims.

While psychopathy research largely focuses on these basic emotion processes, there is substantial evidence that these deficits are moderated by context. Newman and Baskin-Sommers (2011) propose that the context specificity of the psychopathic individual's deficits is associated with a core dysfunction in the adaptive deployment of selective attention, which then interferes with processing information, including emotions. *Selective attention* is a multistage process that influences encoding, processing, and response selection, and basically any and all of our interactions. It is impossible to attend to every stimulus in our environment; therefore, we use selective attention to discern what stimuli are important as events occur (e.g., noticing a loud noise outside while one is talking to a friend). Newman and Baskin-Sommers suggest that a dysfunction at an early stage of selective attention, known as an *early attention bottleneck,* sifts through and evaluates multidimensional information serially rather than simultaneously, thus hindering information processing that either conflicts with goal-directed behavior or requires an efficient evaluation of information embedded within a complex, multifaceted context (Baskin-Sommers, Curtin, & Newman, 2011). For individuals with psychopathy, the bottleneck creates an advantage in many situations that require individuals to filter potential distracters (Hiatt, Schmitt, & Newman, 2004; Mitchell et al., 2006; Wolf et al., 2012; Zeier, Maxwell, & Newman, 2009). For example, Mr. A is able to convince women to pay for housing and provide money and sex because he focuses on his conquests without being affected by the distress of others or inhibitory emotions that prevent many from taking advantage of others. However, this advantage is counterbalanced by the reduced ability of psychopathic individuals to attend to multiple ongoing streams of information (Baskin-Sommers, Curtin, & Newman, 2013; Glass & Newman, 2009; Newman & Kosson, 1986). In the case of Mr. A, the cold logic he described in the moment and upon recounting the murder he committed demonstrates a stark focus on "respect" and order, and ignores the downstream impact murder can have on the victim, on the victim's family (e.g., grief), and on Mr. A (e.g., reincarceration). Consequently, this trade-off results in a tendency to overlook important information, unless it specifically relates to the psychopathic individual's goal-directed focus of attention.

Research using diverse experimental tasks, ranging from those that assess learning about punishment (e.g., passive avoidance) and threat (e.g., instructed fear conditioning) to viewing emotional pictures to make moral decisions, to experiencing regret (e.g., counterfactual reasoning), support the attention bottleneck perspective. These studies demonstrate that psychopathic offenders display normal responses (e.g., behavioral inhibition, fear-potentiated startle, emotion-modulated startle, amygdala activation, electrodermal activity, and affective ratings) to affective information when it is part of their goal-directed task or embedded in a perceptually simple display (Baskin-Sommers et al., 2011, 2013; Baskin-Sommers, Stuppy-Sullivan, & Buckholtz, 2016; Dadds et al., 2006; Decety, Skelly, et al., 2013; Meffert, Gazzola, den Boer, Bartels, & Keysers, 2013; Newman, Curtin, Bertsch, & Baskin-Sommers, 2010; Newman & Kosson, 1986; Sadeh & Verona, 2012). Yet their reactions to the same affective stimuli are deficient, relative to reactions of nonpsychopathic offenders, when their attention has been allocated to an alternative goal or complex aspect of the situation (see Newman & Baskin-Sommers, 2011, for review).

In practical terms, this cognitive–affective deficit in attention to context results in a myopic perspective on decision making and goal-directed behavior. Thus, individuals with psychopathy are adept at using information that is directly relevant to their goal to effectively regulate behavior (modulate behavior and ignore emotions to con someone; e.g., when Mr. A takes advantage of other inmates or women), but they display impulsive behavior (e.g., quitting a job in the absence of an alternative one; when Mr. A moves from one place to another) and egregious decision making (e.g., seeking publicity for a con while wanted by police) when information is beyond their immediate focus of attention.

A recent series of studies investigating fear-potentiated startle (FPS) and amygdala activation provides strong support for the context specificity of psychopathy-related cognitive–affective deficits. The first experimental task in these studies required participants to view and categorize letter stimuli that may also be used to predict the administration of electric shocks. Instructions engaged either a goal-directed focus on threat-relevant information (i.e., the color that predicted electric shocks) or an alternative, threat-irrelevant dimension of the letter stimuli (i.e., an uppercase/lowercase letter or its match/mismatch in a two-back task). The results provided no evidence of a psychopathy-related deficit in FPS under conditions that focused attention on threat-relevant information. However, psychopathy scores were significantly inversely related to FPS under conditions that required participants to focus on a threat-irrelevant dimension of stimuli (i.e., peripheral threat cues).

Although the results from Newman and colleagues (2010) provide some of the strongest evidence to date that the fear deficit in psychopathy is moderated by attention, the study did not specifically define the attentional mechanism underlying this effect. Moreover, several different cognitive–affective processes can influence goal-directed behavior and may involve diverse neural and cognitive systems. Narrowing down the possible mechanisms responsible for psychopathic individuals' attention abnormality provides a more nuanced conceptualization of why psychopathic individuals do what they do and identifies a precise target for intervention.

Baskin-Sommers and colleagues (2011) specified this attention-mediated abnormality in a new sample of offenders by measuring FPS in four conditions that crossed attentional focus (threat vs. alternative) with temporal presentation of goal-relevant cues (early vs. late). First, the authors replicated the key findings reported by Newman and colleagues (2010): Psychopathic individuals' deficit in FPS was virtually nonexistent under conditions that focused attention on the threat-relevant stimuli (i.e., threat-focus conditions), but it was pronounced when threat-relevant cues were peripheral to their primary focus of attention (i.e., alternative-focus conditions). More specifically, the psychopathic deficit in FPS was only apparent in the early alternative-focus condition, in which threat cues were presented after the alternative goal-directed focus was already established. Furthermore, in a separate sample of offenders, using the same task, Larson and colleagues (2013) demonstrated that psychopathic, compared to nonpsychopathic, individuals displayed significantly lower activation in the amygdala in the early alternative-focus condition, but there was no difference in amygdala activation in other conditions. Moreover, higher lateral prefrontal cortex activation, a neural substrate of the attention bottleneck, mediated the relationship between psychopathy and amygdala activation. Combined, these studies show that affective and inhibitory deficits can appear and disappear in psychopathic individuals, depending on the congruence of affective or inhibitory information with their goal (Brazil et al., 2012; Glass & Newman, 2009; Hiatt et al., 2004; Sadeh & Verona, 2008, 2012); that is, the emotion deficits of psychopathic individuals are not pansituational, or fundamental in an absolute sense, but rather are context-specific. By identifying the contexts under which psychopathic individuals do and do not experience emotion provides a target for intervention.

While substantial progress has been made in specifying the types of behaviors that characterize psychopathy and in identifying well-validated measures that assess their underlying etiology, there has been no sustained effort to translate this progress into treatment programs. In some ways, this is due to lingering doubts regarding the amenability of psychopathic individuals to treatment. However, these misgivings are rooted in the failure of traditional therapies to address the relatively unique cognitive–affective dysfunctions associated with this subgroup of offenders. Therefore, if progress in treatment is to be made, interventions must integrate scientific knowledge about the cognitive–affective problems that are specific to psychopathy.

How Can We Apply Knowledge of Cognitive–Affective Mechanisms to Treatment for Psychopathy?

For decades, mental health professionals have struggled with the "one size fits all" approach to treatment. Clinicians have experienced great frustration when delivering treatment to clients who do not respond, or regrettably, even worsen. There has been little cross-fertilization between researchers and clinicians generally, and, with respect to psychopathic individuals, there has been little incentive to focus on innovations for a population deemed largely "untreatable." However, recent technological advances in individualized medicine have opened avenues for innovative approaches that integrate basic research with clinical practice. There is some early evidence that these new approaches may be effective, even in the treatment of psychopathy.

As briefly reviewed earlier, psychopathic individuals have a fundamental problem with attending to contextual cues, whether those are affective, inhibitory, or other forms of information. This dysfunction is located in several neural structures (i.e., amygdala, orbitofrontal cortex, and prefrontal cortex) and manifests in the psychopathic individual's unremitting, cold-blooded, and antisocial behavior. While some consider this picture of psychopathy to be evidence of its unreachability, we maintain that there is promise in taking this information regarding psychopathy-related cognitive–affective dysfunction and integrating it with our understanding of neural plasticity. In other words, treatment of psychopathic individuals may be effective if we recognize the malleability of dysfunctions in the brain and target the specific cognitive–affective mechanisms associated with this particular form of psychopathology.

Cognitive remediation is an intervention rooted in the assumption that if we can identify and understand the mechanisms of behavior, then we can improve functioning. Specifically, it emphasizes the training of individuals in particular cognitive skills—such as sustained attention and working memory—so that behavior can be modified (Klingberg, 2010; Wykes, Huddy, Cellard, McGurk, & Czobor, 2011). For example, in healthy adults, Klingberg and colleagues have shown that working memory training not only improves overall working memory capacity, but it also changes the functioning of dopamine neurotransmission and brain plasticity (see McNab et al., 2009). Research examining the effects of cognitive remediation on disorders with known cognitive abnormalities, such as attention-deficit/hyperactivity disorder and schizophrenia, also have been promising (Stevenson, Whitmont, Bornholt, Livesey, & Stevenson, 2002; Wykes et al., 2003).

In light of the information emerging from the attention bottleneck perspective, we sought to adapt cognitive remediation interventions for the treatment of psychopathy. Baskin-Sommers, Curtin, and Newman (2015) designed a cognitive intervention that targeted the attention to context deficit associated with psychopathy and examined the efficacy of this intervention in a sample of incarcerated, adult male offenders. Participants in the study included 124 substance-dependent inmates who were classified as psychopathic or nonpsychopathic. The overall goal of this study was to evaluate the possibility of measuring the cognitive–affective deficits specific to psychopathy, bring about change in those deficits (i.e., training), and effect generalizable change relevant to other tasks that were not the focus of repeated practice (i.e., pre- and posttasks).

First, all participants completed five different attention, working memory, and emotion tasks that measured behavioral and psychophysiological responses (e.g., instructed fear conditioning, described earlier; Baskin-Sommers et al., 2011). Second, after completion of pretesting, psychopathic and nonpsychopathic offenders were randomly assigned to one of two computerized training packages, utilizing a 2 × 2 crossover design. Each of the training packages consisted of a 1-hour computer-based training session, once a week for 6 weeks, that used three tasks to target a particular deficit. The experimental training targeted the psychopathy-related attention to context deficit, while the control training targeted general affect regulation and cognitive control (deficits not present in psychopathic individuals). At the end of each training task within each session, participants were shown a graph of their progress on relevant task measures. The end-of-session graphs displayed the session number on the x-axis and some measure of behavioral performance for that task (e.g., percent correct) on the y-axis. During the presentation of each graph, the research assistant explained to the participant his score for that session and pointed out how the participant's performance compared to performance on other sessions, as appropriate. If

the participant improved, the research assistant said something to the effect of "You can see that from Session X to this session, you did better. This suggests that your training is helping build the necessary skills to notice and use important information." If the participant's performance was the same, the research assistant would say, "Sometimes when you are learning new skills, you don't always improve on every session." Finally, if the participant's performance declined, the research assistant would state, "Sometimes when you are learning new skills, you don't always improve on every session. In fact, sometimes we do worse before we can do better. But with practice, things will eventually click, and everything will come together. You will have other opportunities to practice these skills." The purpose of these graphs was to address motivational engagement.

Consistent with the research noted earlier on cognitive–affective mechanisms related to psychopathy, the actual training for psychopathy was focused on attending to and integrating contextual information. Each task provided individuals with opportunities to practice attention to peripheral or nonsalient cues and notice changes in contextual information (e.g., rule changes using a reversal learning task, context discrimination using a divided visual field task, and integrating facial information to respond to instructions about the direction of eye gaze). For example, in the reversal learning task, animals appeared on the screen. The participant had to choose one of the animals. After the participant's response, the participant was told whether he was correct (win 100 points) or incorrect (lose 100 points). One animal began as being correct more often, but at some point during the task, that winning animal started losing the participant points, and the previously losing animal started winning him points. Therefore, to do well on this task, the participant had to notice that shift (i.e., context) related to winning and losing animals. In the divided visual field task, participants were suppose to indicate whether a string was all letters, all numbers, or a combination of letters and numbers. But surrounding those strings was a colored box; if the box was green, the participant responded per the instructions, but if it was yellow, the participant was instructed to withhold his response. In other words, to do this task well, the participant needed to pay attention to the color of the box before making a response. Finally, in the gaze task, participants had to respond to whether the eyes on a face were looking left or right, by pressing the button that matched the eye gaze (right gaze, right button; left gaze left button). However, each session, the participant was told that for one of the emotion faces (e.g., anger, happy, fear), he had the press the button that was the opposite of the eye gaze (e.g., if the eyes look left, press the right button). Therefore, if the participant failed to notice the emotion on the face, then he would probably respond incorrectly. The control training package was not designed to target psychopathy but instead focused on providing practice inhibiting behavior and regulating emotion reactions more generally (e.g., incentive salience and cognitive control using a GoStop task, distress tolerance using breath holding, and cognitive control using a Simon task). For example, in the Go-Stop task, participants saw circles and squares and had to press one button for the circle and the other for the square. However, on some trials, participants heard a tone after the square or circle appeared on the screen. When participants heard a tone, they were supposed to withhold their response. After the trial, participants were told whether they were correct (won 5 cents) or incorrect (lost 25 cents). This type of task did not test the attention to and integration of contextual information; rather, the focus was more on learning to inhibit a response in the face of rewards and punishment (processes not related to the core cognitive–affective dysfunctions in psychopathy). The other two control tasks measured distress tolerance and cognitive control, respectively, which also are not deficient processes in psychopathic individuals. Last, following completion of the training session, all participants repeated the pretesting behavioral and psychophysiological assessments.

After 6 weeks of computerized training, psychopathic participants in the attention to context (i.e., the psychopathy-specific) training group demonstrated significant improvement on the three training tasks. Conversely, psychopathic participants in the control condition showed no significant improvement over the course of training on the non-psychopathy-specific tasks. Moreover, psychopathic participants who received the deficit-matched training related to attending to contextual cues showed significant improvement on the pre- and postmeasures, whereas those who received the control training did not improve from pre- to postmeasures; that is, whereas psychopathic individuals previously showed deficits in FPS on instructed fear conditioning, they no longer showed significant deficits on this measure if they received the attention to context training. Together, these results demonstrate that it is possible to identify and target the cognitive–affective deficits associated with psychopathy; specifically, training designed to remedy these deficits resulted in differential improvement on trained and nontrained tasks.

As noted throughout this chapter, Mr. A can be viewed as a prototypical psychopathic individual whose cold, callous, impulsive, and antisocial behavior is best understood as a problem attending to contextual cues. He ignores the feelings of others and the consequences of his behavior not because he does not care or is incapable, but because he has a diminished ability to notice and integrate all pieces of a situation at the same time. Moreover, traditional treatments have failed Mr. A, and this is quite likely because those treatments require noticing cues in a situation or patterns across time that are necessitated by integrating contextual cues. However, Baskin-Sommers and colleagues (2015) demonstrated that it is possible to identify failures in attention to context and modify those failures. For Mr. A, learning to integrate the facial emotion and direction of the eyes, to notice rule changes in a game, and to discriminate between stimuli to determine the best response address his core deficiency. Importantly, Mr. A does not need to be aware of these changes or deliberately engage with them. The advantage of the training is that he just needs to learn how to play the games better, and by extension, is learning to use functions that are normally inadequate for him. Ultimately, this type of training targets the fractionated view Mr. A has of the world around him and trains him to develop a more unified representation of a given context.

These findings represent only a first test of the efficacy of a cognitive remediation approach to the treatment of psychopathy, but they are especially promising because they oppose the common notion that the deficits associated with psychopathy are intractable, and that effective treatment is not possible. However, it is important to remember that these tests were conducted in a laboratory setting, and it would be naive to assume that psychopathy can be treated by playing focused computer games for 6 hours. Therefore, it is essential to test whether this type of cognitive remediation training translates to real-word behavior and settings outside of the lab. Additionally, questions related to durability, efficiency, and portability of the lab-based interventions must be addressed. For example, the use of homework assignments (e.g., vignettes that depict situations relevant to attending to context), booster training sessions, and other assessments may help generalize the training effects to more ecologically valid indices of self-regulation and community adjustment. Despite the substantial work needed to move forward this line of research, our work emphasizes the value of identifying, developing, and testing mechanism-based intervention. Moreover, it highlights the substantial potential to address psychopathic individuals' disinhibited and costly behavior by identifying and targeting the specific cognitive–affective dysfunctions that characterize this form of psychopathology.

Summary

Psychopathy is a multifaceted disorder that has perplexed clinicians for many years. Individuals with psychopathy present as callous, superficial, manipulative, impulsive, and antisocial. To be in a room with a psychopathic individual can feel like the walls are closing in on you, but at the same time you are enjoying your time with this person. The grandiosity, charm, and control psychopathic individuals display leave clinicians feeling overwhelmed and uncertain. These traits, in addition to historically poor treatment outcomes, contribute to the common belief that psychopathy is simply an untreatable disorder. Fundamentally, though, psychopathic individuals are humans: people who have experiences and predispositions that shape them and determine how they engage with the world around them. We invite clinicians to begin to think in interdisciplinary and evidence-based ways to meet the needs of such challenging clients rather than view these individuals as hopeless.

Decades of experimental research have identified that individuals with psychopathy are effectively oblivious to emotional, inhibitory, and punishment cues that contraindicate ongoing goal-directed behavior. Thinking critically about what this means for engaging in treatment, it is not surprising that psychopathic individuals struggle to incorporate treatment skills and information into their real-world behavior. Therefore, traditional treat-

ment approaches may be futile on their own. If, however, the underlying mechanisms of the psychopathy-related attention-to-context deficit are addressed, clinicians may be better able to effectively use treatments designed to help with real-world functioning. Combining cognitive remediation training and traditional therapeutic approaches has the potential to address the cognitive–affective dysfunctions associated with psychopathy from multiple angles. The use of cognitive remediation provides a psychobiologically based approach to target dysfunctions that impact how information in processed by psychopathic individuals and circumvents issues of insight, motivation for change, and treatment engagement. Once key psychobiological substrates are modified, the way in which psychopathic individuals take in information may also change, positioning them to view and use other therapeutic skills in a different, more adaptive manner.

Though research on novel approaches to treating psychopathy is in its infancy, clinicians can take steps to integrate knowledge of the mechanisms underlying psychopathic behavior into their case conceptualization and treatment approach. For instance, clinicians can ask questions that consider attending to contextual cues (e.g., noticing the emotions of others, noting the consequences), they can read available empirical research that extends beyond traditional treatment (e.g., cognitive remediation/computerized training), they can critically evaluate the situations in which therapeutic skills work (e.g., when emotions are self-focused or central to the psychopathic individual's goal) and do not work (e.g., when situations are complex), and they can consider mechanistic reasons for treatment success or failure. Ultimately, it is most likely that the combination of these traditional therapeutic techniques and technology (e.g., cognitive remediation through computerized training) will have the greatest potential for targeting the complex behavior of psychopathic individuals. Regardless of the approach, the key is to be aware of and target the underlying mechanisms.

Psychopathy produces suffering for the individual, for his or her family members, for the community, and for society at large. Importantly, the underlying cognitive–affective mechanisms tell us *why* the psychopathic individual continues to engage in these behaviors, despite the persistence of suffering. Utilizing the approach of knowledge integration from basic science on these cognitive–affective mechanisms to intervention research highlights the path for alleviating this suffering.

References

Anderson, D. A. (1999). The aggregate burden of crime. *Journal of Law and Economics, 42*(2), 611–642.

Baskin-Sommers, A. R., Curtin, J. J., & Newman, J. P. (2011). Specifying the attentional selection that moderates the fearlessness of psychopathic offenders. *Psychological Science, 22*(2), 226–234.

Baskin-Sommers, A. R., Curtin, J. J., & Newman, J. P. (2013). Emotion-modulated startle in psychopathy: Clarifying familiar effects. *Journal of Abnormal Psychology, 122*(2), 458–468.

Baskin-Sommers, A. R., Curtin, J. J., & Newman, J. P. (2015). Altering the cognitive–affective dysfunctions of psychopathic and externalizing offender subtypes with cognitive remediation. *Clinical Psychological Science, 3*(1), 45–57.

Baskin-Sommers, A. R., Neumann, C., Cope, L. M., & Kiehl, K. (2016). Latent-variable modeling of brain gray-matter volume and psychopathy in incarcerated offenders. *Journal of Abnormal Psychology, 125*(6), 811–817.

Baskin-Sommers, A. R., Stuppy-Sullivan, A., & Buckholtz, J. (2016). Psychopathic individuals experience, but do not avoid regret during counterfactual decision making. *Proceedings of the National Academy of Sciences of the USA, 113*(50), 14438–14443.

Berger, K., Rotermund, P., Vieth, E. R., & Hohnhorst, A. (2012). The prognostic value of the PCL-R in relation to the SUD treatment ending. *International Journal of Law and Psychiatry, 35*(3), 198–201.

Brazil, I. A., Verkes, R. J., Brouns, B. H., Buitelaar, J. K., Bulten, B. H., & de Bruijn, E. R. (2012). Differentiating psychopathy from general antisociality using the P3 as a psychophysiological correlate of attentional allocation. *PLOS ONE, 7*(11), e50339.

Chakhssi, F., de Ruiter, C., & Bernstein, D. (2010). Change during forensic treatment in psychopathic versus nonpsychopathic offenders. *Journal of Forensic Psychiatry and Psychology, 21*(5), 660–682.

Craig, M. C., Catani, M., Deeley, Q., Latham, R., Daly, E., Kanaan, R., et al. (2009). Altered connections on the road to psychopathy. *Molecular Psychiatry, 14*(10), 946–953.

D'Silva, K., Duggan, C., & McCarthy, L. (2004). Does treatment really make psychopaths worse?: A review of the evidence. *Journal of Personality Disorders, 18*(2), 163–177.

Dadds, M. R., Perry, Y., Hawes, D. J., Merz, S., Riddell, A. C., Haines, D. J., et al. (2006). Attention to the eyes and fear-recognition deficits in child psychopathy. *British Journal of Psychiatry, 189,* 280–281.

Decety, J., Chen, C., Harenski, C., & Kiehl, K. A. (2013). An fMRI study of affective perspective taking in individuals with psychopathy: Imagining another in pain does not evoke empathy. *Frontiers in Human Neuroscience, 7,* 489.

Decety, J., Skelly, L. R., & Kiehl, K. A. (2013). Brain response to empathy-eliciting scenarios involving pain in incarcerated individuals with psychopathy. *JAMA Psychiatry, 70*(6), 638–645.

Glass, S. J., & Newman, J. P. (2009). Emotion processing in the criminal psychopath: The role of attention in emotion-facilitated memory. *Journal of Abnormal Psychology, 118*(1), 229–234.

Glenn, A. L., Iyer, R., Graham, J., Koleva, S., & Haidt, J. (2009). Are all types of morality compromised in psychopathy? *Journal of Personality Disorders, 23*(4), 384–398.

Hare, R. D. (1996). Psychopathy: A clinical construct whose time has come. *Criminal Justice and Behavior, 23*(1), 25–54.

Hare, R. D. (2006). Psychopathy: A clinical and forensic overview. *Psychiatric Clinics of North America, 29,* 709–724.

Hare, R. D., Clark, D., Grann, M., & Thornton, D. (2000). Psychopathy and the predictive validity of the PCL-R: An international perspective. *Behavioral Sciences and the Law, 18*(5), 623–645.

Hare, R. D., & Neumann, C. S. (2009). Psychopathy: Assessment and forensic implications. *Canadian Journal of Psychiatry, 54*(12), 791–802.

Harris, G. T., & Rice, M. E. (2006). Treatment of psychopathy. In C. J. Patrick (Ed.), *Handbook of psychopathy* (pp. 555–572). New York: Guilford Press.

Hiatt, K. D., Schmitt, W. A., & Newman, J. P. (2004). Stroop tasks reveal abnormal selective attention among psychopathic offenders. *Neuropsychology, 18*(1), 50–59.

Hitchcock, G. L. (1994). *The efficacy of cognitive group therapy with incarcerated psychopaths.* Dissertation, California School of Professional Psychology, Fresno, CA.

Hobson, C. W., Scott, S., & Rubia, K. (2011). Investigation of cool and hot executive function in ODD/CD independently of ADHD. *Journal of Child Psychology and Psychiatry, 52*(10), 1035–1043.

Hughes, G., Hogue, T., Hollin, C., & Champion, H. (1997). First-stage evaluation of a treatment programme for personality disordered offenders. *Journal of Forensic Psychiatry, 8*(3), 515–527.

Hyde, L. W., Byrd, A. L., Votruba-Drzal, E., Hariri, A. R., & Manuck, S. B. (2014). Amygdala reactivity and negative emotionality: Divergent correlates of antisocial personality and psychopathy traits in a community sample. *Journal of Abnormal Psychology, 123*(1), 214–224.

Kiehl, K. A., & Hoffman, M. B. (2011). The criminal psychopath: History, neuroscience, treatment, and economics. *Jurimetrics, 51,* 355–397.

Klingberg, T. (2010). Training and plasticity of working memory. *Trends in Cognitive Sciences, 14*(7), 317–324.

Koenigs, M., Baskin-Sommers, A. R., Zeier, J. D., & Newman, J. P. (2011). Investigating the neural correlates of psychopathy: A critical review. *Molecular Psychiatry, 16*(8), 792–799.

Larson, C. L., Baskin-Sommers, A. R., Stout, D. M., Balderston, N. L., Curtin, J. J., Schultz, D. H., et al. (2013). The interplay of attention and emotion: Top-down attention modulates amygdala activation in psychopathy. *Cognitive, Affective, and Behavioral Neuroscience, 13*(4), 757–770.

Levenston, G. K., Patrick, C. J., Bradley, M. M., & Lang, P. J. (2000). The psychopath as observer: Emotion and attention in picture processing. *Journal of Abnormal Psychology, 109*(3), 373–385.

Lykken, D. T. (1957). A study of anxiety in the sociopathic personality. *Journal of Abnormal and Social Psychology, 55,* 6–10.

Lykken, D. T. (1995). *The antisocial personalities.* Hillsdale, NJ: Erlbaum.

Marsh, A. A., & Blair, R. J. R. (2008). Deficits in facial affect recognition among antisocial populations: A meta-analysis. *Neuroscience and Biobehavioral Reviews, 32*(3), 454–465.

Marsh, A. A., Finger, E. C., Fowler, K. A., Adalio, C. J., Jurkowitz, I. T., Schechter, J. C., et al. (2013). Empathic responsiveness in amygdala and anterior cingulate cortex in youths with psychopathic traits. *Journal of Child Psychology and Psychiatry, 54*(8), 900–1010.

McNab, F., Varrone, A., Farde, L., Jucaite, A., Bystritsky, P., Forssberg, H., & Klingberg, T. (2009). Changes in cortical dopamine D1 receptor binding associated with cognitive training. *Science, 323,* 800–802.

Meffert, H., Gazzola, V., den Boer, J. A., Bartels, A. A., & Keysers, C. (2013). Reduced spontaneous but relatively normal deliberate vicarious representations in psychopathy. *Brain, 136*(8), 2550–2562.

Mitchell, D. G., Fine, C., Richell, R. A., Newman, C., Lumsden, J., Blair, K. S., & Blair, R. J. (2006). Instrumental learning and relearning in individuals with psychopathy and in patients with lesions involving the amygdala or orbitofrontal cortex. *Neuropsychology, 20*(3), 280–289.

Motzkin, J. C., Newman, J. P., Kiehl, K. A., & Koenigs, M. (2011). Reduced prefrontal connectivity in psychopathy. *Journal of Neuroscience, 31*(48), 17348–17357.

Newman, J. P., & Baskin-Sommers, A. R. (2011). Early selective attention abnormalities in psychopathy: Implications for self-regulation. In M. I. Posner (Ed.), *Cognitive neuroscience of attention* (2nd ed., pp. 421–440). New York: Guilford Press.

Newman, J. P., Curtin, J. J., Bertsch, J. D., & Baskin-Sommers, A. R. (2010). Attention moderates the fearlessness of psychopathic offenders. *Biological Psychiatry, 67*(1), 66–70.

Newman, J. P., & Kosson, D. (1986). Passive avoidance learning in psychopathic and nonpsychopathic offenders. *Journal of Abnormal Psychology, 95*(3), 252–256.

Ogloff, J. R., Wong, S., & Greenwood, A. (1990). Treating criminal psychopaths in a therapeutic community program. *Behavioral Sciences and the Law, 8*(2), 181–190.

Olver, M. E., Lewis, K., & Wong, S. C. (2013). Risk reduction treatment of high-risk psychopathic offenders: The relationship of psychopathy and treatment change to violent recidivism. *Personality Disorders: Theory, Research, and Treatment, 4*(2), 160–167.

Olver, M. E., & Wong, S. C. (2009). Therapeutic responses of psychopathic sexual offenders: Treatment attrition, therapeutic change, and long-term recidivism. *Journal of Consulting and Clinical Psychology, 77*(2), 328–336.

Olver, M. E., & Wong, S. (2011). Predictors of sex offender treatment dropout: Psychopathy, sex offender risk, and responsivity implications. *Psychology, Crime and Law, 17*(5), 457–471.

Patrick, C. J. (1994). Emotion and psychopathy: Startling new insights. *Psychophysiology, 31*(4), 319–330.

Patrick, C. J. (2007). Getting to the heart of psychopathy. In H. Herve & J. C. Yuille (Eds.), *The psychopath: Theory, research, and social implications* (pp. 207–252). Hillsdale, NJ: Erlbaum.

Rice, M. E., Harris, G. T., & Cormier, C. A. (1992). An evaluation of a maximum security therapeutic community for psychopaths and other mentally disordered offenders. *Law and Human Behavior, 16*(4), 399–412.

Roche, M. J., Shoss, N. E., Pincus, A. L., & Ménard, K. S. (2011). Psychopathy moderates the relationship between time in treatment and levels of empathy in incarcerated male sexual offenders. *Sexual Abuse, 23*(2), 171–192.

Sadeh, N., & Verona, E. (2008). Psychopathic personality traits associated with abnormal selective attention and impaired cognitive control. *Neuropsychology, 22*(5), 669–680.

Sadeh, N., & Verona, E. (2012). Visual complexity attenuates emotional processing in psychopathy: Implications for fear-potentiated startle deficits. *Cognitive, Affective, and Behavioral Neuroscience, 12*(2), 346–360.

Salekin, R. T., Worley, C., & Grimes, R. D. (2010). Treatment of psychopathy: A review and brief introduction to the mental model mpproach for psychopathy. *Behavioral Sciences and the Law, 28*(2), 235–266.

Seto, M. C., & Barbaree, H. E. (1999). Psychopathy, treatment behavior, and sex offender recidivism. *Journal of Interpersonal Violence, 14*(12), 1235–1248.

Shamay-Tsoory, S. G., Harari, H., Aharon-Peretz, J., & Levkovitz, Y. (2010). The role of the orbitofrontal cortex in affective theory of mind deficits in criminal offenders with psychopathic tendencies. *Cortex, 46*(5), 668–677.

Skeem, J. L., & Cooke, D. J. (2010). Is criminal behavior a central component of psychopathy?: Conceptual directions for resolving the debate. *Psychological Assessment, 22*(2), 433–445.

Stevenson, C. S., Whitmont, S., Bornholt, L., Livesey, D., & Stevenson, R. J. (2002). A cognitive remediation programme for adults with attention deficit hyperactivity disorder. *Australian and New Zealand Journal of Psychiatry, 36*(5), 610–616.

Wolf, R. C., Carpenter, R. W., Warren, C. M., Zeier, J. D., Baskin-Sommers, A. R., & Newman, J. P. (2012). Reduced susceptibility to the attentional blink in psychopathic offenders: Implications for the attention bottleneck hypothesis. *Neuropsychology, 26*(1), 102–109.

Wykes, T., Huddy, V., Cellard, C., McGurk, S., & Czobor, P. (2011). A meta-analysis of cognitive remediation for schizophrenia: Methodology and effect sizes. *American Journal of Psychiatry, 168*(5), 472–485.

Wykes, T., Reeder, C., Williams, C., Corner, J., Rice, C., & Everitt, B. (2003). Are the effects of cognitive remediation therapy (CRT) durable?: Results from an exploratory trial in schizophrenia. *Schizophrenia Research, 61*(2), 163–174.

Zeier, J. D., Maxwell, J. S., & Newman, J. P. (2009). Attention moderates the processing of inhibitory information in primary psychopathy. *Journal of Abnormal Psychology, 118*(3), 554–563.

CHAPTER 18

Sequential Repetitive Transcranial Magnetic Stimulation and Mindfulness–Based Cognitive Therapy for Treatment–Resistant Depression

Rationale and Clinical Illustration
of Evidence-Based Practice in Action

EVAN COLLINS
SUSAN E. ABBEY
NORMAN FARB
JONATHAN DOWNAR
ZINDEL V. SEGAL

Michelle, a 52-year-old white woman who works as a paralegal, has a long-standing history of major depressive disorder (MDD), complicated by degenerative disk disease and chronic pain. She has dated the same man for 20 years, although they live separately in their own apartments. Michelle has struggled with recurrent depression with anxious features since her late teens. Her depressive episodes are associated with sadness, increased sleep and appetite, lack of motivation, and social isolation, as well as generalized anxiety. In the past she has shown mixed responses to different classes of antidepressants managed by her general practitioner (GP), but in the last 3 years, medication trials have only achieved partial response, along with increased sensitivity to adverse effects. Michelle has had one short-term hospitalization for suicidal ideation, although, generally, she says she would not harm herself because of her family, and her pet cats.

The past year Michelle became quite depressed after going on disability because of chronic back pain and impaired mobility. She was referred to a new psychiatrist and tried sequentially two different classes of antidepressant medication plus trials of both an atypical antipsychotic and a psychostimulant as augmentation strategies, all with only modest and fluctuating improvements in mood. There was an attempt to integrate pharmacotherapy with cognitive-behavioral therapy (CBT), and although Michelle seemed to understand and appreciate the model, her lack of motivation limited her ability to make use of the therapy. With a Beck Depression Inventory score of *moderately severe* and a General Anxiety score of *moderate,* she was referred for repetitive transcranial magnetic stimulation (rTMS), an established therapy for treatment-resistant depression (TRD). She completed a 1-month course of rTMS and following this was referred to mindfulness-based cognitive therapy (MBCT) for relapse prevention. In this chapter, we describe our work with Michelle as an example of how we used the principles of evidence-based practice (EBP) to address the important and understudied problem of TRD.

*   *   *

Michelle's experience, unfortunately, is not uncommon. MDD has a chronic and impairing course for most individuals, with relapse and recurrence following recovery being one driver of this disorder's enormous social costs. In fact, MDD is the fifth leading cause of disability-adjusted life years lost in North America (Murray et al., 2012), with U.S. lifetime and 12-month prevalence estimated to be 16.2 and 6.6%, respectively (Kessler et al., 2003). In our jurisdiction of Ontario, Canada, the MDD health burden is greater than all major cancers combined, and double that of all infectious diseases (Ratnasingham et al., 2013).

The magnitude of MDD burden reflects limited treatment options. Longitudinal data from the Sequenced Treatment Alternatives to Relieve Depression (STAR*D) project indicate that antidepressants fail to achieve remission in at least one in three patients with MDD (Rush et al., 2006) leading to residual symptoms in the best of cases and, as Michelle experienced, TRD in the worst. The public health impact of TRD is significant and associated with increased rates of symptom burden, polypharmacy, comorbidity, and disability (Rizvi et al., 2014). Looking outside of pharmacological interventions, the utility of psychotherapeutic interventions to target TRD is mixed (Trivedi, Nieuwsma, & Williams, 2011). Both CBT and the Cognitive Behavioral Assessment System of Psychotherapy (CBASP) have shown some efficacy in this population (Schatzberg et al., 2005; Wiles et al., 2013), but response and remission rates are far from optimal.

The Promise of Neurostimulation for TRD

The need to improve outcomes for patients with TRD has led to the development of a number of new interventions that attempt to leverage the mood-enhancing consequences of targeted neurostimulation. The most established form of neurostimulation is electroconvulsive therapy (ECT), which is highly effective but comes with significant adverse effects, including the impacts of repeated general anesthesia, postseizure confusion, and short-term memory loss (Lisanby, 2007).

A newer form of stimulation, rTMS, involves the application of focused magnetic field pulses to induce changes in the activity of frontal lobe regions involved in regulation of thoughts, emotions, and behavior (Downar & Daskalakis, 2013). Stimulation is applied noninvasively via a handheld magnetic coil, does not require anesthesia, and has been approved as an MDD treatment by North American and European regulatory agencies as a safe and effective treatment for depression, with a minimal burden of adverse effects.

For Michelle, the course of rTMS involved targeting the dorsomedial prefrontal cortex. She underwent 20 sessions of stimulation, each lasting about 15 minutes, given once daily Monday to Friday, with the stimulator coil placed at a specific location along the midline, near the top of the forehead, so as to maximize stimulation of the target region (for technical details, see Bakker et al., 2015). She tolerated the stimulation without any serious adverse effects aside from the typical report of mild pain around the stimulation site during the sessions, although this reduced somewhat as she became acclimated to treatment.

The efficacy of rTMS as an intervention for TRD has been well established by systematic reviews and meta-analyses (Berlim, van den Eynde, Tovar-Persomo, & Daskalakis, 2014; Brunoni et al., 2017; Gaynes et al., 2014). Michelle's experience was consistent with these meta-analytic findings. At first, she found it challenging to come in to treatment 5 days a week, but by the third week she was feeling more energy and motivation, although her mood remained low. By completion of rTMS, she demonstrated an improvement in depressive rating scales from moderately severe to mild-to-moderate depression, although her anxiety scores remained moderate. Following rTMS, she reported that she felt much better in mood and energy, though not 100%. She had significant anxious rumination around the possibility of slipping back into depression.

The Limitations of rTMS

Despite the promise of rTMS for acute intervention, it is not without limitations. The data are consistent with Michelle's question to us about how long she could expect the effects to last. An emerging literature suggests high rates of depressive relapse following treatment response with rTMS; specifically, ≥50% of responders relapse within 6 months of treatment completion

(Janicak et al., 2010; Kedzior, Reitz, Azorina, & Loo, 2015). These findings tempered our enthusiasm for rTMS as a monotherapy for Michelle and highlighted the need for a relapse prevention strategy to complement the acute efficacy of rTMS in order to achieve sustained remission.

We hypothesized that Michelle would need something more than just rTMS to stay well and were intrigued with the promising approach of eschewing monotherapies in favor of sequenced, phase-specific treatments (Guidi, Tomba, & Fava, 2016). Specifically, we began to consider studies that had sequenced pharmacologically induced remission with psychological prophylaxis of relapse/recurrence. This approach took advantage of the cost-efficiency of antidepressant pharmacotherapy in reducing acute symptomatology, while providing a psychological intervention during recovery to reduce the subsequent risk of depressive relapse or recurrence (Guidi, Fava, Fava, & Papakostas, 2011). Prior studies of interpersonal psychotherapy and CBT had demonstrated the potential clinical utility of structured psychotherapies sequenced after antidepressant treatment as a relapse prevention strategy in major depression (e.g., Fava et al., 2004; Frank et al., 1990). Another widely investigated sequential, phase-specific preventive approach is MBCT, an intervention with which our group had deep clinical and research expertise. MBCT is an 8-week, group psychosocial intervention that may have unique benefits deriving from the fact that MBCT is (1) targeted specifically at maladaptive cognitions that drive depression relapse; (2) suitable for use in group settings to maximize accessibility and minimize wait times; and (3) manualized and structured into a formal curriculum, so that therapists may be more easily trained in applying the treatment effectively. MBCT teaches patients how to disengage from depression-related ruminative thought patterns that increase relapse risk (Segal, Williams, & Teasdale, 2013). Given the impracticality of long-term maintenance rTMS and the importance of sustained remission, we considered whether it would be helpful for Michelle—and other patients like her—to follow rTMS with psychotherapy focused on relapse prevention, and specifically with MBCT.

Acquiring and Appraising the Evidence Base

To guide our initial thinking about the use of MBCT following Michelle's course of rTMS,

we gathered a team of collaborators representing expertise in rTMS and the clinical delivery and evaluation of MBCT. To review and appraise the available evidence base, we conducted a search of key words *rTMS* and *MBCT* using Medline, PsycINFO, the Cochrane Library, Health Canada's Clinical Trials database, and the U.S. *clinicaltrials.gov*. We reviewed together the evidence for the efficacy of rTMS. One meta-analysis (Gaynes et al., 2014) shows good-quality evidence for decreasing depression severity (17 trials; $n = 686$) and increasing response rates (15 trials; $n = 643$), and moderate strength of evidence for achieving remission (7 trials; $n = 332$). Another systematic review and meta-analysis (29 trials; $n = 1,371$) showed similar results for response and remission, plus a benign tolerability profile based on examining rates of patient dropout (Berlim et al., 2014). Separate researchers have argued that rTMS has the advantage of being cost-effective through ease of administration and volume of patients treated (Nguyen & Gordon, 2015). This is likely to increase as mechanisms of action are further understood, so that coil placement can occur with greater precision (Silverstein et al., 2015). We were confident that Michelle had received guideline-concordant rTMS and that her experience was consistent with the results reported in the literature.

We also reviewed the evidence for the relapse prevention effects of MBCT, and we concluded that there is strong evidence for efficacy in preventing depressive relapse based on well-conducted randomized controlled trials (RCTs) and meta-analyses, and evidence also for community effectiveness and cost-effectiveness. Specifically, MBCT has been shown to provide significant prophylaxis against MDD relapse following successful treatment with antidepressant medication. A recent meta-analysis ($n = 1,258$) indicated that MBCT reduces risk of relapse by 31% relative to treatment as usual (TAU) over 14-months follow-up, with patients having higher baseline depression receiving greater benefit from MBCT compared with other treatments (Kuyken et al., 2016). A large RCT has confirmed community effectiveness, with MBCT being no less efficacious than maintenance pharmacotherapy (Kuyken et al., 2015).

For treating active symptomatology of depression and anxiety, there are two meta-analyses supporting efficacy (Strauss, Cavanagh, Oliver, & Pettman, 2014; Van Aaldren, Donders, Peffer, & Speckens, 2015) and an RCT supporting community effectiveness (Pots, Meulen-beek, Veehof, Klungers, & Bohlmeijer, 2014). There have been at least three open-label pilot studies suggesting positive results and toler-ability for TRD (Eisendrath et al., 2008; Kenny & Williams, 2007; Pradhan, Parikh, Makani, & Sahoo, 2015). More recently, an RCT in TRD has shown significantly greater reduction in de-pressive symptomatology when compared to an active psychoeducational control (Eisendrath et al., 2016). Putative mechanisms of therapeutic effect for MBCT include both cognitive (Beil-ing et al., 2012; Kuyken et al., 2010) and neuro-biological changes (Barnhofer et al., 2016).

We found limited evidence for using MBCT following rTMS and no RCTs. There is a sugges-tion in a prominent textbook of rTMS indicating that this sequence would be clinically plausible (Fitzgerald & Daskalakis, 2013) and a review article proposing a model that relies on the au-thor's modification of MBCT sequentially fol-lowing rTMS (Pradhan et al., 2015). One small open-label RCT in which rTMS was concur-rently combined with a modified short course of MBCT along with computerized CBT, relax-ation, and other psychological therapies, found no difference between groups and suggested limited benefit (Gill, Clarke, Rigby, Carnell, & Galletly, 2014). There is, however, one case re-port in which CBT administered in conjunction with rTMS suggested some benefit (Vedeniapin, Cheng, & George, 2010). A more recent meta-analysis supports the sequential integration of pharmacotherapy and psychotherapy following somatic therapies for depression (Guidi et al., 2016) and identifies one positive RCT of CBT as a continuation therapy following ECT (Brake-meier et al., 2014). Taken together, these data suggest that MBCT might be promising as an adjunct for those patients who show partial or no response to acute-phase treatments such as rTMS or as a sequenced intervention for patients who show positive response to rTMS but need additional long-term protection from relapse.

As we considered combining rTMS and MBCT more specifically, we grew increasingly interested also in the biological rationale for this combination. Biologically speaking, there is good evidence from the neuroimaging lit-erature to suggest that rTMS and MBCT may synergistically engage a common mechanism for emotional self-regulation within the brain. rTMS appears to exert its therapeutic effects by enhancing the synchronized activity between two specific networks of brain regions, known as the "executive" and "salience" networks,

involved in executive control and signaling motivational salience, respectively (Seeley et al., 2007; reviewed in Downar, Blumberger, & Daskalakis, 2016). Both networks feature core nodes in the prefrontal cortex, including brain regions such as the bilateral dorsolateral and dorsomedial prefrontal cortices in the executive network, and the anterior insula and dorsal an-terior cingulate cortex in the salience network. rTMS appears to act by increasing the syn-chronization of activity between these regions, enhancing cognitive control—the capacity for self-regulation of thoughts, behaviors, and emo-tional states (Dunlop et al., 2015; Salomons et al., 2014). Specifically, rTMS seems to increase inhibitory connectivity between the salience and executive networks, serving as a neural model of prefrontal control over emotion.

Similarly, neuroimaging studies of the effects of MBCT suggest that mindfulness training offers similar enhancement of inhibitory con-nectivity between the executive and salience networks (Farb, Segal, & Anderson, 2013). Specifically, 8 weeks of group-led mindfulness training was associated with the emergence of reciprocal connectivity between the dorsome-dial prefrontal cortex, a hub of the executive network, and regions of the right insula that are associated with the representation of visceral signals from the body. These regions are also core nodes of the salience network, suggesting that mindfulness training may enhance salience network integrity and thereby improve cogni-tive control capacity.

It should be noted that while this reciprocal connectivity between networks represents the normative state of brain connectivity in healthy adults, converging research has linked depres-sion to excitatory rather than inhibitory func-tional connectivity between executive and sa-lience regions (Sheline, Price, Yan, & Mintun, 2010). By contrast, rTMS (Salomons et al., 2014) and mindfulness training (Farb et al., 2013) both normalize prefrontal connectivity. These common neural effects bolster the notion that rTMS and MBCT may act on common regulato-ry mechanisms and therefore have the potential to operate synergistically to reduce depression vulnerability.

Collaborative Clinical Decision Making and Initiating MBCT

We recommended that Michelle consider the eight-session MBCT class following successful rTMS. Michelle was intrigued by the potential benefits of mindfulness, having read about mindfulness in recently published popular books and magazines. Also, given her history of recurrent depression, and anxiety over potential relapse risk with rTMS, she was excited to try something focused on relapse prevention. We decided with her to implement a course of MBCT and used EBP principles to develop, administer, and evaluate this indication of MBCT for Michelle and other patients like her. Specifically, we used the framework of EBP by assessing outcomes from the sequential combination of MBCT following acute-phase response to rTMS in depressed patients. We conducted a clinical pilot of MBCT among outpatients, including Michelle, who had recently completed a course of rTMS for TRD, in order to perform a preliminary evaluation of a sequential treatment strategy that may be theoretically well founded, but is so far untested for its efficacy and tolerability.

We conducted two MBCT groups at the University Health Network in Toronto, where both the rTMS Clinic and a long-standing mindfulness program were affiliated, albeit at different general hospitals in the network. Brochures were produced, explaining the rationale for offering MBCT post-rTMS, and patients were approached by their physician and/or clinic staff. We accepted all patients expressing interest in MBCT whether or not they had improved from rTMS to gain experience in the effects of MBCT in partial and nonresponders. In the screening and orientation session, mention was made of some of the evidence for MBCT improving acute and chronic depressive symptomatology and whether there was sensitivity to any potential difficulty experienced by still depressed participants being mixed with those who had improved with rTMS.

The groups were led by two experienced facilitators of MBCT (Collins and Abbey) in coordination with the head of the rTMS Clinic (Downar), and with guidance from one of the treatment developers of MBCT (Segal). The curriculum used was based on the standard MBCT protocol (Segal et al., 2013). We do not review in detail here the delivery of the MBCT protocol, but we do reflect below on the ways in which our pilot work may inform future delivery of MBCT with this population. Prospective participants were invited to an orientation at which the program was explained and an intake form was completed, detailing past medical and psychiatric history, and symptomatol-

ogy was assessed using a number of symptom rating scales. Intake forms were reviewed and if there were any clinical concerns, or need for clarification, participants were contacted and screened further. Following orientation, eight weekly sessions of 2.5 hours each were offered, along with an optional 5-hour day of silent mindfulness practice between Sessions 6 and 7. In keeping with the original curriculum, emphasis was placed on home practice, with participants encouraged to do at least 45 minutes a day of practice in between sessions.

Michelle was one of 38 post-rTMS patients expressing interest in MBCT, of which 30 attended orientation and 29 started the program. Of the 29 starting, 11 had no or minimal depressive symptoms, suggesting good response to rTMS; 10 patients, Michelle included, had mild to moderate symptoms suggestive of a partial response to rTMS, and eight patients had more severe symptoms at baseline, suggesting no response. The cohort had an average age in their mid-40s, was three-quarters female and predominantly white, and the majority were retired or off work and living alone. About half the group reported past experience with CBT, and around 40%, with mindfulness in one form or another. When Michelle began the first MBCT session, it had been 5 weeks since her final rTMS session. She continued to feel somewhat improved in mood, although she had days of low mood accompanied with anxiety.

Monitoring Clinical Outcomes: Engagement and Symptom Severity

With rTMS showing a moderate ability to reduce TRD, but not maintaining these gains for well over half the treated patients, there are a number of vital clinical and research questions to address. Can MBCT delay relapse for those who have responded to rTMS? Can MBCT improve depressive symptoms in those showing partial or no response to rTMS? What do treatment responders reveal about pathways of relapse vulnerability? Despite the importance of these questions, it was not likely that they could be answered through our modest clinical pilot with Michelle and other patients like her. Thus, we decided to pose more proximal, and clinically pragmatic, questions. Specifically, we asked:

1. Would MBCT following rTMS be of interest to these patients? Given that the ratio-

nale behind neurostimulation treatments stresses that MDD is a biological disorder that is amenable to somatic intervention, how might patient expectations interact with participating in an intervention that is psychological in nature?

2. Was MBCT following rTMS safe and clinically tolerated?
3. Did MBCT following rTMS show short-term symptomatic benefits?

To address our first question about patient interest, we explored patient reasons for joining the group. Overall, there was strong interest, although, as might be expected, patient motivation and expectations for the course differed. Most patients talked about learning coping strategies, or tools, to deal with depression or anxiety, and some just said they wanted to feel better. Like Michelle, a number specifically mentioned relapse prevention as an objective. Some patients said they wanted to learn to relax, and others had no expectations and/or were taking the course because the rTMS Clinic had recommended it. A few participants had taken either mindfulness-based stress reduction (MBSR) or MBCT courses in the past and cited wishing to consolidate their understanding of mindfulness and reestablish a regular meditation practice.

With respect to our second question regarding engagement, Michelle was clearly interested in improving upon treatment gains realized through rTMS as a tool that might prevent relapse to future depressive episodes. Although Michelle attended seven of eight sessions of the course, and the all-day session, among the other 28 participants who started, seven dropped out before the third session (early dropouts) and three dropped out before the fifth session (late dropouts). This translates into an early dropout rate of 24%, a late dropout rate of 10%, and a total dropout of 35%. Nineteen participants completed the program, 13 women and six men. Comparing demographic and historical factors between completers and dropouts, there were no differences except that completers had a greater likelihood of having had previous experience with CBT and mindfulness. Baseline depression, anxiety, and quality-of-life scores differed between completers and dropouts, and both early and late dropouts had higher mean levels of depression and anxiety, and lower quality of life, at baseline, but none of these differences were significant.

Of the seven early dropouts, five were reached for exit interviews, four claimed logistical reasons for needing to drop out (scheduling, travel distance, work, school pressures), and one stated that the course was "not for me." Two early dropouts did not respond to requests for exit interviews and declined to say why. Of the three late dropouts, all reported deriving benefit from the course but stated that circumstances prevented them from continuing. One had not responded to rTMS at all and had the opportunity to enter into a course of ECT. Another had only a partial response to rTMS and had a family emergency that prevented him or her from continuing. The third late dropout was also a partial responder to rTMS and said the timing was not right due to a need to return to work. All three asked to be considered for a future MBCT group.

Finally, although the real value of MBCT will be whether it can delay relapse in those who have responded to rTMS, there is some potential value in tracking symptomatology to assess the gross benefit of MBCT as a measure of tolerability, and as a potential treatment for those who had partial or no response to rTMS. For purposes of clinical monitoring, we administered the Beck Depression Inventory–II (BDI-II), the Patient Health Questionnaire–9 (PHQ-9), the General Anxiety Disorder–7 (GAD-7) scale, the Quality of Life Enjoyment and Satisfaction Questionnaire (Q-LES-Q), and the Mindful Attention Awareness Scales (MAAS) assessing dispositional mindfulness at baseline, midway and course end. Aside from the MAAS, the other scales were standard in the rTMS Clinic to measure baseline and response. In addition, participants completed a precourse assessment asking about expectations, a midcourse three-item feedback questionnaire, and a postcourse assessment evaluating their experience, how useful they found the program, and suggestions for improvement. We report here broad changes in the scales of the cohort, and the specific experiences of Michelle.

Of the 19 participants who completed the program, aggregate scores evidenced three participants who were *very much improved*; six participants who were *much improved*; six participants who were *minimally improved*; three who had *no change*; and one participant who was *minimally worse*. It should be noted that the one participant who rated minimally worse on depression and quality-of-life ratings reported a major life event during the group and also showed minimal improvements in anxiety and dispositional mindfulness scores. This person also rated the course as *extremely positive* and *extremely useful* and asked to take the course again.

Aggregate scores of BDI-II showed a mean group reduction from moderate to mild depression scores, and these differences were statistically significant. PHQ-9 scores improved from low end of moderate to high mild scores but showed no statistical significance. GAD-7 scores improved from moderate scores to mild and showed significance. Group Q-LES-Q scores measuring quality of life and life satisfaction improved a statistically nonsignificant 6 points, and MAAS increased a statistically significant 9 points, suggesting improvements in dispositional mindfulness.

Michelle showed an improvement in her two depressive and one anxiety rating scores from moderate to mild. These improvements were commensurate with improvements quality of life and life satisfaction, and dispositional mindfulness. She rated the course as somewhat helpful in managing current depressive symptoms and the risk of future relapse. Michelle found most helpful the skill to disengage from negative thinking and to see depression recurrence as a spiral that might be prevented. Of note, midcourse she reported her sister being diagnosed with breast cancer. Michelle reflected that normally she would find this highly stressful and that it would precipitate debilitating anxious and depressive rumination and withdrawal, but in this case, she was better able to manage these thoughts and be more available to support her sister. She stated that she still felt sadness for her sister, and worry about her own health, but was able to "hold these feelings without them spiralling out of control."

Global evaluations of the MBCT program provided by patients were very encouraging. Participants completed a 0- to 10-point Likert scale indicating how negative or positive their experience was, and how unhelpful or helpful the course was for them. Mean ratings showed a *somewhat* to *extremely* positive experience, and as to utility or helpfulness, a mean rating of *somewhat* helpful. Positive statements elicited from participants that supported their ratings on these two dimensions included "Less rumination," "Extremely supportive environment," "It's been a life changer," "Realizing I am not my depression is liberating," and "My psychiatrist has noticed a real improvement in my mood." Like a number of participants, Michelle described how supportive it was to be among other people who had experienced lifelong depression, and had gone through rTMS. She reflected that this normalized depression for her and allowed her to see it "more as an illness and less as a moral failing."

In contrast to Michelle, some participants described negative responses, such as "Practicing at home remains difficult," "I feel bad I am not doing it on my own even though the facilitators have normalized this," "I find the meditation of turning toward the difficult scary and brings my mood down," "I still don't understand why in some meditations we observe our thoughts when thoughts are my problem." When Michelle was asked about potential negative aspects of her experience, she reported, "I continue to struggle to practice formally, but the 3-minute breathing space and mindful walking practices really help. I can commit to those most days." She also reported that she wanted to seek out additional mindfulness courses to further consolidate her learning, and she was exploring a mindfulness-based chronic pain course to focus on addressing her pain.

Does MBCT Need to Be Adapted for Patients with TRD?

One of the key strengths of the EBP framework is that it supports ongoing dialogue between clinical practice and research. Our initial pilot groups provide a dynamic illustration of this dialogue in action. We implemented the standard MBCT curriculum (Segal et al., 2013) with no formal modifications in the two pilot groups. However, we monitored outcomes and the subjective experiences of both patients and providers, and we use those data to reflect on future changes to the MBCT curriculum that might be tested in future research and practice.

Although the focus remained on prevention of depressive relapse, some of the participants had achieved little or no response to rTMS. This seemed to be a key issue in the first group, in which some rTMS nonresponders expressed difficulty in hearing others talk glowingly about their response to rTMS and how much better they felt. It also contributed to at least one late dropout in the first pilot group. Michelle herself commented that she was grateful for the improvement brought by rTMS, but she also reported feeling envious of those who appeared to her to be "all better" given that she experienced some residual symptoms of depression. In the second group it was less of an issue, probably because patients in that group had significantly higher baseline depression and anxiety at baseline than the first group. Although this led to a good deal of affective expression during the course, especially when exploring the *Territory of Depression* and *Identifying Relapse Signatures* modules of the MBCT curriculum, participants were highly engaged in the course and reported benefit.

In each session, participants' experience with home practice was discussed. The facilitator's impression was that home practice was somewhat more of a struggle for these participants compared to other groups of depressed patients treated with MBCT, and that levels of anxiety and depression correlated with difficulties in practice. Although it is an integral part of the MBCT curriculum to normalize this, to identify how judgmental thoughts about the practice compound the difficulties, and to encourage recommitment to next week's practice, this needed to be emphasized more than in other MBCT groups conducted by the facilitators. In some instances, shorter practices, like the 3-minute breathing space, or shorter meditation periods, were encouraged, and in a few cases, it was conceded that no formal practice was being done but there was still value in informal mindfulness practices at home and formal practices in class. Michelle herself found it challenging to do home practice; however, over time, she reported an ability to see this as "just the way it is" and not something to personalize and judge herself around.

With respect to patient attrition, our dropout rate seems high compared to what has been previously reported in the literature. Patients who did drop out had higher levels of depressive symptoms, possibly making it difficult for them to engage fully in the mindfulness practices. We reflected together on the fact that our figures are higher than those reported in a recently completed RCT of MBCT for TRD—here the dropout rate was 12.7% (Eisendrath et al., 2016), although patients in this study were not receiving rTMS, but rather optimization of their initial antidepressant pharmacotherapy. Further clinical delivery of MBCT in this population will allow us to determine whether the nature of TRD in post-rTMS patients requires additional orientation and retention strategies throughout the 8-week program. Despite the dropout rate,

and one participant having minimally worse ratings postcourse, MBCT appeared to be well tolerated, with no adverse reactions.

Conclusions

Our clinical impression is that MBCT was a useful intervention in this post-rTMS population, as illustrated by the case of Michelle. The particular sequential approach of offering MBCT following rTMS was of interest to the patient population and valued by participants as both a positive experience and useful to them in dealing with depression, and it was feasible, safe and tolerated well, and seemed to show short-term therapeutic benefit. From the perspective of our pilot work, we would conclude that MBCT shows promise as a sequential therapy with rTMS but that further, more structured evaluation is needed to define its positioning within routine clinical practice. Data from controlled evaluations will also be needed to assess its value for relapse prophylaxis. Obviously, to answer the question of whether MBCT can improve relapse rates of depression post-rTMS, there will need to be RCTs that our pilot work can inform.

There are some clinical considerations that might need to be addressed in future groups relating to mixing responders and nonresponders, as well as modifications to the curriculum to account for the high baseline levels of symptomatology even after rTMS, the experience of having lived with TRD potentially triggering curriculum elements such as the *Territory of Depression* and *Relapse Signatures,* and potential difficulties with home practice. Given that there seemed to be some distress created from mixing robust rTMS responders with those showing only a partial, or nonresponse, there may be some value in conducting different groups for relapse prevention versus persistent TRD. For the latter, one consideration would be to utilize some of the adaptations to MBCT suggested by Eisendrath, Chartier, and McLane (2011) in their work with TRD, including modifying the language to emphasize dealing with current depression versus prevention of relapse, pointing to the state dependency of mood and thought linkages, and employing select practices from acceptance and commitment therapy. An example of the latter would be demonstrating the woven bamboo finger trap (Hayes, 2007), in which participants learn that pulling one's fingers away only tightens the grip, and only by relaxing and moving one's fingers closer together can one release the trap. This illustrates the metaphor of turning toward the difficult and acceptance of depression as a management strategy.

As an example of EBP, we see our work as demonstrating how an intervention can be introduced to a new population in which there is rationale for its benefit but little formal research evidence. EBP in action provides a way to approach adaptations to new populations by asking specific questions, critically appraising and applying the available evidence, assessing the impact and tolerability of the intervention using rating scales and other measures outside of a formal research context, and modifying future application accordingly. This is especially relevant to psychotherapies such as mindfulness-based interventions, whose increasing popularity is leading to widespread application to new populations and clinical problems, with only preliminary evidence to support its use. Our work has the potential to model how mindfulness-based interventions such as MBCT can be adapted to new patient populations for which good evidence is lacking. Given the exponential growth of "therapeutic" mindfulness in a wide range of populations and clinical conditions, there is a need for more rigorous, evidence-based approaches to adapting these modalities for new uses while waiting for higher levels of evidence to accrue through research (Dimidjian & Segal, 2015). For the clinical problem of depression, and in particular TRD, which is a tremendous personal and public health burden, our work with Michelle and with patients like her, provides a guide for how to explore new treatment approaches in ways that are methodologically rigorous, conceptually sound, and evidence based.

References

Bakker, N., Shahab, S., Giacobbe, P., Blumberger, D. M., Daskalakis, Z. J., Kennedy, S. H., et al. (2015). rTMS of the dorsomedial prefrontal cortex for major depression: Safety, tolerability, effectiveness, and outcome predictors for 10 Hz versus intermittent theta-burst stimulation. *Brain Stimulation, 8*(2), 208–215.

Barnhofer, T., Huntenburg, J. M., Lifshitz, M., Wild, J., Antonova, E., & Margulies, D. S. (2016). How mindfulness training may help to reduce vulnerability for recurrent depression: A neuroscientific perspective. *Clinical Psychological Science, 4*(2), 328–343.

Beiling, P. J., Hawley, L. L., Bloch, R. T., Corcoran, K. M., Levitan, R. D., Young, L. T., et al. (2012). Treatment specific changes in decentering following mindfulness-based cognitive therapy versus antidepressant medication or placebo for prevention of depressive relapse. *Journal of Consulting and Clinical Psychology, 80*(3), 365–372.

Berlim, M. T., van den Eynde, F., Tovar-Perdomo, S., & Daskalakis, Z. J. (2014). Response, remission and drop-out rates following high-frequency repetitive transcranial magnetic stimulation (rTMS) for treating major depression: A systematic review and meta-analysis. *Psychological Medicine, 44*, 225–239.

Brakemeier, E. L., Merkl, A., Wilbertz, G., Quante, A., Regen, F., Bührsch, N., et al. (2014). CBT as a continuation therapy after electroconvulsive therapy in depression: A randomized controlled trial. *Biological Psychiatry, 3*, 194–202.

Brunoni, A. R., Chaimani, A., Moffa, A. H., Razza, L. B., Gattaz, W. F., Daskalakis, Z. J., et al. (2017). Repetitive transcranial magnetic stimulation for the acute treatment of major depressive episodes: A systematic review with network meta-analysis. *JAMA Psychiatry, 74*(2), 143–152.

Dimidjian, S., & Segal, Z. (2015). Prospects for a clinical science of mindfulness-based intervention. *American Psychologist, 70*(7), 593–620.

Downar, J., Blumberger, D. M., & Daskalakis, Z. J. (2016). The neural crossroads of psychiatric illness: An emerging target for brain stimulation. *Trends in Cognitive Sciences, 20*(2), 107–120.

Downar, J., & Daskalakis, C. J. (2013). New targets for rTMS in depression: A review of convergent evidence. *Brain Stimulation: Basic, Translational, and Clinical Research in Neuromodulation, 6*, 231–240.

Dunlop, K., Woodside, B., Lam, E., Olmsted, M., Colton, P., Giacobbe, P., et al. (2015). Increases in frontostriatal connectivity are associated with response to dorsomedial repetitive transcranial magnetic stimulation in refractory binge/purge behaviors. *NeuroImage: Clinical, 2*(8), 611–618.

Eisendrath, S. J., Chartier, M., & McLane, M. (2011). Adapting mindfulness-based cognitive therapy for treatment-resistant depression: A clinical case study. *Cognitive and Behavioral Practice, 18*(3), 362–370.

Eisendrath, S. J., Delucchi, K., Bitner, R., Fenimore, P., Smit, M., & McLane, M. (2008). Mindfulness-based cognitive therapy for treatment-resistant depression: A pilot study. *Psychotherapy and Psychosomatics, 77*(5), 319–320.

Eisendrath, S. J., Gillung, E., Delucchi, K. L., Segal, Z. V., Nelson, J. C., McInnes, L. A., et al. (2016). A randomized controlled trial of mindfulness-based cognitive therapy for treatment-resistant depression. *Psychotherapy and Psychosomatics, 85*(2), 99–110.

Farb, N. A., Segal, Z. V., & Anderson, A. K. (2013). Mindfulness meditation training alters cortical representations of interoceptive attention. *Social Cognitive and Affective Neuroscience, 8,* 15–26.

Fava, G. A., Ruini, C., Rafanelli, C., Finos, L., Conti, S., & Grandi, S. (2004). Six-year outcome of cognitive behavior therapy for prevention of recurrent depression. *American Journal of Psychiatry, 61*(10), 1872–1876.

Fitzgerald, P. B., & Daskalakis, Z. J. (2013). *Repetitive transcranial magnetic stimulation treatment for depressive disorders: A practical guide.* New York: Springer.

Frank E., Kupfer D. J., Perel J. M., Cones C., Jarrett D. B., Mallingher A. G., et al. (1990). Three-year outcomes for maintenance therapiers in recurrent depression. *Archives of General Psychiatry, 47,* 1093 1099.

Gaynes, B. N., Lloyd, S. W., Lux, L., Gartlehner, G., Hansen, R. A., Brode, S., et al. (2014). Repetitive transcranial magnetic stimulation for treatment-resistant depression: A systematic review and meta-analysis. *Journal of Clinical Psychiatry, 75,* 477–489.

Gill, S., Clarke, P., Rigby, A., Carnell B., & Galletly, C. (2014). Transcranial magnetic stimulation and psychological therapies: Considering the benefits of a combined treatment approach for depression. *World Journal of Medical Research, 3,* 46–53.

Guidi, J., Fava, G. A., Fava, M., & Papakostas, G. I. (2011). Efficacy of the sequential integration of psychotherapy and pharmacotherapy in major depressive disorder: A preliminary meta analysis. *Psychological Medicine, 41*(2), 321–331.

Guidi, J., Tomba, E., & Fava, G. A. (2016). The sequential integration of pharmacotherapy and psychotherapy in the treatment of major depressive disorder: A meta-analysis of the sequential model and a critical review of the literature. *American Journal of Psychiatry, 173*(2), 128–137.

Hayes, S. C. (2007). Hello darkness: Discovering our values by confronting our fears. *Psychotherapy Networker, 31*(5), 46–52.

Janicak, P. G., Nahas, Z., Lisanby, S. H., Solvason, H. B., Sampson, S. M., McDonald, W. M., et al. (2010). Durability of clinical benefit with transcranial magnetic stimulation (TMS) in the treatment of pharmacoresistant major depression. *Brain Stimulation, 3,* 187–199.

Kedzior, K. K., Reitz, S. K., Azorina, V., & Loo, C. (2015). Durability of the antidepressant effect of the high-frequency repetitive transcranial magnetic stimulation (rTMS) in the absence of maintenance treatment in major depression: A systematic review and meta-analysis. *Depression and Anxiety, 32,* 193–203.

Kenny, M. A., & Williams, J. M. (2007). Treatment-resistant depressed patients show a good response to mindfulness-based cognitive therapy. *Behaviour Research and Therapy, 45*(3), 617–625.

Kessler, R. C., Berglund, P., Demler, O., Jin, R., Koretz, D., Merikangas, K. R., et al. (2003). The epidemiology of major depressive disorder: Results from the National Comorbidity Survey Replication (NCS-R). *Journal of the American Medical Association, 289*(23), 3095–3105.

Kuyken, W., Hayes, R., Barrett, B., Byng, R., Dalgleish, T., Kessler, D., et al. (2015). Effectiveness and cost-effectiveness of mindfulness-based cognitive therapy compared with maintenance antidepressant treatment in the prevention of depressive relapse or recurrence (PREVENT): A randomised controlled trial. *Lancet, 386,* 63–73.

Kuyken, W., Warren, F. C., Taylor, R. S., Whalley, B., Crane, C., Bondolfi, G., et al. (2016). Effect of MBCT in prevention of depressive relapse: An individual patient data meta-analysis from randomized trials. *JAMA Psychiatry, 73,* 565–574.

Kuyken, W., Watkins, E., Holden, E., White, K., Taylor, R. S., Byford, S., et al. (2010). How does mindfulness-based cognitive therapy work? *Behaviour Research and Therapy, 48*(11), 1105–1112.

Lisanby, S. H. (2007). Electroconvulsive therapy for depression. *New England Journal of Medicine, 357*(19), 1939–1945.

Murray, C. J., Vos, T., Lozano, R., Naghavi, M., Flaxman, A. D., Michaud, C., et al. (2012). Disability-adjusted life years (DALYs) for 291 diseases and injuries in 21 regions, 1990–2010: A systematic analysis for the Global Burden of Disease Study 2010. *Lancet, 380,* 2197–2223.

Nguyen, K. H., & Gordon, L. G. (2015). Cost-effectiveness of rTMS versus antidepressant therapy for treatment-resistant depression. *Value Health, 18*(5), 597–604.

Pots, W. T., Meulenbeek, P. A., Veehof, M. M., Klungers, J., & Bohlmeijer, E. T. (2014). The efficacy of mindfulness-based cognitive therapy as a public mental health intervention for adults with mild to moderate depressive symptomatology: A randomized controlled trial. *PLOS ONE, 9,* e109789.

Pradhan, B., Parikh, T., Makani, R., & Sahoo, M. (2015). Ketamine, transcranial magnetic stimulation, and depression specific yoga and mindfulness-based cognitive therapy in management of treatment resistant depression: Review and some data on efficacy. *Depression Research and Treatment, 2015,* Article No. 842817.

Ratnasingham, S., Cairney, J., Manson, H., Rehm, J., Lin, E., & Kurdyak, P. (2013). The burden of mental illness and addiction in Ontario. *Canadian Journal of Psychiatry, 58,* 529–537.

Rizvi, S. J., Grima, E., Tan, M., Rotzinger, S., Lin, P., Mcintyre, R. S., et al. (2014). Treatment resistant depression in primary care in Canada. *Canadian Journal of Psychiatry, 59*(7), 349–357.

Rush, A. J., Trivedi, M. H., Wisniewski, S. R., Nierenberg, A. A., Stewart, J. W., Warden, D., et al. (2006). Acute and longer-term outcomes in depressed outpatients requiring one or several treatment steps: A STAR*D report. *American Journal of Psychiatry, 163,* 1905–1917.

Salomons, T. V., Dunlop, K., Kennedy, S. H., Flint, A., Geraci, J., Giacobbe, P., et al. (2014). Resting-state cortico-thalamic-striatal connectivity predicts response to dorsomedial prefrontal rTMS in major depressive disorder. *Neuropsychopharmacology, 39,* 488–498.

Schatzberg, A. F., Rush, A. J., Arnow, B. A., Banks, P. L., Blalock, J. A., Borian, F. E., et al. (2005). Chronic depression: Medication (nefazodone) or psychotherapy (CBASP) is effective when the other is not. *Archives of General Psychiatry, 62*(5), 513–520.

Seeley, W. W., Menon, V., Schatzberg, A. F., Keller, J., Glover, G. H., Kenna, H., et al. (2007). Dissociable intrinsic connectivity networks for salience processing and executive control. *Journal of Neuroscience, 27,* 2349–2356.

Segal, Z. V., Williams, M., & Teasdale, J. (2013). *Mindfulness-based cognitive therapy for depression* (2nd ed.). New York: Guilford Press.

Sheline, Y. I., Price, J. L., Yan, Z., & Mintun, M. A. (2010). Resting-state functional MRI in depression unmasks increased connectivity between networks via the dorsal nexus. *Proceedings of the National Academy of Sciences of the USA, 107,* 11020–11025.

Silverstein, W. K., Noda, Y., Barr, M. S., Vila-Rodriguez, F., Rajji, T. K., Fitzgerald, P. B., et al. (2015). Neurobiological predictors of response to dorsolateral prefrontal cortex rTMS in depression: A systematic review. *Depression and Anxiety, 32*(12), 871–891.

Strauss, C., Cavanagh, K., Oliver, A., & Pettman, D. (2014). Mindfulness-based interventions for people diagnosed with a current episode of an anxiety or depressive disorder: A meta-analysis of randomised controlled trials. *PLOS ONE, 9*(4), e96110.

Trivedi, R. B., Nieuwsma, J. A., & Williams, J. W., Jr. (2011). Examination of the utility of psychotherapy for patients with treatment resistant depression: A systematic review. *Journal of General Internal Medicine, 26*(6), 643–650.

Van Aaldren, J. R., Donders, A. R., Peffer, K., & Speckens, A. E. (2015). Long-term outcome of mindfulness based cognitive therapy in recurrently depressed patients with and without a depressive episode at baseline. *Depression and Anxiety, 32,* 563–569.

Vedeniapin, A., Cheng, L., & George, M. S. (2010). Feasibility of simultaneous cognitive behavioral therapy and left prefrontal rTMS for treatment resistant depression. *Brain Stimulation, 3*(4), 207–210.

Wiles, N., Thomas, L., Abel, A., Ridgway, N., Turner, N., Campbell, J., et al. (2013). Cognitive behavioural therapy as an adjunct to pharmacotherapy for primary care based patients with treatment resistant depression: Results of the CoBalT randomised controlled trial. *Lancet, 2,* 375–384.

CHAPTER 19

Beyond Specialty Mental Health

*Rationale and Clinical Application
of Behavioral Activation in Primary Care*

SAM HUBLEY
CHRISTOPHER R. MARTELL
JENNIFER N. CARTY

Tony is a 37-year-old, married, Mexican American man with two young children. One thing to know about Tony is that he has good hands. Before he had a family, Tony had two big passions in life—cars and football. On most weekends as a kid, you could find Tony in his dad's garage working on someone's broken-down car or at the nearby park playing pickup football with neighborhood friends. He had early aspirations for a pro football career and excelled as a slot receiver through high school, but Tony decided in his junior year to become a mechanic and work on race cars. It was also during this time that Tony experienced depression for the first time, and he nearly got kicked off the football team for skipping school and declining grades.

Tony recovered from this episode of depression without medical or psychological treatment only to experience a more severe episode later that year, for which he eventually received antidepressant medication from his primary care provider (PCP). As the oldest of eight children, Tony's parents provided little support to him during these episodes and instead focused on his younger siblings and their own jobs. His father took an especially hard line: "Next to me, you are the man of this family, so start acting like it. Your mother and I work very hard for you and your brothers and sisters, and we don't have time to baby you.

Unless you're hurt or sick, we expect you to pass your classes and stay on the football team. Got it?"

Despite continued struggles with depression, Tony graduated high school and immediately found work at a local garage owned by a family friend who specialized in rebuilding engines for race cars. He experienced one to two episodes of depression per year, which he learned to "muscle" through by forcing himself to work every day despite feeling like he was "coming apart," and he had little energy most of the time. Even when not depressed, Tony often felt stressed out and like he was not living up to his potential. He found some degree of comfort in alcohol and food, which evolved into a habit of making two stops on his way home from work every day—first, to buy a pint of vodka at a liquor store, and second, to buy a supersize soda from his favorite fast-food restaurant, into which he poured half that vodka.

Several years of this routine culminated in a diagnosis of type 2 diabetes at age 26. Tony described that, initially, he did not follow medical recommendations to manage his type 2 diabetes by exercising more and making healthier food choices. Tony thought that, like his depression, diabetes was something he could just "muscle" through. By the time Tony turned 31, he had developed several secondary problems due to poorly controlled type 2 diabetes. In addition to increasing fatigue and troubles with his vision, most distressing to Tony was severe chronic neuropathic pain, which was unremitting despite myriad trials of multiple medications and medical procedures. Tony's depression had also gotten progressively worse in tandem with increasing pain, such that through the better part of his 30s, Tony was experiencing five episodes of depression annually.

Currently, Tony is out of work and spends much of his day watching television. He no longer drinks but still reports difficulty with eating healthily. Due to progressive neuropathic pain, he no longer exercises and even has difficulty walking from one room to the other. Tony describes multiple ways in which depression and chronic pain are interfering with his life and highlights in particular that he feels worthless. Having experienced little benefit from previous interventions, he understandably feels hopeless. He often asks himself rhetorically, "What kind of man am I if I can't provide for my family or even throw a football with my kids?"

*   *   *

Tony's experience of depression, diabetes, and chronic pain is common in the primary care setting. In fact, 78% of individuals with depression present for treatment in the primary care setting, and these patients have an average of 2.5 chronic medical comorbidities (Young, Klap, Sherbourne, & Wells, 2001). Not only is there a high co-occurrence between behavioral health disorders and medical conditions (Barnett et al., 2012), but the presence of a behavioral health disorder adversely impacts the course and prognosis of co-occurring medical conditions in ways that increase the likelihood for disability, poor outcomes, and extraneous costs (Merikangas et al., 2007; Olfson, Blanco, Wang, Laje, & Correll, 2014). The question of how best to care for patients like Tony has been a focus of intense national attention (Baird et al., 2014; Kazak, Nash, Hiroto, & Kaslow, 2017; National Center for Quality Assurance, 2014). Although national, epidemiological surveys indicate that most people with behavioral health disorders never receive treatment (Wang et al., 2005), people with behavioral health disorders are more likely to visit a primary care clinic than a behavioral health clinic (National Center for Health Statistics, 2015) and those who do receive treatment are just as likely to be seen in general medical versus specialty mental health

sectors (Petterson, Miller, Payne-Murphy, & Phillips, 2014; Wang et al., 2005).

There is a growing trend for delivering behavioral health interventions within primary care (Butler et al., 2008; Kwan & Nease, 2013). The Agency for Healthcare Research and Quality (AHRQ) Lexicon for Behavioral Health and Primary Care (Peek, 2013) defines integrated behavioral health and primary care (IBHPC) as

> a practice team of primary care and behavioral health clinicians working together with patients and families, using a systematic and cost-effective approach to provide patient-centered care for a defined population. This care may address mental health and substance abuse conditions, health behaviors (including their contribution to chronic medical illnesses), life stressors and crises, stress-related physical symptoms, and ineffective patterns of health care utilization. (p. 2)

Within this model, behavioral health providers (BHPs) function as consultants to PCPs and patients by providing brief (15–30 minutes) consultations and short-term psychotherapy (five to six visits). Focusing on brief consultation and psychotherapy allows BHPs to be available to a larger portion of patients on a clinic's panel, in addition to protecting time for other important administrative tasks (e.g., developing registries, implementing quality improvement and research initiatives, and working with clinic leadership to obtain federal and local reimbursement designations) and clinical functions (e.g., precepting, accepting "warm handoffs," and conducting shared medical appointments with PCPs). Though it can be tempting to function as the "in-house psychotherapist" due to the high need for mental and behavioral health interventions within the primary care setting, providing brief episodes of care allows BHPs to function as an integral member of the primary care team as opposed to a "co-located" therapist (i.e., *co-location* involves providing psychotherapy only in the same location, but with little engagement within the clinic otherwise).

In this chapter, we emphasize the clinical functions of BHPs in the primary care setting by using our work with Tony to illustrate our selection of an empirically supported treatment, behavioral activation (BA), and our methods of adapting it to fit within the integrated behavioral health and primary care model. There are multiple examples of researchers and clinicians successfully adapting empirically supported behavioral health interventions to the primary care setting (e.g., Roy-Byrne et al., 2010; Wiles et al., 2013). We have emphasized BA in our work with Tony and patients like him given a strong conceptual and pragmatic rationale for the ways in which BA "fits" in the context of integrated behavioral health and primary care settings. We conclude the chapter by reflecting on implications for clinical practice in primary care settings and highlighting future research and quality improvement initiatives to address gaps in the evidence base.

An Invitation to Behavioral Health

Tony's PCP, Dr. Williams, had known Tony for only a couple of years and inherited him as a patient when Tony's previous PCP retired. While discussing new options for addressing his pain in a particularly difficult visit, Tony leveled with her, "Honestly Doc, I'm not even sure I want to go down that road. Just like everything else you've tried, it probably won't work and I'll just go on being useless to my family." Dr. Williams had suspected that in addition to long-standing chronic neuropathic pain secondary to type 2 diabetes, Tony also suffered from depression. She felt discouraged about following up on this issue because, in previous visits, Tony had stonewalled her attempts to discuss the relationship between stress, depression, and pain: "I was raised to be tough and not complain about how I feel."

Dr. Williams requested a 2-minute consultation with one of our clinic's BHPs (Carty, third author) before Tony's next visit. In the minutes before his next visit, the BHP and Dr. Williams met in the precepting room and developed a plan to validate Tony's frustration and skepticism about treatment, while also normalizing the process of addressing mental health concerns. The BHP suggested, "Some patients are more open to the idea that stress caused by pain is completely normal, and there are effective treatments for stress that have nothing to do with being weak. If you can get a window, ask if he will answer some more questions or agree to meet me for a brief intro."

When Dr. Williams asked if Tony was still feeling depressed, Tony said he did not want to talk about his feelings. She acknowledged his upbringing and preference to not discuss his feelings but also suggested that uncontrolled pain and the stress it causes can get the better of even the toughest and most self-reliant men.

Tony softened a bit and agreed that it was very stressful to be in so much pain. She went on to describe that she has a set of questions she asks patients about stress, and Tony agreed to complete the Patient Health Questionnaire–9 (PHQ-9; Kroenke, Spitzer, & Williams, 2001). After reviewing his score of 22 out of 27, Tony's initial surprise gave way to choking up as he admitted he was miserable and did not know what to do. Dr. Williams asked him to accept a referral to the clinic's integrated behavioral health service.

To initiate the referral to behavioral health, Dr. Williams explained that a BHP worked closely with her in the clinic and that she could set up an initial visit. Tony got cold feet and started saying he was not so sure he wanted to follow through with the meeting, as he did not see the point of complaining about his problems. Dr. Williams acknowledged his viewpoint and agreed that therapy focused on talking about feelings is not very everyone. She clarified also that the nature of the behavioral health service feels more like learning and problem solving. Still sensing Tony's reluctance, she suggested that she introduce Tony to the BHP right away for a brief meeting and Tony could decide later if he wanted to follow up with her for a longer visit. Tony agreed to this arrangement, so Dr. Williams found the BHP in the precepting room and requested a meeting with Tony and his wife at the end of his medical appointment to review his PHQ-9 score and chronic pain concerns, and gauge his interest in engaging in behavioral health treatment. She explained to the BHP that Tony was reluctant about engaging with behavioral health because "Real men don't cry." That phrase triggered the BHP to recall her multicultural training, which emphasized how culture-specific attitudes, behaviors, and norms transmitted through generations influence health care decision making (Shiraev & Levy, 2010; Sue & Sue, 1999). The BHP suspected that Tony might benefit from integrating a behavioral health perspective into his medical treatment plan, but that there was a risk that he might not engage if she appeared too focused on a diagnosis of depression or emphasized talking about feelings as their primary intervention.

Due to the integrated, rather than co-located, nature of the clinic, the BHP was immediately available to meet Tony on the same day as his medical appointment and provided a 5-minute introduction and description of the behavioral health service. Tony was quiet during this interaction, but his wife thanked the BHP for stopping in and expressed significant concerns about the fact that Tony "wasn't himself." In particular, she said that he was spending many hours watching TV as opposed to engaging with their children or hobbies that were normally important parts of Tony's life, and she knew that he needed help but had not known how to help him. Tony nodded during this part of the conversation and said that he felt terrible about being a burden and not contributing more to his family. The BHP normalized how hard it is to live with chronic pain, and how there is a whole set of stressors to deal with because of chronic pain. Tony agreed emphatically but then expressed frustration that he was stuck and nothing helped his pain. The BHP took this opportunity to say that she might not be able to help Tony reduce his pain, but she could help identify ways to reduce the stress caused by the pain; she asked him if he would agree to meet with her one time so that she could hear more about his story and discuss some potential options. Tony agreed to follow up with her in the primary clinic the following week. To facilitate communication between the medical teams, the BHP added a note in the electronic medical record describing the content of her conversation with Tony and his wife and, later in the day, caught up with Tony's PCP in the lunchroom to update her on the plan for follow-up with Tony.

Reviewing the Data and Selecting an Approach

In preparing for her work with Tony, the BHP deliberated over using a cognitive-behavioral, interpersonal, or BA approach. There is a strong evidence base supporting each of these approaches in the treatment of depression (e.g., Barth et al., 2013). Given that Tony's score on the PHQ-9 indicated severe depression and that he was engaging in multiple avoidant behaviors (e.g., prolonged episodes of TV watching, reduced time spent with children, abandonment of previously enjoyed activities such as working on cars and playing sports), the BHP seriously considered the choice of BA. Five considerations informed her choice.

First, the theoretical foundation for BA is based on the idea that in response to feeling distressed or overwhelmed with difficult life situations, many people respond with avoidant coping behaviors. Avoidant coping behaviors, such as "comfort" eating, prolonged sedentary

activity (e.g., watching TV, Internet browsing), and tobacco, alcohol or substance, misuse, are conceptualized as negatively reinforcing behaviors because they temporarily function to reduce distress despite carrying long-term negative consequences.

Second, the evidence base for BA in general was compelling. Jacobson and colleagues (1996) conducted a seminal dismantling study of cognitive-behavioral therapy (CBT) to compare the relative contributions of BA and CBT. In this study, adults with major depression were randomly assigned to one of three treatment conditions: BA only, BA plus automatic thought modification, and the full CBT package. Results suggested comparability between BA and the full CBT package in terms of acute efficacy (Jacobson et al., 1996) and relapse prevention (Gortner, Gollan, Dobson, & Jacobson, 1998). Following development of BA into a stand-alone treatment (Jacobson, Martell, & Dimidjian, 2001; Martell, Addis, & Jacobson, 2001; Martell, Dimidjian, & Herman-Dunn, 2013) and a self-help manual (Addis & Martell, 2004), BA was subsequently tested in a randomized controlled clinical trial (RCT) comparing BA, CBT, antidepressant medication (ADM), and a placebo control (Dimidjian et al., 2006). Results of this study similarly suggested comparability of CBT and ADM, the "gold standards" of depression treatment, in terms of acute efficacy (Dimidjian et al., 2006) and relapse prevention (Dobson et al., 2008). BA also appeared to outperform CBT for more severely depressed patients (Coffman, Martell, Dimidjian, Gallop, & Hollon, 2007), and lost fewer patients to attrition and was more cost-effectiveness than ADM (Dimidjian et al., 2006). This study provided a strong empirical base for BA that continues to grow rapidly. In fact, the number of BA-relevant articles has grown sharply in the past decade, now numbering several hundred compared to an estimated cumulative total of 50 articles before 2000 (Dimidjian, Barrera, Martell, Muñoz, & Lewinsohn, 2011). Meta-analytic summaries of over 30 trials (Cuijpers, van Straten, & Warmerdam, 2007; Ekers, Richards, & Gilbody, 2008; Mazzucchelli, Kane, & Rees, 2009) and national treatment guidelines (e.g., National Institute for Health and Clinical Excellence, 2009) provide further support for the important role of BA in the treatment of depression.

Third, the evidence base for BA also was compelling in its application with Latino patients (Kanter, Santiago-Rivera, Rusch, Busch, & West, 2010), and patients with comorbid medical conditions such as cancer (Hopko, Bell, Armento, Hunt, & Lejuez, 2005; Hopko et al., 2011), obesity (Pagoto, Bodenlos, Schneider, Olendzki, & Spates, 2008), and diabetes (Schneider et al., 2011). The breadth of this work suggests that BA may be particularly well suited as a treatment framework for a wide variety of people, especially when a focus on explicit behavioral change is desired.

Fourth, BA, a parsimonious psychotherapy that is amenable to delivery within primary care settings, is consistent with integrated behavioral health and primary care models that emphasize brief, patient-centered behavioral interventions geared toward functional improvement. There exist multiple examples of transporting BA to unique settings such as primary care using both mental health specialists (Gros & Haren, 2011; Uebelacker, Weisberg, Haggarty, & Miller, 2009) and nonspecialists (Ekers, Dawson, & Bailey, 2012; Ekers, Richards, McMillan, Bland, & Gilbody, 2011). Similarly, Hopko and colleagues (2011) have demonstrated effectiveness of BA for depressed cancer patients in oncology clinics, and Dimidjian and colleagues (2017) recently completed an RCT of BA delivered by obstetric nurses and behavioral health providers for antenatal depression.

Finally, the BHP's decision making was informed by the focus on clinician expertise and patient preferences in the delivery of evidence-based practice (EBP) (see Spring, Marchese, & Steglitz, Chapter 1, this volume). Specifically, the BHP's supervisor (Hubley) was an expert in BA and knew that she would have access to high-quality supervision in adapting the delivery of BA for integrated care. Also, among the available treatments for depression, the BHP thought that the choice of BA seemed most resonant with the concerns and preferences expressed by Tony's wife, with whom he at least offered some nonverbal agreement in the initial contact. This was particularly important considering Tony's initial reluctance in meeting with the BHP because it felt too "touchy feely" and he did not want to be "analyzed." During that first visit, the BHP surmised that a psychodynamic or acceptance and commitment therapy approach would require substantial discussion of emotion and the importance of increasing awareness of difficult emotional experiences, which was not consistent with Tony's stated preferences; also, she wondered if a CBT approach would feel too

analytical. With BA, she felt confident that she could reassure Tony that they would take a very practical approach that would help them (1) understand why he was stuck in this vicious cycle of depression and chronic pain and (2) identify concrete strategies for improving his mood and engagement with life.

Visit 1: Creating a Map

Tony and his wife arrived for his first visit at the primary care clinic with the BHP. Due to Tony's physical limitations, they were taken into an exam room close to the waiting room and commented on the convenience of receiving behavioral health treatment in a clinic in which they were already familiar with the location and check-in process. While walking back to the exam room, Tony also commented how hard it was for him to make this appointment and that he had contemplated canceling but decided against doing so, since he thought the BHP was kind to him during their initial introduction. In the first minute of their visit, the BHP thanked Tony for coming and praised him for trying something new with an open mind. She considered exploring in more detail his hesitancy to engage with her and decided that discussing his attitudes and feelings "right off the bat" was too closely aligned with his belief that "therapy is too touchy feely." She therefore made a mental note to return to this topic at the end of this visit, then jumped right in, explaining the nature of the behavioral service and collecting basic background information about Tony and his presenting problems.

From the referral from the PCP, the BHP knew that Tony had struggled with depression since adolescence, but that his most recent episode was triggered after the loss of his job due to the severity of his diabetes, and that his primary concern was his inability to interact with or provide for his family in a meaningful way. She had multiple questions in mind, though, that she wanted to answer in this first interaction with Tony. Specifically, she was interested in multiple contextual factors, such as Tony's biological predisposition to depression and chronic pain, the frequency and intensity of adverse child events, and his current stressors. She was also interested in a more personalized understanding of his experience of depression and chronic pain. In addition to assessing the extent to which these experiences were difficult for him to tolerate and how much they interfered with his pursuit of short- and long-term goals, the BHP also knew that knowing Tony as a person would be critical in terms of adapting BA to increase compatibility with his cultural values (Barrera & Castro, Chapter 8, this volume; Bernal, Jiménez-Chafey, & Domenech Rodríguez., 2009). Based on the limited information she knew about Tony, the BHP had already decided to not initiate discussion on his reluctance to engage with behavioral health until the end of the visit. She also resolved to refocus any discussion of masculinity away from generalized discussions of *machismo* and toward ways in which his physical and mental health problems interfered with acting like the father, the husband, and the man he would like to be. This approach (1) acknowledged prior work demonstrating that authoritarianism, emotional restrictiveness, and controlling behavior represent only a minority of Latino men and that there is significant variation with which *machismo* is reflected in modern Latino male identity (Torres, Solberg, & Carlstrom, 2002) and (2) converged with previous examples of considering social role functioning and viewing oneself in relation to others (i.e., *allocentrism*) in the adaptation of evidence-based interventions for Latinos (La Roche, Batista, & D'Angelo, 2011).

Accomplishing all of these objectives in 45 minutes was unrealistic, so the BHP decided against assessing each of these constructs with individual measures and instead conducted a functional assessment of Tony's physical and psychological symptoms using the BA framework. Accordingly, Tony responded to questions to describe triggers to his current symptoms, his emotional and physical experience of depression and chronic pain, and the ways in which these triggers and symptoms affected his behavior. The BHP referred to this process of case conceptualization as creating a "map" to help Tony better understand the problems for which he was seeking help:

BHP: First, I really want to acknowledge how happy I am that you were able to make it in today, Tony. I can imagine that your pain can make it difficult to even leave the house.

TONY: You have no idea. Most days it is hard to even leave the couch to get to the bathroom.

BHP: Wow, so coming in today was a really big deal for you and shows how important this is for you.

TONY: Well, yeah, I'm here.

BHP: Well, what I want to do today is spend some time getting to know you. I want to understand when all of this began for you, how it has affected you, and what you are and aren't doing anymore as a result. My hope is that by the end of today, we'll have a better sense of how all these pieces fit together, and we'll use that understanding to put our heads together and come up with some ideas for how to help get you unstuck. I also want your feedback today because it is really important to me that I understand things from your perspective, so if I don't get something right, please let me know.

TONY: Yes, Doc.

BHP: Great! So, let's start from the beginning. I'll be taking a lot of notes to create a kind of "map" of the problems you're experiencing, and after we talk for a while we'll look at it together. Does that sound OK?

TONY: Yes.

At this point, the BHP is collaborating with Tony to develop a case conceptualization that will also help him make sense of the strategies employed over time. BA BHPs work with clients to identify possible changes in their lives that have led to decreases in life's rewards or increases in difficulties that are associated with the onset or continuation of their depression. From the perspective of the BA model, depression is seen as a result of an interaction between the client's life circumstances and his or her emotional and behavioral response to them rather than a problem within the person. Put simply, depression is not something one has but is a combination of environmental, emotional, and behavioral relationships. In particular, the natural response of individuals to try to escape from or avoid emotional pain, or life's hassles, ultimately keeps them stuck in a downward cycle of depression.

BHP: Tell me when did you begin having problems with pain and what was going on in your life then?

TONY: Well, about 5 or 6 years ago, I started noticing a lot of pain and tingling in my feet, but I kinda just chalked it up to working long hours at the garage. I was a mechanic before I had to quit. And, you know, I am the kind of guy that, you know, takes a lot of pride in providing for my family and I didn't want my wife to think she needed to work, so I just ignored the pain and worked through it.

BHP: For you, your family is so important to you that you're willing to do whatever is necessary to provide for them, even if it means being in a lot of pain. Tell me more about the pain.

TONY: Yeah, exactly. The pain, it's just . . . it started just tingling, like when your foot starts to fall asleep, but then it got worse and worse, and now it's like this sharp pain and all the time. . . . I just . . . it never stops.

BHP: So with this pain that's happening all the time at this level, how did that start?

TONY: Well my doctor says it's because of the diabetes and that my blood vessels and nerves in my feet are shot.

BHP: Yes, your doctor told me the same thing. Tell me more about how your pain impacts your life.

TONY: What do you mean?

BHP: Well, one thing I'm interested in is how your pain affects how you spend your time. If before, you worked long hours to support your family, what do you do now?

TONY: I just don't want to do anything but find relief from my pain.

BHP: And it's been really hard for you to do things you enjoy . . .

TONY: Yeah, like I don't play ball with my kids anymore and I feel guilty for that, and because now my wife has to work because I can't be on my feet for more than 5 to 10 minutes a time. It's depressing. I mean, what kind of man makes his wife work while he stays at home? It's pathetic.

BHP: It's easy for you to feel inadequate when you can't contribute to your family in the ways that you want to. Tell me about some of the other things that you aren't doing anymore because of your pain.

TONY: I don't see my friends as much, and I miss a lot of family events and my kids' sports.

BHP: Wow, your pain is making it really difficult to do a lot of the things that are really important to you as a man and a father, so you naturally find yourself doing less of those things. Help me understand how your pain has contributed to you doing more of other activities.

According to the BA model, life events, either recent or cumulative over a person's development, result in low rates of response-contingent positive reinforcement or high rates of punishment or aversive control of behavior. To unpack all that jargon, some peoples' natural response to life, or to sudden changes in life, is to feel overwhelmed, fatigued, blue, and so forth. In other words, they begin to experience the affective and physiological aspects of depression. Life then is not reinforcing or rewarding, either because the person is in such a troubled state that he or she is not able to experience reward in the same way as he or she did previously (i.e., response-contingent positive reinforcement), or the person tries to escape from the negative feelings by withdrawing from typically pleasant activities (i.e., aversive control). The cycle continues and the person feels badly and stops engagement in activities that once made life enjoyable, and the depression persists or worsens.

TONY: Not much, really. It mostly gets in the way of spending time with my kids and family. But I do see more of my one friend. He comes over a lot during the day to hang out.

BHP: And that totally makes sense—you are in so much pain all the time that it makes it really, really hard to be the husband and father you want to be. Plus, it sounds like all of this has impacted your mood as well. What kinds of things are you finding yourself doing more of in an effort to get rid of the pain or distract yourself from your low mood?

TONY: Oh, well, I spend most of my day either watching TV or sleeping. I try to help out with the kids and their homework, you know, when they get home. But mainly, yeah, mainly I spend a lot of time on the couch because my feet hurt so bad.

BHP: I can imagine that you'd be trying to do whatever you can to get some relief from the pain, even if it's just a short distraction while watching TV or catching a nap.

TONY: Exactly. I'm just in pain and bummed out all the time and worried about my family and my health. I've tried so much to make it better, but nothing seems to work.

BHP: How frustrating. I see a lot of patients who have this very problem of trying to get relief from pain and also feeling really depressed about not contributing to their families as much as they used to. OK if I share my thoughts with you?

TONY: Yeah, I'm willing to do whatever at this point.

BHP: I really appreciate your openness. So here is what I've been writing down for the last 10 minutes (see Figure 19.1). I organized your story into three sections: (1) things that have happened to you—I call these "triggers"; (2) how these triggers make you feel, both physically and mentally—I call this your "experience"; and (3) how these triggers and feelings influence your behavior—I call these "behaviors." So you received this diagnosis of type 2 diabetes in your late 20s and didn't think much of it, and you kept focusing on providing a good living for your family. Eventually the tingling turned into pain, which got progressively worse until it was too much and you had to stop working. When you went to the doctor, you found out that you have neuropathic pain in your feet and legs due to poorly controlled diabetes. Because you are such a family man, you didn't make too many changes to your life and tried to keep working, but eventually you had to stop working. Since then you are noticing that you don't spend as much quality time with your kids and family, as you spend more time trying to cope with the pain and depression. All of this is having a really big impact on you. You struggle with depression and are worried about your family and your health. You feel kinda helpless and guilty. Is that a good summary?

TONY: Yeah, exactly. I feel like you are the first person to really understand this, besides my wife.

BHP: I'm glad we're on the same page! But let me know if I miss anything or am not getting something quite right. So because of all the pain and depression and worries, you do less of the things that are really important to you and more of the things that are aimed toward coping with your pain.

TONY: Yeah, I don't spend as much time with my kids or my wife, and I never get into the garage to work on my cars. And I feel like I just spend all of my time going to the doctors and trying to do things to make my pain go down.

BHP: And it sounds like you feel kinda stuck there.

TONY: Yeah.

BHP: I hear this from a lot of my patients, that they start getting sick or depressed and it gets in the way of the things they enjoy doing or that are important to them. And then that tends to make the pain or depression worse, which then makes it even harder to do the things that are important to you. It all just starts to become this really vicious cycle and downward spiral. Does that sound familiar to you?

TONY: That is exactly what happens.

Tony's response here is similar to many we have heard from clients after presenting this model as it relates to their circumstances. Occasionally, however, clients have an initially negative reaction to seeing this cycle written out and make statements about it being "depressing." BHPs can minimize this by emphasizing the hope that BA strategies address this very process, as can be seen in the following exchange.

BHP: What I want to suggest is that we start identifying some ways to reverse this cycle. We'll start small and I'm here to help you problem-solve. So to get us started, let's pick one activity to start experimenting with this week. Which of these sounds most promising in terms of breaking this cycle between experiencing a lot of pain, both physically and emotionally, and doing less?

TONY: It would be great to be more active with my kids, I just don't know if I can do that.

BHP: Right! We will likely have to get creative here given that you probably can't play with them for hours like you used to. This might be hard, but I agree that this is a worthwhile place to begin. So that's a great idea. For now, I want you to take these notes home with you and look for other ways that you might inadvertently keeping yourself stuck in this depression and pain trap by focusing mostly on activities that aim to relieve or distract from pain, and less on activities that are truly important to you. How does that sound?

TONY: I can do that.

BHP: Great! Last thing before we end today, I'm curious about your experience working with me today. Would you say that today's visit was helpful, unhelpful, or it's too early to tell?

TONY: Oh it was fine. A lot of this make sense

TRIGGERS	EXPERIENCE	BEHAVIORS
(What happened?)	(How do I feel?)	(What do I do?)

TRIGGERS	EXPERIENCE	BEHAVIORS
Mid-20s: Diagnosed with type II diabetes, didn't take it serious	Minor tingling in feet, no pain. Mood okay.	No major lifestyle changes, work through the tingling
Late 20s/early 30s: Worsening type II diabetes	Tingling turns into pain, frustrated with pain.	Working through pain
Late 30s: Poorly controlled type II diabetes	Severe neuropathic pain and depression. Difficulty standing for more than 5–10 minutes. Low mood, feels worthless and guilty.	Stopped working, less time with family and friends. More time watching TV and taking naps.

Short-term consequences = distraction from pain and depression, small bit of immediate "relief"

Long-term consquences = no improvement with pain or depression, increased guilt, new problems

FIGURE 19.1. BA case "map."

to me, so we'll just have to see if doing this actually helps.

BHP: That makes sense to me. I appreciate your honesty because I know that it can be difficult for a lot of people to get started with this type of work. Is there anything I could do differently to make this more engaging or more effective?

TONY: No, you're good. I thought this would be really weird or embarrassing or something, but it was all pretty straightforward and I like how you laid everything out.

BHP: OK, good. And remember that the door is open for us to look at the way we're working together and to make changes if necessary.

I'm really looking forward to seeing you back in 2 weeks.

At the end of the first session, the BHP's impression was that Tony was falling into a typical pattern of avoidance that is common in patients with chronic pain and depression (and many other conditions). Given the central role that avoidance appeared to be playing in the maintenance and exacerbation of Tony's pain and depression, the BHP felt confident in her initial idea that using BA was a promising approach. Tony's pain contributed to difficulties working, spending less time with his family, and focusing almost exclusively on seeking pain relief, instead of doing things that are important to him, and this formulation was consistent with the BA framework. In fact, it appeared that it his efforts to find relief were contributing to his depression and likely making his pain worse in the long run. This was particularly evident Tony's negative feelings toward himself and feeling guilty for not contributing more to his family. Thus, in the subsequent sessions, the BHP's goal was to help the patient identify behaviors that functioned to alleviate pain or depressive symptoms in the short term but carried negative long-term consequences and interfered with problem solving to increase value-based activities, particularly those involving his family. The BA BHP invites clients to use self-monitoring to begin to tease out the behaviors and activities that may bring more enjoyment to life, or that the client is experiencing as depressogenic.

Visit 2: Small Steps

Tony returned to clinic 4 weeks later, after canceling his 2-week follow-up appointment due to difficulty with transportation. In the second 30-minute visit, Tony began with a review of events that contributed to his elevated PHQ-9 score (20/27). The BHP wanted to strengthen their bond by empathizing with Tony about a difficult experience before switching focus to further explore his avoidance pattern related to his chronic pain, with specific examples in his life and coming up with small steps Tony could be making to reengage in important activities in his life.

BHP: Good to see you back, Tony! I'd like to continue to our conversation from our last meeting about how your pain and mood is getting in the way of doing the things that are important to you, and to come up with some strategies to make those things easier. I noticed your PHQ-9 score is still pretty high, so that tells me you're still experiencing quite a bit of stress. Is there anything else you noticed between our last session and now that you wanted to share, or anything you wanted to add to our agenda today?

TONY: Well, I've been feeling pretty frustrated lately. Something happened with my dad the other day that just made me so mad.

BHP: OK, let's talk about that first, and then we'll get back to the other conversation. Tell me about what happened.

TONY: Well. My dad got really sick while I was

over at his house, so I had to call the ambulance for him. When they got there, they immediately started making assumptions that he was on drugs and that's why he was passed out. And my dad doesn't use drugs, but they just wouldn't believe me. I'm still so mad about it.

BHP: Absolutely. That would make anyone angry to have someone making negative assumptions like that about their family.

Tony and the BHP spent 5 more minutes discussing the incident. Using a validating and matter-of-fact approach, the BHP listened to Tony's story and commended him for "being there" for his father at a critical time. The BHP then transitioned the conversation to discussing a key aspect of the BA model: how strong negative emotions or physical sensations increase the likelihood of avoidant behaviors that temporarily reduce distress yet can develop into "vicious cycles" of withdrawal and worsening symptoms.

BHP: Tony, I'm curious what you do in other situations when you feel strong emotions like anger.

TONY: Well, I don't ever want to make the situation worse, so I just hold back my feelings. I used to go out to my garage and work on my cars when I'd get mad, but now I can't do that.

BHP: Kinda like how you stopped doing some of the things that are important to you, you also tend to avoid those strong emotions. And now the best coping skill you had isn't available to you because of your pain.

TONY: I've never thought of it like that, but yeah, I just try to not feel those emotions, but it's harder now because I don't have an outlet. I mean, I just sat on the couch all afternoon watching TV. Normally, I would've worked on my cars to get my mind off of everything.

BHP: And it is important to have some kind of outlet for those feelings. If you try to suppress those emotions, they tend to come back and get you in some way anyway—they might make your pain worse or you might lash out at your family.

TONY: I actually got into it with my son later that evening when he wanted to play video games but wasn't done with his homework. I kinda came down on him too hard. I shouldn't have done that. . . . Sometimes I just let it build up and then I yell at my kids, even when they haven't really done anything wrong.

BHP: And what's the consequence of that?

TONY: Well, I feel even worse after.

BHP: Exactly. When we suppress our emotions or avoid doing the things we enjoyed because we're in pain or angry, it has a way of making things worse in the long run.

TONY: Yeah, I can see that.

BHP: OK, great. So let's start there. First, let's map out this situation with your dad to better understand how your behavior functioned to provide immediate relief to feeling so angry, but might increase the chances of getting short with your kids later in the day and saying something you regret.

In BA, the emphasis is on the consequence of an activity, whether it results in the client engaging further in it under similar circumstances or in the client being less likely to engage in the activity. The BHP and client work together to systematically increase activities that will result in further activation and engagement in life, decrease escape and avoidance behaviors, and either improve the client's life situation or mood, or both. By acting as a coach and validating the client's emotional reactions and experience, the BA BHP works to structure activities that the depressed client will be able to accomplish, regardless of mood, and to slowly increase the complexity and frequency of the activities.

The BHP then guided Tony through "mapping out" the encounter with his father according the BA model (see Figure 19.2). In particular, it was important to point out the immediate positive effect of Tony's decision to "hold back" in the moment so as not to interfere with his father's immediate health care needs. The BHP also described how it made sense for Tony to try distracting himself from feeling so angry, but it unfortunately contributed to yelling at his son.

BHP: What could be a way that you express your emotions, rather than suppressing them, in a way that would be healthy for you, in a way that doesn't make you pay a price later?

TONY: I know that I should talk with someone about it. . . . It's just hard.

BHP: It can be uncomfortable to do something that seems against the grain for you, but I wonder if you'd be willing to give it a try, because I think it would be really interesting to learn what happened if you did share your emotions with someone else.

TONY: I can do it. I know I have to do something different than what I have been doing.

BHP: Who could be a good person in your life to talk about your anger or other emotions with?

TONY: I have a good buddy, Joe, who comes to my house a lot to check on me, and he's always asking me how I'm doing. Usually I just tell him I'm fine, but maybe I could tell him more.

BHP: I think that is a fantastic plan! So, the next time you see him, maybe you could share some of your emotions with him. What do you think you want to share?

TONY: I could tell him about the thing that just happened with my dad, and how I am angry about it.

BHP: Great plan! And I'll be curious to see how expressing your emotions instead of shoving them down impacts your pain and your mood. I've also heard you talk a lot about your kids and how important they are to you. I wonder if there is a goal we can set for you to do with your kids, too.

TONY: I think that would be really helpful.

BHP: Great! What is one small thing that you want to start doing with your kids that has been hard lately?

TONY: I used to take my kids out to the garage, and I would show them how to work on the cars like I would like to be doing. Maybe I can do that more.

BHP: Fantastic! That is wonderful that you are already doing that! And what a creative way to get to still engage in something you really enjoy and spend time with your kids. I think that is a wonderful plan to do that more often. How often could you do this?

TONY: Maybe twice next week for an hour.

BHP: Great plan. Let's have you keep track of how often you do this and see what kind of impact is has on your pain and mood. How does that sound?

TONY: Good, sounds good.

BHP: Wonderful. So we will check-in on this the next time we meet in 2 weeks.

To keep Tony's PCP apprised of their progress, the BHP forwarded all her brief progress notes to the PCP through the secure electronic

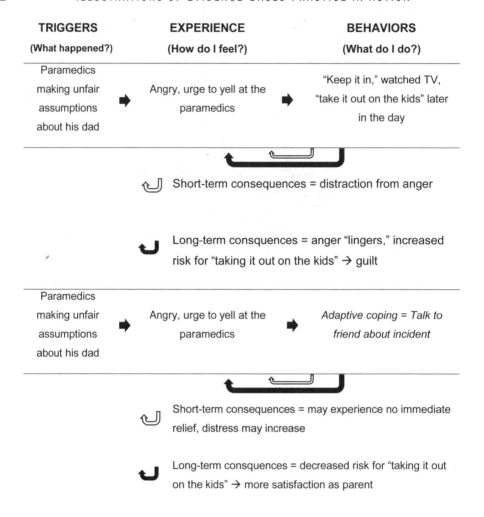

FIGURE 19.2. BA conceptualization for specific avoidant behavior.

medical record. They also briefly caught up about Tony's progress one afternoon in the clinic between seeing their individual patients.

PCP: Thank you for sending your notes on Tony and sharing his progress. I am seeing him for a follow-up appointment next week. Can you tell me a little bit more about how you are thinking about his conditions?

BHP: Of course! Tony and I have been talking about what a large role avoidance plays in his depression, diabetes, and pain. Tony has fallen into a classic cyclical pattern where he might be experiencing pain in his feet, which causes him to stay on the couch all day instead of doing things he enjoys or that are important to him, which then leads him to feel

bad about himself. This pattern continues on and exacerbates each of his conditions—his diabetes gets worse because he feels unable to move due to the pain; he does not want to exercise or even walk more than a few feet because of his pain, which makes his diabetes and depression worse; and so on. So, we've been setting small goals for Tony to start re-engaging in the important aspects of his life, like spending more time with his kids and sharing his difficulties with a close friend.

PCP: That makes a lot of sense. I've tried encouraging him to exercise in the past, but it hasn't worked. How can I help to support him now?

BHP: I'm not sure how you've tried approaching him in the past, so this might be similar to what you've said to him, but we've been focusing on identifying his values and what he is missing out on because of his medical conditions, and from there we have been setting small, achievable goals. Right now his goal is to show his kids ways to work on cars for an hour twice a week. I wonder if when you see him this week, you could check in on how that is going for him?

PCP: I will definitely ask him how that is going and touch base with you afterward.

Visit 3: Troubleshooting Barriers to Activation

Tony returned to the clinic 2 weeks later to follow up on his progress with using emotional expression rather than suppression, and engaging in teaching his children how to work on cars. During this session, the BHP planned to check on Tony's progress and help him further problem-solve around any possible difficulties with engaging in the homework assignment. Prior to the session, the BHP predicted Tony would report that on at least some occasions, his feet were hurting too much to spend time with his children in the garage. Thus, during this session the BHP wanted to reiterate the importance of engaging in pleasant activities based in the client's values (i.e., family) in a modified way rather than complete avoidance.

BHP: So good to see you again, Tony! I thought today we could start by checking on how your homework assignment went and work to problem-solve any difficulties you had. How does that sound?

TONY: Good.

BHP: Anything else you want to make sure we talk about today?

TONY: No, that sounds like a good plan to me.

BHP: OK, great. Why don't you start by telling me how it went over the past couple of weeks sharing your emotions with your friend?

TONY: It actually went better than I expected.

BHP: Great, tell me more about that!

TONY: Well, Joe was really open to what I had to say, even though I was nervous that he would think I was just complaining. And I felt bit more relaxed after.

BHP: So, even though it was uncomfortable at first, you found benefit in sharing your emotions. That is really great. How do you think you want to handle this going forward?

TONY: I want to keep doing it, I think. I think it's going to help me.

BHP: Wonderful, and I agree that it is going to help! I'd also like to hear how things went with your kids.

TONY: It was OK.

BHP: Just OK? Tell me what made it hard.

TONY: There were some days that my pain was just so bad that I couldn't move, even though I knew I was supposed to.

BHP: And it can be really, really hard on those days to want to do anything!

TONY: Right.

BHP: And how did not moving impact your pain and mood on those days?

TONY: Well, it didn't help really. I just felt bad all day.

BHP: Right, so even though you tried to just rest on those days, you didn't really see any improvement on your pain or mood. And how did it feel on those days to not get to spend as much time with your kids?

TONY: I mean, it was hard. . . . I hate that I can't be more involved with them.

BHP: I can see how hard that is for you. What about the days that you were able to do something with your kids, even if it wasn't as much as time as you were hoping for. How did that go?

TONY: It was still really hard because my feet always hurt so bad, but usually after a little bit I had moments of not noticing the pain as much and I was definitely happy that I was spending at least some time with my kids.

BHP: Yeah, yeah, so it still was the case that the pain was there but there were moments when it didn't hurt as bad, and you felt better about yourself because you could see your kids. Did I get that right?

TONY: Exactly.

BHP: Good. Well, this is a really important point to make. There are times when the pain—whether it's emotional or physical—is so bad that all you want to do is rest. In this particular case, resting didn't seem to help very much with the physical pain, but it almost functioned to make your emotional pain worse because you were feeling guilty about not spending as much time with your kids. We also have an example where you followed through with your plan to spend time with your kids even though you were feeling a good amount of pain. In that case, the pain didn't get worse, and you even had some moments when you didn't notice it as much. Better yet, you felt better about yourself for spending time with your kids compared to days where you spend most of the time on the couch. The question we have to ask ourselves now is, what can we do to make it easier for you to still spend time with them, even on the days the pain feels bad?

TONY: I just don't know.

BHP: I think we can figure this out, especially since spending time with your kids is so important to you!

TONY: OK.

BHP: Let's spend a little more time talking about the day you were able to spend time with the kids in the garage. Tell me a little bit about what you are doing when you do teach them about car mechanics.

TONY: Well, I take them out to the garage because I have an old car that I am working on. And I usually am standing up with them, showing them what I am doing, and then having them try, as long as it is safe for them. But I started to get frustrated because it was hard for me to bend over enough to get to the brake fluid without being in pain. And the kids weren't understanding me. So sometimes it just felt like a waste.

BHP: Yeah, you are trying so hard to be active and with your kids and it's just over their head, so that does sound frustrating. Remember the main goal here—you are doing this to spend quality time with them, not to turn them into expert mechanics. So, in some ways, it really doesn't matter how they understand, but rather that you get to spend some time sharing something you really enjoy with them. And like you just said, when you spend more time with them, your mood is usually better.

The goal in BA is to help clients to increase activities that will ultimately be rewarded in their natural environment (Martell et al., 2013) or that may prove to be "antidepressant behaviors" (Martell et al., 2013). Often the potential activities will be those that result in an improvement in the client's mood as the BHP here points out to Tony, or that are highly valued.

Tony clearly valued time with his children and found activities that allowed him to spend time with them to be meaningful. Not only did these activities function to limit the amount of time Tony spent passively coping (e.g., television, sleeping) or ruminating, they also aligned with his desire to feel more active in contributing as a father and husband by spending quality time with his children doing something he inherently enjoyed.

TONY: Yeah, I forgot about that part, but you're right, the times I was able to spend with them was much more enjoyable than just watching TV or playing video games.

BHP: Exactly! And that's what we're aiming for, time with your kids that keeps you active and contributes to your sense that you're still being the kind of dad you want to be, even though the pain makes it hard sometimes. And that's the challenge, the pain will want to tell you to "give up" or not even get started in the first place. Here's where we get to be creative in finding ways to follow through with plans, even in the face of pain. Tell me how long were you standing while you were in the garage?

TONY: I'll stand for about 20 minutes, but that's when the pain starts to really get to me, so then I usually just call it quits and go back inside.

BHP: So another part of this is that the pain gets bad, and that adds to the frustration. What if we tried something a little different? How could we get you to spend a good chunk of time with your kids in the garage in ways that also respect the difficulties you have with being on your feet for too long?

TONY: I don't know. What if I took a chair and sat down whenever my feet started to hurt?

BHP: That's a great idea! There's a strategy called "pacing," where you estimate how long you could stand before your feet really start to hurt and then make a plan to sit down before that even happens. Maybe something like you'd plan to sit down for a quick break every 10 minutes, regardless of your pain level. How would that work?

TONY: Yeah, I think I could try that. And then maybe I can be out there for longer and not get so frustrated.

BHP: That would be exactly what we're going

for! And what do you want to teach them that might easier for them to understand?

TONY: Last time I tried showing them how to change fuses and they didn't understand what the fuses were for, and I started getting worried about it maybe being too dangerous for them.

BHP: And your priority it making sure they are safe. What is something that would be safer?

TONY: Hmm . . . well it's not very exciting, but they could help add windshield wiper fluid.

BHP: Oh, that is a great idea! I love it. When do you want to try that with them?

TONY: I can do it this weekend.

BHP: Perfect! Remember the two things you are going to do a little different this time: (1) Remember it's not about how much they understand, but just spending time with them, and (2) you are going to take a break every 10 minutes to reduce your pain. How does that sound?

TONY: Well, it's worth a shot. I am not really looking forward to it.

Activity structuring and scheduling are the main strategies used to increase patients' engagement with life. During activity structuring, BHPs and patients determine activities to experiment with between clinic visits. Then, they determine the intensity for each activity or how difficult the first and subsequent attempts will be. For example, a patient who has had difficulty keeping up with basic housekeeping may "structure" housekeeping by defining making a bed in the morning several times a week as the first step that he or she can successfully complete while progressively developing a more comprehensive cleaning plan. At first, patients begin with lower intensities such as scheduling the activity for only certain mornings. In this way, patients are invited to practice acting according to a plan (i.e., making the bed scheduled for Tuesday and Thursday at 9:00 A.M.) rather than a mood (i.e., waking up feeling miserably blue on those days and just leaving the bed in a mess). Part of activity structuring and scheduling for Tony was the inclusion of 10-minute breaks. This attests to the functional nature of BA—BHPs are not just trying to get patients busy with activities that feel good; they collaborate with patients to engage in activities in a manner that works for them.

Visit 4: Fine-Tuning Activation and Long-Term Planning

Due to scheduling and transportation difficulties, Tony returned to the clinic 3 weeks later. During this session, the BHP planned to follow up on how Tony's homework assignment went and to add additional areas in which Tony could increase his level of activation.

BHP: I am happy to see you again, Tony. I want to hear about how things went with the plans we made last time we met, and I also want to talk about next steps for continuing this work with someone in your community who has expertise with the types of problems you're dealing with. Is there anything else you'd like to add to our agenda for today?

TONY: No that sounds good. I have to tell you that I wasn't totally confident about our plan, but I have to admit that I did much better this time with teaching my kids about cars.

BHP: That is so great, Tony! What do you think went differently this time?

TONY: Well, I focused less on making sure things went perfectly and more on just enjoying the time I had with them. I still had a lot of pain, but I felt more proud of myself afterward.

BHP: Wonderful! And that is kinda what we might expect. We might not be able to change your pain, but if we can keep you active and doing things that are important to you, you are going to feel better overall. How did it go with taking time for breaks?

TONY: I did take one break, but it got hard to remember to take the breaks once I got really excited. I didn't do the break at 10 minutes because I was feeling pretty good. But then, later on, I felt this tingling in my left foot, which usually means that it's going to get worse. I asked the kids to go get some water from the house while I sat down for a few minutes. It's like we didn't really miss a bit.

BHP: Yeah, sometimes when we really get into an activity, it's hard to remember to take breaks. It's a new skill to learn that activity pacing and taking breaks can be really, really helpful with pain, so just remember to be mindful about that. Since this was so successful, how do you want to continue doing this moving forward? Either when you're spending time with your kids or in other situations?

This exchange regarding the break is a good example of a patient acting according to a mood not a goal. Although Tony was continuing because he enjoyed the activity, his activity schedule incorporated 10-minute breaks to keep him from getting fatigued. BA BHPs must attend to mood-dependent activity whether the mood is gloomy or upbeat. The idea is that following a plan and schedule while trying to make therapeutic gains will prevent patients from being tossed about, metaphorically, by the whims of emotion.

TONY: I was thinking about this the other day, and I think that teaching them something about cars once a week would be really doable for me.

BHP: Great plan! And tell me, since I am not an expert in car mechanics like you, how many activities are there that you can teach kids your age?

TONY: There are a few, but I guess now that you are saying that I might run out of things in a few weeks.

BHP: Can you think of some other activities you'd like to do with them?

TONY: I used to really love playing football with them and playing catch, but I just can't stand for that long.

BHP: So kind of like what happened with working on the cars, you stopped playing sports with your kids because it's hard to stand for too long. How could you alter how you play sports with them to still be active but not make the pain too overwhelming?

TONY: I could just bring my chair with me again and sit to throw the ball with them. Then I'm still moving around and playing but not making my feet hurt worse.

BHP: I think that is a perfect plan! You can still take breaks and sit when you need to, probably every 10 minutes again, and you can still be involved with your kids.

TONY: Yeah, it just feels weird to be sitting down while playing sports. I mean I was such a good athlete when I was younger.

BHP: That's exactly right. It can be a big adjustment making new plans to accommodate the physical limitations of your body. In the end, though, we know that it's worth it because

at the end of the day, your kids and family are really important to you, and even though you might not be able to do everything you used to be able to do, you still have so much to offer, and we want to make sure you keep doing those things that are important to you.

After four sessions of BA in the integrated primary care clinic, Tony and his BHP determined that he would benefit from continued BA therapy and was referred to a BHP within the community who could continue this work with BA for chronic pain and depression. The BHP met with Tony for four sessions (due to the brief therapy model employed in integrated primary care), far fewer than BA treatment durations that have been studied in clinical trials (i.e., 10–24 sessions). Despite having only four sessions, Tony began to make progress. Specifically, he was beginning to spend more time with his children, he and had a slight reduction in his PHQ-9 score, which dropped from 23 points during his initial visit down to 18 points. His PCP also commented that she was seeing a shift in his thinking surrounding his pain medication—in the past, his goal was to was to get medication to completely alleviate the pain, but now he was commenting that his goal was to get back some of his functioning, even if that meant being in pain.

Two months after the referral, the BHP called the outpatient psychotherapist to whom she had referred Tony and left her a message inquiring about Tony's progress. The BHP learned that Tony had missed several of his initial sessions but was now attending regularly and had made some preliminary progress. She reported that he was spending more time playing with his children, she addressed some medication concerns with his physician, and noted that by taking a more active role in his children's lives, his medical condition was improving, as were his mood and sense of self-efficacy.

Case Summary

Tony's story of receiving BA for depression, chronic pain, and type 2 diabetes via IBHPC is an example of EBP in action. It also highlights some of the limitations in implementing EBP within medical settings that typically have higher patient volumes and faster workflows than outpatient mental health settings. Within the integrated behavioral health and primary care consultation model, the BHP prioritized developing a case conceptualization, highlighting the pitfalls of persistent avoidance patterns, and using the BA model to help Tony develop more adaptive coping responses to his pain and low moods. Key successes with Tony included engaging an initially reluctant man in an evidence-based psychotherapy; conducting a functional assessment of a primary care patient's physical and mental health comorbidity; initiating interventions that simultaneously address both sets of problems in collaboration with his PCP; and facilitating a referral to long-term outpatient psychotherapy. It is possible that had this primary care clinic operated without a BHP, Tony might have continued to receive care that did not adequately address the full range of his health care needs.

It is also important to recognize suboptimal features of Tony's care in this setting. Tony met with the BHP only four times, far less than the dose of BA (~12–24 sessions) studied in clinical trials (e.g., Dimidjian et al., 2006). Meeting with patients for a limited number of visits allows BHPs to remain available to the whole population of patients under a clinic's care, which often numbers in the thousands. Less contact with patients requires BHPs to condense evidence-based interventions, which typically entail creating modified versions of detailed treatment protocols with specific implementation recommendations. As in Tony's case, these adapted versions typically emphasize a rapid assessment and case conceptualization process, and quick transition to targeted interventions. Efficiency and brevity can come at the expense of more thorough explorations of important topics. For Tony, it may have been beneficial to engage him in a more in-depth discussion of his views and the origins of those views on manhood and parenting. A more detailed examination of the similarities and discrepancies between the parenting style he was exposed to as a child and the parenting style he wanted to implement with his own children may have provided additional context that often facilitates more engagement with treatment planning and follow through.

In ideal circumstances, there is also greater integration of treatment plans across behavioral health, primary care, and specialty care (including outpatient psychotherapy). For example, in many clinics, co-consultations are common where a patient's PCP and a BHP conduct joint visits to ensure compatibility of behavioral health and medical treatment plans, and dem-onstrate a unified commitment to the patient and the importance of their treatment plans. In Tony's case, the joint visit did not occur because both the BHP and the PCP were experiencing high patient volume, and they agreed that they would consider scheduling a joint visit if Tony had sustained difficulty engaging with the BHP. Similarly, stronger coordination with Tony's outpatient psychotherapist would have likely helped increase the consistency and effectiveness of messages to support Tony in following through with his treatment goals and long-term plans.

Building Behavioral Health Expertise in Primary Care

Specialty mental health operating independently of the larger health care context will continue to play a vital role for many decades, but the health care landscape is undergoing a remodeling that emphasizes multidisciplinary teams. Mental health providers from all disciplines (i.e., psychiatry, psychology, social work, nursing, counseling) will see increasing opportunity to work alongside medical health providers in providing "whole-person," patient-centered care. Within primary care, the Behavioral Joint Principles published in the *Annals of Family Medicine* recommend proactively and comprehensively integrating BHPs into all processes of primary care, from patient workflows to meeting accreditation requirements, to implementing sustainable financial models (Baird et al., 2014). That these recommendations are ratified into national standards for assessing primary care quality (National Center for Quality Assurance, 2014) highlights the growing recognition of need for effective BHPs within the primary care setting.

Increase Competence in Providing Integrated Care

To meet increasing demand for BHPs within primary care, there are several training resources to draw on for competence evaluation and development. Core competencies for interprofessional collaborative practice seek to prepare students in all health professions to work together effectively to promote more effective, patient-centered, and population-oriented health care (Interprofessional Education Collaborative Expert Panel, 2011). More specific to

BHPs in primary care, an expert national panel defined six domains of core competencies: science, systems, professionalism, relationships, application, and education (McDaniel et al., 2014). Each domain is further delineated with additional *essential components* and *behavioral anchors* that provide substantial guidance on the range of knowledge, attitudes, and skills of highly competent BHPs. Longer training guides go into more detail on the most common problems that present in primary care and recommend suggestions for structured treatment approaches (Hunter, Goodie, Oordt, & Dobmeyer, 2009; Robinson & Reiter, 2007). Additionally, the Agency for Healthcare Quality and Research hosts a website called the Academy for Integrating Behavioral Health and Primary Care (*https://integrationacademy.ahrq.gov*), which presents a suite of resources for developing, implementing, and sustaining IBHPC.

In-person trainings and national conferences also provide excellent opportunities to further develop competence. Faculty members at the University of Massachusetts–Worcester who were integral to early efforts to advanced integrated behavioral and primary care (e.g., Blount, 2003) created and continue to host an intensive workshop. On the West Coast, the University of Washington also conducts regular training at the Center for Advancing Integrated Mental Health Solutions (*https://aims.uw.edu*). High-quality professional conferences are sponsored annually by organizations vital to promoting integrated care, such as the Association for Psychologists in Academic Health Centers, the Collaborative Family Healthcare Association, the North American Primary Care Research Group, the Society of Behavioral Medicine, and the Society of Teachers in Family Medicine. A combination of literature review, formal training and supervision, and ongoing continuing education is highly recommended.

Develop Training Opportunities

Put simply, there are not enough mental health providers to meet the full demand for integrated BHPs, which in part reflects the deficit of training opportunities to prepare mental health providers to work in integrated primary care. For example, Beacham and colleagues (2017) estimated that to meet the projected need for BHPs in primary care settings, 90% of the 93,000 clinically trained psychologists in the United States would have to migrate to this setting.

Even if a large majority of mental health providers wanted to pursue careers in primary care, it is unlikely that our existing training programs have adequately prepared such a workforce. To take psychology as an example again, only two doctoral psychology programs offer training in integrated primary care as a major area of study (American Psychological Association, 2013a). Similarly, a related 2013 report also highlighted the low number of internship and postdoctoral programs offering two or more major rotations in integrated primary care (American Psychological Association, 2013b, 2013c). In order for the field to be positioned to respond to integration opportunities, we need a well-prepared workforce that can provide the type of services required for whole-person care.

To develop integrated primary care training opportunities, readers may consult the Frank, McDaniel, Belar, Schroeder, Hargrove, and Freeman (2004; McDaniel et al., 2004) model for curricula and practicum structure. Early exposure to primary care settings is critical given the "culture shock" experienced by many who transition from specialty mental health to integrated primary care (e.g., Blount, 1998). In the absence of formal training opportunities, activities such as clinical shadowing, participating in primary care-based research projects, and contributing to quality improvement initiatives function to acclimate trainees to this new environment. Learning from, observing, and contributing to treatment planning and decision making with colleagues from other health care disciplines begins to socialize trainees to provide primary care even if they are not contacting patients directly. Effectively integrating into primary care requires not only knowledge about how to adapt common mental health interventions to the primary care setting but also the ability to understand the professional worlds of PCPs in terms of their knowledge, assessments and interventions, and attitudes. Formal, *in vivo* learning opportunities can facilitate the acquisition of this knowledge.

Finally, important training activities are not restricted to targeting mental health trainees as the learners. Mental health clinicians can facilitate integration by improving the capacity of allied health professionals to work alongside BHPs. Formal and informal didactics, as part of residency education and during "learning lunches" or in the precepting room, can help non-behavioral health specialists acquire basic behavioral health assessment and intervention skills, and better appreciate the role BHPs play on the primary care team.

Gaps in the Evidence Base and Future Directions

The evidence for the effectiveness of integrated behavioral health and primary care is emerging. A comprehensive review commissioned by the AHRQ indicated that, in general, IBHPC improves outcomes but that there is significant heterogeneity in study design and quality (Butler et al., 2008). Kwan and Nease (2013) provided an updated review that confirms the general findings of the AHRQ report but also highlights four major gaps in the evidence base. First, the majority of studies have focused on the treatment of depression in primary care using a variety of evidence-based psychotherapies such as BA, CBT, and problem-solving therapy (Gilbody, Bower, Fletcher, Richards, & Sutton, 2006); this has occurred, however, at the expense of attention to other commonly occurring mental illnesses and behavioral health disorders. It will be important for future research studies to maximize external validity and give special attention to multimorbid presentations.

Second, the evidence base rests largely on RCTs conducted within large academic, health care settings. The extent to which these findings generalize to settings outside of academic settings in urban areas is uncertain. Furthermore, alternative research designs to the RCT are used less frequently but may be of particular relevance to evaluating IBHPC because IBPHC models are complex and varied, and it would be unwieldy to evaluate each combination of various components of IBHPC. For example, the AHRQ Lexicon (Peek, 2013) definition of IBHPC we referenced earlier contains six *defining clauses* and 12 *parameters* that outline the ways in which IBPHC models can vary. Quasi-experimental design for quality improvement evaluation, qualitative analyses of patient and provider experiences, observational studies to explore correlations between care structures and processes and outcomes, and mixed-methods approaches can complement the traditional RCT approach and provide important data on the effectiveness and value of IBPHC.

Third, some studies have demonstrated associations between structural factors such as strategies for screening and referral, compositions of care teams, and the implementation of treatment protocols (Craven & Bland, 2013), but less attention has been paid to other factors, such as the effective use of data management and information technology, training background and clinical competency, clinic policies and practices, and physical space factors.

Finally, the prevailing fee-for-service financial models can constrain BHPs to focus on billable activities (i.e., direct patient care) at the expense of the range of associated activities required of BHPs (i.e., care coordination, program development and evaluation), which can limit the full potential of the behavioral health service (Hubley & Miller, 2016). Further research is needed to determine which alternative payment models, such as pay for performance and global payments, permit more flexibility for aligning with what works best for a given population treated by a tailored treatment team in a unique context (Miller et al., 2017).

Summary

BHPs have considered holistic, nondualistic approaches to care for decades, but progress in integrating behavioral and physical care in most medical settings has been slow. Tony's case is a prime example of how the use of BA can address both physical and mental health concerns that patients frequently experience and report in the primary care context. Recognizing the importance of using integrated BHPs and PCPs to address simultaneously the varied medical conditions and mental illnesses treated in primary care is an at all time high. Increased demand for competent mental health providers to function as BHPs in primary care is reflected in the expansion of requirements for the integration of BHPs in primary care stipulated by national standards for primary care accreditation (National Center for Quality Assurance, 2014). During this period of rapid expansion, leaders in the field will have increasing opportunities to shape the approaches, conceptualization, and treatment of problems presented in primary care. The flexibility and efficiency of BA is an important reason BHPs might consider BA as a front-line treatment when patients present with clear patterns of behavioral avoidance. Initial BA work in a primary care setting may be sufficient or may motivate patients to pursue further BA treatment or another psychotherapeutic approach if further treatment is required. This practical therapy appeals to many patients and provides a good fit for the busy world of primary care.

References

Addis, M. E., & Martell, C. R. (2004). *Overcoming depression one step at a time: The new behavioral activation approach to getting your life back.* Oakland, CA: New Harbinger.

American Psychological Association. (2013a). Directory of doctoral training programs with training opportunities in primary care psychology. Retrieved from *www.apa.org/ed/graduate/doctoral-directory. pdf.*

American Psychological Association. (2013b). Directory of internship programs with training opportunities in primary care psychology. Retrieved from *www.apa.org/ed/graduate/internship-directory.pdf.*

American Psychological Association. (2013c). Directory of postdoctoral training programs with training opportunities in primary care psychology. Retrieved from *www.apa.org/ed/graduate/postdoc-directory. pdf.*

Baird, M., Blount, A., Brungardt, S., Dickinson, P., Dietrich, A., Epperly, T., et al. (2014). Joint principles: Integrating behavioral health care into the patient-centered medical home. *Annals of Family Medicine, 12*(2), 183–185.

Barnett, K., Mercer, S. W., Norbury, M., Watt, G., Wyke, S., & Guthrie, B. (2012). Epidemiology of multimorbidity and implications for health care, research, and medical education: A cross-sectional study. *Lancet, 380,* 37–43.

Barth, J., Munder, T., Gerger, H., Nüesch, E., Trelle, S., Znoj, H., et al. (2013). Comparative efficacy of seven psychotherapeutic interventions for patients with depression: A network meta-analysis. *PLoS Medicine, 10*(5), e1001454.

Beacham, A. O., Van Sickle, K. S., Khatri, P., Ali, M. K., Reimer, D., Farber, E. W., et al. (2017). Meeting evolving workforce needs: Preparing psychologists for leadership in the patient-centered medical home. *American Psychologist, 72,* 42–54.

Bernal, G., Jiménez-Chafey, M. I., & Domenech Rodríguez, M. M. (2009). Cultural adaptation of treatments: A resource for considering culture in evidence-based practice. *Professional Psychology: Research and Practice, 40*(4), 361–368.

Blount, A. E. (1998). *Integrated primary care: The future of medical and mental health collaboration.* New York: Norton.

Blount, A. (2003). Integrated primary care: Organizing the evidence. *Families, Systems, and Health, 21*(2), 121–133.

Butler, M., Kane, R. L., McAlpine, D., Kathol, R. G., Fu, S. S., Hagedorn, H., et al. (2008). *Integration of mental health/substance abuse and primary care.* Rockville, MD: Agency for Healthcare Research and Quality.

Coffman, S. J., Martell, C. R., Dimidjian, S., Gallop,

R., & Hollon, S. D. (2007). Extreme nonresponse in cognitive therapy: Can behavioral activation succeed where cognitive therapy fails? *Journal of Consulting and Clinical Psychology, 75*(4), 531–541.

Craven, M. A., & Bland, R. (2013). Depression in primary care: Current and future challenges. *Canadian Journal of Psychiatry, 58*(8), 442–448.

Cuijpers, P., Van Straten, A., & Warmerdam, L. (2007). Behavioral activation treatments of depression: A meta-analysis. *Clinical Psychology Review, 27*(3), 318–326.

Dimidjian, S., Barrera, M., Jr., Martell, C., Muñoz, R. F., & Lewinsohn, P. M. (2011). The origins and current status of behavioral activation treatments for depression. *Annual Review of Clinical Psychology, 7,* 1–38.

Dimidjian, S., Goodman, S. H., Sherwood, N. E., Simon, G. E., Ludman, E., Gallop, R., et al. (2017). A pragmatic randomized clinical trial of behavioral activation for depressed pregnant women. *Journal of Consulting and Clinical Psychology, 85*(1), 26–36.

Dimidjian, S., Hollon, S. D., Dobson, K. S., Schmaling, K. B., Kohlenberg, R. J., Addis, M. E., et al. (2006). Randomized trial of behavioral activation, cognitive therapy, and antidepressant medication in the acute treatment of adults with major depression. *Journal of Consulting and Clinical Psychology, 74*(4), 658–670.

Dobson, K. S., Hollon, S. D., Dimidjian, S., Schmaling, K. B., Kohlenberg, R. J., Gallop, R. J., et al. (2008). Randomized trial of behavioral activation, cognitive therapy, and antidepressant medication in the prevention of relapse and recurrence in major depression. *Journal of Consulting and Clinical Psychology, 76*(3), 468–477.

Ekers, D., Dawson, M., & Bailey, E. (2012). Dissemination of behavioural activation for depression to mental health nurses: Training evaluation and benchmarked clinical outcomes. *Journal of Psychiatric and Mental Health Nursing, 20*(2), 186–192.

Ekers, D., Richards, D., & Gilbody, S. (2008). A meta-analysis of randomized trials of behavioural treatment of depression. *Psychological Medicine, 38*(5), 611–623.

Ekers, D., Richards, D., McMillan, D., Bland, J. M., & Gilbody, S. (2011). Behavioural activation delivered by the non-specialist: Phase II randomised controlled trial. *British Journal of Psychiatry, 198*(1), 66–72.

Frank, R. G., McDaniel, S. H., Bray, J. H., & Heldring, M. E. (2004). *Primary care psychology.* Washington, DC: American Psychological Association.

Gilbody, S., Bower, P., Fletcher, J., Richards, D., & Sutton, A. J. (2006). Collaborative care for depression: A cumulative meta-analysis and review of longer-term outcomes. *Archives of Internal Medicine, 166*(21), 2314–2321.

Gortner, E. T., Gollan, J. K., Dobson, K. S., & Jacobson, N. S. (1998). Cognitive-behavioral treatment for depression: Relapse prevention. *Journal of Consulting and Clinical Psychology, 66*(2), 377–384.

Gros, D. F., & Haren, W. B. (2011). Open trial of brief behavioral activation psychotherapy for depression in an integrated veterans affairs primary care setting. *Primary Care Companion to CNS Disorders, 13*(4), Article No. 11m01136.

Hopko, D. R., Armento, M. E., Robertson, S., Ryba, M. M., Carvalho, J. P., Colman, L. K., et al. (2011). Brief behavioral activation and problem-solving therapy for depressed breast cancer patients: Randomized trial. *Journal of Consulting and Clinical Psychology, 79*(6), 834–849.

Hopko, D. R., Bell, J. L., Armento, M. E. A., Hunt, M. K., & Lejuez, C. W. (2005). Behavior therapy for depressed cancer patients in primary care. *Psychotherapy: Theory, Research, Practice, Training, 42*(2), 236–242.

Hubley, S. H., & Miller, B. F. (2016). Implications of healthcare payment reform for clinical psychologists in medical settings. *Journal of Clinical Psychology in Medical Settings, 23*(1), 3–10.

Hunter, C. L., Goodie, J. L., Oordt, M. S., & Dobmeyer, A. C. (2009). *Integrated behavioral health in primary care: Step-by-step guidance for assessment and intervention*. Washington, DC: American Psychological Association.

Interprofessional Education Collaborative Expert Panel. (2011). *Core competencies for interprofessional collaborative practice: Report of an expert panel*. Washington, DC: Author.

Jacobson, N. S., Dobson, K. S., Truax, P. A., Addis, M. E., Koerner, K., Gollan, J. K., et al. (1996). A component analysis of cognitive-behavioral treatment for depression. *Journal of Consulting and Clinical Psychology, 64*(2), 295–304.

Jacobson, N. S., Martell, C. R., & Dimidjian, S. (2001). Behavioral activation treatment for depression: Returning to contextual roots. *Clinical Psychology: Science and Practice, 8*(3), 255–270.

Kanter, J. W., Santiago-Rivera, A. L., Rusch, L. C., Busch, A. M., & West, P. (2010). Initial outcomes of a culturally adapted behavioral activation for Latinas diagnosed with depression at a community clinic. *Behavior Modification, 34*(2), 120–144.

Kazak, A. E., Nash, J. M., Hiroto, K., & Kaslow, N. J. (2017). Psychologists in patient-centered medical homes (PCMHs): Roles, evidence, opportunities, and challenges. *American Psychologist, 72*(1), 1–12.

Kroenke, K., Spitzer, R. L., & Williams, J. B. (2001). The PHQ-9: Validity of a brief depression severity measure. *Journal of General Internal Medicine, 16*(9), 606–613.

Kwan, B. M., & Nease, D. E., Jr. (2013). The state of the evidence for integrated behavioral health in primary care. In M. R. Talen & A. Burke Valeras (Eds.), *Integrated behavioral health in primary care* (pp. 65–98). New York: Springer.

La Roche, M. J., Batista, C., & D'Angelo, E. (2011). A content analyses of guided imagery scripts: A strategy for the development of cultural adaptations. *Journal of Clinical Psychology, 67*(1), 45–57.

Martell, C. R., Addis, M. E., & Jacobson, N. S. (2001). *Depression in context: Strategies for guided action*. New York: Norton.

Martell, C. R., Dimidjian, S., & Herman-Dunn, R. (2013). *Behavioral activation for depression: A clinician's guide*. New York: Guilford Press.

Mazzucchelli, T., Kane, R., & Rees, C. (2009). Behavioral activation treatments for depression in adults: A meta-analysis and review. *Clinical Psychology: Science and Practice, 16*(4), 383–411.

McDaniel, S. H., Grus, C. L., Cubic, B. A., Hunter, C. L., Kearney, L. K., Schuman, C. C., et al. (2014). Competencies for psychology practice in primary care. *American Psychologist, 69*, 409–429.

McDaniel, S. H., Hargrove, D. S., Belar, C. D., Schroeder, C. S., Freeman, E. L., & Frank, R. G. (2004). Recommendations for education and training in primary care psychology. In K. R. Merikangas, M. Ames, L. Cui, P. E. Stang, T. B. Ustun, M. Von Korff, et al. (2007). The impact of comorbidity of mental and physical conditions on role disability in the US adult household population. *Archives of General Psychiatry, 64*(10), 1180–1188.

Miller, B. F., Ross, K. M., Davis, M. M., Melek, S. P., Kathol, R., & Gordon, P. (2017). Payment reform in the patient-centered medical home: Enabling and sustaining integrated behavioral health care. *American Psychologist, 72*(1), 55–68.

National Center for Health Statistics. (2015). *Health, United States, 2014: In brief.* Hyattsville, MD: U.S. Department of Health and Human Services.

National Center for Quality Assurance. (2014). Patient Centered Medical Home (PCMH 2014) Standards Parts 1 and 2 Training. Retrieved from *www.ncqa. org/programs/recognition/relevanttoallrecognition/ recognitiontraining/pcmh2014standards.aspx*.

National Institute for Health and Clinical Excellence. (2009). *Depression in adults with a chronic physical health problem: Treatment and management* (Clinical Guideline 91). London: Author.

Olfson, M., Blanco, C., Wang, S., Laje, G., & Correll, C. U. (2014). National trends in the mental health care of children, adolescents, and adults by office-based physicians. *JAMA Psychiatry, 71*(1), 81–90.

Pagoto, S., Bodenlos, J. S., Schneider, K. L., Olendzki, B., & Spates, R. C. (2008). Initial investigation of behavioral activation therapy for co-morbid major depressive disorder and obesity. *Psychotherapy Theory Research and Practice, 45*, 410–415.

Peek, C. J. (2013). Lexicon for behavioral health and primary care integration: Concepts and definitions developed by expert consensus. Retrieved from *http://integrationacademy.ahrq.gov/sites/default/ files/lexicon.pdf.*

Petterson, S., Miller, B. F., Payne-Murphy, J. C., & Phillips, R. L., Jr. (2014). Mental health treatment in the primary care setting: Patterns and pathways. *Families, Systems, and Health, 32*, 157–166.

Robinson, P. J., & Reiter, J. T. (2007). *Behavioral consultation and primary care: A guide to integrating services*. New York: Springer.

Roy-Byrne, P., Craske, M. G., Sullivan, G., Rose, R. D., Edlund, M. J., Lang, A .J., et al. (2010). Delivery of evidence-based treatment for multiple anxiety disorders in primary care: A randomized controlled trial. *Journal of the American Medical Association, 303,* 1921–1928.

Schneider, K. L., Pagoto, S. L., Handschin, B., Panza, E., Bakke, S., Liu, Q., et al. (2011). Design and methods for a pilot randomized clinical trial involving exercise and behavioral activation to treat comorbid type 2 diabetes and major depressive disorder. *Mental Health and Physical Activity, 4*(1), 13–21.

Shiraev, E. B., & Levy, D. A. (2010). *Cross-cultural psychology: Critical thinking and contemporary applications* (4th ed.). Boston: Allyn & Bacon.

Sue, D. W., & Sue, D. (1999). *Counseling the culturally different: Theory and practice* (3rd ed.). New York: Wiley.

Torres, J. B., Solberg, V. S. H., & Carlstrom, A. H. (2002). The myth of sameness among Latino men and their machismo. *American Journal of Orthopsychiatry, 72*(2), 163–181.

Uebelacker, L. A., Weisberg, R. B., Haggarty, R., & Miller, I. W. (2009). Adapted behavior therapy for persistently depressed primary care patients: An open trial. *Behavior Modification, 33*(3), 374–395.

Wang, P. S., Lane, M., Olfson, M., Pincus, H. A., Wells, K. B., & Kessler, R. C. (2005). Twelve-month use of mental health services in the united states: Results from the National Comorbidity Survey Replication. *Archives of General Psychiatry, 62,* 629–640.

Wiles, N., Thomas, L., Abel, A., Ridgway, N., Turner, N., Campbell, J., et al. (2013). Cognitive behavioural therapy as an adjunct to pharmacotherapy for primary care based patients with treatment resistant depression: Results of the CoBalT randomised controlled trial. *Lancet, 381,* 375–384.

Young, A. S., Klap, R., Sherbourne, C. D., & Wells, K. B. (2001). The quality of care for depressive and anxiety disorders in the United States. *Archives of General Psychiatry, 58*(1), 55–61.

CHAPTER 20

E–Behavioral Activation in Primary Care for Depression
A Measurement-Based Remission-Focused Treatment

JOSEPH M. TROMBELLO
MADHUKAR H. TRIVEDI

Linda appeared on the computer screen wearing a gray scarf and a Dallas Cowboys baseball cap, hiding much of her short, black hair. She smiled tentatively as she greeted the teletherapist for the first time with a slight wave of her hand and a quiet "hello." Her large, brown eyes were turned downward, and she fumbled at the threads in her scarf as the therapist began to introduce himself and explain the nature of the day's meeting as one that would be different than any other session going forward, as he would ask many questions in order to better understand Linda and how they might work together to help her feel better.

Haltingly, as she responded to the therapist's initial question of what brought her in, Linda, a 42-year-old Latina, described that her mood had declined precipitously over the previous 2 years, especially worsening 1 year earlier, after she moved to Texas from Alabama, where most of her family still resides. A job loss precipitated the move: Linda had previously worked as a receptionist but lost her job 2 years earlier due to her chronic pain, low mood, and poor concentration that left her often calling in sick and unable to work or, when she was at work, performing her job duties poorly. She briefly sought other employment but reported that she began to feel "hopeless" about securing other employment: "Who would hire me, in my condition?" In order to save money, Linda

moved in with her sister, with whom she had an often contentious relationship, as they had never gotten along, even growing up together. Linda's sister was self-assured, consistently employed, and, per Linda's report, often hypercritical of Linda's inability to work and persistently staying in her room, isolated from others.

Linda described that she was struggling with depression, as she also had 10 years earlier. Softly, and at times tearfully, she reported current depressive symptoms, including frequent crying and sadness; difficulty falling asleep; loss of interest and motivation to visit friends, spend time with her two children, and play board games; fatigue; poor concentration, which made reading or watching her favorite soap operas nearly impossible; and worthlessness. She denied any suicidal ideation (SI). We asked her to complete a number of self-report questionnaires to understand better her depressive/anxious symptoms, and their severity. Her score of 13 on the Patient Health Questionnaire–9 (PHQ-9), a nine-item measure of depression severity, indicated moderate depressive symptoms, while her score of 12 on the General Anxiety Disorder–7 (GAD-7), a seven-item measure of anxiety symptoms, indicated a moderate level of anxiety symptoms. Finally, her score of 14 on the Irritability subscale of the Concise Associated Symptoms Tracking (CAST) scale also indicated a moderate level of irritability. Linda not only struggled with depression, but she also described impairing chronic pain in her hip, back, knees, and foot, and rheumatoid arthritis in her left hand. Linda grimaced often as she moved around in her chair, the pain evident on her face. She also presented with hypertension and type 2 diabetes, which were being well managed by her primary care provider (PCP) through medication and psychoeducation. She reported taking tramadol for her chronic pain, alongside 30 mg of duloxetine.

Linda noted several close relationships with friends in Dallas and Alabama, and with her two children. She reported spending much of the day alone in her room, with very little activity or social interaction, while her children were at school. She denied engaging in regular physical activity due to chronic pain. She reported seeking care because she wanted to reduce her depressive symptoms and enhance her ability to engage in pleasurable activities, especially with her children: "I'm just ready to get back to playing with my kids, going out, connecting with friends. Just being me."

By the end of the intake, it was clear to the therapist that Linda would be an excellent candidate for behavioral activation (BA), as her depression likely stemmed, at least in part, from her lack of engagement in activities that promoted pleasure and accomplishment. Spending the majority of her day in her room stood in stark contrast to the vibrant woman Linda had described in happier times, when she was working, active, walking daily, and socializing with family and friends. Given the exacerbation of her mood in regard to her job loss, activities that would help to build a sense of accomplishment and productivity were also likely to be important for her. However, it was also clear that given Linda's extensive chronic medical conditions and her current relationship with a PCP prescribing antidepressant medication, close consultation with the PCP would be important to help to facilitate progress. The therapist therefore planned for biweekly consultations with Linda's PCP in order to ensure that psychotherapy plus medication would be effective for Linda, to communicate to the PCP any medication nonadherence/side effects, to work with the PCP to suggest any changes to medication following established algorithms, and to consult with the PCP regarding what level of physical activity would be indicated for Linda, so as not to exacerbate her chronic pain but to enable some

activity that would likely be helpful for both her mental and physical health.

*   *   *

A core guiding principle of our work is reflected in our initial contacts with Linda and our reliance on measurement of her presenting symptoms to guide her care. The framework of measurement-based care (MBC) in depression arose out of several large-scale, national trials of depression treatment, including the Texas Medication Algorithm Project (TMAP) and Sequenced Treatment Alternatives to Relieve Depression project (STAR*D), and other empirical and review articles (Culpepper & Trivedi, 2013; Gaynes et al., 2008; Harding, Rush, Arbuckle, Trivedi, & Pincus, 2011; Kurian, Grannemann, & Trivedi, 2012; Kurian, Trivedi, et al., 2009; Morris, Toups, & Trivedi, 2012; Morris & Trivedi, 2011; Trivedi, 2009, 2013; Trivedi & Daly, 2007; Trivedi & Kurian, 2010; Trivedi et al., 2006, 2007; Warden et al., 2014). The primary focus of MBC is to tailor treatment decisions at each clinical encounter based on specific clinical status. MBC uses a highly structured approach to antidepressant treatment, best delivered in the context of several visits to a physician or clinician within a specified period of time. These visits occur on a relatively specified interval structure and require the patient to fill out a number of self-report forms, including depressive symptom severity, medication adherence/experienced side effects (if medication is the chosen treatment), and critical associated symptoms such as SI, insomnia, irritability, and mania.

Following a review of these self-report measures and a clinical interview, clinicians/physicians use a detailed stepwise algorithm to decide whether antidepressant medication dosages should be continued or increased, or whether medications should be augmented or switched, psychotherapeutic approaches need to be modified, or exercise or repetitive transcranial magnetic stimulation (rTMS) parameters need to be reevaluated. These algorithms presuppose follow-up visits with patients every 2–4 weeks and also presume patient adherence to medication, with side effects that do not interfere with adherence. After each follow-up visit, providers are faced with several treatment options, including maintenance of the current dosage (recommended if patients have not been on the medication for 4 consistent, adherent weeks), increasing the dosage (recommended if minimal symptom reduction has occurred after 4 weeks of adherence, and the dosage has not yet been maximized), or switching or augmenting the medication (recommended if the initial medication has already been maximized in terms of dosage, or if side effects or other factors make adherence intolerable). A similar decision support approach has also been used in trials examining cardiovascular exercise as an augmentation treatment for major depressive disorder (Trivedi, Greer, et al., 2011). These critical decisions in turn are designed to ensure that the treatment strategy and tactics are guiding patient status toward remission of symptoms, and diminution of adverse events and residual symptoms of depression.

In this chapter, we draw on the conceptualization and interventions suggested in MBC to detail using a combined approach of pharmacotherapy and empirically supported psychotherapy, BA. In addition, we describe an innovative program in which we deliver these treatments through brief teletherapy with low-income, primarily underserved or no-pay patients referred by PCPs from resource-strapped primary care clinics. Through the detailed case example of Linda, we describe our teletherapy BA program and detail how decisions informed by MBC can enhance the psychotherapy interventions to help patients achieve depression remission in the context of ongoing pharmacotherapy. We begin with a review of the literature on MBC in psychiatry because this work provides the rationale for our overall framework of care. We then extend this literature review to the use of measurement approaches in the practice of psychotherapy and describe the creation and implementation of our teletherapy BA program, illustrated through our work with Linda.

Why Practice MBC in Psychiatry?

A substantial amount of research has focused on the use of measurement-based care to guide psychiatry practice and, specifically, to treat depression within primary or specialty care. Several review articles (Kurian et al., 2012; Morris et al., 2012; Morris & Trivedi, 2011; Trivedi, 2009; Trivedi & Kurian, 2010) have discussed key elements of MBC, which include assessment instruments to measure depressive symptoms; medication adherence and side effects; and treatment emergent symptoms such as mania, irritability, or suicidality; a regimented, set visit schedule with providers for follow-up care to monitor improvements or changes in symptoms; and an algorithm to enumerate critical decision points, or established visits when medication increases, augmentations, or changes may be needed if patients are not responding well to antidepressant medication (i.e., adherence is low, side effects are intolerable, depressive symptoms are little changed). Table 20.1 summarizes these principles.

Multiple literature reviews support the efficacy and effectiveness of MBC. In a seminal review, Trivedi (2009) demonstrated how to use depressive symptom severity levels at critical decision points within a fixed schedule of follow-up visits to formulate a detailed treatment algorithm. Several phases of antidepressant treatment were recommended, including an initial, acute phase (6–12 weeks), a continuation phase for patients achieving depression remission (approximately 4–9 months), then

---

TABLE 20.1. Principles of MBC for Depression

1. Monitor depressive symptoms through established self-report measures.

2. Monitor antidepressant medication adherence and side effects through self-report measures.

3. Monitor any symptoms such as mania or suicidality that might emerge with antidepressant treatment through established self-report measures.

4. Establish a set follow-up visit schedule to regularly monitor changes in symptoms, side effects, and treatment-emergent symptoms.

5. At follow-up visits, make use of an algorithm to enumerate and employ critical decision points at which medication changes or changes in modality of treatment are considered, based on symptom improvement or nonresponse.

6. Treat to depression remission, and engage in continuation and maintenance treatment following successful acute treatment of depression.

---

long-term maintenance care (approximately 12 months beyond continuation to, potentially, lifetime, depending on relapse risk factors). This initial review also argued for the importance of assessment and problem solving relative to medication nonadherence; if such nonadherence is due to side effects, such symptoms can be measured, monitored, and addressed (through psychoeducation about the relative short-term nature of some side effects, or making changes to medication to ameliorate more troubling or longer-term symptoms). However, nonadherence may be due to other factors, such as stigma or forgetfulness, which can also be targeted through validation, psychoeducation, and problem-solving how to achieve medication compliance. A second important review article (Morris & Trivedi, 2011) elaborated on the earlier review to discuss the importance of assessing for baseline and changes in SI using an array of self-report and clinician-based assessments, including the Concise Health Risk Tracking and Concise Associated Symptoms Tracking scales (Trivedi, Wisniewski, et al., 2011). This review also elaborated on initial medication decisions and recommended a detailed analysis of any past medication history and current symptoms to consider factors such as prospective medication cost, feasibility, tolerability, and associated side effect or symptom profiles that may actually be beneficial to the patient, depending on individual needs. Other reviews have focused on the problematic nature of residual symptoms in depression treatment and have suggested the use of MBC and psychoeducation to facilitate treating and minimizing residual symptoms such as fatigue and cognitive dysfunction (Culpepper, Muskin, & Stahl, 2015; McIntyre, 2013) and to improve antidepressant efficacy (Kurian, Greer, & Trivedi, 2009).

These review articles have primarily stemmed from findings of two landmark research studies that inform our approach to working with patients like Linda. The TMAP (Crismon et al., 1999; Rush et al., 1999; Trivedi et al., 2004) and STAR*D (Trivedi et al., 2006) merit a brief discussion because they have been so influential in clinical practice. Several noteworthy reviews of the major findings of these studies also are available (Adli, Bauer, & Rush, 2006; Cain, 2007; Trivedi & Daly, 2007). First, TMAP's design involved the use of medication algorithms to treat schizophrenia, bipolar disorder, and major depressive disorder in outpatient clinics (Rush et al., 2003); however, the study's

intervention involved more than simply the use of algorithms. The algorithm package also incorporated other key elements that are consistent with an MBC approach: trained clinical coordinators to assist study physicians, ongoing education for physician and coordinators, assessment and documentation of symptoms and side effects at each follow-up visit, and a program of patient/family psychoeducation. Some clinics received the algorithm package and others received only treatment as usual (Adli et al., 2006). Patients at clinics receiving the algorithm package experienced greater improvement on depressive symptoms and overall mental health functioning compared to patients at clinics receiving only treatment as usual, especially during the first 3 months of treatment (Trivedi et al., 2004).

Building off of TMAP, STAR*D also included trained clinical coordinators and family/patient education. However, unlike TMAP, STAR*D focused exclusively on depression treatment and involved 23 psychiatric or 18 primary care clinics across the United States. Participants with single or recurrent nonpsychotic major depressive disorder were initially prescribed citalopram for 12 weeks, then could be switched or augmented by up to three additional levels of treatment that involved other antidepressant medications or cognitive therapy. Visits were scheduled at Weeks 2, 4, 6, 9, and 12, and following the principles of MBC, assessment of depressive symptoms and side effects was completed at each visit and the goal was treatment to remission. Patients who achieved remission were then followed for 12 additional months (Adli et al., 2006; Rush et al., 2003). Noteworthy findings included similar rates of remission and response in both primary and specialty care (Gaynes et al., 2008). MBC also was associated with reductions in disparities in the use of mental health care based on race, gender, insurance status, and education, suggesting important public health and policy implications in the use of MBC (Gaynes et al., 2009; Kashner et al., 2009). More recent research has replicated and extended these results to a sample of Chinese outpatients (Guo et al., 2015). Taken together, both the TMAP and STAR*D studies suggest successful rates of depression treatment to remission using the principles of MBC.

In addition to these seminal studies, additional researchers have used facets and extensions of MBC to improve patient outcomes. These studies were important in guiding our decision making with Linda because nonadherence to or ineffective use of antidepressant medication could have impeded her general treatment progress and slowed time to achieve depression remission. In a large-scale study using MBC in 15 primary and specialty care clinics, rates of patient medication nonadherence to monotherapy and combination antidepressant therapy were relatively low, with 71.6% of patients across 12 weeks of treatment being nonadherent less than 10% of the time. Furthermore, medication nonadherence was not associated with differences in remission, response, or symptom severity over 12 weeks, perhaps due in part to the relatively low rates of medication nonadherence (Warden et al., 2014). These findings compare favorably to other research, including a systematic review, indicating median adherence rates to depression interventions to be 63%, with a median observation period of 12 weeks (Pampallona, Bollini, Tibaldi, Kupelnick, & Munizza, 2002). The results of Warden and colleagues (2014) therefore indicate that provider education, frequent follow-up visits, and the use of MBC principles are associated with low rates of antidepressant medication nonadherence. Chang and colleagues (2014) tested usual care versus an intervention to provide monthly feedback of depressive symptom severity via study personnel faxing results of patient symptom severity questionnaires to treating physicians; antidepressant use was 85% greater for those in the intervention arm versus usual care, suggesting that more frequent depression measurement and communication of symptoms to physicians are associated with greater antidepressant medication adherence. In addition, this intervention was associated with a greater likelihood of treatment response and remission compared to the treatment-as-usual group (Yeung et al., 2012). Additional research has extended aspects of MBC to additional populations, including elderly adults (Mavandadi, Benson, DiFilippo, Streim, & Oslin, 2015) and children/adolescents (Elmquist, Melton, Croarkin, & McClintock, 2010).

The Design and Delivery of an MBC Teletherapy Program

Despite the strong support for MBC in psychiatry, studies indicate that its use is not widespread. Among a survey of over 300 psychiatrists in the United States (Zimmerman & McGlinchey,

2008), more than half, 50.8%, reported that they *never* or *rarely* use standardized depression severity scales to measure patient outcomes. The most common reasons provided for not using such measures included lack of training in the use of such measures (34.3% of respondents) or that the measures took too much time (33.9% of respondents). These results highlight the importance of developing programs that are guided by MBC principles and feasible to implement in the specialty and primary care settings in which psychiatric management is typically provided.

Our work has focused on designing and delivering an MBC program of teletherapy. This program is an offshoot of a larger program, called VitalSign[6], to introduce screening and MBC treatment of depression within primary care. VitalSign[6] aims to make depression screening the sixth vital sign within primary care, in addition to body temperature, heart rate, respiratory rate, blood pressure, and weight.

VitalSign[6] was introduced within primary care for multiple reasons, most notably the high patient volume in primary care as opposed to specialty care, the preponderance of depression in primary care (Katon & Schulberg, 1992) alongside the lack of mental health screening in these settings, and the comorbidity between depression and physical health concerns, as is true in Linda's case. Problems such as hypertension, diabetes, and aspects of the metabolic syndrome are common among patients with depression who present within primary care (Kessler, Ormel, Demler, & Stang, 2003; Moussavi et al., 2007). While PCPs typically attempt to treat these underlying chronic physical health concerns, depression is a key barrier to adherence to a variety of recommendations—including proper diet, exercise, medication adherence, and other positive health-related behaviors—commonly provided by physicians (DiMatteo, Lepper, & Croghan, 2000). These results suggest that treating comorbid depression may yield positive benefits in terms of diet, exercise, and lifestyle changes that can ameliorate the symptoms of the common chronic physical diseases listed earlier.

VitalSign[6] works as follows. Using a Web-based software delivered through iPads, patients at affiliated primary care clinics within the Dallas–Fort Worth metroplex complete the two-item Patient Health Questionnaire (PHQ-2) at their initial primary care visit; if patients screen positive (i.e., a score of 3 or higher), they are administered the PHQ-9 (Kroenke, Spitzer,

& Williams, 2001). Providers view self-report results through either the iPad or a secure desktop website and conduct a diagnostic interview to confirm or rule out a diagnosis of major depressive disorder or related disorders, such as adjustment disorder with depressed mood or persistent depressive disorder. Providers make a formal diagnosis within the VitalSign[6] software and are then prompted to select a follow-up treatment option, including initiating MBC through pharmacology. Providers and primary care clinic staff members receive comprehensive training in the use of the application, as well as diagnosis, assessment, and treatment of depression through antidepressant medications, including the need for acute, continuation, and maintenance phases of pharmacotherapy.

Once a formal depressive disorder has been identified and MBC through medication has been initiated, patients are asked to return on a set schedule of visits (i.e., Weeks 4, 6, 8, 10, and 12), which are guided by treatment algorithms, as previously mentioned. These algorithms also specify parameters under which medication dosages should be maintained, increased, switched, or augmented. Patients fill out additional questionnaires through the VitalSign[6] application at subsequent visits. At these visits, in addition to continual monitoring of depressive symptoms through the PHQ-9, patients also complete measures including the GAD-7 (Spitzer, Kroenke, Williams, & Lowe, 2006), the Patient Adherence Questionnaire (Rush et al., 2011), and the Frequency, Intensity, and Burden of Side Effects Rating scale (FIBSER; Wisniewski, Rush, Balasubramani, Trivedi, & Nierenberg, 2006) to determine antidepressant medication adherence and side effects. They also complete the Concise Associated Symptom Tracking scale (CAST; Trivedi, Wisniewski, Morris, Fava, Kurian, et al., 2011) to monitor the presence of treatment-emergent signs and symptoms, including mania, irritability, insomnia, and panic. SI is frequently assessed through not only the final item in the PHQ-9 but also an optional measure, the Propensity Index of the Concise Health Risk Tracking scale (CHRT; Trivedi, Wisniewski, Morris, Fava, Gollan, et al., 2011), for individuals who endorse any SI at baseline. Additional measures include a single measure, the four-item Pain Frequency, Intensity and Burden Scale (dela Cruz et al., 2014) and two single items that screen for potential alcohol and drug misuse. These measures have been selected because of the comorbidity between

depression and chronic pain/substance misuse, the negative impact of comorbid substance use/chronic pain on baseline symptoms and treatment response (Davis et al., 2006, 2010; Friedman et al., 2009; Howland et al., 2009; Leuchter et al., 2010), and the need to rule out substance use or general medical conditions, including substantial chronic pain, before making a formal diagnosis of major depressive disorder.

Teletherapy through videoconferencing has been offered to a subset of clinics using the VitalSign[6] application, thereby extending the principles of MBC in psychiatry to the practice of psychotherapy. These clinics were selected because they lacked their own behavioral health clinicians or a strong mental health referral system. Teletherapy was chosen as the medium of treatment delivery in order to offer an innovative service that removes barriers in access to care, as patients are accustomed to visiting their primary care clinics and often lack the financial and emotional resources to visit a new facility, at a new location, with a new provider. Therapy services have been offered in English and Spanish given the high volume of patients in Texas whose first and/or primary language is Spanish. The program initially planned for a 45-minute intake appointment and 30-minute follow-up sessions given the limited availability of therapy providers at each clinic and the need to create as many therapy appointment times as possible. However, additional session time was deemed necessary based on several factors, including patients often coming late to sessions, the need to complete various VitalSign[6] questionnaires, and setting up the videoconferencing software, all of which further cut into session time. Thus, this vast majority of the program's sessions have been 60 minutes for the intake appointment and 45 minutes for psychotherapy. The program has allowed for the intake, eight follow-up psychotherapy sessions, ideally once per week, and biweekly or once-a-month booster sessions, as needed, for approximately the next 3 months. With patient consent, therapy providers routinely send therapy session notes to and engage in periodic consultative phone calls with PCPs to further enhance the continuity of care between primary care clinics and the VitalSign[6] staff. Relationships with local community and public mental health agencies were harnessed for patients who required more extensive psychotherapy beyond this brief program of care.

The teletherapy program was designed to primarily focus on BA given the emphasis on treating depression in primary care with limited time constraints, and our review of the psychotherapy evidence base indicated the value of BA as a brief form of depression psychotherapy. BA is an empirically supported treatment for major depressive disorder (Dimidjian, Barrera, Martell, Muñoz, & Lewinsohn, 2011; Dimidjian et al., 2006; Hopko, Lejuez, Ruggiero, & Eifert, 2003; Soucy Chartier & Provencher, 2013), including various subtypes, such as atypical depression (Weinstock, Munroe, & Miller, 2011). BA is also effective when compared to cognitive therapy and antidepressant medication in preventing the relapse and recurrence of depression (Dobson et al., 2008).

BA as a modality of psychotherapy operates from the conceptualization that the symptoms and behaviors associated with depression stem from an inability to experience positive rewards, including pleasure from daily life events. Critical BA interventions focus on working with those with depression to select and engage in small, daily activities that enhance their experience of pleasure and engagement with activities and other people. We believed that the focus on activity monitoring in BA provided a strong practical match with the principles of MBC. Although MBC has typically been identified with psychotropic medication interventions, aspects of measurement commonly occur within psychotherapy. Mood check-ins are an integral part of cognitive-behavioral therapy (CBT) generally, in order to begin the session, consider changes in symptoms from the prior session, and to help set the agenda for the remainder of the psychotherapy session. CBT clinicians therefore frequently inquire, through either verbal means or the use of self-report symptom rating scales such as the Beck Depression Inventory, about a patient's symptom severity from week to week (Beck, 2011). Patient ratings beyond standardized self-report measures are used throughout cognitive and behavioral interventions, for example, to rate a subjective level of distress to design a fear exposure hierarchy or to rate the percentage that a particular thought is believed to be true both before and after cognitive restructuring interventions. Patient ratings are also frequently used specifically within BA to determine changes in mood, pleasure, and achievement/mastery before and after completing an activity (Martell, Dimidjian, & Herman-Dunn, 2013).

In the model, we deliver BA teletherapy services, roughly 1 day per week, from two providers (the first author, Trombello, who is also a licensed psychologist, and a bilingual licensed master social worker supervised by a licensed clinical and doctoral-level social worker). Providers received BA training by reading *Behavioral Activation for Depression: A Clinician's Guide* (Martell et al., 2013) and completing the University of Washington's IMPACT training module on BA.

The intake session includes psychoeducation about BA, the introduction of activity scheduling, and handouts about depression (and, if necessary, anxiety) to read for homework. Subsequent sessions include a discussion of therapy goals and, at each session, working through a pleasant activity tracking form to identify several small behavioral activities to be completed each week. The strength of depressive symptoms, the pleasure of the event, and the achievement experienced from completing the event are rated before and after activity completion. Given that patients endorse mood boosts for both pleasurable and accomplishment/productivity tasks, it is often important to help patients set a mix of both kinds of activities. Progress on behavioral task completion is discussed at each session, with problem-solving barriers to activity completion occurring as necessary. Final sessions augment standard BA with a brief introduction to the cognitive model and the discussion of cognitive biases within depression and anxiety, as we have found that some of our patients' barriers to BA have been cognitive in nature (i.e., thoughts/self-talk such as "I'm not motivated to do this activity," "This won't help me feel better," or "I'm worthless"), as will be shown in Linda's case example. Cognitive work in our program is also employed primarily when depressiogenic thinking (i.e., "I'm worthless." "This activity will never work for me") or low self-esteem are clearly impairing activity setting and completion. Cognitive work has also been used frequently for our patients with primary anxiety disorders, in order to teach them that cognitive biases—primarily overestimating the likelihood of feared/worst-case scenarios occurring and underestimating their ability to cope even if the worst-case scenario occurred—are common barriers to task completion (i.e., behavioral exposure to feared stimuli). The final two sessions involve openly discussing the termination process and completing a detailed relapse prevention handout to concretize gains made in the areas of pleasant and social activities, exercise, thinking styles, relaxation, and social/professional support. This approach helps patients continue to be their own therapist and problem-solve on their own, as well as summarizing gains made and skills learned. A discussion of either booster sessions or transferring to a higher level of care also is initiated before termination.

Although there is a set structure to the teletherapy program, it is also designed to be flexible and incorporate facets of other modalities, as appropriate for each person's needs. Therefore, at times, the cognitive model and cognitive restructuring work are introduced earlier (previously discussed) and additional material, including diaphragmatic breathing for relaxation, sleep hygiene psychoeducation, problem solving, and interpersonal effectiveness skills from dialectical behavior therapy (Linehan, 1993) are discussed when our clinicians collaborate with patients to tackle these issues. For example, for some patients, fatigue and poor sleep are common barriers to BA task completion, which merits sleep psychoeducation and behavioral work; for others, such as Linda, interpersonal conflict and psychosocial stressors are key elements that maintain patient inertia, and therefore depression, which suggests a need for interpersonal effectiveness/communication training to augment BA work. Review of the aforementioned assessment instruments within the VitalSign[6] application occurred before every session, in accordance with MBC principles, and this review of symptoms also informed interventions used (i.e., with clinicians noting that patients who are high in insomnia may be offered sleep behavioral training; that those with elevations in anhedonia merit BA work). Psychoeducational handouts and other materials were drawn from the Centre for Clinical Interventions, the University of Washington's IMPACT program, *therapistaid.com,* and *psychologytools.org.*

All sessions make use of a standard BA/CBT format: formal mood check-in (through reviewing VitalSign[6] questionnaires), a bridge from the previous session, agenda setting, homework review, agenda progression, setting homework, and soliciting patient feedback. Readers may review Chapter 3, specifically page 45, of *Behavioral Activation for Depression: A Clinician's Guide* (Martell et al., 2013) for additional details as to the session structure. Sessions also frequently made use of Socratic questioning techniques, helping to guide the patient through self-discovery and agenda progression by asking specific open-ended questions rather than simply providing the "answers" or offering advice to patients; this follows relatively recent research on the importance of Socratic questioning for clinical outcomes (Braun, Strunk, Sasso, & Cooper, 2015). Additional details about the structure of therapy can be found in Trombello and colleagues (2017).

Linda was treated in the context of the BA teletherapy program, and her course of treatment provides a clear illustration of how aspects of measurement-based care guide clinical decision-making and intervention for psychotherapy and pharmacotherapy, as well as overlay her chronic physical health conditions and concerns such as chronic pain/rheumatoid arthritis and hypertension/diabetes. A summary of our work with Linda is supplied in Table 20.2, and Figure 20.1 denotes specific principles that can be applied when symptoms fail to improve after a period of a few weeks.

Intake

After conducting the psychodiagnostic interview and reviewing Linda's scores with her (moderate levels of depression, anxiety, and irritability as assessed by the PHQ-9, GAD-7, and CAST), the first author (Trombello) ended the intake by describing to Linda the therapy program, including a conceptualization of her symptoms through the BA model—that her lack of engagement in activities promoting pleasure and mastery was related to her low mood, anhedonia, feelings of worthlessness, and fatigue. They then discussed how increasing Linda's engagement in activities would not only help with her depressive symptoms but also improve her self-esteem, increase her fitness to improve her glucose and blood pressure numbers, and reduce Linda's focus on her chronic pain. Finally, they discussed the need for regular homework to practice skills.

THERAPIST: Linda, thanks so much for answering all my questions today, both verbally and on the iPad. That really helps me to understand you better. Both your answers to my questions, and to those on the iPad, indicate that currently you have a moderate level of depression, anxiety, and irritability. I'll ask you to fill out these questionnaires each week, so that we can begin to measure change and progress, and so that we can also know if certain symptoms are improving: This would suggest that we need to target them more fully, perhaps through specific interventions, for example, to help you sleep better or com-

TABLE 20.2. Outline of Evolution of BA Treatment with Linda: Target PHQ-9 ≤ 5

Session	PHQ-9 score	Interventions used	Homework assigned
Intake	13	• Depression and BA model education • Assessed targets of behavior inactivation	• Read handouts about depression and anxiety • Track time through activity scheduling
1	12	• Scheduled BA activities • Sleep and insomnia education	• Complete one activity (walking with mother) • Practice two specific behavioral sleep changes
2	21	• Reviewed BA activity completion • Scheduled new BA activities • Discussed how napping less led to increased energy	• Proceed with new BA activities (playing cards, reading book, writing letter) • Practice reducing daytime napping
3	19[a]	• Empathy and reflective listening • Thought stopping • Designed BA activities	• Complete new BA activities • Practice thought stopping
4	8	• Reviewed cognitive and behavioral homework • Discussed barriers to activity completion • Cognitive restructuring to complete BA activities	• Complete new BA activities • Practice cognitive coping statements to motivate when energy is low
5	6	• Interpersonal effectiveness and assertiveness education • Interpersonal effectiveness role play • Set upcoming BA activities	• Practice assertiveness skills • Complete new BA activities
6	6	• Discussed new apartment move • Introduced cognitive model • Reviewed alternative thoughts to self-motivate • Set BA activities	• Begin moving process (set budget) • Practice cognitive restructuring skills to self-motivate • Complete BA tasks
7	7	• Reviewed cognitive and BA homework • Discussed additional steps toward moving • Set BA activities	• Review relapse prevention handout • Complete BA tasks
8	4	• Completed relapse prevention handout • Consolidated treatment gains • Processed therapeutic relationship ending	• Practice cognitive, behavioral, relaxation, communication, and support-seeking skills

[a]The patient reported filling out the PHQ-9 incorrectly, as she said she forgot the ordering of the anchors. This score represents the new PHQ-9 upon readministration after the therapy session concluded.

municate more effectively with your sister. Also, to enhance your care, your PCP and I will be speaking every other week about how your medication and therapy are doing, and if either I or your PCP might benefit from making any changes to what we are doing. How does this sound?

LINDA: It all sounds good. Thanks for taking so much time to help me.

THERAPIST: No, it's my pleasure. Thank you. I also want to tell you that our therapy will be different than other forms of therapy, as we'll be meeting each week for up to 8 weeks. We'll be working together each week on is-

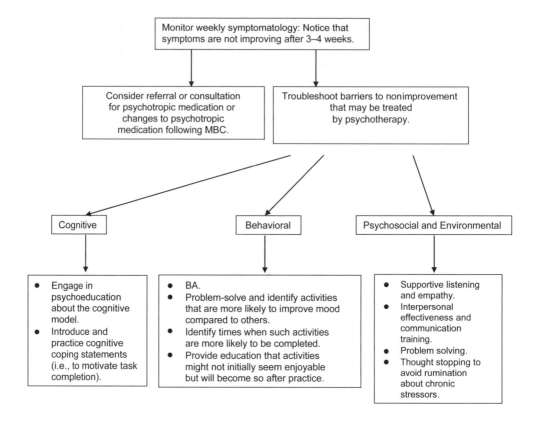

FIGURE 20.1. Depiction of how to problem-solve barriers to psychological treatments when depressive symptoms change little or not at all.

sues that we identify together, but we'll also go through some of the skills in this folder. We focus primarily on behavioral activation for depression, which just means that when folks feel depressed or stressed, they stop doing things that used to be fun for them, such as going out with family or friends, or working out. The less they do, the less they want to do, and the worse they feel. Does this describe you?

LINDA: Yes, that absolutely fits me.

THERAPIST: Yes, I think it does, too. The good news is that just as these negative cycles of inactivation occur, we can start to interrupt these cycles to help you, little by little, do activities that you find enjoyable and that accomplish goals that you have. In this way, you'll start to feel better over time. And, this likely will improve not only your mental health but also your physical health because if we can help get you more physically active, this will likely help to manage your hypertension and diabetes. We'll work together to help set physical activities that are doable for you given your chronic pain, and we might even want to talk with your PCP, too, for her input in this process. How does this sound?

LINDA: Good. I think it's doable. I just want to get better.

THERAPIST: I know you do. I want that for you, too. In order to help with that, actually, as I'll only be with you less than an hour per week, and you're with yourself the rest of the time, it's really important that you and I work together at the end of each session to help set some tasks that you can do at home, and that we'll discuss next week. This will help you to practice the skills and make progress faster. Are you willing to do this?

LINDA: Yes, I'll do my best to practice each week.

THERAPIST: Good. We'll work together to help you set tasks that are realistic, and we'll talk about them either way. I want to set this up as a no-lose proposition. If you're able to do the homework, that's great. If not, that's perfectly fine, too: We'll talk about it either way and help you problem-solve what happened the week before in order for you to persevere with homework going forward.

As the session concluded, Linda and the therapist set homework of reading psychoeducational handouts about the symptoms and treatment of depression and anxiety and completing an activity scheduling form to track how she was spending her time, in order to better inform what activities should be increased and reduced. Finally, the therapist solicited feedback at the end of the intake session, and Linda reported feeling excited to begin treatment and comfortable talking to the therapist.

Session 1

The therapist reviewed Linda's questionnaires through the desktop application connected with VitalSign[6] software: Her PHQ-9 scores were little changed over the prior week's scores, with a total score of 12; her GAD-7 score of 11 was also nearly identical to the prior week's score, as was her Irritability score of 12 from the CAST. She endorsed specific symptoms at higher levels, including fatigue, anhedonia, and insomnia. The Patient Adherence Questionnaire indicated that Linda was taking her antidepressant medication daily as prescribed, while the FIBSER indicated no side effects. As SI was not present at intake, the therapist did not administer the CHRT at any follow-up interval. They reviewed her activity scheduling form, which indicated that she was sleeping often throughout the day and night. She also reported, however, that her low mood and energy while sleeping/napping stood out in contrast to other times throughout the week, when she was more activated. Therefore, they collaboratively designed a specific behavioral assignment—walking with her mother at a specific time on the following Sunday morning. They also discussed the value of being as specific as possible with action plans given that more concrete and specific activities are more likely to be completed. They also selected walking, as it is a low-impact exercise that would not exacerbate her chronic pain but would offer cardiovascular benefit to help with

her diabetes and hypertension. The therapist noted that if the pain ever got too intense, she could stop, and he and Linda would discuss this at the next session. Before setting the assignment, the therapist had also consulted with her PCP to ensure that walking was an appropriate exercise given her chronic pain. Finally, given her hypersomnia and fatigue, the therapist provided Linda with psychoeducation about sleep and how daytime napping can make it difficult to fall asleep at night. Linda agreed to work on two specific sleep goals over the next week: reducing daytime sleeping and getting out of bed to engage in a quiet activity if she could not fall asleep after 20 minutes.

Session 2

Linda reported a substantial increase in her depressive symptoms in Session 2; her PHQ-9 score was 21, indicating a severe level of depressive symptomatology. She reported that this elevation was due to a conflict with her sister an hour before the visit. After validating this recent difficult encounter, and the tendency for mood symptoms to be influenced by recent events, they discussed the importance of completing the session-by-session questionnaires about the entirety of the preceding 2 weeks, so as not to have a recent life event bias future PHQ-9 administrations. The verbal assessment indicated that her PHQ-9 was likely inflated due to the life event, and that her functioning before this interaction had been better. A review of the PHQ-9 indicated frequent concerns with low mood, sleep difficulties, feeling like a failure, poor concentration, and psychomotor retardation. Linda's GAD-7 score of 15 also indicated a severe level of anxiety and represented an increase over the prior week's symptoms. The majority of the session focused on reviewing her behavioral homework and setting up new activities for her to complete over the forthcoming week. Time constraints prevented the therapist from problem-solving the specific interaction Linda had with her sister, but the therapist did note in the conceptualization that interpersonal conflicts seemed common in this relationship, and that likely Linda would need some additional skills building in interpersonal communication in a future session(s) if conflicts continued. As part of the homework review, Linda reported having engaged in pleasurable activities several times over the prior week, including going for walks and playing cards with her family. She described clearly that her level of depressive symptoms was reduced, and her level of pleasure and achievement was increased after completing these activities. She rated a higher level of benefit from playing cards with her children compared to going for a walk; given this information, the therapist decided to continue and, in fact, to increase her time playing cards in the future. They scheduled additional activities for the next week, including writing a letter to Linda's friend in another state on Tuesday, and reading a book at her mother's house on Wednesday. They also reviewed various behavioral interventions for insomnia, as discussed in the previous session; as a result of this psychoeducation and discussion the previous week, Linda reported taking naps less frequently throughout the day. Through the use of Socratic questioning, the therapist fostered a conversation about how napping less frequently is associated with improved energy and the ability to engage in activities during the day, and more ease falling asleep at night.

THERAPIST: Linda, what did you notice about your napping this week? I remember that was a goal from our session last week.

LINDA: Well, I tried to nap less often during the day. I think I only napped one day, on Friday.

THERAPIST: OK, and how did you feel after you took a nap on Friday?

LINDA: Well, actually I still felt tired. And then I also felt bad about myself because I didn't get any of the activities done I had wanted to accomplish.

THERAPIST: OK, that's really useful information. How about Thursday, a day you didn't nap? What was your mood and energy like then?

LINDA: It's funny, but I actually felt better and more energized that day. I cleaned part of the apartment and went outside for a short walk.

THERAPIST: Hmm, that's interesting. So if we were to compare Thursday and Friday, what did you notice?

LINDA: Well, actually, I felt better and had more energy on Thursday, when I was doing activities and not napping, versus Friday, when I was napping and lying around and not doing very much.

THERAPIST: Exactly right! What do you think this means about how you want this coming week to proceed?

LINDA: I think I want to have more days like Thursdays and less like Fridays (*laughing*).

THERAPIST: (*laughing, too*). Yes! I imagine you would. So let's help you keep setting activities to do during the day and trying your best to avoid napping when you're tired. How does that sound?

LINDA: Really good.

They concluded the session by summarizing homework and processing session feedback: Linda reported especially enjoying the mood comparison between Thursday and Friday to support her decision to take fewer naps.

Session 3

Linda's depressive and anxious symptoms had declined notably from the prior session per self-report (a PHQ-9 score of 6 and a GAD-7 score of 10) but the Irritability subscale from the CAST had increased (subscale score of 20). Medication adherence continued to be good, with no side effects. However, during the mood check-in, Linda reported an especially difficult and stressful week due to notable family stress and tension. She was also frequently tearful during the mood check-in. Although Linda was not directly in front of the therapist, due to the videoconferencing nature of their sessions, the therapist still was able to provide empathic and supportive interventions by lowering his voice, speaking slowly and softly, reflecting her emotions/feelings, and giving her the space and time to express her feelings and emotions, including tearfulness. (Interestingly, we have found that we use the same nonspecific therapy skills to heighten and/or respond to affect whether conducting sessions in person or through teletherapy.) The marked shift in her affect and self-reported distress, in contrast to her reduced scores on self-report measures, led the therapist to gently inquire about this discrepancy. Linda commented that she must have answered the self-report questions incorrectly, as she thought that higher responses on the scales indicated fewer symptoms. The therapist therefore suggested that she redo the measure at the end of the session (score at that time: 19), in order not to further exhaust the session's limited time.

In response to Linda's reported stressors and tearfulness, the therapist used empathy and supportive listening interventions, as well as reflecting that it must have been very difficult to complete behavioral activities if she wanted to avoid, hide, and escape her family stress. In the context of such validation, the therapist also highlighted the data gathered in prior weeks, calling attention to the ways in which Linda's mood was elevated when engaging in pleasurable activities, and he also noted that a key therapy goal was to reduce daytime sleeping. The therapist and Linda collaboratively designed three specific activities to be completed for homework, and he also introduced thought stopping to help Linda avoid thinking about family stress. Following the somewhat flexible nature of treatment, the therapist introduced cognitive work (i.e., thought stopping to prevent rumination) earlier than usual into the BA program, as it was clear that Linda's substantial rumination on family stress was preventing activity completion. This intervention represents an example of engaging in cognitive work to promote BA. As Linda endorsed frequent rumination on negative feedback that she heard from her mother and sister, and believing that she was "worthless" and "lazy," they discussed thought stopping to provide a more instant form of relief and distraction from those negative thoughts that impaired Linda's motivation and activity completion. However, additional interventions were employed beyond thought stopping: They also discussed how activity completion itself could also distract Linda from her problems with her family, and they worked together to develop a mantra ("I need to do my activity even if I don't feel like doing it, as it will help me feel better") that she could use to motivate herself when she noticed herself ruminating, being stuck, or reflecting on conflict with her family. They decided that thought stopping might be more effective at this point than a more time-consuming intervention such as interpersonal effectiveness and communication training, but they left open the possibility of using these interventions in future sessions, when more time could be allotted to them.

Session 4

Linda's affect was noticeably brighter during the mood check-in, as the therapist observed her laughing and smiling more frequently on the video, and her voice reflected a greater degree of energy and enthusiasm. She reported that her depressive and anxious symptoms were substantially lower and noted that thought stopping was highly effective to help her move on

from reflections about chronic family stressors. Such improvements were also confirmed on her self-report assessments, with a PHQ-9 score of 8 and a GAD-7 score of 4, indicating significant declines from prior weeks. Irritability was also markedly decreased (CAST subscale: 8), with robust medication adherence and minimal medication side effects. They reviewed/reinforced thought stopping and discussed Linda's behavioral activities. She reported having engaged in several pleasurable activities over the prior week, including playing cards with her children, calling a friend, and going for a walk. Ratings of her mood, pleasure, and achievement before and after these events were used to set new activities over the following week. They discussed potential barriers to task completion, including feeling tired and wanting to sleep, and reinforced cognitive strategies to increase her motivation (i.e., her "I need to do my activity even if I don't feel like doing it, as it will help me feel better" mantra). Finally, the therapist reminded Linda of an initial aspect discussed in the BA overview, namely, that sometimes getting started with a task leads to increased energy and motivation later. Linda reported that this information was very helpful, and that she would challenge herself to get started on activities even if she did not feel like doing them. In this way, they engaged in problem-solving potential barriers to activity completion.

Session 5

Linda reported that her mood was a bit better than last week; her PHQ-9 score of 6 indicated a mild level of depression, while her GAD-7 score of 4 indicated no or minimal levels of anxiety. Her depressive symptoms were confined to only "several days" over the last 2 weeks, with no item greater in frequency or intensity than this level on the PHQ-9. She reported substantial psychosocial stressors and arguments with her sister, with whom she lived, that could not always be ameliorated through her thought-stopping techniques (reminding herself to stop thinking about the conflict that occurred). Given the chronicity of these interpersonal stressors and the need for additional intervention beyond thought stopping, the therapist also incorporated interpersonal effectiveness/communication training to attempt to resolve the conflicts. Using "DEAR MAN" (Describe, Express, Assert, Reinforce, Mindful, Appear confident, Negotiate) skills (Linehan, 1993), they worked together to help Linda describe her need for her sister to be more respectful toward her, as well as express in emotional terms the importance of this behavioral change and reinforce how this change would benefit her sister. In addition to direct psychoeducation about the skills, Linda and the therapist practiced these skills together through role play, with the therapist playing Linda's sister and demonstrating different ways that she might respond. During the feedback portion of the session, Linda reported that the skills and role play to practice how to respond to various ways her sister might react were especially helpful. As in all sessions, completion of existing behavioral activities was reviewed, and creation of new activities over the upcoming week were collaboratively discussed.

Session 6

Linda's symptoms were at a similar level as in previous weeks (a PHQ-9 score of 6 and a GAD-7 score of 7). These scores are good but not quite to remission level (below 5 for both measures), indicating that additional work was needed to get her there. (The fact that Linda was not yet fully in remission after over 4 weeks of being on the same dosage of medication also merited additional consultation with her PCP to recommend a medication dosage increase.) At the beginning of the session, when setting the agenda, Linda had noted that she wanted to talk about a new goal: "I've begun thinking that I really do need to get my own place. This would help me move away from some of my family who gets me down and also help me to feel more in control and on my own." In response to this agenda item, the therapist problem-solved Linda's moving into her own apartment by helping her think about the very first thing she needed to accomplish (setting her budget), and setting some time aside during the week to think about how much she could spend. The therapist reviewed Linda's BA activities, most of which she was able to complete, and which she noted were helpful in improving her mood. Linda commented that, at times, she was unable to motivate herself when her children were at school. In response to this barrier to activity completion, aspects of cognitive therapy, including the cognitive model, were introduced in a discussion of how automatic thoughts ("The kids are gone to school; there's nothing for me to do") were related to feeling sad and sleeping during the day. These thoughts were contrasted with alternative thoughts ("This is an opportunity for me to do

something active") that might be related to feeling happier and being more likely to engage in a pleasurable activity. New activities were designed over the upcoming week, including calling her best friend Monday evening, writing a letter to another friend Saturday afternoon, and listening to relaxing music for 20 minutes each night before bed. Linda also agreed to practice introducing alternative thoughts to respond to negative automatic thoughts.

Session 7

Linda's symptoms were similar to those of the prior week (PHQ-9 and GAD-7 scores of 7). She reported that cognitive restructuring work helped her to get out of bed and stay motivated, and that BA work was also helpful. Specifically, she said, "I think I'm really getting the hang of how important it is for me to stay active and busy and to stop thinking about negative stuff about myself or my family that just gets me down." Linda also commented that she had mostly been ignoring her sister and did not yet practice the assertiveness skills. The therapist talked about specific steps she could take to move into her apartment (i.e., identifying the area in which she wanted to live, locating various apartments, beginning to discuss her plans with friends who might be able to physically help her move). Linda expressed excitement about this potential move and raised concerns about potential barriers, such as her children needing to change schools. They brainstormed some potential alternatives to these barriers, including involving her children in the school selection process, discussing ways to save a bit more money to acquire furniture and other needed items, and so forth. In the latter part of the session, the therapist reminded Linda that the next week would be the final therapy session, and Linda agreed to read a handout on relapse prevention for part of her homework. Additional activities were also assigned, including going for a walk on Saturday and playing cards with her daughter Friday night.

Session 8

Linda's mood was improved compared to prior weeks, including a PHQ-9 score of 4 and a GAD-7 score of 3. She reported slightly increased anxiety due to the stress about looking for a new apartment; however, she also reported making substantial process in the search process and significant excitement about being able to live on her own. She and the therapist discussed the relapse prevention plan, with specific items for each of the elements written down. She discussed positive coping thoughts, such as "I'll feel better after I complete an activity" or "Stop thinking that way"; pleasurable and social activities, including playing cards with her family and visiting/calling friends; relaxing activities, including listening to music and taking a bath and exercising by walking around her front lawn; and social support, including several close friends in and beyond Dallas. They processed the end of their therapy relationship by noting that they would miss each other, yet both were excited by her progress. The therapist suggested continued medication management through her PCP given that depression remission had just occurred, and he also offered his number should she ever wish to have a "booster" session.

Summary

The work with Linda illustrates several important points about how to apply the principles of MBC to the practice of BA therapy delivered via videoconferencing teletherapy and combined with pharmacotherapy. First, the use of measurements at every visit is essential to monitor progress toward therapy goals and track progress. In each session, measurements were confirmed by diagnostic interview or the patient's subjective report, and any discrepancies were reconciled. Measurements also offer the clinician an indication of what should be prioritized, or whether any interventions need to be modified. For example, paying attention to elevations or decreases in symptoms with Linda provided valuable information about what interventions should be continued (specific behavioral activities; e.g., playing cards with her children), and when new interventions were needed (i.e., cognitive interventions and interpersonal effectiveness training to combat chronic stressors that served as a barrier to activity completion). Linda's medication adherence and side effect profiles were very stable, and thus required less explicit time and attention than would be the case for a patient with more complex medication management issues. Even for Linda, though, it was important to consistently review the symptom and side effect measures to determine the efficacy of antidepressant medication and whether any changes might be recommended.

The structured psychotherapy program of BA served as a kind of treatment algorithm, akin to that of MBC for antidepressant medications; however, some flexibility was allotted by clinician judgment, and such flexibility was essential toward adding in new interventions of different modalities that were highly effective. Adhering to a set schedule for psychotherapy—ideally, on a weekly basis—allowed for rapid progress and amelioration of symptoms, even within a brief course of only eight, 30-minute psychotherapy sessions (which we also have expanded to 45 minutes). The use of psychotherapy homework to practice skills and activities was also essential to treatment progress, as was the use of nonspecific therapy skills such as empathy, genuineness, and warmth. Rapport with Linda was surprisingly easy to build and maintain even when psychotherapy was conducted over the Internet through videoconferencing.

In this chapter, we have reviewed the literature on MBC in psychiatry and discussed how such principles have been applied to psychotherapy. We encourage all readers, especially trainees in mental health, to distill from this chapter several key points: (1) the importance of regularly using self-report measures before each psychotherapy session, in order to consistently monitor symptoms and follow any changes in symptoms, including analyzing when specific symptoms have not yet ameliorated and may require a more thorough focus; (2) to be consistently collaborative with patients in identifying session-by-session goals and working toward them; (3) to consistently set and review homework; (4) to maintain a warm, empathic, and Socratic style of therapy; (5) to be thoughtful about when patients are not making progress and consider new intervention approaches; and (6) to engage in regular supervision or consultation with supervisors, colleagues, or other medical professionals treating the patient, especially for cases that are difficult, or when a patient is not improving. Our chapter and its accompanying program of teletherapy also lend themselves to several research questions, which we plan to analyze and publish in the future. These include questions such as the following:

1. How many sessions are necessary for optimal symptom reduction to occur?
2. What specific intervention strategies are associated with symptom reduction?
3. Does one consistent intervention, such as BA, need to be regularly applied, or can

other intervention approaches also show benefit for specific situations?

4. How can we consistently engage patients in follow-up care; that is, how can we reduce no-shows and the preponderance of patients who never actually complete a psychotherapy session?

Preliminary research with our data has indicated that the majority of patients receiving at least one psychotherapy session achieved depression remission at some point during the course of psychotherapy, and that approximately one-third of patients only attended the intake session (Trombello et al., 2017).

Finally, in describing our work with Linda, we have illustrated the use of MBC principles to develop and deliver a novel and brief form of BA. This teletherapy program has expanded access to care among low-income, primary care patients and provides an example of how to use scientific evidence to guide clinical innovation. We are excited by our program's innovative use of technology to reduce the barriers to care access, as well as its use of a specific, empirically supported approach to treat depression and anxiety within primary care, thereby beginning to address a major public health problem.

References

Adli, M., Bauer, M., & Rush, A. J. (2006). Algorithms and collaborative-care systems for depression: Are they effective and why?: A systematic review. *Biological Psychiatry, 59*(11), 1029–1038.

Beck, J. S. (2011). *Cognitive behavior therapy: Basics and beyond* (2nd ed.). New York: Guilford Press.

Braun, J. D., Strunk, D. R., Sasso, K. E., & Cooper, A. A. (2015). Therapist use of Socratic questioning predicts session-to-session symptom change in cognitive therapy for depression. *Behaviour Research and Therapy, 70,* 32–37.

Cain, R. A. (2007). Navigating the Sequenced Treatment Alternatives to Relieve Depression (STAR*D) study: Practical outcomes and implications for depression treatment in primary care. *Primary Care: Clinics in Office Practice, 34*(3), 505–519.

Chang, T. E., Jing, Y., Yeung, A. S., Brenneman, S. K., Kalsekar, I. D., Hebden, T., et al. (2014). Depression monitoring and patient behavior in the Clinical Outcomes in MEasurement-Based Treatment (COMET) trial. *Psychiatric Services, 65*(8), 1058–1061.

Crismon, M. L., Trivedi, M., Pigott, T. A., Rush, A. J., Hirschfeld, R. M., Kahn, D. A., et al. (1999). The Texas Medication Algorithm Project: Report of the Texas Consensus Conference Panel on Medication

Treatment of Major Depressive Disorder. *Journal of Clinical Psychiatry, 60*(3), 142–156.

Culpepper, L., Muskin, P. R., & Stahl, S. M. (2015). Major depressive disorder: Understanding the significance of residual symptoms and balancing efficacy with tolerability. *American Journal of Medicine, 128*(9, Suppl.), S1–S15.

Culpepper, L., & Trivedi, M. H. (2013). Using measurement-based care with patient involvement to improve outcomes in depression. *Primary Care Companion for CNS Disorders, 15*(6).

Davis, L. L., Frazier, E., Husain, M. M., Warden, D., Trivedi, M., Fava, M., et al. (2006). Substance use disorder comorbidity in major depressive disorder: A confirmatory analysis of the STAR*D cohort. *American Journal on Addictions, 15*(4), 278–285.

Davis, L. L., Wisniewski, S. R., Howland, R. H., Trivedi, M. H., Husain, M. M., Fava, M., et al. (2010). Does comorbid substance use disorder impair recovery from major depression with SSRI treatment?: An analysis of the STAR*D level one treatment outcomes. *Drug and Alcohol Dependence, 107*(2–3), 161–170.

dela Cruz, A. M., Bernstein, I. H., Greer, T. L., Walker, R., Rethorst, C. D., Grannemann, B., et al. (2014). Self-rated measure of pain frequency, intensity, and burden: Psychometric properties of a new instrument for the assessment of pain. *Journal of Psychiatric Research, 59,* 155–160.

DiMatteo, M. R., Lepper, H. S., & Croghan, T. W. (2000). Depression is a risk factor for noncompliance with medical treatment: Meta-analysis of the effects of anxiety and depression on patient adherence. *Archives of Internal Medicine, 160*(14), 2101–2107.

Dimidjian, S., Barrera, M., Jr., Martell, C., Muñoz, R. F., & Lewinsohn, P. M. (2011). The origins and current status of behavioral activation treatments for depression. *Annual Review of Clinical Psychology, 7,* 1–38.

Dimidjian, S., Hollon, S. D., Dobson, K. S., Schmaling, K. B., Kohlenberg, R. J., Addis, M. E., et al. (2006). Randomized trial of behavioral activation, cognitive therapy, and antidepressant medication in the acute treatment of adults with major depression. *Journal of Consulting and Clinical Psychology, 74*(4), 658–670.

Dobson, K. S., Hollon, S. D., Dimidjian, S., Schmaling, K. B., Kohlenberg, R. J., Gallop, R. J., et al. (2008). Randomized trial of behavioral activation, cognitive therapy, and antidepressant medication in the prevention of relapse and recurrence in major depression. *Journal of Consulting and Clinical Psychology, 76*(3), 468–477.

Elmquist, J. M., Melton, T. K., Croarkin, P., & McClintock, S. M. (2010). A systematic overview of measurement-based care in the treatment of childhood and adolescent depression. *Journal of Psychiatric Practice, 16*(4), 217–234.

Friedman, E. S., Wisniewski, S. R., Gilmer, W., Nierenberg, A. A., Rush, A. J., Fava, M., et al. (2009). Sociodemographic, clinical, and treatment characteristics associated with worsened depression during treatment with citalopram: Results of the NIMH STAR(*)D trial. *Depression and Anxiety, 26*(7), 612–621.

Gaynes, B. N., Rush, A. J., Trivedi, M. H., Wisniewski, S. R., Balasubramani, G. K., McGrath, P. J., et al. (2008). Primary versus specialty care outcomes for depressed outpatients managed with measurement-based care: Results from STAR*D. *Journal of General Internal Medicine, 23*(5), 551–560.

Gaynes, B. N., Warden, D., Trivedi, M. H., Wisniewski, S. R., Fava, M., & Rush, A. J. (2009). What did STAR*D teach us?: Results from a large-scale, practical, clinical trial for patients with depression. *Psychiatric Services, 60*(11), 1439–1445.

Guo, T., Xiang, Y. T., Xiao, L., Hu, C. Q., Chiu, H. F., Ungvari, G. S., et al. (2015). Measurement-based care versus standard care for major depression: A randomized controlled trial with blind raters. *American Journal of Psychiatry, 172*(10), 1004–1013.

Harding, K. J., Rush, A. J., Arbuckle, M., Trivedi, M. H., & Pincus, H. A. (2011). Measurement-based care in psychiatric practice: A policy framework for implementation. *Journal of Clinical Psychiatry, 72*(8), 1136–1143.

Hopko, D. R., Lejuez, C. W., Ruggiero, K. J., & Eifert, G. H. (2003). Contemporary behavioral activation treatments for depression: Procedures, principles, and progress. *Clinical Psychology Review, 23*(5), 699–717.

Howland, R. H., Rush, A. J., Wisniewski, S. R., Trivedi, M. H., Warden, D., Fava, M., et al. (2009). Concurrent anxiety and substance use disorders among outpatients with major depression: Clinical features and effect on treatment outcome. *Drug and Alcohol Dependence, 99*(1–3), 248–260.

Kashner, T. M., Trivedi, M. H., Wicker, A., Fava, M., Wisniewski, S. R., & Rush, A. J. (2009). The impact of nonclinical factors on care use for patients with depression: A STAR*D report. *CNS Neuroscience and Therapeutics, 15*(4), 320–332.

Katon, W., & Schulberg, H. (1992). Epidemiology of depression in primary care. *General Hospital Psychiatry, 14*(4), 237–247.

Kessler, R. C., Ormel, J., Demler, O., & Stang, P. E. (2003). Comorbid mental disorders account for the role impairment of commonly occurring chronic physical disorders: Results from the National Comorbidity Survey. *Journal of Occupational and Environmental Medicine, 45*(12), 1257–1266.

Kroenke, K., Spitzer, R. L., & Williams, J. B. (2001). The PHQ-9: Validity of a brief depression severity measure. *Journal of General Internal Medicine, 16*(9), 606–613.

Kurian, B. T., Grannemann, B., & Trivedi, M. H. (2012). Feasible evidence-based strategies to manage depression in primary care. *Current Psychiatry Reports, 14*(4), 370–375.

Kurian, B. T., Greer, T. L., & Trivedi, M. H. (2009). Strategies to enhance the therapeutic efficacy of antidepressants: Targeting residual symptoms. *Expert Review of Neurotherapeutics, 9*(7), 975–984.

Kurian, B. T., Trivedi, M. H., Grannemann, B. D., Claassen, C. A., Daly, E. J., & Sunderajan, P. (2009). A computerized decision support system for depression in primary care. *Primary Care Companion to the Journal of Clinical Psychiatry, 11*(4), 140–146.

Leuchter, A. F., Husain, M. M., Cook, I. A., Trivedi, M. H., Wisniewski, S. R., Gilmer, W. S., et al. (2010). Painful physical symptoms and treatment outcome in major depressive disorder: A STAR*D (Sequenced Treatment Alternatives to Relieve Depression) report. *Psychological Medicine, 40*(2), 239–251.

Linehan, M. M. (1993). *Skills training manual for treating borderline personality disorder.* New York: Guilford Press.

Martell, C. R., Dimidjian, S., & Herman-Dunn, R. (2013). *Behavioral activation for depression: A clinician's guide.* New York: Guilford Press.

Mavandadi, S., Benson, A., DiFilippo, S., Streim, J. E., & Oslin, D. (2015). A telephone-based program to provide symptom monitoring alone vs symptom monitoring plus care management for late-life depression and anxiety: A randomized clinical trial. *JAMA Psychiatry, 72*(12), 1211–1218.

McIntyre, R. S. (2013). Using measurement strategies to identify and monitor residual symptoms. *Journal of Clinical Psychiatry, 74*(Suppl. 2), 14–18.

Morris, D. W., Toups, M., & Trivedi, M. H. (2012). Measurement-based care in the treatment of clinical depression. *Focus: The Journal of Lifelong Learning in Psychiatry, 10,* 428–433.

Morris, D. W., & Trivedi, M. H. (2011). Measurement-based care for unipolar depression. *Current Psychiatry Reports, 13*(6), 446–458.

Moussavi, S., Chatterji, S., Verdes, E., Tandon, A., Patel, V., & Ustun, B. (2007). Depression, chronic diseases, and decrements in health: Results from the World Health Surveys. *Lancet, 370,* 851–858.

Pampallona, S., Bollini, P., Tibaldi, G., Kupelnick, B., & Munizza, C. (2002). Patient adherence in the treatment of depression. *British Journal of Psychiatry, 180,* 104–109.

Rush, A. J., Crismon, M. L., Kashner, T. M., Toprac, M. G., Carmody, T. J., Trivedi, M. H., et al. (2003). Texas Medication Algorithm Project, phase 3 (TMAP-3): Rationale and study design. *Journal of Clinical Psychiatry, 64*(4), 357–369.

Rush, A. J., Rago, W. V., Crismon, M. L., Toprac, M. G., Shon, S. P., Suppes, T., et al. (1999). Medication treatment for the severely and persistently mentally ill: The Texas Medication Algorithm Project. *Journal of Clinical Psychiatry, 60*(5), 284–291.

Rush, A. J., Trivedi, M. H., Stewart, J. W., Nierenberg, A. A., Fava, M., Kurian, B. T., et al. (2011). Combining medications to enhance depression outcomes (CO-MED): Acute and long-term outcomes of a single-blind randomized study. *American Journal of Psychiatry, 168*(7), 689–701.

Soucy Chartier, I., & Provencher, M. D. (2013). Behavioural activation for depression: Efficacy, effectiveness and dissemination. *Journal of Affective Disorders, 145*(3), 292–299.

Spitzer, R. L., Kroenke, K., Williams, J. B., & Lowe, B. (2006). A brief measure for assessing generalized anxiety disorder: The GAD-7. *Archives of Internal Medicine, 166*(10), 1092–1097.

Trivedi, M. H. (2009). Tools and strategies for ongoing assessment of depression: A measurement-based approach to remission. *Journal of Clinical Psychiatry, 70*(Suppl. 6), 26–31.

Trivedi, M. H. (2013). Evaluating and monitoring treatment response in depression using measurement-based assessment and rating scales. *Journal of Clinical Psychiatry, 74*(7), e14.

Trivedi, M. H., & Daly, E. J. (2007). Measurement-based care for refractory depression: A clinical decision support model for clinical research and practice. *Drug and Alcohol Dependence, 88*(Suppl. 2), S61–S71.

Trivedi, M. H., Greer, T. L., Church, T. S., Carmody, T. J., Grannemann, B. D., Galper, D. I., et al. (2011). Exercise as an augmentation treatment for nonremitted major depressive disorder: A randomized, parallel dose comparison. *Journal of Clinical Psychiatry, 72*(5), 677–684.

Trivedi, M. H., & Kurian, B. T. (2010). Major depressive disorder: A measurement-based care approach. In C. B. Taylor (Ed.), *How to practice evidence-based psychiatry* (pp. 183–193). Washington, DC: American Psychiatric Publishing.

Trivedi, M. H., Rush, A. J., Crismon, M. L., Kashner, T. M., Toprac, M. G., Carmody, T. J., et al. (2004). Clinical results for patients with major depressive disorder in the Texas Medication Algorithm Project. *Archives of General Psychiatry, 61*(7), 669–680.

Trivedi, M. H., Rush, A. J., Gaynes, B. N., Stewart, J. W., Wisniewski, S. R., Warden, D., et al. (2007). Maximizing the adequacy of medication treatment in controlled trials and clinical practice: STAR(*)D measurement-based care. *Neuropsychopharmacology, 32*(12), 2479–2489.

Trivedi, M. H., Rush, A. J., Wisniewski, S. R., Nierenberg, A. A., Warden, D., Ritz, L., et al. (2006). Evaluation of outcomes with citalopram for depression using measurement-based care in STAR*D: Implications for clinical practice. *American Journal of Psychiatry, 163*(1), 28–40.

Trivedi, M. H., Wisniewski, S. R., Morris, D. W., Fava, M., Gollan, J. K., Warden, D., et al. (2011). Concise Health Risk Tracking scale: A brief self-report and clinician rating of suicidal risk. *Journal of Clinical Psychiatry, 72*(6), 757–764.

Trivedi, M. H., Wisniewski, S. R., Morris, D. W., Fava, M., Kurian, B. T., Gollan, J. K., et al. (2011). Concise Associated Symptoms Tracking scale: A brief self-report and clinician rating of symptoms associated with suicidality. *Journal of Clinical Psychiatry, 72*(6), 765–774.

Trombello, J. M., South, C., Cecil, A., Sanchez, A., Sanchez, K., Kahalnik, F., et al. (2017). Efficacy of a behavioral activation teletherapy intervention to treat depression and anxiety in primary care. *Primary Care Companion for CNS, 19*(5), 17m02146.

Warden, D., Trivedi, M. H., Carmody, T., Toups, M., Zisook, S., Lesser, I., et al. (2014). Adherence to antidepressant combinations and monotherapy for major depressive disorder: A CO-MED report of measurement-based care. *Journal of Psychiatric Practice, 20*(2), 118–132.

Weinstock, L. M., Munroe, M. K., & Miller, I. W. (2011). Behavioral activation for the treatment of atypical depression: A pilot open trial. *Behavior Modification, 35*(4), 403–424.

Wisniewski, S. R., Rush, A. J., Balasubramani, G. K., Trivedi, M. H., & Nierenberg, A. A. (2006). Self-rated global measure of the frequency, intensity, and burden of side effects. *Journal of Psychiatric Practice, 12*(2), 71–79.

Yeung, A. S., Jing, Y., Brenneman, S. K., Chang, T. E., Baer, L., Hebden, T., et al. (2012). Clinical Outcomes in Measurement-based Treatment (COMET): A trial of depression monitoring and feedback to primary care physicians. *Depression and Anxiety, 29*(10), 865–873.

Zimmerman, M., & McGlinchey, J. B. (2008). Why don't psychiatrists use scales to measure outcome when treating depressed patients? *Journal of Clinical Psychiatry, 69*(12), 1916–1919.

CHAPTER 21

A "Real–Life" Biopsychosocial Psychotherapy Case

CHRISTINE M. NEZU
ARTHUR M. NEZU
MEGHAN M. COLOSIMO

Richard, 67 years old, was referred to our outpatient psychotherapy practice for a primary concern of dizziness that occurred daily, accompanied by a loss of balance and shaking. He had seen numerous physicians to determine the cause of the dizziness, and, in fact, Richard reported to us that he had undergone "every medical test known to man." No medical explanation for his dizziness was identified, and no medications were found to provide satisfactory relief. He was diagnosed with somatic symptom disorder during a recent visit to a large southwestern health system that referred him to our practice.

Richard reported a long history of significant motion sickness, noting that he typically experienced an improvement in these symptoms when he was driving a vehicle. Approximately 7 years earlier, he experienced an episode of sudden hearing loss and tinnitus in his left ear, which reportedly resolved with a course of steroidal treatment. He recounted an occasion about 1 year later in which he stood up from a recliner and suddenly experienced intense external spinning, vertigo, nausea, imbalance, and motion intolerance. Subsequently, Richard was taken by ambulance to a nearby emergency department. The spinning, which reportedly resolved if he remained perfectly still, was treated with medication (clonazepam), and the symptoms completely subsided by the following day. Since that time, he has experienced only one other, similar episode of vertigo, which occurred 2 years ago. Richard reported that he first started experiencing ongoing dizziness about 6 months after his first episode of vertigo. He described it as feeling "like a hat was on too tight," accompanied by a subjective sense of unsteadiness and shakiness, but no sensation of spinning. This feeling of head "fullness" and imbalance had progressively worsened in severity over the past 2 years and had increased in frequency to become a chronic daily occurrence.

Richard stated that the dizziness started in the morning and persisted most of the day, indicating that it has been worse the past 6–12 months, and particularly so in the past month. The symptoms were aggravated by motion and visually complex stimuli (e.g., grocery stores and crowds) and reportedly improved when he was sitting or lying down. He noted that "bed is the real escape." Richard indicated that "meditation music" had occasionally been helpful in reducing his symptoms; however, he recalled that the dizziness returned afterward. Additionally, he noted that he occasionally became so involved in activities that he realized that he was temporarily unaware of the dizziness and was not impacted by it. He described the activities as those that "you really have to focus and concentrate on," such as using the computer.

Richard also described psychological symptoms of anxiety and depression, which he related to his physical distress. Richard indicated that he had experienced "lifelong" anxiety, noting that he had a "Type A personality" and was a self-described "worrier," "pessimist," and "control freak." He reported increasing anticipatory anxiety about his physical symptoms, including fear of the dizziness returning even when he was not experiencing symptoms. His symptoms had negatively impacted his life over the past few years, including preventing him from participating in many activities that he found pleasurable. He enjoyed staying busy and formerly had been much more active, reporting that he is no longer able to weed the garden, mow the lawn, sit on his porch swing, ride his motorcycle, or drive his antique sports car, with symptoms so severe some days that he spends much of the day in bed. This loss of previous functioning levels has contributed greatly to his persistent demoralization about his present situation and associated depressive symptoms, which, in turn, have resulted in his lowered and generalized interest in certain activities (e.g., he states that now does not "even feel like sitting on the porch"). Richard describes feeling embarrassed and "like I am holding [my wife] back from enjoyment of life." He reported occasional thoughts of suicide, but denies any intent. Richard also has reported sleep disturbances, including daily early awakening and frequently fitful sleep.

Richard's clear priority for treatment was reducing the dizziness; however, he also shared concerns about problems with erectile dysfunction (ED) that began around the same time as the dizziness, although he was unsure which came first. He recalled a brief period of ED symptoms when he and his wife were first sexually intimate approximately 42 years ago, but described no problems until the time of the dizziness. He believed that his sexual concerns might be related to his parents' frequent arguments about sex in front of him during his childhood. He also believed his medications might be a causal factor, although he noted that he had been taking many of them before, with the exception of clonazepam (Klonopin). Additionally, Richard suggested that he and his wife have different sex drives and that she is "more prudish"; however, he denied any change in her sex drive, indicating that it has always been the same, with him being the "instigator." He was quick to note that "she does everything she can," reporting that when he initiates, she "goes along with it about 70–80% of the time." Moreover, he indicated that he has less difficulty achieving an erection after waking from sleep because his "mind is clear" but noted that when he did have an erection, he was reluctant to initiate sex because he believed "it's not going to work and I will lose it." Although he had difficulty engaging in sexual intercourse with his wife, he reported that they shared other forms of intimacy together, including "snuggling, talking, and sharing thoughts." A joint interview with Richard's wife, Clara, revealed that addressing his ED was not a priority for her and she described her experience of a postmenopausal reduction of interest in intercourse. She also explained that she believed the ED was a result of other problems on Richard's mind (i.e., dizziness) and a decrease in his confidence.

Finally, although Richard's top concern was the dizziness, followed by the ED, he also shared that he had experienced lifelong "stomach problems." At the time of his referral, his digestive difficulties included diarrhea and intestinal polyps, for which he received colonoscopies every 6 months. He also reported experiencing frequent gas, indigestion, and heartburn. Richard had one-third of his colon removed 3 years earlier and simultaneously his gallbladder. He reported experiencing a weight loss of 30 pounds in the first 6 months of this year. Although his weight was currently stabilized, Richard reported having no appetite, necessitating that he drink Ensure and "make myself eat" in order to maintain his weight. He was required to adhere to a specific diet, eliminating foods such as corn and nuts, to help control his digestive symptoms.

When Richard called to set up an initial appointment, he focused on his medical history and frustration with what he considered poor outcome regarding multiple medical treatments for his symptoms. He stated that although he was following through with a referral to a psychologist, he and his wife believed that that he should not give up searching for a medical explanation and treatment. He also expressed continued frustration with the various physicians he had seen, as well as a psychiatrist, who appeared to Richard to minimize the physical pain and discomfort that he experienced. Richard rated this discomfort on a subjective scale of 0–10 as a "7" on good days and a "10" on bad days.

*   *   *

Our clinical practice assumes a careful and evidence-based approach to the treatment of a wide breadth of adults, couples, and family patients. We do this by embracing a case formulation model (C. M. Nezu, Nezu, Ricelli, & Stern, 2015) that seeks to "practice what we preach" by incorporating a problem-solving-based approach that conceptualizes the development of a treatment plan as, essentially, our own therapeutic problem to solve. This type of case conceptualization, which focuses on the functional relationship of instrumental and ultimate outcomes, has a long history in evidence-based care and was originally described by Rosen and Proctor (1981). Our assessment process, which informs the case formulation, is comprehensive and typically includes conducting several clinical interviews, a mental status examination, meeting with the patient (and family, as relevant) to gather a family and social history, and obtaining a psychiatric and medical history. In addition, we administer various psychological measures that are tied to the specific presenting problems. These may include rating scales, questionnaires, life history forms, and standardized tests. Finally, we seek records and input from other professionals engaged in the patient's care. We then integrate all of this information to develop the case formulation. The metamessage regarding our assessment and treatment approach is that a clinical issue well defined is essential to finding effective evidence-based solutions. As such, after 30 years in clinical practice, we are convinced that additional time in both clinical and more standardized assessment sets the stage for the most effective and well-matched interventions.

Richard's assessment took place over two 90-minute evaluation sessions. He also was provided with self-report questionnaires to complete at home. It was explained in the initial consultation session that the purpose of the assessment was to understand his life story and unique symptoms and experiences, so that an individualized treatment plan respectful of his specific history, health, relationships, and psychological and emotional factors could be developed and shared with him for his input. This case formulation approach appeared especially important for Richard, who was hopeful that there was a medical diagnosis and cure for his symptoms. In addition to the clinical interviews and measures we administered, it was important to obtain medical records from a large multispecialty health care system where Richard had undergone extensive medical examinations and follow-up appointments with numerous physicians he visited after multiple emergency room (ER) visits.

Mental Status Examination at Intake

Richard arrived early to the initial appointment, accompanied by his wife Clara. He was neatly dressed and well groomed, with physical appearance, eye contact, and posture all within normal limits. He was alert and oriented as to person, place, and time. His immediate memory appeared intact. However, he reported some difficulty with his long-term memory, particularly regarding negative events. His attitude toward the interviewer was cooperative and pleasant, and both his speech and psychomotor activity were within normal limits. Richard exhibited a full range of affect, and his overall mood was anxious, frustrated, and depressed. He reported suicidal thoughts but denied any current urge or intention regarding suicidal or self-injurious behavior, noting that that he is "not one to give up," "too narcissistic to kill myself," and that he has "some hope for the future." Although he appeared outwardly calm and balanced for most of the intake, he stated that although he projects himself as "controlled" to people, he is "screaming on the inside." One exception was when he related very intense anger toward the psychiatrist he had previously seen, who suggested that his symptoms were "all in his head." His thought processes were generally organized and goal-directed, and there was no evidence of formal delusions or hallucinations. Richard appeared to have some insight regarding the role of his psychological state in his physical symptoms, acknowledging that the symptoms "must be" related to his mind because no physical cause had yet been identified. However, he stated that he and his wife will not "give up hope" that cause and cure for his symptoms may still be discovered and he will "be myself again." He denied the use of alcohol and other substances.

Family and Social History

Richard was born and raised in a rural Southwestern region of the United States. His father was a foundry worker, whom he described as very easygoing, and his mother was a housewife, whom he described as controlling, having a quick temper with others, and "often happiest when mad at someone." He reported that his father worked "all the time," and because of this, Richard spent much more time with his mother and developed a closer relationship with her. He stated that both his parents treated him well growing up, and that they disciplined him with "spankings." Additionally, Richard indicated that he was able to confide in his parents, primarily his mother.

He reported that there was very little emotion or affection shown between his parents or toward him, noting that his parents had frequent arguments, many of which he thought were about sex. For example, he reported that his father would try to initiate sex with his mother, and she would deny him and belittle him for it. Richard recalled a traumatic incident during one of these arguments, when his mother said to his father, "All you ever think about is sex," then proceeded to raise her dress and expose herself to both his father and to him. Richard viewed these upsetting experiences as contributing to a fear of "forcing myself on someone," and he attributed his problems with ED to them.

Richard also stated that both his mother and his maternal grandmother were "hypochondriacs," who spent much time seeking diagnoses from physicians. In addition to his mother's concern over her own health, he reported that she frequently took Richard to doctors and hospitals during his youth. This practice occurred despite his account that he was in good health growing up and was unaware of having any illnesses, except once for appendicitis.

Richard's mother died at age 70 years due to cancer, and his father died at 71 years due to a stroke. Richard reported that he had one sibling, a sister who was 12 years older, who died of cancer at 71 years of age, and he expressed a degree of fatalism regarding the likelihood of his life ending in several years at a similar age.

Richard met his wife Clara while he was living in the Southwest, and they had been married 47 years and have one son, who is now 45 years old and living in Indiana. Richard noted that he has a "good" relationship with his son, although at times he wishes he had been more affectionate with him. He and his wife both verbally reported being "very satisfied" with their marriage. When interviewed separately, however, each partner reported discomfort with both intimacy and sexual activities. For example, Clara stated that she had experienced a postmenopausal loss of libido and avoided sex. Richard indicated an ongoing issue pertaining to the "quality time" he and his wife spend together before bed every night, during which they share their "thoughts and feelings about the day." Richard reported that sometimes when he goes to bed, Clara tells him she will finish what she is doing and

join him at a certain time, but she comes to bed much later than promised. He stated that he feels angry, rejected, and disappointed at these times and experiences thoughts such as "what she's doing is more important than our quality time" and "she doesn't think enough about me to make the time." Richard reported that this was a frequent occurrence throughout the duration of their marriage, indicating that it "upsets me quite a bit."

Richard completed high school and, after some college, left school to work for a large local company, until he retired 7 years earlier, along with his wife, who had done secretarial work. Currently, Richard reports that he enjoys doing things on his own, although he used to enjoy socializing and being helpful to others. For example, he used to have breakfast with his friends every morning, and he notes that he would spend 1½ hours doing so each day, but he now limits himself to only occasional visits due to his symptoms. He reports, "I don't want my buddies to notice me stumbling," and he finds it upsetting when his friends ask how he is feeling. He states that he has "always been self-sufficient," and it is difficult for him to accept help from, or be dependent in any way on other people. Because of this, he does not discuss his difficulties with his friends, instead telling them that he is "doing fine." He also reports that he fears that if he began a social exchange and became dizzy, he would not be able to admit that he needs to lie down and leave the social interaction. He states that he enjoys many solitary activities, some of which he used to do with Clara, including sewing, embroidering, quilting, painting, and building furniture; however, he currently engages in these activities at only a minimal level.

Psychiatric and Medical History

Richard reported a long-standing history of anxiety, describing himself as a "worrywart." With the onset of the dizziness, his anxiety worsened, and Richard also developed depressive symptoms. He reported seeking treatment with a psychiatrist approximately 4–5 years earlier, noting that it was an unpleasant experience. He stated that the psychiatrist told him "it's all in your head" and prescribed medications that were no help in alleviating his symptoms. He became visibly aroused and angry when speaking about this psychiatrist.

He had undergone a number of additional medication trials with other doctors for his dizziness and associated anxiety and mood symptoms, most of which were ineffective or resulted in adverse side effects. Richard also reported seeing a therapist a few years back, and described the treatment as involving "tapping." From his description, it may have been a type of "emotional freedom technique" (EFT) directed at reducing unpleasant emotions (Craig, 2011). These techniques have reportedly mixed results regarding effectiveness (Guidano, Brown, & Miller, 2012). Richard reported seeing this therapist "for a while," stating that it was of some help, but he could not remember the therapist's name.

Richard was not receiving psychological treatment currently, but he reported that he was prescribed the following psychoactive medications: clonazepam (Klonopin; 1–2 mg daily in the morning or as needed, up to 4 mg daily, for "anxiety and shaking") and trazodone (Desyrel; 100 mg at bedtime for sleep). Although the clonazepam appeared initially somewhat helpful with increasing sleep, he reported that his symptoms of "dizziness," "jitteriness" and agitation returned during waking hours and that he was, once again, frustrated with the lack of a clear medical solution for his chronic dizziness. Other medications he was currently prescribed were focused on his comorbid medical challenges and included: levothyroxine (Levoxyl; 137 mµg) once daily for hypothyroidism, simvastatin (Zocor; 40 mg) once daily for high cholesterol, nifedipine (Nifedical XL; 60 mg) once daily for hypertension, metformin (Glumetza; 1,000 mµg) twice daily for diabetes, and lansoprazole (Prevacid; 30 mg) twice daily for gastroesophageal reflux. All of these medications were prescribed by the Richard's family physician, Jane Medical, MD.

We obtained a signed release for communication with his physician. We saw this communication as essential, as Richard reported that Dr. M increased clonazepam doses when Richard became frustrated, discussed going to a hospital ER for help, or actually went to the hospital with complaints. It seemed possible that Richard's physician might have experienced a sense of helplessness to provide any other type of treatment, and may have viewed medication as the sole means of addressing his symptoms.

Richard reported a history of migraine headaches in both his late teens and mid-30s for a few years each. The migraines were characterized by recurrent, severe, throbbing and unilateral head pain accompanied by nausea, vomiting, photophobia, and motion intolerance, which occurred up to once every 2 weeks. After treatment with medications, as well as stopping the consumption of alcohol in his 30s, the migraines resolved and he has not experienced any episodes since his late 30s. Richard also reported a past history of melanoma, minor surgeries, and current medical comorbid diagnoses that included fatigue, insomnia, hypertension, hypothyroidism, type 2 diabetes, gastroesophageal reflux disease, hyperlipidemia, and irritable bowel syndrome. He denied use of alcohol or cigarettes; however, he presently used a nicotine replacement (electronic cigarette) since he quit smoking 2 years prior, after 50 years.

Administered Self-Report Questionnaires

Richard's evaluation also consisted of several measures that were administered to confirm or disconfirm the information gleaned from his initial interview, to develop further clinical hypotheses, and to begin to prioritize areas to target in treatment. A list of all measures and the clinical decision making to support them for this patient is provided in Table 21.1. A summary of the findings from the administered questionnaires indicated the following information.

Richard's responses on the Psychiatric Diagnostic Screening Questionnaire (PDSQ) indicated that he scored above the clinical cutoff for agraphobia (for which he substituted the word *dizzy* for *anxiety* when endorsing these items), and at the clinical cutoff for somatization disorder and hypochondriasis. He also endorsed critical items, but did not pass the full clinical criterion in the domains of major depressive disorder, agoraphobia, and generalized anxiety disorder. Richard's self-report on the Outcome Questionnaire–30 (OQ-30) was at a similar level of symptomatology as that reported by mixed outpatient samples and significantly greater than the level of symptomatology reported by a community sample. This confirmed that he was in significant distress. With regard to the Social Problem-Solving Inventory—Revised (SPSI-R; D'Zurilla, Nezu, & Maydeu-Olivares, 2002) assessment, Richard's responses indicated that he had strengths on several problem-solving dimensions. Specifically, he did not appear impulsive or avoidant, and he had strong planful problem-solving skills, with particular

TABLE 21.1. Assessment Choices for Richard's Clinical Evaluation

Measure	Description	Rationale for including in assessment
Multimodal Life History Inventory (Lazarus & Lazarus, 1991)	A self-report data collection questionnaire—divided into sections that include general information, personal and social history, description of presenting problems, and expectations regarding therapy.	To inform case formulation and treatment design that is tailored to specific client needs. It addresses seven important areas: behaviors, feelings, physical sensations, images, thoughts, interpersonal relationships, and biological factors.
Psychiatric Diagnostic Screening Questionnaire (PDSQ; Zimmerman & Mattia, 2001)	A brief self-report scale designed to screen for the most common DSM-IV Axis I disorders encountered in outpatient mental health settings.	To provide a screening for confirmation or disconfirmation of several possible psychiatric syndromes.
Outcome Questionnaire–30 (OQ-30.2; Lambert et al., 1996)	A brief symptom assessment questionnaire that is sensitive to what happens during any session. It should be administered prior to, or at the very beginning of any therapeutic visit.	To continually assess for critical symptoms, such as suicide, and to have an ongoing measure of therapy progress.
Social Problem-Solving Inventory—Revised: Long Form (SPSI-R:L; D'Zurilla, Nezu, & Maydeu-Olivares, 2002)	Assesses strengths and weaknesses in one's problem-solving abilities, so that deficits can be addressed and progress monitored. Problem-solving ability has implications for all areas of life, including interpersonal and work-related relationships.	To develop a problem-solving profile of the patient's strengths and weaknesses for the purpose of both case formulation and to determine where to best target treatment.
Young Schema Questionnaire—Long Form (YSQ-L; Young & Brown, 1994)	A self-report measure to assess schemas. Questionnaire items are grouped by schema.	To assess the presence of early maladaptive schemas, and to confirm or disconfirm initial therapeutic hypotheses gleaned from the clinical interview. Additionally, to aid in the discovery of patient coping styles when schemas are triggered (surrender, avoidance, or overcompensation).

strengths noted in his ability to creatively *generate alternative solutions*. His overall score, however, indicated the presence of a lower than average ability to solve day-to-day and interpersonal problems. The lowered score appeared most related to a significant *negative orientation* and degree of pessimism particularly concerning his medical complaints and perceptions of rejection regarding his wife, Clara. From his responses on this questionnaire, it appeared that when Richard faced specific problems accompanied by strong feelings (e.g., problems associated with his medical complaints), he had a decreased ability to use his problem-solving strengths. This is a pattern that has been ob-

served in patients with chronic pain (Allen & Woolfolk, 2010).

Richard's responses to the Young Schema Questionnaire (YSQ; Young & Brown, 1994) indicated strong and pervasive maladaptive schemas in the areas of *unrelenting standards* (a belief in high standards of behavior to avoid criticism), and *self-sacrifice* (going above and beyond to meet the needs of others), as well as moderately strong schemas concerning *emotional inhibition* (overly suppressing spontaneous emotional expression), *Approval seeking* (placing an excessive amount of importance on recognition, attention, or approval from others), and *negativity/pessimism* (a consistent underlying focus on the perceived negative parts of life; e.g., death, pain, suffering, or betrayal). These were assessed as long-term schemas and often linked to each other when triggered by stressful problems. Richard's behavior reflected an attempt, though often not on a conscious level, to either surrender (in the case of the first two) or avoid, and/or overcompensate (in the case of the last three) for the negative feelings associated with their activation. Such reactive modes are predictable concerning the triggering of early maladaptive schemas (Young, Klosko, & Weishaar, 2003). Finally, with some patients, we also administer the Millon Clinical Multiaxial Inventory–III (MCMI-III; Millon, Millon, Davis & Grossman, 2009) to obtain a standardized and comprehensive assessment that is likely to detect the presence of a range of personality disorders and syndromes, although this was not a feature of our work with Richard due to the wealth of other data available to us.

Initial Case Formulation

We provided Richard with the following case formulation as means of psychoeducation and explanation of how he came to react the way he does, developed certain patterns of thought, and currently reacts to stressful problems (i.e., his emotional triggers and how he has learned to respond to these triggers). Additionally, the consequences of his learned psychological, emotional, and behavioral reactions were explained. Finally, the therapist proposed her evidence-based therapeutic plan based on this formulation. A visual graphic representation that is referred to as a *clinical pathogenesis map* (CPM) in the case formulation model co-developed by two of the coauthors (A. M. Nezu & C. M. Nezu) was used to illustrate the case formulation, as illustrated in Figure 21.1 (see A. M. Nezu, Nezu, & Cos, 2007; A. M. Nezu, Nezu, & Lombardo, 2004; C. M. Nezu et al., 2015). Through the use of a graphic representation, we integrated complex information in a way that communicated important therapeutic targets and represented our best evidence-based hypotheses regarding what would most effectively address Richard's reasons for seeking treatment.

Sharing a case formulation in this way also allowed us to frame Richard's therapy-interfering beliefs and behaviors (e.g., going the ER whenever in distress) as understandable choices given his unique learning history and the emo-

tional schemas that were present in his reactions. It was helpful to the therapeutic alliance for us to communicate with Richard that, under these circumstances, he was clearly "doing the best he could." His therapist then laid out a plan within the context of sharing what new learning experiences were needed for Richard to have the tools that would be useful to improve management of his symptoms, particularly when his urge to "run to" the ER intensified.

In sharing Figure 21.1 with Richard, we clarified that his ultimate outcome goals for treatment included reduced dizziness, associated anxiety, and depressive symptoms, and improved intimate functioning. After discussing the various factors associated with Richard's ED, it was clarified that Richard's concerns were more focused on intimacy and emotional support from his wife than on actual sexual activity. Additionally, both Richard and his wife acknowledged that Clara's avoidance of sex often resulted in avoidance of all forms of intimacy. As such, increased nonsexual intimacy was a goal that both Richard and Clara shared. While collaboratively sharing with Richard his case formulation, we shared our understanding of his current distress (as described in the next paragraph), the specific mental health diagnoses for which he met clinical criteria, and the specific interventions that could be helpful in achieving his goals. We shared this information collaboratively, inviting Richard to share his agreement, input, and/or suggested changes.

Understanding Current Distress

We began with sharing our hypotheses regarding Richard's early learning history as a context for understanding his current distress. We suggested that Richard's experience of his mother as "controlling" and as having a "quick temper" likely contributed to his development of the schemas of unrelenting standards, self-sacrifice, and approval seeking, in an attempt to satisfy her and avoid her anger. Additionally, we hypothesized that since she was the parent with whom he identified the most, he may have adopted some of her negative and pessimistic views of problems. We spoke with Richard about the unrelenting standards schema, which he endorsed in a self-report inventory, and ways it may be related to his desire to control his experiences and relationships. We raised the possibility with Richard that this need for control, while historically useful to him in some career-

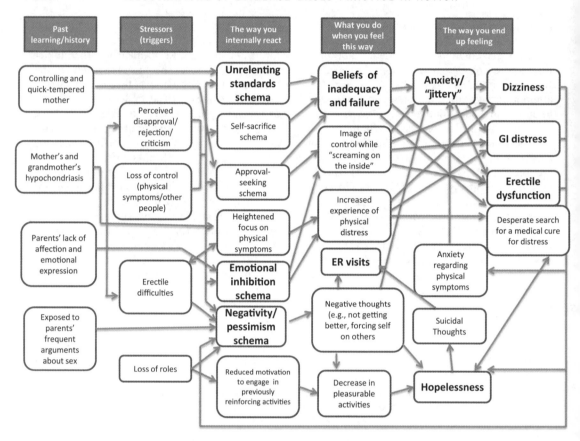

FIGURE 21.1. CPM: Graphic depiction of Richard's case formulation.

related tasks, might be exacerbating much of the anxiety he was experiencing. Additionally, we highlighted his reports consistent with a schema of emotional inhibition and theorized that this may be linked to his parents' lack of both affection and emotional expression when he was growing up, as well as his need for control. The sum total of these experiences may have taught him to project himself as "calm and controlled" to others and not displaying emotions, causing him to keep hidden his anxiety (manifesting as in his own words, "screaming on the inside"). By placing such stressful demands on himself, we hypothesized, Richard's body was likely to react—contributing to and worsening his physical symptoms (i.e., dizziness, gastrointestinal distress, sense of "jitteriness").

We also highlighted Richard's reports of his mother's and grandmother's hypochondriacal behavior and hypothesized with him that he may have developed a heightened sensitivity to any physical sensations, and these triggered

fears of illness. Moreover, a sense of being cared for may have reinforced the trips to the hospital. Heightened anxiety exacerbated his physical symptoms, creating a perpetual cycle of anxiety, physical symptoms, and care seeking that was occasionally interrupted for brief periods when Richard was intensely focused on an activity, such as driving. When this occurred, his attention and concentration were temporarily displaced from his physical sensations to the activity in which he was engaging, resulting in transient periods of symptom relief.

Richard's unrelenting standards contributed to rigid beliefs that he must be self-reliant and successful. Predictably, these symptoms began shortly after he retired. When his dizziness prevented him from participating in activities, this further loss of roles triggered a sense of failure and dependence on others that he perceived as beyond his control, resulting in feelings of depression. Moreover, his depression led to a decreased interest in certain activities, adding to his reduction in pleasurable activities. This withdrawal from what made life rewarding for Richard exacerbated his depressive symptoms. The common strategy he employed in such circumstances was to desperately search for the cure in a medication or a specific technique that would provide him with control over his symptoms. When no such "cure" was evident or available, he became hopeless and engaged in suicidal thinking and statements. Moreover, Richard's firm beliefs as the person who helps (vs. needs) others prevented him from benefiting from his social supports, resulting in suppression of both thoughts and feelings, and virtually no outlets for his distress. The only means of coping he had was to share his feelings with his wife during their "quality time"; however, there had been little direct conversation about the impact of his retirement or the process of aging in general.

It was explained to Richard that his ED appeared to be associated with his increasing sense of rejection and triggering of a fear of forcing himself on his wife, a response he learned from repeatedly observing his parents argue about sex during his youth. However, when Richard learned that Clara's avoidance of their time alone together at night was more related to her own loss of sexual interests and her own fears of disappointing him by not having intercourse, he and Clara were able to share a goal of emotional and intimacy without requiring intercourse. This did much to reduce his performance concerns about his own ED or requirement of intercourse for intimacy satisfaction. Finally, it was suggested that the large number of medications and the possible impact of these medications with regard to sexual functioning would need to be explored with his physician.

Richard's assessment revealed that he strived to be seen as proper and conventional in spite of the ambivalent feelings under his controlled surface. We discussed his strong sense of responsibility and duty that often led him to be inflexible in his pattern of denying and hiding negative feelings. As Richard stated when questioned about an episode of worsening symptoms, "I just feel like it's time to end it all when I can't control this damn dizziness and I'm no good to Clara or anyone." He held very pessimistic beliefs about the opportunities for himself and his relationship with Clara as he looked ahead to aging. As such, he experienced significant barriers to sharing reports of symptoms

until they increased to point of desperation. It was suggested to him that the therapeutic relationship would require him taking a risk to become more emotionally aware and wise, in order to achieve maximum benefit from treatment. For example, his therapist explained to Richard, "I know that in the past you believed that feelings were sort of useless, in that if you told Clara or others about your feelings, they might feel sorry for you. To avoid that, you go straight to trying to 'fix' your dizziness, and remove your negative feelings, by denying them. You end up feeling as though you failed at successfully ridding yourself of the dizziness. It's a little scary, but allowing some negative feelings in and asking others for their support and help, while uncomfortable, is one approach that you have not given a chance."

DSM-5 Diagnosis

We shared our diagnostic impression with Richard, which included the following diagnoses: somatic symptom disorder (persistent, moderate), major depressive disorder (single episode, moderate, currently in remission), ED (acquired, moderate), and the presence of possible side effects of multiple medications. When providing Richard with our diagnostic impressions, it was important for us to share with him the case formulation, framed as his "life story" in a user-friendly way. In this way, we were able to solicit his opinions and collaboration regarding the combination of factors that we believed were causally related to the diagnoses associated with the symptoms he was experiencing. These were explained to him regarding how his life history had impacted the ways he reacted to and coped with stressful problems, and how this led to his patterns of emotional triggers, thoughts, and behavior. This explanation provided a nonstigmatized explanation of his symptoms as "learned" (vs. as evidence of mental illness). Finally, interventions could be explained as ways to introduce new learning experiences in which he could "train his brain and body" to do something different.

Treatment Plan

Using the clinical CPM (Figure 21.1), important factors were identified as instrumental to making changes to achieve Richard's ultimate goals for treatment. The instrumental targets that were assessed as directly and indirectly impacting his ultimate treatment goals included (1) awareness, acceptance, and increased tolerance of negative emotions; (2) changing schema-driven reactive responses associated with unrelenting standards, self-sacrifice, approval seeking, emotional inhibition, and negativity/pessimism; (3) decreasing hopelessness; (4) decreasing ER visits; and (5) increasing positive experiences. Major barriers to these areas of change focused on (1) his emotional inhibition schema, (2) his relentless attempt to hide or control all distress, (3) his self-sacrifice and avoidance of any demands on other people as a means of gaining approval, and (4) his continued belief that his internal medicine provider, Dr. M, or the hospital ER would provide him with a full cure. This last barrier was significant, as we describe below.

Figure 21.2 provides a graphic depiction of the therapist's selection of treatment techniques, adopted from multiple evidence-based treatment approaches, in order to demonstrate a strategic approach to therapeutic intervention

of these target areas. It has been our experience that the most effective treatment protocols that are currently available do not result in significant improvement for 100% of the patients for which they are prescribed. From a philosophy of an individualized approach to treatment, one size clearly does not fit all. Moreover, we view the "art" of psychotherapy as being able to systematically apply the "science" that is available. Hence, our approach to evidence-based care adopts a "principle-based" method of identifying the target in need of change (vs. adopting a full protocol for one diagnostic area in need of change), then making a decision about the best match of what specific strategy or technique to use with a given patient. These are selected from various empirically supported protocols. The use of case formulation and a principles-based approach is documented in the literature (Barlow et al., 2010; Persons, 2012; Tarrier & Johnson, 2015).

Through a review of the CPM, the therapist identified areas of needed change that appeared

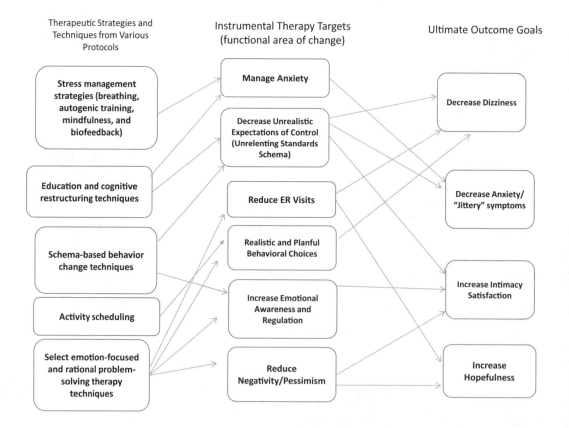

FIGURE 21.2. Therapeutic goal attainment (strategic treatment plan).

to have the most promise of direct and indirect effects on either the ultimate treatment targets or other, instrumental treatment targets. The CPM provides a picture of where the functional relationships of these effects are the most prominent for a given patient. Next, we selected techniques or combinations of strategies. Overall, the treatment plan aimed to address the clinical targets described earlier by integrating techniques from schema therapy, cognitive therapy, contemporary problem-solving therapy, and various stress management training strategies (deep breathing, biofeedback-assisted relaxation, autogenic training imagery, and mindfulness-based techniques). These choices were made through a cost–benefit analysis that included an assessment of the factors specific not only to Richard (i.e., those described previously and his stated preferences for care) but also the therapist (i.e., our clinical expertise with the technique and our interpretation of the scientific literature). Whereas other clinicians may select a specific treatment protocol associated with a primary diagnosis, such as somatoform disorder, our commitment to an individualized approach is to follow a treatment based on identification of specific, functional mediating factors in need of change as instrumental to the symptoms and incorporate those techniques that match the particular patient's needs. Empirically supported, protocol-driven treatments are important and form the base from which we draw in our work; however, in treating clients like Richard, rarely is there a "one size fits all" protocol available that takes into account all of the relevant characteristics that need to be considered in treatment planning, including age, culture, comorbid diagnoses, interpersonal context, and so forth.

Summary of Treatment

During our work with Richard, we focused on several important tools for the first 8-10 months. Although he was a willing participant who mostly cooperated with the homework required to learn several of these tools, and experienced consistent progress concerning moments of greater intimacy and some improved management of gastrointestinal symptoms, Richard continued to experience anxiety, hopelessness, and dizziness. Improvement in these areas was not realized until much later in treatment (10–15 months).

In beginning treatment, we adopted a positive orientation that included an optimistic and mindful awareness of clinical decision making; however, two issues that were present at the start served as a personal challenge for the therapist. First, Richard had an overwhelming focus on medical symptoms and persistence that "there must be a medical condition to explain all of this," and that if he continued to see more physicians, he would finally find an answer. Clara also supported this medical model, and despite the therapist's repeated attempts to provide an educative and user-friendly biopsychosocial explanation, Richard stated that he would try the treatment plan, as it reflected things he might learn to better cope with his symptoms, but he did not really "buy into" the view that psychological and emotional factors might actually be causally linked to his medical symptoms.

This first challenge was related to the second, namely that it is important to be aware of our own emotional reactivity when confronted with an internal medicine physician who ignores best faith attempts to reach out, to share the case formulation and treatment plan (with Richard's permission), and to express concerns regarding her treatment approach with Richard. Despite a lack of physical findings, Dr. M repeatedly reinforced Richard's hope for finding physical explanations and pharmacological treatments. Moreover, an initial clinical dilemma occurred, as our reading of the literature suggested that both trazodone and clonazepam (especially in combination with numerous other prescribed medications) were capable of producing concerning side effects relevant to Richard's symptom presentation. As medication advice was beyond the scope of our practice, we were confronted with the inability to suggest a decrease in medications for Richard. It seemed that when Richard's frustration with his symptoms would intensify, the direct result was for Dr. M to increase his medications. This seemed to reinforce Richard's perceptions that he "just needed more medication." Regardless of our attempts to reach out to Dr. M and offer to work collaboratively with her toward an improvement in Richard's symptoms, she was nonresponsive and unavailable to us.

Initially, we sought to target Richard's specific interactions with the medical system that increased his sense of hopelessness. For instance, his hopelessness seemed functionally related to his crisis visits to the ER. Richard would make approximately two visits per month to the hospital ER, stating that everything he tried "wasn't working," and these visits would be followed by expression of suicidal thoughts (although intent was low). Examples included statements such as "I don't know what else to do, so what good is living if this never gets any better." These were depressive overgeneralizations, as Richard did experience periods of improvement. Unfortunately, this would trigger a tendency to overextend himself with ambitious attempts at activities. When the symptoms returned, he reported that he just wanted to get a shot or some medication at the ER that would put him to sleep. He then would spend long hours waiting to see a doctor and being told to take an additional clonazepam, and schedule a follow-up visit with his physician. He would return to home, depleted, hungry, angry and depressed. Occasionally, an ER physician would suggest yet more tests or consultations that yielded no benefit. Although Richard's actual suicidal intention was low to minimal, his therapist was concerned regarding his surge in hopelessness at these times, and aware of the increased rates of suicide in older white men (Centers for Disease Control and Prevention, 2014).

In order to address this barrier, Richard agreed to the following plan. Specifically, because the conversations with his therapist around this hopelessness would occur after Richard went to the ER, it was suggested that he contact his therapist when these suicidal thoughts and urges to go to the ER were starting to "take him down the hopeless road." Consistent with the planful problem-solving skills that he was learning, the therapist explained that such instances provided a real-life, distressful problem to solve. Richard agreed to this approach. After the resulting telephone conversations took place, which included reviewing Richard's immediate goal (usually getting relief from intensified dizziness symptoms), his barriers to the goal (no immediate cure, frustration, anger, hopelessness), and possible alternative courses of action (going to the ER as planned, lying down to rest, persevering in his use of a stress management strategy, recognizing the absence of facts that would support the likelihood of an ER cure, etc.), Richard would usually decide to stay home. As an alternative choice, he would typically go to bed, use his breathing techniques, and turn on the television in his room.

Richard's is initial treatment also focused on increasing his emotional awareness and expression, as well as the communication of his emotions with his wife when he experienced relationship distress. The reduction of Richard's emotional inhibition led to considerable improvements in Richard's symptoms; however, the emergence of additional stressors in Richard's environment also occurred (e.g., the increased emotional awareness and disclosure often led to discussions of challenges to their relationship). While helpful in understanding some of the long-term problems between them, Richard experienced insight regarding his own behavior, including a tendency to invalidate and control his wife's feelings. This not only motivated him to be more appreciative and loving, but it also resulted in self-criticism, that, while constructive, was stressful. At such times, he experienced predictable worsening of symptoms. These calls typically occurred on weekends, when Richard compared himself to others who were out and about, and when Clara had plans. Schema-focused cognitive therapy strategies were helpful in addressing Richard's underlying schemas and problematic negative beliefs, and resulted in an increase in his willingness to accept time to get needed rest, a reduction of the times when he pushed himself too hard, and engagement in limited pleasant activities. This contributed to increased motivation and feelings of worth, both of which improved his mood.

Richard reported significant improvements in his dizziness and gastrointestinal distress when he engaged in enjoyable or distracting activities, noting that he felt better and his physical symptoms were more tolerable. However, Richard had a tendency to continue to place a substantial amount of pressure on himself, and he occasionally pushed himself too hard when he was feeling better, which typically caused an exacerbation of his physical symptoms, triggering feelings of hopelessness. Techniques from problem-solving therapy were helpful in reducing these feelings of hopelessness, as well as suicidal ideation.

The remaining barrier that interfered with therapy progress was Richard's continued search for the "cure" of his dizziness. Progress toward this barrier occurred rather serendipitously. One evening, Richard went to the ER because he was experiencing symptoms that appeared consistent with a possible stroke. He decided not to call the therapist, in keeping with the agreed-upon intervention, because these symptoms were not related to his dizziness or hopelessness, but they were symptoms he had not experienced previously. At this visit, it was suspected that Richard may have experienced a mild transient ischemic attack (TIA), and a neurologist was called in to consult. The neurologist, who confirmed that Richard had not experienced a TIA, expressed extreme concern regarding the medications that had been prescribed by Dr. M and urged Richard to change his primary care physician. This doctor opined that Richard's original dizziness was a somatic symptom that was probably a somatoform disorder, but that more recent difficulties were likely related to an addiction that had developed to his long-term and high-dose clonazepam (Klonopin) prescription. He urged Richard to work with a new doctor on a withdrawal plan and continue to work with his psychologist for help with learning less harmful ways to cope with life. This experience led to the insight that marked our next session.

RICHARD: (*after explaining all that transpired*) When I heard this from the neurologist, I got home and I made a goal to come off this stuff. I discovered lots of websites and chat groups that talk about how nasty this Klonopin is—I can see that I'm addicted and that Dr. M is my "pusher." I need to come off this stuff. All the while, you have been saying that there is no cure, but I kept looking and looking, and Dr. M kept giving me prescriptions—I thought about suing, but I realize that I wanted to believe there was a cure so bad, that I didn't really buy what you were telling me all this time.

THERAPIST: Wow, Richard. It takes incredible courage to face this. What kept you from buying the whole mind–body model?

RICHARD: I think if I let myself believe it, then I would have to give up hope that I would never be the same as I used to be. I just kept taking the drugs she was pushing on me.

THERAPIST: I couldn't have said it any better myself. In this case, your concerns about aging, retirement, sexual functioning, and the initial stress-related dizziness were understandable. But your avoidance of accepting the changes in your life associated with aging, as well as the consequences of your learned ways of reacting, led you to make some very emotional decisions. What do you see as the next step? Do you see the tools that we have been working with as being helpful?

RICHARD: I think I'm going to have to use these tools to get off this nasty crap. The breathing, the imagery, sharing my feelings with Clara, and not pushing myself too hard. . . . How's that for problem solving? (*Laughs.*)

THERAPIST: I think these are excellent ideas. It will also be especially important for you to practice patience and have more reasonable expectations for how quickly you can do this—your unrelenting standards can really work against you here.

RICHARD: Oh, I know that this will take time . . . but I'm committed. . . . I know now that there is no "magic pill." It will take hard work and me getting through each step of bringing down the dose until I'm off completely. When the withdrawal is bad, I'll just have to 'tough it out.'

THERAPIST: I can see we still have some work to do during this. . . . Rather than "tough it out," how about reframing that as "abiding and tolerating the distress, using the tools to get me through?"

Richard experienced significant improvement and excellent therapy outcome following his recognition of how his learned way of thinking served as an obstacle to his improvement. This left us with the following clinical insight. Regardless of our evidence-based clinical toolbox of techniques and interventions that have been evaluated as effective, there are communication and relationship aspects that are essential to each case. In Richard's case, he had an educated understanding of the interventions offered, and respect for the therapy and therapist. However, he did not have full "buy-in" of the situation he was facing—that no medical explanation, pill, surgery, or other cure was around the corner. The implicit cognition was that no cure was equal to no hope. Ironically, of course, the very acceptance of no cure was the *only* road to hope through the use of stress management, pain distraction, self-acceptance, and problem-solving coping strategies that could improve his life 5, 10, or even 50%. Moreover, if he learned greater flexibility, accepting that there were people and circumstances he could not change, and if he became more forgiving and kind to himself, there was much reason to have hope. For the next few months, Richard worked with a new physician, who titrated his clonazepam dosage gradually, until he was no longer taking it. As he reflected on this process, Richard stated that his "take-away" message was acceptance and adjustment to his aging process, and knowing there are few magic pills to remove the required adjustment to the changes that are part of the process. Moreover, a powerful sense of control can paradoxically result from "letting go" of past learning and schema-driven behavior when practicing new skills.

Summary

In this chapter, we have selected a clinical case from our practice that is representative of the complex and multifaceted nature of real-life, evidence-based practice in action. We conducted an extensive assessment process to develop a case formulation to guide our selection of treatment interventions based on each individualized target of needed change. Actual strategies and techniques from various empirically supported treatments were chosen through a decision-making process that took into account each area of needed change, what was most acceptable to the patient and consistent with available evidence, as well as other factors, including our training and expertise, in an overall cost–benefit analysis.

Our "lessons learned" as Richard's therapists were many. Richard began treatment with some openness to the idea that we might be able to offer him some tools to cope with an underlying (if not currently medically definable) disease, and *not* a way out of the disease. This is not uncommon for individuals experiencing distressing, real, stress-related physical symptoms for which there is no medical explanation (A. M. Nezu, Nezu, & Lombardo, 2001) and was heavily reinforced by Richard's wife and his physician. Initially, we agreed with a plan that treatment would focus less on cure and more on all of the challenging decisions Richard had before him, including management of the array of medication prescriptions, medical opinions, the variability of his physical distress, and ways to cope with all psychological and emotional factors that might possibly be associated with his very stressful (yet unexplainable) physical symptoms. Psychotherapy interventions for individuals with medically unexplained physical symptoms represent an extremely challenging application of evidence-based treatment because it requires an initial strategic component of establishing a "buy-in" from patients who have been seeking relief from many different physicians regarding symptoms that have significantly interfered with their lives. It requires

the therapist to find effective metaphors and other user-friendly explanations to develop this "buy-in." One of our colleagues, who was departmental head of a large and well-known behavioral medicine consultation service, often told patients that their symptoms could be considered analogous to a raging forest fire spreading out of control and threatening homes and life. In such a case, continually trying to identify what started the fire was not nearly as important as managing its potentially destructive path and containing it.

In working with Richard, we also were reminded of the value of tuning in more closely to the inherent role transitions and loss of control involved in aging and the importance of embedding treatment in a developmental context. Despite Richard's stated intellectual, verbal acceptance of the aging process, we realize that articulating the specific goal of adjustment and coping with these transitions in a more deliberate manner was critical for his progress. Richard's shift in openness to a psychosocial understanding of his symptoms seemed to occur simultaneous with the insight that his fear that not finding a cure was equal to acceptance of his aging process and loss of control.

Finally, we saw clearly the importance of being persistent in developing a strong multidisciplinary treatment team when working with a patient receiving conjoint psychotherapy and pharmacotherapy. Although we experienced a sense of frustration with Dr. M, we thought it was important to assume a stance of objectivity and monitor our own emotionally laden cognitions concerning her lack of responsiveness. In hindsight, our desire to remain neutral and objective, while likely empowering Richard by respecting his choices, may ultimately have reinforced his physician's continued tendency to prescribe large doses of benzodiazepines and delayed improvement of his symptoms. Fortunately, a more willing partner in the medical system appeared later in the course of treatment and prompted greater openness from Richard to understanding the benefits of psychosocial intervention.

References

Allen, L. A., & Woolfolk, R. L. (2010). Cognitive behavioral therapy for somatoform disorders. *Psychiatric Clinics of North America, 33,* 597–593.

Barlow, D. H., Farchione, T. J., Fairholme, C. P., Ellard,

K. K., Boisseau, C. L., Allen, L. B., et al. (2010). *Unified protocol for transdiagnostic treatment of emotional disorders: Therapist guide*. New York: Oxford University Press.

Centers for Disease Control and Prevention. (2014). Fatal injury report. Retrieved from *www.cdc.gov/injury/wisqars/fatal_injury_reports.html*.

Craig, G. (2011). *Emotional freedom techniques: The manual* (2nd ed.). Santa Rosa, CA: Energy Psychology Press.

D'Zurilla, T. J., Nezu, A. M., & Maydeu-Olivares, A. (2002). *Social Problem-Solving Inventory—Revised (SPSI-R)*. North Tonawanda, NY: Multi-Health Systems.

Gaudiano, B., Brown, L., & Miller, I. (2012). Tapping their patients' problems away?: Characteristics of psychotherapists using energy meridian techniques. *Research on Social Work Practice, 22*(6), 647–655.

Lahmann, C., Henningsen, P., Brandt, T., Strupp, M., Klaus, J., Dieterich, M., et al. (2015). Psychiatric comorbidity and psychosocial impairment among patients with vertigo and dizziness. *Journal of Neurology, Neurosurgery, and Psychiatry, 86*, 302–308.

Lambert, M. J., Burlingame, G. M., Umphress, V., Hansen, N. B., Vermeersch, D. A., Clouse, G. C., et al. (1996). The reliability and validity of the outcome questionnaire. *Clinical Psychology and Psychotherapy, 3*(4), 249–258.

Lazarus, A. A., & Lazarus, C. N. (1991). *Multimodal Life History Inventory*. Champaign, IL: Research Press.

Millon, T., Millon, C., Davis, R. D., & Grossman, S. (2009). *Millon Clinical Multiaxial Inventory–III (MCMI-III): Manual*. Minneapolis, MN: Pearson/PsychCorp.

Nezu, A. M., Nezu, C. M., & Cos, T. A. (2007). Case formulation for the behavioral and cognitive therapies. In T. D. Eells (Eds.), *Handbook of psychother-apy case formulation* (2nd ed., pp. 349–378). New York: Guilford Press.

Nezu, A. M., Nezu, C. M., & Lombardo, E. R. (2001). Cognitive-behavior therapy for medically unexplained symptoms: A critical review of the treatment literature. *Behavior Therapy, 32*(3), 537–583.

Nezu, A. M., Nezu, C. M., & Lombardo, E. R. (2004). *Cognitive-behavioral case formulation and treatment design: A problem-solving approach*. New York: Springer.

Nezu, C. M., Nezu, A. M., Ricelli, S., & Stern, J. B. (2015). Case formulation for the cognitive and behavioral therapies: A problem-solving perspective. In C. M. Nezu & A. M. Nezu (Eds.), *The Oxford handbook of cognitive and behavior therapies* (pp. 62–78). New York: Oxford University Press.

Persons, J. B. (2012). *The case formulation approach to cognitive-behavior therapy*. New York: Guilford Press.

Rosen, A., & Proctor, E. K. (1981). Distinctions between treatment outcomes and their implications for treatment evaluation. *Journal of Consulting and Clinical Psychology, 49*(3), 418–425.

Tarrier, N., & Johnson, J. (Eds.). (2015). *Case formulation in cognitive behaviour therapy: The treatment of challenging and complex cases*. Hove, UK: Routledge.

Young, J. E., & Brown, G. (1994). Young Schema Questionnaire. In J. E. Young (Ed.), *Cognitive therapy for personality disorders: A schema-focused approach* (pp. 63–76). Sarasota, FL: Professional Resource Exchange.

Young, J. E., Klosko, J. S., & Weishaar, M. E. (2003). *Schema therapy: A practitioner's guide*. New York: Guilford Press.

Zimmerman, M., & Mattia, J. I. (2001). A self-report scale to help make psychiatric diagnoses: The Psychiatric Diagnostic Screening Questionnaire. *Archives of General Psychiatry, 58*(8), 787–794.

CHAPTER 22

Clinical Decision Making in Combined Pharmacotherapy and Psychotherapy with Complex Clients

Adopting an Evidence-Based Approach in a Partial Hospitalization Setting

CATHERINE D'AVANZATO
MARK ZIMMERMAN

Beth, a middle-aged, twice-divorced European American female, was referred to our program by a physician for treatment of depressive and anxiety symptoms. She was referred for psychiatric evaluation and treatment at the Rhode Island Hospital Adult Partial Hospitalization Program. Beth was born and raised, along with her three siblings, in Providence, Rhode Island, and describes her childhood as "mostly bad." She reported significant physical and emotional abuse, as well as neglect, by her father, who struggled with alcoholism. Beth recalled often going hungry and not having enough food and clothing. She had a close relationship with her mother, who had to work multiple jobs to support the family and was home infrequently. She described disliking high school due to difficulties making new friends and fitting in; however, she kept one or two friends throughout much of her childhood. After graduating high school, Beth worked various jobs as a cashier and receptionist.

Shortly after graduating high school, Beth married her first husband. She reported a history of physical, emotional, and sexual abuse for over a decade by him, with whom she had a daughter. She had another child in her second marriage of approximately a decade, denying abuse in that relationship, which ended amicably. Beth presently lives with a roommate, with whom she has been friends for some time. However, in recent months, she has described conflict with her roommate related to her alcohol use and not following through on household chores and responsibilities.

Upon intake, Beth's primary complaint was "I've been in a depression for quite some time, and I'm having difficulty finding a job." Her depressive symptoms, which started several months earlier, had been worsening in the context of multiple ongoing stressors, including financial strain, family tension, and caretaking for her elderly mother. Beth attributed the worsening in her depression first and foremost to relationship strain with her daughter, as well as conflict with her siblings stemming from her perception that she was taking on a disproportionate share of caretaking responsibilities for their elderly mother. She had been fired from her previous job 1 year earlier, which she attributed to an unstable boss with a history of conflicts with employees, and she had not yet found employment. Beth endorsed the following depression symptoms: depressed mood, anhedonia, weight loss and loss of appetite (i.e., loss of at least 10 pounds throughout the present episode), reported and observed physical agitation, insomnia, constant feelings of worthlessness and guilt, low energy and fatigue, and worsening of her concentration difficulties. She had experienced multiple depressive episodes since her teen years and reports that most of the episodes were similar to how she has been feeling of late.

When we first met Beth, she also was struggling with active suicidal thoughts, as well as a plan, which she refused to disclose. Although she reported that she did not intend to act on her plan due to concern for her family, she also described persistent hopelessness, as well as a prior suicide attempt several years ago.

At the time of her intake, Beth was already prescribed the following medications by her outpatient psychiatrist: clonazepam (1 mg), Adderall XR (20 mg), duloxetine (60 mg), and tramadol (50 mg). She reported that duloxetine and clonazepam initially were beneficial, but no longer adequately addressed her symptoms. Previously, she had tried at least two other selective serotonin reuptake inhibitors (SSRIs), one of which she reported was of no benefit, and the other, which she was on for nearly a decade, was discontinued, as it was not adequately addressing her symptoms. She had also tried desvenlafaxine for at least a few months but did not recall whether it helped. Beth reported seeing multiple therapists dating back to her first divorce; however, up until 5 years ago, she had a history of dropping out of therapy and expressed doubt about whether it benefited her. She had nearly 10 hospitalizations, including a couple inpatient admissions and several partial hospitalizations, but typically did not persist with therapy following discharge from the hospital. While Beth began to change this pattern 5 years ago, once again she had begun complaining of not benefiting from therapy and questioning whether to drop out.

*   *   *

Despite demonstrating partial, temporary benefit at points in her treatment history, Beth's treatment to date had been inadequate in addressing her symptoms and functional impairment, as well as in preventing rehospitalization. It was unclear to her providers what to do next: Should Beth switch and try a new medication? Switch therapists or therapy approaches? Or was this a matter of motivational and behavioral factors that would likely persist regardless of the specific treatment approach? For this reason, she was referred to a partial hospitalization program (PHP) to address gaps in her conceptualization and refine her treatment plan. Our purpose in this chapter is to outline our steps in

answering these questions and to provide recommendations for how providers from diverse disciplines, working together as a multidisciplinary team, can inform their decision making with science to avoid common clinical pitfalls, which may contribute to impasses in cases such as Beth's.

Beth was a strong candidate for partial hospitalization because of the severity of her depression and anxiety symptoms, her suicidal ideation, and her impairment in several areas of her life. The daily visits with her therapist and psychiatrist, as well as the structure provided by the PHP, allowed us to monitor her safety more closely and to achieve more rapid progress in treatment than would be possible with weekly outpatient visits. The challenge we faced was how to make the best use of Beth's stay in the PHP as guided by the clinical research that was most relevant to her care. One of the primary questions was how much to emphasize medication changes during her stay in the PHP, as opposed to focusing exclusively on behavioral interventions (e.g., whether to adjust the dosages of her current medications, augment or remove medications, or switch medications). We also asked whether there may have been gaps or errors in Beth's diagnostic formulation and case conceptualization to date, and what tools we might use to achieve clarification. Also, we asked ourselves, what was the most promising behavioral intervention for Beth, based on the best available science?

Our clinical research group has had the unique opportunity to transform an existing PHP, which previously operated within an eclectic therapy orientation, into a new program based on empirically supported third-wave behavioral therapies, with the goal of providing high-quality care for patients like Beth. This new program includes empirically supported diagnostic and outcome monitoring tools, and supports integrated clinical research and practice. Through our work, we have learned a great deal about how to integrate empirically supported approaches into a truly "real-world" clinical setting. Importantly, PHP and other acute care settings present many challenges for the implementation of evidence-based practice (EBP), chief among which is how best to provide combined pharmacological and behavioral intervention approaches. Although empirically supported treatments (ESTs) have been criticized for not being generalizable to real-world clinical settings such as PHP and other acute care settings, we have demonstrated that EBP can be effectively implemented in such settings and is highly relevant for and well received by clients like Beth.

Our aim in this chapter is to describe our decision-making and strategies to address the challenge of delivering EBP in routine acute care settings. We do so by describing our work with Beth. First, we outline how we utilized evidence-based approaches in Beth's initial diagnosis and case conceptualization, using the five-step model described by Spring, Marchese, and Steglitz (see Chapter 1, this volume). We next discuss some of the challenges that arose in treatment planning, with a focus on typical challenges that arise in working with clients with complex and severe presentations. Our discussion highlights decision-making processes that guide determining when pharmacological approaches may be indicated and how to weigh advantages and disadvantages of a combined versus monotherapy intervention strategy. Finally, we illustrate the ways in which we use ongoing data collection to inform the application of treatment, including outcome evaluation, treatment planning, and delivery as needed.

Step 1: Considerations of EBP in Assessment and Diagnosis

Comprehensive, evidence-based assessment is the foundation of EBP. In our practice, we utilize an evidence-based approach to two aspects of assessment: (1) initial diagnosis and case conceptualization and (2) routine outcome assessment throughout the course of treatment. Semistructured interviews, such as the Structured Clinical Interview for the Diagnosis of DSM-5 Disorders (SCID-5; First, Williams, Karg, & Spitzer, 2015) or Anxiety Disorders Interview Schedule for DSM-5 (ADIS-5; T. Brown & Barlow, 2014), are considered to be "gold standard" diagnostic tools, yet unstructured interviews based heavily on clinical judgment are the norm in typical clinical care settings. In comparison to unstructured intake interviews, semistructured interviews increase accurate detection of mood and anxiety disorders and reduce false-positive diagnoses, such as mistakenly diagnosing major depression in the case of adjustment disorder (Shear et al., 2000). Moreover, these tools have been shown in prior studies to increase accurate detection of comorbid diagnoses, including anxiety disorders (Zimmerman & Chelminski, 2003), which are commonly missed in unstructured intake interviews. Accurate diagnosis is critical because it guides treatment selection. Diagnostic errors are likely to interfere with selecting interventions that are best suited to a particular client.

Beth is among a subgroup of approximately 30% of patients attending our program who was administered a SCID-5. The remaining patients who are not eligible to receive a SCID-5 in our practice complete a standard unstructured diagnostic intake combined with validated self-report measures. While all clients would ideally receive a SCID-5, this is often not feasible in routine clinical practice due to restrictions on insurance reimbursement and clinicians' time. An additional obstacle in short-term treatment settings is the sizable proportion of clients presenting for only one or two sessions and prematurely terminating (G. Brown & Jones, 2005), which some experts have advocated may warrant curtailing the intake in order to begin intervention in the very first session to maximize the therapeutic impact of these initial sessions (Strosahl, Robinson, & Gustavson, 2012). The following guidelines may be helpful to mental health professionals who cannot feasibly conduct semistructured interviews with all clients, but who nonetheless would like to integrate empirically supported practices to improve diagnostic accuracy.

In most settings, the decision about whether to administer a semistructured interview is determined in part by insurance coverage. For patients like Beth, often the case may be made that semistructured interviews can help to reduce rates of diagnostic error given complex presentations and diagnostic ambiguity. In acute care settings, identification of clients with complex presentations may be based on information obtained from the referring provider. This information helps to flag particular patients to receive a semistructured interview. Occasionally, clients in our setting may request a comprehensive diagnostic evaluation, such as in cases in which prior misdiagnosis is being explored as a factor accounting for multiple prior failed interventions.

When it is not possible to conduct semistructured interviews, due to time or other resource constraints, diagnostic screening questionnaires, such as the Psychiatric Diagnostic Screening Questionnaire (PDSQ; Zimmerman & Mattia, 2001), may be administered. The PDSQ is a 125-item self-report questionnaire that assesses current and recent (e.g., the past 6 months) symptoms of 13 DSM-IV Axis I disorders in five areas: mood (major depressive disorder), anxiety (obsessive–compulsive disorder [OCD], panic disorder, agoraphobia, generalized anxiety disorder, and social phobia), eating (binge eating and bulimia), substance use (alcohol abuse/dependence and non-alcohol drug abuse/dependence), somatization and hypochondriasis, as well as psychosis. The PDSQ was designed to maximize sensitivity to ensure that most individuals with a disorder are detected; in the most recent study, it demonstrated a sensitivity of 85% and negative predictive value of 97% averaged across all 13 subscales, with a specificity rate of 69% (Zimmerman & Chelminski, 2006). Such tools can save clinicians substantial time by alerting them to symptom areas that require more comprehensive assessment (D'Avanzato & Zimmerman, 2017).

In our work with Beth, the SCID-5 revealed extensive comorbidity beyond recurrent major depression that had not previously been diagnosed by her outpatient providers, as has been documented in prior research (Zimmerman & Mattia, 1999). Beth met criteria for generalized anxiety disorder, panic disorder without agoraphobia, and a specific phobia. She endorsed posttraumatic stress symptoms stemming from a history of multiple traumatic events, including most notably witnessing abuse of siblings by a caretaker in childhood and long-term physical, emotional, and sexual abuse by her first husband during their marriage.

The accurate detection of anxiety comorbidity should be considered in treatment planning, as it is likely to impact outcomes. We conducted a review of 39 antidepressant efficacy trials that demonstrated significant variability across trials, as well as lack of generalizability, in inclusion and exclusion criteria (Zimmerman, Chelminski, & Pasternak, 2004). As anxiety comorbidity is a frequent exclusion criterion in such trials, the efficacy of antidepressants among depressed individuals with comorbid anxiety disorders may be lower than that suggested by such trials. Likewise, there are many reasons to predict that failure to account for anxiety comorbidity during treatment of depression may negatively impact outcomes. Approximately 50% of individuals with major depressive disorder meet criteria for a comorbid anxiety disorder (Howland et al., 2009), and anxiety comorbidity is associated with greater psychosocial morbidity and poorer treatment outcomes (Petersen, Andreotti, Chelminski, Young, & Zimmerman, 2009). As a result, modifications to standard EBP for depression may be needed in order to optimize treatment outcome. If a clinician misses a comorbid anxiety disorder, he or she is less likely to provide adequate treatment to address it. For example, in a depressed client with comorbid OCD, a psychiatrist who did not detect OCD may not prescribe an SSRI, which is considered the first-line pharmacological treatment in this case. Similarly, had Beth's comorbid posttraumatic stress disorder (PTSD) been a primary concern that was missed, particularly if it played a role in the course of her depression, treatment might be less successful in helping her achieve remission from her depression, as it would not include critical treatment components (e.g., exposure) to reduce her PTSD. In fact, clients' opinions regarding the importance of anxiety appear to converge with empirical findings. A survey of depressed clients presenting for treatment in our outpatient clinic indicated that the majority of clients reported that it was important that their anxiety be addressed during treatment (Zimmerman & Chelminski, 2003). While some studies have found that anxiety moderates treatment response to different antidepressants, most of the research has not been supportive (Uher, Payne, Pavlova, & Perlis, 2014). Nonetheless, clinicians indicated that anxiety is the symptom that most commonly influences their choice of antidepressant in depressed patients (Zimmerman, Posternak, et al., 2004). Importantly, Beth viewed her anxiety as excessive and a significant concern warranting treatment. She expressed the most concern about her worry, stating, "I worry about anything and everything, and I wish it would stop because it keeps me from doing the things that I'm worried about." She sought help to cope better with her anxiety, as it was a source of distress each day and was causing her to withdraw further from her relationships and activities.

Steps 2 and 3: Case Conceptualization and Treatment Planning with Complex Clients

Pharmacotherapy Conceptualization: When to Utilize Medication versus Therapy or a Combined Approach

Beth's diagnostic profile presented us with a challenging decision: Was it in her best interest to recommend combined psychotherapeutic and pharmacological interventions or a mono-therapy approach? If we were going to recommend a monotherapy approach, which made more sense—pharmacotherapy or psychotherapy? Because psychotherapy is a substantial component of care for all clients in our program (as described in detail below), practically, the question facing us was whether to supplement psychotherapy with medication or to augment or switch medications already prescribed to clients entering the program. This question poses a challenge for many therapists working in more traditional outpatient settings as well. What clients should be referred to a psychiatrist or primary care provider for further evaluation and consideration of starting medication upon intake? If a decision is made to delay referral for pharmacotherapy, at what point in the course of psychotherapy should this referral again be considered? That is, how does one gauge when a combined approach would be superior to therapy alone based on a client's presentation, severity, or response to treatment?

To aid in making the decision on whether to add or switch medications, it is important to consult original peer-reviewed research, as well as treatment guidelines published by professional organizations (e.g., American Psychiatric Association and American Psychological Association), being aware of the strengths and limitations of each source (as described in this volume by Kraemer & Periyakoil, Chapter 4; Cuijpers & Cristea, Chapter 5; Hollon, Chapter 6).

We began our examination of the literature with a focus on treatment guidelines regarding EBP, but we did not stop there. We also focused on identifying relevant meta-analyses in high-quality peer-reviewed journals because such reports save time and aid in synthesizing results across studies. In addition, we did not want to rely too heavily on a single study or a small number of studies, results of which may not be generalizable to Beth's specific case. Meta-analysis offers a number of additional advantages in interpreting research, such as estimating the impact of publication bias on the effects and clarifying the magnitude of effects. For us, this was an important consideration, as relying solely on published studies may result in an inflated estimate of an intervention's efficacy given that null results often are not published. Given Beth's history of unsuccessful treatments, we wanted to have as much confidence as possible in our recommendations. An advantage of consulting original peer-reviewed research, as opposed to relying solely on treatment guidelines, is that guidelines may not be updated frequently enough, nor may they be comprehensive enough, to adequately reflect the most recent research. Additionally, whereas the American Psychiatric Association has issued clear guidelines regarding which treatments are evidence based and the sequence in which to initiate various treatment options, the American Psychological Association and other leading psychology organizations have been slower to issue analogous guidelines for psychotherapy interventions, though efforts are under way (Gaudiano, Dalrymple, D'Avanzato, & Bunaciu, 2016).

In Beth's case, our review of the literature suggested that results have been mixed regarding both the superiority of a combined versus monotherapy intervention strategy and when medication or therapy may be preferred. Specifically, the American Psychiatric Association (2010) guidelines indicate that either medication or an evidence-based psychotherapy alone may be considered first-line treatments for mild depression. When electing to prescribe an antidepressant, SSRIs, serotonin–norepinephrine reuptake inhibitors (SNRIs), bupropion, or mirtazapine are recommended as first-line agents, and practitioners are advised to tailor their decision on particular medications within these classes based on individual patient characteristics, such as side effect profile, risks, prior response, cost and patient preference. Either treatment alone or a combined medication and therapy approach is recommended for moderate depression. Practitioners are advised to weigh anticipated benefits and costs for a particular client when deciding whether to utilize a pharmacotherapy approach. Factors to be considered include symptom severity, magnitude of response (e.g., a greater magnitude of response may be seen in moderate or severe cases), speed of response (i.e., typically faster response with antidepressant treatment than psychotherapy), severity and tolerability of side effects and medical risks, and records or report regarding past medication adherence. For example, for a client with mild depressive symptoms and difficulty tolerating the side effects of an antidepressant, the costs of starting medication may outweigh the benefits in light of prior research questioning the specific efficacy of antidepressants for mild depression (e.g., see meta-analysis by Kirsch et al., 2008). However, Fournier and colleagues (2010) recently argued that a significant limitation of the Kirsch and colleagues (2008) meta-analysis (as is also the case with most prior randomized controlled trials [RCTs]) is that only one of 35 studies included had a sample with a mean depression severity on the Hamilton Depression Rating Scale (HDRS) of less than 23 (which corresponds to *very severe* depression on the HDRS). This is likely due to the strict inclusion criteria typically used in U.S. Food and Drug Administration (FDA) registered RCTs, and the authors concluded that the results therefore cannot be generalized to a typical treatment-seeking outpatient population (Fournier et al., 2010). In their more recent mega-analysis (i.e., which employed more rigorous and powerful meta-analytic techniques based on patient-level data) of six large-scale placebo-controlled trials using a more representative range of depression severity levels, which included minor depression, they found that medication did not separate from placebo at either the mild, moderate, or lower end of the severe range, only crossing the threshold of clinical significance for HDRS scores above 25 (i.e., corresponding to *very severe*). This study illustrates the limitations of relying exclusively on professional organization treatment guidelines or single RCTs alone, and it also points to the importance of critically evaluating the methodology and inclusion criteria of meta-analyses. In contrast, for severe depression, the American Psychiatric Association guidelines state that an antidepressant medication or electroconvulsive therapy (ECT) "definitely should be provided," with the option of augmenting either treatment with psychotherapy. Thus, for a client with moderate to severe depressive symptoms accompanied by serious suicidal ideation (SI) and plan, the benefits of prescribing an antidepressant or a combined intervention are argued to outweigh the additional costs. Few guidelines are given regarding when to augment medication with therapy, though it is recommended to consider adding therapy in cases in which interpersonal difficulties or maladaptive personality traits appear to play a prominent role in an individual's presenting concerns.

In consideration of both treatment guidelines and the most recent science, it was clear that we needed to conceptualize the severity of Beth's presentation and to go beyond relying solely on treatment guidelines. In our view, her depression could be classified as moderate to severe. This classification was based on the number

and severity of DSM-5 depression symptoms, as well as an assessment of suicidal risk. Beth's scores on both depression and anxiety severity measures placed her at the low end of the severe range. However, she endorsed strong current SI, past suicidal gestures, and criteria for all DSM symptoms of a major depressive episode, which may indicate that Beth should be considered severely depressed. While meeting each of the DSM symptoms for depression, the severity of each individual symptom endorsed was mild, and she experienced only moderate daily functional impairment. In light of these factors, we considered Beth to be at the border between the moderate and severe ranges. In addition, she firmly denied intent to act on the suicide plan and endorsed a number of protective factors lowering her risk, including her engagement in treatment, insight, future orientation and desire to get better, supportive friends, and a strong motivation to stay alive for the sake of her family relationships. Thus, a medication and/or therapy focus might be justified.

A recent meta-analysis of 21 clinical trials demonstrated that a combined medication and therapy approach may produce superior outcomes to pharmacotherapy alone among individuals with depression (Oestergaard & Moldrup, 2011), thus experts in the treatment of depression are increasingly advocating consideration of a combined approach. It is important to note, however, that some studies have not found evidence of superiority of a combined approach (Melvin et al., 2006; Singh & Reece, 2014). In a large multisite trial, Hollon and colleagues (2014) found no differences in remission rates or time to remission between combination medication plus cognitive therapy treatment and medication alone. However, participants in the combined treatment condition achieved recovery (i.e., 26 weeks without a relapse) at significantly higher rates, particularly among individuals with severe and nonchronic depression (Hollon et al., 2014). As Beth's depression could be classified as severe, yet chronic, and the Hollon and colleagues article did not include a psychotherapy-only arm, the results of this study do not provide definitive guidance regarding a combined versus monotherapy approach. In addition, there are a number of methodological limitations of prior studies that have compared pharmacological, psychotherapy, and combined approaches that prevent firm conclusions about the superiority of any approach. With the exception of the study by Hollon and colleagues, one limitation of the existing literature is the lack of long-term follow-up data (Moradveisi, Huibers, & Arntz, 2015), which is a significant gap in light of the frequently recurrent and/or chronic course of depression. Also, compared to individuals who received only antidepressant medication, evidence-based psychotherapy (e.g., cognitive-behavioral therapy [CBT] and behavioral activation) appears to result in superior long-term outcomes in a number of studies (e.g., Dobson, Hollon, & Dimidjian, 2008). When psychotherapy is compared to individuals receiving medication alone who continue their medication, however, results are more mixed. Combination treatment in the study by Dobson and colleagues (2008) demonstrated superiority to medication alone, even though participants in this study continued their medications. Likewise, one recent meta-analysis found a statistical trend toward superiority of behavioral therapy compared to antidepressant medication, even when participants continued their medication (Cuijpers et al., 2013); however, further research is needed.

Taken together, when conducting treatment planning with individuals with recurrent depression, it may be worthwhile to consider the likelihood that a particular client will discontinue medication against the recommendation of his or her psychiatrist. In Beth's case, discontinuation of medication was less of a concern, as she reported adhering to her antidepressant and anxiolytic medication throughout the past several years. Likewise, she remained with the same psychiatrist and therapist for the past several years prior to the present PHP admission. Prior to that, she had been on sertraline for 10 years, with no reported difficulties with adherence. Nevertheless, Beth's depression course was marked by frequent recurrences since her teenage years, leading to multiple partial and inpatient hospitalizations, despite her report of minimal depressive symptoms between episodes. Thus, her high risk for relapse and recurrence warrants a treatment strategy emphasizing long-term, in addition to acute, gains. Given that Beth reported at least some benefit from her current medication, denying side effects, the decision was made to keep her on antidepressant and anxiolytic medications. The question regarding whether to change, increase, or augment her current medications, however, remained.

More recent studies have sought to achieve a more nuanced understanding of the mechanisms through which pharmacotherapy and psychotherapy approaches influence short- and long-term outcomes in order to better match treatment approaches with particular individuals. The precise targets of a treatment and the mechanisms through which it exerts its impact may be useful to consider when deciding among medication, therapy, or their combination. One mechanism through which psychotherapy has been hypothesized to result in more durable treatment gains in the prior studies we reviewed is through imparting new skills and behaviors that may protect against recurrence well beyond treatment termination (Strunk, DeRubeis, Chiu, & Alvarez, 2007).

Another hypothesized mechanism through which interventions may differentially affect outcomes is through shaping clients' attributions of what causes improvement. Specific attributions regarding change, independent of skills and new behaviors, may confer additional long-term benefits. In support of this hypothesis, in a recent study of 100 depressed individuals randomized to either antidepressant medication or behavioral activation, Moradveisi and colleagues (2015) found that antidepressant medication and behavioral activation led to different attributional patterns in depressed clients. Individuals in the pharmacotherapy arm reported greater attribution of their gains to medication efficacy, whereas individuals undergoing therapy endorsed greater attribution of their gains to their coping ability, as well as greater tendency to attribute gains to internal factors. In addition, the authors found that attributing treatment gains to coping and internal factors partially mediated their finding of superior 1-year follow up treatment outcomes, as indicated by the Beck Depression Inventory (BDI) and HDRS, in the therapy-only condition. It was hypothesized that an attributional style that credits coping skills and internal variables for progress may motivate individuals to engage in healthy actions, which in turn protect against relapse. Taken together, beginning with therapy alone as a way of building efficacy and responsibility for actions, as well as shaping internal attributions, might be considered for a client with a tendency to underestimate his or her role in the process of change, particularly when changing behavioral or interpersonal patterns appears necessary to prevent recurrence. Alternatively, there are likely to be different ways for psychiatrists to introduce and discuss medication that may be more likely to encourage internal attributions for change. This would be an important topic for future research. In addition, as no studies to our knowledge examined attributions for change and related impact on outcomes in a combined treatment arm, this would be critical to examine in future studies. Our prediction based on our own clinical experience would be that individuals receiving combined treatment may be more likely to attribute gains to medication, though, again, this has yet to be tested.

In applying this logic to treatment planning with Beth, we hypothesized that a tendency to discount internal factors may have played a role in maladaptive behavior patterns maintaining her long-standing emotional difficulties, despite her compliance with the medication regimen. Of note, Beth attributed the current episode to worsening strain in her relationship with her daughter, as well as ongoing stress related to caretaking for her mother, which was also leading to disagreements with her siblings. She was initially vague regarding the source of tension in these relationships and tended to attribute disagreements to her family members' actions. As treatment progressed, maladaptive emotion regulation and related interpersonal behaviors became increasingly evident, supporting our hypothesis that they might play a role in Beth's disorder. Likewise, some inconsistency and difficulty in relationships with therapy providers was evident. She had had only one brief experience in therapy decades ago, which was court-ordered during a divorce. "It was a waste," Beth said, and she had had no additional therapy since that time. With her current therapist of 5 years, she had reported increasing sense of "disappointment," again providing vague reasons as to why. Thus, in order to gain more information regarding the role of interpersonal and emotion regulation difficulties, a family meeting was held with Beth's daughter, who confirmed our observations. In the meeting, her daughter asked if Beth could step out of the room, noting that she was concerned that Beth was so highly sensitive to feedback or perceived minor criticism that she worried about hurting her or damaging their relationship further. Her daughter highlighted strong ruminative tendencies, as well as a tendency to overanalyze, jump to conclusions, and misinterpret others' nonverbal expressions, which had led family members to withdraw from her to some degree. Thus, it appeared that Beth had not sufficiently addressed these behavioral factors throughout the course

of her treatment to date. After discussing feedback on these observations and the family meeting with one another and the multidisciplinary team, it was decided in collaboration with Beth that it made most sense to focus on psychotherapy, foregoing the option to increase her duloxetine and/or augment her medication (e.g., with an atypical antipsychotic, which had been considered in light of her anxiety). We reasoned that a change in medications was not only unlikely to sufficiently address these interpersonal patterns, but that it would also be important to highlight Beth's agency, efficacy, and sense of responsibility for making these important behavioral changes.

An additional factor that is increasingly emphasized in evidence-based treatment planning, coinciding with the movement within the field toward patient-centered care, is client preferences. There is growing evidence that client preferences have important implications for treatment planning. Clients who are not matched with their preferred treatment modality have been found to demonstrate poorer treatment outcomes (Swift, Callahan, & Vollmer, 2011). This is a significant concern, as high drop-out rates are seen in both pharmacotherapy and psychotherapy, but particularly pharmacotherapy, for depression and related disorders (Cuijpers, van Straten, van Oppen, & Andersson, 2008; Fernandez, Salem, Swift, & Ramtahal, 2015; Olfson, Marcus, Tedeschi, & Wan, 2006). A recent meta-analysis of 34 studies of client preference indicated that patients with depression and/or anxiety tended to prefer psychotherapy over medication alone by a ratio of approximately 3 to 1, and that young individuals, and women in particular, tended to favor therapy (McHugh, Whitton, Peckham, Welge, & Otto, 2013). Not surprisingly, individuals who attribute their symptoms to biological causes may be more likely to favor medication (Aikens, Nease, & Klinkman, 2008), whereas attributions to social factors were associated with favoring therapy (Houle et al., 2012). Attempts to match patients' preferences regarding particular interventions have been tied to superior treatment adherence, retention, and, in turn, outcomes in some studies (Kwan, Dimidjian, & Rizvi, 2010; Swift et al., 2011), though results have not uniformly supported matching treatment to preferences, and more research clarifying the relation between preference with adherence and outcome is needed (Steidtmann et al., 2012). At a minimum, in cases in which different treatment options being considered demonstrate comparable efficacy (e.g., antidepressants vs. therapy for moderate depression) and there are no other contraindications, it may be ideal to offer the client's preferred treatment option. Unfortunately, few studies have investigated client preferences for and acceptability of combined antidepressant treatment and psychotherapy. However, recent studies that included a combined therapy arm have generally found that clients prefer it to a medication-only approach and have therefore advocated considering greater utilization of combined therapy in cases in which the advantages may justify the increased cost (Steidtmann et al., 2012). In Beth's case, we had a good degree of flexibility, as she expressed openness to both pharmacological and psychotherapeutic interventions; therefore, we moved forward with our plan to emphasize psychotherapy.

Psychotherapy Conceptualization: An Acceptance and Commitment Therapy Approach

Our next decision was *which* therapy model to select. A significant advantage of acceptance and commitment therapy (ACT) in Beth's case, in light of her comorbidity and complexity, is its flexible, transdiagnostic approach. An ACT approach offered the ability to target the most problematic avoidance behaviors and processes, cutting across different diagnoses, as opposed to being constrained by focusing on one specific disorder at a time. This was a key consideration in Beth's case given that she wanted to address multiple areas of concern simultaneously (i.e., her depression, chronic worry, and PTSD) during her PHP admission. A second consideration influencing our decision to use ACT was Beth's prior nonresponse to treatment and history of not following through with therapy long term. This may be related to her strong and longstanding avoidance tendencies. Recent research has demonstrated the effectiveness of ACT in individuals who did not adequately respond to traditional behavioral therapies (e.g., Gloster et al., 2015). Individuals with intransigent avoidant behavior patterns, who may not be willing to engage sufficiently with their emotions, as is required in prolonged exposure for PTSD, may be a particularly good match for an ACT approach, which may help them more gradually to build the required openness and willingness needed to proceed with exposure-based work (Orsillo & Batten, 2005). ACT's emphasis on values clarification, which we discuss further

as applied to Beth's case, may play an important role in motivation building among clients such as Beth, who are struggling with ambivalence about change.

Our next step was to complete a full conceptualization of Beth grounded in ACT principles. To aid in developing a psychosocial conceptualization of a client, we find treatment guides to be very helpful (see Hayes, Strosahl, & Wilson, 2011; Westrup, 2014). In particular, Strosahl and colleagues' (2012) guide on conducting brief ACT-based interventions and rapid case conceptualization, focused ACT (FACT), has been particularly useful in our setting given that treatment planning must typically be completed within the first session.

ACT case conceptualizations highlight six core psychological processes contributing to psychological inflexibility, which represents a central feature of the full spectrum of psychological concerns. Clients are conceptualized along each of these dimensions (i.e., acceptance, values, committed action, mindfulness, cognitive defusion, and self-as-context). Strosahl and colleagues further distill these processes into three pillars of psychological flexibility: openness, awareness, and engagement. Openness comprises the core processes of *defusion,* or learning to detach from thoughts, rigid cognitive rules, and stories that can interfere in change, and *acceptance,* or the willingness to fully experience emotions, thoughts, and challenging content. Awareness includes the core processes of mindfulness and self-as-context, which broadly involve building the ability to observe, acknowledge, and maintain attention on one's present-moment experience. Finally, engagement work targets core processes of *valuing,* or clarifying important personal values and life directions, as well as *committed action,* the continual engagement and reengagement in values-based actions.

With regard to openness, we first sought to identify avoidance behaviors toward which Beth often gravitated, as well as to understand *how* specifically they function in her effort to control difficult emotions and content. Of note were her tendencies to ruminate, worry, isolate from others, and suppress her thoughts and feelings for fear of judgment by others, interfering in effective communication and contributing to not having her emotional needs met. Next, we explored the specific consequences of these behavior patterns in contributing to Beth's suffering, and the particular values from which she became disconnected. As became evident during a family meeting with Beth and her daughter, her rumination and problematic interpersonal behaviors appeared to cause significant strain in her relationships. The remaining emphasis of therapy was on clarifying important life directions on which Beth wanted to focus going forward. She highlighted her daughter and other family members as her reason for living; thus, the focus in therapy was on ways to shape her interactions in order to strengthen these relationships and live more consistently with her ideals in this domain. Last, it was important to assess barriers to engagement pertaining to openness and awareness to prioritize during therapy, which was done primarily with experiential exercises to build mindfulness skills and skills to detach from unhelpful thoughts and interpersonal interpretations.

As in traditional behavior therapies, in ACT, it is also important to conduct a thorough diagnostic assessment and functional analysis to fully capture problem areas for Beth and understand how they are interrelated. These steps aid in tailoring ACT exercises and integrating psychoeducation content to particular situations with which the client is struggling most. For example, in Beth's case, we determined that her depression was the primary concern, and generalized anxiety was a secondary concern. She noted minimal impairment or distress related to her residual PTSD symptoms, and while she reported distress associated with her panic attacks occurring about once per week, she noted minimal functional impairment and avoidance related to her panic. Thus, we tailored acceptance and mindfulness exercises to address problematic avoidance in Beth's interpersonal relationships, which appeared to play a central role in her depression, but we highlighted throughout treatment how she might also apply these principles to other problem areas moving forward. In addition, mindfulness and defusion techniques to address her rumination and worry were a central focus. Had PTSD been a primary concern that had been missed, for example, in the absence of doing a comprehensive diagnostic assessment, we have found in our clinical experience that this may slow or interfere in treatment progress. For example, another client was referred to the PHP to address panic symptoms; however, throughout the course of her stay in the program, we discovered that PTSD was in fact the primary concern. It was hypothesized that progress in addressing her panic had been poor

due to her PTSD not having being addressed. In fact, once we began focusing exercises on her PTSD and integrating psychoeducation related to PTSD, she began improving. Last, but importantly in our experience, the client's preference with regard to which problem areas to begin with should be considered and honored when possible in order to ensure engagement in and readiness for treatment. Beth was in agreement with us that addressing her depression and worry were her primary goals.

Steps 4 and 5: Applying Treatment, Analyzing Effects, and Adjusting Practice

Not only is initial assessment a cornerstone of EBP, but ongoing assessment of the client's outcome is also critical in guiding therapists' decision making about when to modify the treatment plan. Just as with initial assessment, the use of evidence-based standardized assessment tools is rare in routine clinical practice (Zimmerman & McGlinchey, 2008). Instead, treatment outcome tends to be determined by unstructured interviewing and clinical judgment alone. However, the use of well-validated standardized assessment tools is considered the "gold standard," as it more finely attunes the clinician to a client's symptoms and status. This prevents missing or delaying modifications to the treatment plan, reducing rates of nonresponse or inadequate response. For example, based on elevated depression symptoms on a symptom measure, a psychiatrist may be alerted more quickly to the need to augment or switch medications, or to recommend adding therapy. While more controlled research is needed to clarify the precise impact of routine outcome monitoring on treatment outcome, a number of studies have demonstrated improved outcomes associated with the integration of routine outcome questionnaires (Guo et al., 2015; Lambert, 2007).

One of the most challenging questions facing clinicians is *which aspects* of treatment outcome to measure. Early studies of the impact of adding routine outcome monitoring on treatment outcome were limited by the use of one or few item measures of general distress, which likely do not provide sufficient information to clinicians to support decision making on the particular treatment plan modifications that would be most beneficial. Therefore, more recent research has focused on the use of symptom measures specific to the client's primary disorder or primary treatment target. Information on specific symptoms with which the client is struggling (e.g., insomnia) may alert the clinician to consider treatment modifications, such as augmentation with additional medication or therapy. On a related note, experts in the pharmacological treatment of depression now advocate for complete or near-complete symptomatic remission given that residual symptoms of depression (Rush, Kraemer, & Sackeim, 2006), and more recently anxiety (D'Avanzato et al., 2013), are associated with greater psychosocial morbidity and risk for relapse. This reality was clearly evident in Beth's illness course. She reported a history of multiple depressive episodes dating back to childhood. Despite reporting benefit from her medication, Beth reported that some depressive symptoms (e.g., low self-esteem, low energy, and concentration difficulty related to rumination), as well as her chronic anxiety and panic attacks, have persisted outside of depressive episodes during times throughout her life when she was doing relatively well compared to her baseline. In addition, she has persistently experienced impairment in functioning in her interpersonal relationships and work functioning, despite fluctuations in her symptoms. The use of scales specific to depression is necessary to detect residual symptoms, which are less likely to be picked up by unstructured questions, such as "How is your mood today?" Such scales also reduce clinicians' bias in gauging patient outcome (i.e., reducing their tendency to overestimate the impact of their intervention). Thus, in our PHP, Beth, along with all patients, completed three daily symptom measures: a measure of depression, the Clinically Useful Depression Outcome Scale (CUDOS; Zimmerman, Chelminski, McGlinchey, & Posternak, 2008), a measure of anxiety (Clinically Useful Anxiety Outcome Scale [CUXOS]; Zimmerman, Chelminski, Young, & Dalrymple, 2010), and a measure of anger in development, the Clinically Useful Anger Outcome Scale (CUANGOS). These scales were selected for their thorough coverage yet brevity, patient acceptability, and ease of both completion and interpretation, which are key considerations when selecting an outcome measure for regular use in "real-world" clinical settings. For example, sample CUDOS items include "I felt sad or depressed," "I was not as interested in my usual activities," and "I had problems concentrating" (see Zimmerman et al., 2008, Appendix A, for

the complete scale); sample CUXOS items include "I felt nervous or anxious," "I worried a lot that bad things might happen," and "I felt keyed up or on edge" (see Zimmerman et al., 2010, for the full scale); sample CUANGOS items include, "I felt very angry or irritable," "I yelled or argued," and "I had the urge to hit or hurt someone."

On the other hand, some experts in the intervention of depression and anxiety, particularly within the ACT community, have raised questions about the exclusive use of symptom measures to assess treatment outcome. As previously discussed, acute symptom change may not always coincide with long-term symptom change, let alone other outcomes, which some argue may be just as important, such as functioning, quality of life, healthy coping, and adaptive behavior. For this reason, it may not be advisable to aim for symptomatic remission among clients, such as Beth, treated within a PHP. ACT experts have questioned a narrow conceptualization of treatment outcome within the field that neglects mechanisms or principles of change. A criticism of "second-wave" behavioral therapies, such as traditional CBT, is that their development outpaced scientific evidence supporting the theorized principles of change (e.g., that cognitive change is necessary in order to achieve behavioral change) (Hayes, Luoma, Bond, & Lillis, 2006). Hayes and colleagues point to mixed findings in dismantling studies supporting the incremental utility of cognitive restructuring and other cognitive interventions, above and beyond behavioral components, such as exposure and behavioral activation, although other authors point out a similar lack of data on the incremental utility of particular modules of third-wave therapies such as dialectical behavior therapy (DBT) (Rosen & Davison, 2003). While CBT for depression, for instance, has well-documented efficacy, as many as 50% of individuals do not respond adequately, and recurrence rates are high (Blackburn & Moore, 1997; Gloaguen, Cottraux, Cucherat, & Blackburn, 1998). While hundreds of therapy manuals targeting a continually expanding range of psychological disorders and concerns are available, the failure to root intervention development in evidence-based mechanisms of change may hinder the field from achieving substantive improvements in treatment response rates and treatment efficiency (Rosen & Davison, 2003).

There are also potential clinical consequences of a symptom-focused approach that fails to consider mechanisms. One example relates to the core ACT process of experiential avoidance. A central tenet of ACT is that at the root of many diverse psychological problems, and human suffering in general, are common maladaptive cognitive and behavioral processes that contribute to psychological rigidity. ACT theorists question whether the field's, and our culture's, emphasis on acute symptom relief (and complete symptomatic remission) may inadvertently feed into clients' tendency to respond to negative emotions and stressors with experiential avoidance (e.g., Harris, 2008). The emphasis on feeling better *now* may lead clients to view symptoms and emotional discomfort as "bad"; thus, they continue struggling to get rid of this content in ways that maintains suffering long term, as opposed to focusing on more adaptive, approach-driven behavior. For Beth, this was evident in her pattern of not persisting with therapy focused on behavioral changes, while instead continuing to search for a new medicine or treatment that would reduce her anxiety and depression short term. For this reason, ACT practitioners have placed greater emphasis on identifying and targeting mechanisms of change (i.e., the six core processes), with the goal of helping clients to achieve more meaningful and durable change.

As a result, in our PHP, we include daily and pre- and posttreatment measures of functioning and ACT-relevant mechanisms of change to track whether our intervention is, in fact, altering these mechanisms and building psychological flexibility. Beth filled out measures of mindfulness (Five-Factor Mindfulness Questionnaire [FFMQ]; Baer et al., 2008), experiential avoidance (Acceptance and Action Questionnaire-II [AAQ-II]; Bond et al., 2011), and approach-driven behavior in important valued directions (Valuing Questionnaire [VQ]; Smout, Davies, Burns, & Christie, 2014) at pre- and post- treatment, as well as completing daily a brief ad hoc measure of ACT processes that our team developed, containing items derived from these scales. The therapist often reviewed Beth's responses to particular items on the daily ACT process measure at the beginning of the therapy session. In addition, when administering symptom measures, we were careful to discuss these with Beth in such a way as to avoid sending the message that anxiety or sadness indicates "failure." For example, reductions in avoidance and increases in valued action were reinforced, and fluctuations

in anxiety were discussed as normal reactions that could be expected in light of beginning to confront anxiety-provoking situations that she had been avoiding for some time. From intake to discharge, Beth reported approximately a 50% reduction in symptom severity on both the CUDOS (intake score: 50, discharge score: 20) and CUXOS (intake score: 63, discharge score: 36), falling from the severe range to the moderate range on these scales (see the graph of Beth's daily symptom scores throughout her 9-day admission in Figure 22.1). The increase in anxiety reported on Beth's last day in the program compared to the prior day reflects a common pattern we have seen that may possibly be due to anxiety about discharge. Her reported anger on the CUANGOS also decreased throughout her admission, from a 22 at intake to a 5 on her day of discharge. Importantly, Beth's scales also demonstrated significant improvements in all ACT processes throughout her 9-day admission, consistent with the majority of patients attending the PHP. Specifically, she demonstrated increased psychological flexibility and willingness, indicated by the AAQ (pretreatment score: 6.3, posttreatment score: 4.3), increased mindfulness (FFMQ pretreatment score: 1.8, posttreatment score: 2.8), and increased values-consistent actions as indicated by the VQ (pretreatment score: 3.1, posttreatment: 4.3). Research to date, including data on our PHP, has demonstrated that ACT results in significant changes in the targeted core processes of change (e.g., Levin, Luoma, & Haeger, 2015). More research is needed to determine whether, in fact, changes in these targeted mechanisms mediate therapy outcomes, and whether ACT's emphasis on mechanisms produces superior results compared to traditional behavioral interventions. In addition, measures of targeted ACT mechanisms, such as the AAQ, the FFMQ, and the VQ, are newer, and concerns with their validity remain. For instance, concerns regarding discriminant and construct validity of the AAQ and other ACT process measures have been raised (Francis, Dawson, & Golijani-Moghaddam, 2016). Further research is needed to demonstrate the psychometric properties of these tools in "real-world" clinical populations and to address issues that have been raised. Efforts are under way to develop new and improved measures (e.g., Francis et al., 2016).

Our research group has also found that clients' own perceptions of what is important in treatment, as well as their progress, are valu-

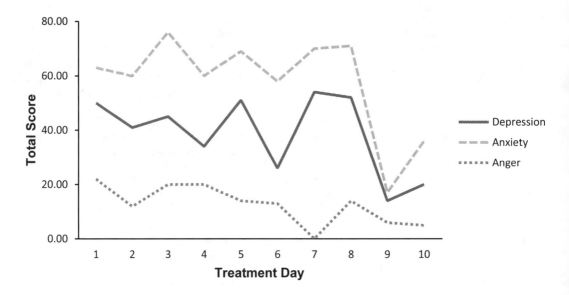

FIGURE 22.1. Beth's daily symptom severity as indicated by the CUDOS, CUXOS, and CUANGOS throughout her 9-day PHP admission. Day 1 was the day her SCID was administered, and Days 2–10 were treatment days.

able in gauging outcome and adjusting our own practice (Zimmerman et al., 2006). Thus, Beth filled out measures of satisfaction daily after each group therapy session, as well as a measure on her last day in treatment assessing all aspects of the program, including her satisfaction with therapy sessions, psychiatry sessions, and each of the four therapy groups offered daily. Because we choose to ask clients to complete these questionnaires anonymously in order to ensure honest feedback, we did not have access to Beth's feedback specifically. However, a point was made in therapy sessions to check in with her regularly on whether she agreed with the treatment goals and focus, and whether she would recommend any adjustments to the therapy sessions to benefit more. Likewise, when clients in the program give negative feedback or suggest a change, we do our best to accept this feedback in an open, nonjudgmental, even encouraging way that makes clients feel comfortable in sharing their feedback openly. Anonymous satisfaction data aggregated across all clients attending the PHP were discussed at weekly staff meetings and used to make adjustments to the program. For example, based on such data, an additional, optional mindfulness group was added, based on feedback from clients indicating that they found great benefit in

having more opportunities for hands-on practice of these skills.

Summary and Conclusions

In combined psychotherapy and psychopharmacology intervention approaches, empirical evidence informs decision making at all stages of treatment, beginning with initial assessment and treatment planning, and continuing throughout the duration of the implementation and outcome evaluation phases. In the case of Beth, the incorporation of evidence-based diagnostic practices enabled us to achieve a more comprehensive and accurate diagnosis. We have consistently found that a comprehensive, accurate diagnosis impacts our clinical decision making in ways that likely contribute to more favorable outcomes. Importantly, the integration of both professional treatment guidelines for EBP and our own literature review and discussion among our multidisciplinary team members informed the decision to emphasize the use of a specific empirically supported psychotherapy, forgoing the option to increase or augment Beth's medication. An ACT-based intervention targeting interpersonal and cognitive avoidance patterns, which appeared to play a central role in her recurrent depression and worry, was associated with a significant reduction in Beth's depression, anxiety, and anger severity, as well as improvement in functioning and ACT-relevant mechanisms of change over her 9-day stay. This is particularly noteworthy in light of the recurrent and treatment-resistant nature of her depression, as well as the brevity of our program. Beth's favorable outcome, consistent with program-level outcome data demonstrating efficacy, lends support to the feasibility and effectiveness of implementing EBPs in challenging, "real-world" clinical settings similar to our own. Our primary future aim is to measure long-term outcomes of clients, as more research discerning the long-term impact of various monotherapy versus combined intervention options is needed.

It is our hope that providers from diverse disciplines will be able to draw from Beth's case in informing their clinical decision making. First, we would reassure providers from all disciplines who deliver therapy, including social work, counseling, nursing, and psychiatry, that it is possible to learn and integrate EBP into their own practices. Beth was successfully treated by a multidisciplinary team of providers—including psychologists, social workers, and psychiatrists—with varying levels of formal training and experience with ACT. There are many opportunities for those who are new to EBP to become more familiar with these therapies, by reading books, attending workshops and conferences, and consulting with colleagues. Second, an immediate way that providers of all disciplines can integrate EBP to improve outcome is by employing evidence-based diagnosis and treatment outcome monitoring. For example, we hope that readers will consider integrating some of the measures reviewed in this chapter in their practices. Finally, our experience with Beth reveals the importance of conducting a complete and thorough case conceptualization that is informed by the latest science. In her case, arriving at a complete, evidence-based diagnosis, case conceptualization, and treatment plan, as well as evaluating and revising the treatment plan, required true multidisciplinary collaboration. We would encourage providers of all disciplines to approach all phases of treatment with an open, flexible, and client-centered approach. Beth demonstrates how the decision to emphasize medicine, versus therapy, and which therapy to select will vary from client to client and ideally depend on consultation of multiple

sources of the most recent scientific evidence. In summary, we hope to convey through our experience working with Beth and thousands of clients each year who come through our program that providers from all disciplines play a critical role in integrating EBP into the "real-world" clinical settings in which they work. There are several avenues through which EBP can be integrated into an ever-expanding range of clinical settings, and it is our hope that readers will feel encouraged to begin this important work in their own practices.

References

Aikens, A., Nease, D. E., & Klinkman, M. S. (2008). Explaining patients' beliefs about the necessity and harmfulness of antidepressants. *Annals of Family Medicine, 6*(1), 23–29.

American Psychiatric Association. (2010). *Practice guideline for the treatment of patients with major depressive disorder* (3rd ed.). Washington, DC: Author.

Baer, R. A., Smith, G. T., Lykins, E., Button, D., Krietemeyer, J., & Sauer, S. (2008). Construct validity of the five facet mindfulness questionnaire in meditating and nonmeditating samples. *Assessment, 15,* 676–688.

Blackburn, I. M., & Moore, R. G. (1997). Controlled acute and follow-up trial of cognitive therapy and pharmacotherapy in outpatients with recurrent depression. *British Journal of Psychiatry, 171,* 328–334.

Bond, F. W., Hayes, S. C., Baer, R. A., Carpenter, K. M., Guenole, N., Orcutt, H. K., et al. (2011). Preliminary psychometric properties of the Acceptance and Action Questionnaire–II: A revised measure of psychological flexibility and experiential avoidance. *Behavior Therapy, 42,* 676–688.

Brown, G., & Jones, E. (2005). Implementation of a feedback system in a managed care environment: What are patients teaching us? *Journal of Clinical Psychology, 61,* 187–198.

Brown, T. A., & Barlow, D. H. (2014). *Anxiety and Related Disorders Interview Schedule for DSM-5 (ADIS-5)—Adult and Lifetime Version.* New York: Oxford University Press.

Cuijpers, P., Hollon, S. D., van Straten, A., Bockting, C., Berking, M., & Andersson, G. (2013). Does cognitive behaviour therapy have an enduring effect that is superior to keeping patients on continuation psychotherapy?: A meta-analysis. *BMJ Open, 3,* e002542.

Cuijpers, P., van Straten, A., van Oppen, P., & Andersson, G. (2008). Are psychological and pharmacologic interventions equally effective in the treatment of adult depressive disorders?: A meta-analysis of comparative studies. *Journal of Clinical Psychiatry, 69*(11), 1675–1685.

D'Avanzato, C., Martinez, J., Attiullah, N., Friedman, M., Toba, C., Boerescu, D., et al. (2013). Anxiety symptoms among remitted depressed outpatients: Prevalance and association with quality of life and psychosocial functioning. *Journal of Affective Disorders, 151*(1), 401–404.

D'Avanzato, C., & Zimmerman, M. (2017). The diagnosis and assessment of mood disorders. In R. J. DeRubeis & D. R. Strunk (Eds.), *The Oxford handbook of mood disorders* (pp. 95–107). New York: Oxford University Press.

Dobson, K. S., Hollon, S. D., & Dimidjian, S. (2008). Randomized trial of behavioral activation, cognitive therapy, and antidepressant medication in the prevention of relapse and recurrence in major depression. *Journal of Consulting and Clinical Psychology, 76*, 468–477.

Fernandez, E., Salem, D., Swift, J. K., & Ramtahal, N. (2015). Meta-analysis of dropout from cognitive behavioral therapy: Magnitude, timing and moderators. *Journal of Consulting and Clinical Psychology, 83*(6), 1108–1122.

First, M. B., Williams, J. B. W., Karg, R. S., & Spitzer, R. L. (2015). *Structured Clinical Interview for DSM-5 Disorders, Clinician Version (SCID-5-CV)*. Arlington, VA: American Psychiatric Association.

Fournier, J. C., DeRubeis, R. J., Hollon, S. D., Dimidjian, S., Amsterdam, J. D., Shelton, R. C., et al. (2010). Antidepressant drug effects and depression severity: A patient-level meta-analysis. *Journal of the American Medical Association, 303*(1), 47–53.

Francis, A. W., Dawson, D. L., & Golijani-Moghaddam, N. (2016). The development and validation of the Comprehensive Assessment of Acceptance and Commitment Therapy processes (CompACT). *Journal of Contextual Behavioral Science, 5*(3), 134–145.

Gaudiano, B. A., Dalrymple, K. L., D'Avanzato, C., & Bunaciu, L. (2016). The need for quality improvement in behavioral health. In W. T. O'Donahue, C. Snipes, & A. Maragakis (Eds.), *Quality improvement and behavioral health* (pp. 33–54). Cham, Switzerland: Springer.

Gloaguen, V., Cottraux, J., Cucherat, M., & Blackburn, I. M. (1998). A meta-analysis of the effects of cognitive therapy in depressed patients. *Journal of Affective Disorders, 49*, 59–72.

Gloster, A. T., Sonntag, R., Hoyer, J., Meyer, A. H., Heinze, S., Strohle, A., et al. (2015). Treating treatment-resistant patients with panic disorder and agoraphobia using psychotherapy: A randomized controlled switching trial. *Psychotherapy and Psychosomatics, 84*(2), 100–109.

Guo, T., Xiang, Y-T., Xiao, L., Hu, C-Q., Chiu, H. F. K., Ungvari, G. S., et al. (2015). Measurement-based care versus standard care for major depression: A randomized controlled trial with blind raters. *American Journal of Psychiatry, 172*(10), 1004–1013.

Harris, R. (2008). *The happiness trap*. Boston: Trumpeter.

Hayes, S. C., Luoma, J. B., Bond, F. W., & Lillis, J. (2006). Acceptance and commitment therapy: Model, process and outcomes. *Behaviour Research and Therapy, 44*(1), 1–25.

Hayes, S. C., Strosahl, K. D., & Wilson, K. G. (2011). *Acceptance and commitment therapy: The process and practice of mindful change* (2nd ed.). New York: Guilford Press.

Hollon, S. D., DeRubeis, R. J., Fawcett, J., Amsterdam, J. D., Shelton, R. C., Zajecka, J., et al. (2014). Effect of cognitive therapy with antidepressant medications vs antidepressants alone on the rate of recovery in major depressive disorder. *JAMA Psychiatry, 71*(10), 1157–1164.

Houle, J., Villaggi, B., Beaulieu, M., Lesperance, F., Rondeau, G., & Lambert, J. (2012). Treatment preferences in patients with first episode depression. *Journal of Affective Disorders, 147*, 94–100.

Howland, R. H., Rush, A. J., Wisniewski, S. R., Trivedi, M. H., Warden, D., Fava, M., et al. (2009). Concurrent anxiety and substance use disorders among outpatients with major depression: Clinical features and effect on treatment outcome. *Drug and Alcohol Dependence, 99*(1–3), 248–260.

Kirsch, I., Deacon, B. J., Huedo-Medina, T. B., Scoboria, A., Moore, T. J., & Johnson, B. T. (2008). Initial severity and antidepressant benefits: A meta-analysis of data submitted to the Food and Drug Administration. *PLoS Medicine, 5*(2), e45.

Kwan, B. M., Dimidjian, S., & Rizvi, S. L. (2010). Treatment preference, engagement, and clinical improvement in pharmacotherapy versus psychotherapy for depression. *Behaviour and Research Therapy, 48*, 799–804.

Lambert, M. J. (2007). Presidential address: What have we learned from a decade of research aimed at improving psychotherapy outcome in routine care? *Psychotherapy Research, 17*(1), 1–14.

Levin, M. E., Luoma, J. B., & Haeger, J. A. (2015). Decoupling as a mechanism of change in mindfulness and acceptance: A literature review. *Behavior Modification, 39*(6), 870–911.

McHugh, R. K., Whitton, S. W., Peckham, A. D., Welge, J. A., & Otto, M. W. (2013). Patient preference for psychological vs pharmacologic treatment of psychiatric disorders: A meta-analytic review. *Journal of Clinical Psychiatry, 74*(6), 595–602.

Melvin, G. A., Tonge, B. J., King, N. J., Heyne, D., Gordon, M. S., & Klimkeit, E. (2006). A comparison of cognitive-behavioral therapy, sertraline, and their combination for adolescent depression. *Journal of the American Academy of Child and Adolescent Psychiatry, 45*(10), 1151–1161.

Moradveisi, L., Huibers, M. J. H., & Arntz, A. (2015). The influence of patients' attributions of the immediate effects of treatment of depression on long-term effectiveness of behavioural activation and antidepressant medication. *Behaviour Research and Therapy, 69*, 83–92.

Oestergaard, S., & Moldrup, C. (2011). Optimal duration of combined psychotherapy and pharmacotherapy for patients with moderate and severe depression: A meta-analysis. *Journal of Affective Disorders, 131,* 24–36.

Olfson, M., Marcus, S. C., Tedeschi, M., & Wan, G. J. (2006). Continuity of antidepressant treatment for adults with depression in the United States. *American Journal of Psychiatry, 163*(1), 101–108.

Orsillo, S. M., & Batten, S. V. (2005). Acceptance and commitment therapy in the treatment of posttraumatic stress disorder. *Behavior Modification, 29*(1), 95–129.

Petersen, T., Andreotti, C. F., Chelminski, I., Young, D., & Zimmerman, M. (2009). Do comorbid anxiety disorders impact treatment planning for outpatients with major depressive disorder? *Psychiatry Research, 169,* 7–11.

Rosen, G. M., & Davison, G. C. (2003). Psychology should list empirically supported principles of change (ESPs) and not credential trademarked therapies or other treatment packages. *Behavior Modification, 27*(3), 300–312.

Rush, A. J., Kraemer, H. C., & Sackeim, H. A. (2006). Report by the ACNP Task Force on response and remission in major depressive disorder. *Neuropsychopharmacology, 31*(9), 1841–1853.

Shear, M. K., Greeno, C., Kang, J., Ludewig, D., Frank, E., Schwartz, H. A., et al. (2000). Diagnosis of nonpsychotic patients in community clinics. *American Journal of Psychiatry, 157,* 581–587.

Singh, N., & Reece, J. (2014). Psychotherapy, pharmacotherapy, and their combination for adolescents with major depressive disorder: A meta-analysis. *The Australian Educational and Developmental Psychologist, 31*(1), 47–65.

Smout, M., Davies, M., Burns, N., & Christie, A. (2014). Development of the Valuing Questionnaire (VQ). *Journal of Contextual Behavioral Science, 3*(3), 164–172.

Steidtmann, D., Manber, R., Arnow, B. A., Klein, D. N., Markowitz, J. C., Rothbaum, B. O., et al. (2012). Patient treatment prefernece as a predictor of response and attrition in treatment for chronic depression. *Depression and Anxiety, 29,* 896–905.

Strosahl, K. D., Robinson, P., & Gustavson, T. (2012). *Brief interventions for radical change: Principles and practice of focused acceptance and commitment therapy.* Oakland, CA: New Harbinger.

Strunk, D. R., DeRubeis, R. J., Chiu, A. W., & Alvarez, J. (2007). Patients' competence in and performance of cognitive therapy skills: Relation to the reduction of relapse risk following treatment for depression. *Journal of Consulting and Clinical Psychology, 75*(4), 523–530.

Swift, J. K., Callahan, J. L., & Vollmer, B. M. (2011). Preferences. *Journal of Clinical Psychology, 67*(2), 155–165.

Uher, R., Payne, J. L., Pavlova, B., & Perlis, R. H. (2014). Major depressive disorder in DSM-5: Implications for clinical practice and research of changes from DSM-IV. *Depression and Anxiety, 31*(6), 459–471.

Westrup, D. (2014). *Advanced acceptance and commitment therapy: The experienced practitioner's guide to optimizing delivery.* Oakland, CA: New Harbinger.

Zimmerman, M., & Chelminski, I. (2003). Clinician recognition of anxiety disorders in depressed outpatients. *Journal of Psychiatric Research, 37,* 325–333.

Zimmerman, M., & Chelminski, I. (2006). A scale to screen for DSM-IV Axis I disorders in psychiatric outpatients: Performance of the Psychiatric Diagnostic Screen Questionnaire. *Psychological Medicine, 36*(11), 1601–1611.

Zimmerman, M., Chelminski, I., McGlinchey, J. B., & Posternak, M. A. (2008). A clinically useful depression outcome scale. *Comprehensive Psychiatry, 49*(2), 131–140.

Zimmerman, M., Chelminski, I., & Pasternak, M. A. (2004). Exclusion criteria used in antidepressant efficacy trials: Consistency across studies and representativeness of samples included. *Journal of Nervous and Mental Disease, 192*(2), 87–94.

Zimmerman, M., Chelminski, I., Young, D., & Dalrymple, K. L. (2010). A clinically useful anxiety outcome scale. *Journal of Clinical Psychiatry, 71*(5), 534–542.

Zimmerman, M., & Mattia, J. I. (1999). Psychiatric diagnosis in clinical practice: Is comorbidity being missed? *Comprehensive Psychiatry, 40*(3), 182–191.

Zimmerman, M., & Mattia, J. I. (2001). The Psychiatric Diagnostic Screening Questionnaire: Development, reliability and validity. *Comprehensive Psychiatry, 42*(3), 175–189.

Zimmerman, M., & McGlinchey, J. B. (2008). Why don't psychiatrists use scales to measure outcome when treating depressed patients? *Journal of Clinical Psychiatry, 69*(12), 1916–1919.

Zimmerman, M., McGlinchey, J. B., Posternak, M. A., Friedman, M., Attiullah, N., & Boerescu, D. (2006). How should remission from depression be defined?: The depressed patient's perspective. *American Journal of Psychiatry, 163*(1), 148–150.

Zimmerman, M., Posternak, M. A., Friedman, M., Attiullah, N., Baymiller, S., Boland, R., et al. (2004). Which factors influence psychiatrists' selection of an antidepressant? *American Journal of Psychiatry, 161*(7), 1285–1289.

PART IV

TRAINING, SUPERVISION, AND CONSULTATION TO PROMOTE EVIDENCE-BASED PRACTICE

CHAPTER 23

Mental Health Training

Implications of the Clinical Science Model

ROBERT W. LEVENSON

Growing concerns about the slow pace of progress in reducing the burden of mental illness are creating new opportunities to rethink the way we approach the development, evaluation, and dissemination of treatments and assessments, and the way we train the next generation of mental health professionals. Of course, we cannot know with certainty what the future will bring. Nonetheless, there are clear trends that argue in favor of thinking about mental health and mental illness in new ways: embracing greater integration of biological, behavioral, and computational approaches; adopting multidisciplinarity as the norm rather than the exception; reaffirming the value of evidence-based practice (EBP); and realizing that there are significant gaps in our scientific knowledge. In this chapter, I review some of these trends and the implications they have for training future generations of mental health professionals for careers as scientists, practitioners, and the many hybrids that combine both.

The Clinical Science Model: Not Just for Clinical Psychology; Not Just for Scientists

Although the clinical science model (Baker, McFall, & Shoham, 2008; Levenson, 2007; McFall, 1991, 2006) was promulgated by clinical psychologists largely to address perceived problems in clinical psychology, its principles, mandates, and proposed solutions are clearly relevant to all of the mental health professions. Central to the clinical science model is the notion that science must be fully infused into all aspects of the training and careers of mental health professionals. Moreover, it envisions scientific evidence as having the deciding vote when adjudicating among available theories, etiological models, diagnostic approaches, clinician intuitions, client viewpoints, and therapeutic practices (Levenson, 2017). While sharing a commitment to the importance of science, the clinical science model differs in important ways from the older "scientist–practitioner" or "Boulder" model (Committee on Training in Clinical Psychology, 1947). In the scientist–practitioner model, research training typically proceeds in *parallel* with training in other areas (i.e., general psychology, dynamics of human behavior, related disciplines, diagnostic methods, therapy). In the clinical science model, science is fully *integrated* in all areas of training (Levenson, 2017). Having this full integration counters the "two-hat" epistemological problem (Levenson, Cowan, & Cowan, 2010) in which mental health professionals use one set of standards of evidence in the clinic (i.e., wearing the "clinical hat") and another in the laboratory (i.e., wearing the "scientist hat"). The clinical science model advocates for one hat that is worn in all settings.

Importantly, just as the clinical science model is not limited to clinical psychology, it is also not limited to the training and professional lives of scientists on the faculty at research-oriented universities and medical schools. Rather, the ability to understand, evaluate, and apply scientific knowledge is critical to all mental health professionals, regardless of whether they are primarily engaged in direct provision of mental health services, teaching, dissemination, program administration, or scientific discovery. In the coming decades, new treatments and assessment tools are likely to come from both expected and unexpected places, reflecting the wide range of disciplines and cross-disciplinary collaborations that are increasingly involved in mental health research and practice. Clinical science provides the common metric for separating the wheat from the chaff, making sure that the best and most effective discoveries are identified, translated, disseminated, and applied to address the enormous unmet mental health needs of the public.

A Hunger for Treatment, Prevention, and Cures

Even a casual observer cannot help but notice the growing number of federal grant program announcements and national conferences in recent years that emphasize developing new treatments and disseminating information concerning existing treatments. One reason for this may be the plethora of data indicating the enormity of mental illness as a public health concern. The 1999 Surgeon General's report estimated that the annual indirect cost of mental illness was $79 billion. According to a 2004 World Health Organization report, major depressive disorder was the leading cause of disability in the United States and Canada among those ages 15–44. A 2010 survey conducted by the Substance Abuse and Mental Health Services Administration (2011) found that 11 million adults in the United States (approximately 5% of the population) have a serious mental illness.

The federal appropriation for the National Institute of Mental Health (NIMH) has ranged from $1.3 to 1.5 billion annually between 2003 and 2010 (according to congressional appropriation records). This is a huge investment, but it is dwarfed by estimates of the costs of mental illness. And how are we doing in the battle with mental illness? This question begets two related ones: (1) Are we making progress in reducing the prevalence of mental illness (by prevention, curative treatments, etc.)? and (2) Are we making progress in reducing the disability and costs associated with mental illness (by treatments and rehabilitation programs that improve functioning and reduce disability)?

It turns out that answering the first of these questions is surprisingly difficult. Attempts to compare mental health prevalence data that were collected at different times and by different investigators are confounded by inconsistencies in the ways that disorders were diagnosed and reference samples were constructed. One of the best sources of information on changes in rates of mental illness over time comes from the National Comorbidity Survey, which was conducted from 1990 to 1992, then repeated a decade later from 2001 to 2003 using the same diagnostic criteria (Kessler, Chiu, Demler, & Walters, 2005). The results from these surveys are not encouraging. Examining the prevalence of DSM-IV disorders in the United States (i.e., people between ages 18 and 54 who met DSM-IV criteria for a disorder during the preceding 12-month period), there is no indication that the nation's mental health improved. Rather, the prevalence actually increased over the decade (from 29.4 to 30.5%).

In terms of the second question, reducing disability and improving function, there have been enormous problems with treatment dissemination. In one study (also based on the National Comorbidity Survey), the delay between the onset of symptoms and receiving appropriate treatments was 6–8 years for mood disorders and 9–23 years for anxiety disorder (Wang et al., 2005). Although inequities in access and utilization of mental health services undoubtedly play a significant role in explaining these delays, they also reflect the continuing challenges involved in getting community-based practitioners to utilize empirically supported treatments (McHugh & Barlow, 2010; Weisz, Ng, & Bearman, 2014; Weisz et al., 2009). With these extremely sobering numbers and the attendant increases in public pressures, the growing emphasis on treatment development and dissemination is not surprising.

Caught between Two Worlds: The DSM and Research Domain Criteria

The Delaware Project on Clinical Science Training was held in October 2011 to advance a redefinition of clinical science training in psychology. The National Institutes of Health (NIH) model for treatment development (Onken, Carroll, Shoham, Cuthbert, & Riddle, 2014) was presented at the outset of the meeting to underscore the importance of training students to be able to develop and disseminate new treatments. Ironically, this model affords little attention to the assessment of mental illness. This is probably because the model was formulated under the assumption that the DSM would continue to serve as the primary basis for organizing treatment development in the future. Thus, the targets of treatment development and dissemination would largely be Axis I (e.g., bipolar disorder) and Axis II (e.g., borderline personality disorder) disorders. However, by the time this model was presented at the Delaware Project meeting, there clearly was an 800-pound gorilla in the room. Many of the attendees were already familiar with the new NIMH Research Domain Criteria (RDoC) project (Cuthbert & Insel, 2010b; Cuthbert & Insel, 2013), having participated in the various RDoC planning meetings. RDoC (discussed in greater detail below) does not focus on DSM clinical syndromes such as bipolar disorder or borderline personality disorder. Rather it focuses on behaviors, neural circuits, biomarkers, and dimensions of functioning. In an RDoC-centric world, a treatment development model would place major emphasis on assessment, including developing, evaluating, and disseminating new assessment methods that could be used to identify targets for intervention and to evaluate the effectiveness of treatments.

Clinical Science Training in an RDoC-Centric World

RDoC (Cuthbert & Insel, 2010b; Cuthbert & Insel, 2013) aims to provide a new way of classifying mental disorders that is based on "dimensions of neurobiology and observable behavior." This approach is quite different from that found in the current psychiatric diagnostic systems (e.g., the American Psychiatric Association's DSM-5, the World Health Organization's ICD-11), which seek to identify particular syndromes on the basis of presenting signs and symptoms. Although the framers of RDoC carefully noted that it was designed as a research classification system rather than one intended for routine clinical use (Cuthbert & Insel, 2013), it may be difficult to maintain this distinction. If RDoC generates a new body of exciting, clinically relevant research findings, the "just for research" mantra will likely be drowned out by questions concerning "What can this do to help relieve the burden of mental illness?" Regardless, clinical scientists and practitioners are going to want to be deeply involved in this new approach to understanding mental illness. Thus, their students will need to be trained in ways that enable them to conduct science and deliver and evaluate services productively in an RDoC-centric world.

The problems inherent in the DSM have been well documented over the decades (Cuthbert & Insel, 2010a; Widiger & Sankis, 2000). Although significant progress has been made in increasing the reliability of certain diagnoses, the ultimate validity and utility of these diagnoses is undercut by a host of factors, including (1) high levels of comorbidity across disorders, (2) lack of specificity in etiology, (3) lack of specificity in pharmacological and behavioral treatments, (4) particular symptoms (e.g., fear) appear in multiple disorders, and (5) broad syndromes (e.g., schizophrenia, major depression), have multiple variants that could be better characterized as different disorders and multiple symptoms that could be better studied and treated separately.

Moreover, as the tools for assessing the genes, molecules, and neural circuits that determine behavior have become dramatically more precise and refined in recent years, attempts to link them with the broad heterogeneous DSM syndromes have seemed increasingly misguided. In addition, increases in the reliability of DSM diagnosis have not produced attendant improvements in the sobering public health statistics described earlier related to the prevalence of mental illness, the associated burden, and the problems associated with developing treatments and applying them to improve the lives of the mentally ill. Finally, even the best of our evidence-based treatments appear to be losing their effectiveness over time (e.g., declining symptom reduction and remission rates for treatment of depression by cognitive-behavioral therapy between 1978 and 2013; Johnsen & Friborg, 2015). For all these reasons, momentum is building for trying a different approach.

RDoC: The Basic Framework

RDoC focuses on behavior and neurobiology. It begins by asking what range of behaviors has the brain evolved to carry out and what neural systems are responsible for implementing these behaviors (Cuthbert & Insel, 2013). Thus, for a behavior to be included in RdoC, there must be a plausibly associated brain circuit. Because the granularity of RDoC is constrained by the state of current neurobiological knowledge, the behavioral units are called *constructs,* leaving the door open for additional validation and revision on the basis of future knowledge.

RDoC next specifies the range of variation in each behavioral construct from normal to abnormal. Thus, behaviors in RDoC are inherently neither good nor bad, but rather represent dimensions that encompass a range of normal and abnormal functioning. Moreover, these dimensions are not necessarily unipolar. For many behaviors, abnormality is associated with both extremes (e.g., having too much or having too little fear are both problematic).

The October 2012 iteration of RDoC (Cuthbert & Insel, 2013) dramatically illustrates how it differs from DSM syndromes. In this version, five domains are elaborated along with their associated behavioral constructs: (1) negative valence systems (acute threat, potential threat, sustained threat, loss, frustrative nonreward); (2) positive valence systems (approach motivation, initial responsiveness to reward, sustained responsiveness to reward, reward learning, habit); (3) cognitive systems (attention, perception, working memory, declarative memory, language behavior, cognitive control); (4) systems for social processes (affiliation and attachment, social communication, perception and understanding of self, perception and understanding of others); and (5) arousal/modulatory systems (arousal, biological rhythms, sleep–wake cycles).

RDoC also provides a framework for examining behavioral constructs at multiple levels of analysis, including genes, molecules, cells, physiology, behavior, and self-reports. Importantly, it also specifies the laboratory paradigms that are used to assess these constructs. Thus, RDoC would apply precise behavioral and biological measures developed in the laboratory to clinical phenomena that have traditionally been assessed using clinician and caregiver observations and patient reports.

Clinical Practice in an RDoC-Centric World: An Imaginary Scenario

What would things look like if RDoC caught on and became the basis for clinical practice? To help illustrate this, imagine the following scenario:

Jim, a 50-year old man with no prior history of major psychiatric illness, is experiencing what he describes as emotional "numbness." This is manifested in a general low level of enthusiasm and lack of enjoyment for work and family activities, once sources of great joy. He has been able to work effectively and his family has remained intact, but he expresses concerns about how his problems ultimately will affect his work and family in the future.

Jim makes an appointment at the Psychological Services Center at a major university for evaluation and treatment. He participates in a daylong assessment that includes structured clinical interviews, functional and structural neuroimaging, genotyping, and laboratory-based observational tests of emotional and cognitive functioning. The results of Jim's assessment are reviewed by a multidisciplinary team that represents psychology, psychiatry, pharmacology, neurology, affective science, and cognitive science. The team concludes that (1) the emotional deficits are characterized by blunted responding in facial expressive behavior, but autonomic responding is at normal levels; (2) the emotional deficits are more pronounced in experienced affect than in anticipated affect; (3) there are pervasive deficits in executive functioning, especially in the realm of measures of cognitive flexibility; (4) volumetric analysis of structural brain scans indicates that brain regions involved in emotion generation and regulation show no evidence of accelerated neurodegeneration; (5) diffusion tensor imaging indicates that major frontal–subcortical networks are intact; (6) genetic analyses reveal a pattern of allelic variations in serotonin and dopamine genes, consistent with high levels of environmental sensitivity; and (7) the medical history includes a cardiac arrhythmia that is currently being treated with a high dose of a broad spectrum beta-blocker.

In consultation with the multidisciplinary team, Jim's primary mental health provider formulates a treatment plan that includes (1) systematic evaluation of the extent to which the current cardiac medication is contributing to the depressed emotional functioning and medication changes, if indicated; (2) careful examination of the patients' home and work environments to identify contextual triggers and reinforcers that are contributing to reduced emotional reactivity, and creation of a plan for modifying these environmental factors; (3) a targeted intervention that focuses on enhancing moment-to-moment emotional experience and expression; and (4) a training program designed to improve low-level executive functioning.

The plan is to treat Jim for 3 months, then, if there is no significant improvement, refer him for evaluation of suitability for two new treatments for emotional blunting, one using a targeted drug delivery system that increases serotonin levels in brain areas critical to emotion generation and the other using deep-brain stimulation to activate these same brain areas, combined with transcranial magnetic stimulation to inhibit emotion regulatory centers in the dorsolateral prefrontal cortex.

Implications for Training

The foregoing scenario is, of course, fictional. It attempts to extrapolate from the RDoC framework and current scientific trends to envision what clinical practice might look like in a not-too-distant future. How accurately this scenario portrays that future remains to be seen, but this kind of a science-based, multidisciplinary approach to assessment, case formulation, and treatment is already being used in some areas of medicine and could certainly be applied in mental health domains as well.

If we assume that this envisioning of the post-RDoC world is at least partially accurate, it raises the question of whether mental health professionals are currently being trained in ways that will enable them to play major roles in advancing science and practice or that their training will cause them to become increasingly marginalized or even irrelevant. For those with long memories, predictions of an imminent revolution in mental health service delivery, along with an associated tsunami of changes rippling through traditional training programs, may seem familiar (e.g., Albee, 1970). Are we

in fact on the verge of a true revolution? Or will this be yet another instance that proves the adage "the more things change, the more they remain the same"? The ultimate answer to this question will only be revealed over time; but for now, I believe that there is value in seriously entertaining the possibility that the changes that will occur in mental health assessment, treatment, and research in the future are going to be pervasive and profound. If this does prove to be the case, then shouldn't we be doing everything possible to ensure that the graduates of our training programs are well prepared for the changes that lie ahead?

Coursework

In an RDoC-centric world, trainees would need to take substantial coursework in genetics, physiology, anatomy, and neuroscience, areas that are not typically required in most curricula. They also will need to take courses in the other areas that are most relevant to RDoC domains, including cognition, emotion, social processes, development, learning, and personality. Such courses will need to provide in-depth exposure to the newest paradigms, theories, and methods. These requirements are a far cry from the "broad and general" exposure historically required for accreditation of doctoral-level training of mental health professionals by the American Psychological Association (Commission on Accreditation, 2009). In addition, rather than having separate courses that cover "normal" and "abnormal" behavior, all courses would need to address the full range of functioning. In many training programs, such courses do not currently exist, creating challenges in curriculum development for faculty in both clinical and nonclinical areas.

Research Training

Programs that provide doctoral-level training for students will need to consider the level of expertise their students should have in the various subareas that are relevant to mental health research. If the goal is to train students who are capable of assuming leadership roles in the multidisciplinary research teams that will work on these complex multilevel problems, then it will be critical that they gain hands-on experience working on these kinds of problems in these kinds of teams. Work in the laboratory of the primary mentor will need to be augmented with experiences working with other mentors and in other laboratories if students are to obtain the necessary breadth and depth of research experience.

In the current version of clinical science training, students often struggle to find time to conduct research with a single mentor amid the demands of required courses, teaching assistantships, clinical work, and other obligations. In this new era, as clinical science students engage in multiple training rotations and pursue demanding, time-intensive research projects, it will be critical to find ways to make more time available for research training.

Practicum Training

Practicum training will also need to change in this new era. Opportunities will need to be developed that allow for extensive observation and direct exposure to a range of patients with different kinds and severity of dysfunction. Because many forms of dysfunction will be identified and treated in laboratory settings, a significant amount of experience with clinical assessment and treatment may be obtained in these kinds of settings as opposed to more traditional clinical training sites. With the increasing importance afforded to underlying neural circuits, trainees will benefit from extensive exposure to neuropathology, in addition to psychopathology. Particularly valuable will be experience with neurological disorders that produce psychiatric-like syndromes (e.g., affective blunting in frontotemporal dementia, hallucinations in Lewy body disease, depression in Parkinson's disease, and affective dysregulation in amyotrophic lateral sclerosis) (Levenson & Miller, 2007; Olney et al., 2011).

The new era will be characterized by different treatment options, some traditional and others not. In terms of the former, behavioral and psychosocial treatments will continue to play an important role, but they may be oriented toward smaller units of dysfunction (e.g., reward prediction errors) rather than larger problems (e.g., anhedonia) or syndromes (e.g., schizoaffective disorder). Other treatments will be more biological, targeting the neural circuits and genes that underlie specific areas of functioning. Already, there are treatments that target neural circuits using deep brain stimulation (Holtzheimer et al., 2012), transcranial magnetic stimulation, and biofeedback. As new drug delivery systems become available, pharmacological treatments

may become more targeted, more effective, and have fewer side effects. New research on gene expression and new methods for controlling the action of genes (Deisseroth et al., 2006) represent another frontier for new treatment approaches.

Treatment will always be a moving target. As new understanding of dysfunction and new approaches to its alleviation are developed, new treatments will come online. Thus, training that emphasizes problem-centered learning, with the goal of developing expertise in the entire process of treatment development and dissemination, will continue to be critical.

Assessment Training

Students will need to gain experience with a broad range of new assessment techniques, including genetic assays, structural and functional neuroimaging, observational coding of behavior, and laboratory-based paradigms (e.g., for testing executive functioning, emotion regulation, and reward estimation). Clinical scientists will be expected to play an increasingly important role in the development of new, effective assessment methods that can be moved from the laboratory to the research clinic, and ultimately into the hands of community practitioners.

Obstacles to Overcome

When it comes to mental health, change will not come easily. Any change in how mental illness is conceptualized, classified, or treated will have profound effects on practitioners, scientists, educators, insurers, advocacy groups, drug companies, patients, families, and many, many others. As compelling as the RDoC approach might seem, it is bound to encounter obstacles.

Inertia in Academia

The scope of changes envisioned here would have profound implications both for training programs and for their parent academic departments. Many faculty members, trained in accordance with more traditional models, may feel unprepared to teach and supervise research and practica in these new ways. Getting consensus for these kinds of changes will be an enormous challenge. Although a "wait and see" approach may have its appeal, this may be a once-in-a-generation opportunity for training programs that embrace the clinical science model to assume leadership roles in moving their departments and broader mental health systems in important new directions.

The DSM

The DSM-5 has numerous improvements and refinements that should help improve the reliability of diagnosis. However, as noted earlier, there are many reasons to doubt that it represents the best approach for guiding future research, assessment, and clinical practice. Here again, change will not come easily. Every diagnosis in the DSM has an associated cottage industry of measures, theories, treatments, paradigms, affordances, reimbursements, streams of research funding, and careers that create a huge vested interest in maintaining some version of the status quo.

Accreditation

Accreditation in all mental health-related fields plays a major role in shaping training program curricula, practicum requirements, and the allocation of faculty and student time and resources. Training programs in clinical psychology, for example, currently have two accreditation options (Levenson, 2017). The newer option is the Psychological Science Accreditation System (PCSAS), which, as of this writing, has accredited 39 doctoral programs in clinical psychology that follow the clinical science model (Baker et al., 2008). PCSAS accreditation places heavy emphasis on "outcomes," carefully examining whether graduates are creating and applying science in their careers. Because it affords less emphasis on "process," it allows programs maximal flexibility in the ways they train their students and utilize available resources to produce the desired outcomes. This flexibility would greatly facilitate the changes in training necessary in an RDoC-centric world.

The older option is the American Psychological Association's Commission on Accreditation, which, as of this writing, has accredited 396 doctoral programs in clinical, counseling, and school psychology. Compared with PCSAS, American Psychological Association accreditation places far greater emphasis on the training "process" (e.g., particular courses, topics, and practicum experiences). In recent years, Ameri-

can Psychological Association accreditation has recognized alternative training models (including clinical science); however, the core requirements for curriculum and practicum experiences were the same for all models (Commision on Accreditation, 2009). In the newest version of the American Psychological Association (2015) accreditation policy, there is a single unified "health service psychology" model.

An area of increasing contention in recent years has been the requirement that students receive "broad and general" training (Zlotlow, Nelson, & Peterson, 2011) through graduate-level coursework in a number of designated areas of psychology (e.g., human development, biological aspects of behavior, cognitive and affective aspects of behavior, history and systems). For clinical science programs, and especially in an RDoC-centric world, it makes more sense to have students take more "focused and specific" courses that cover the specialized, cutting-edge knowledge in the other areas of psychology (Berenbaum & Shoham, 2011).

I expect that in the other mental health disciplines, there are similar concerns as to whether requirements for accreditation facilitate or impede needed changes. It is my hope that these concerns can be addressed and needed changes are implemented in collaborative rather than acrimonious ways.

An Unfortunate Firewall

Within psychology, historically, mental illness has largely been the exclusive province of clinical psychology. In fact, students from other areas of psychology are often actively excluded from receiving clinical training and from being exposed to clinical phenomena. A strong movement at the NIMH in recent years toward a greater investment in mission-critical research and the related increased emphasis on translational science has encouraged scientists from nonclinical areas of psychology to work on problems related to mental health and illness. These trends could be strengthened by providing some applied clinical training and exposure to clinical phenomena for students in nonclinical areas. Broadening training in this way across the mental health disciplines would dramatically increase the number of scientists who work on issues related to mental illness in the future. Fresh eyes combined with new energy, methods, and insights can help lead to the scientific breakthroughs that are sorely needed in treatment development and other areas of mental illness research. RDoC, with its stated agnosticism regarding existing DSM diagnoses, its focus on behaviors that have well-established neural underpinnings, and its interest in behaviors that have normal and abnormal manifestations, seems particularly well suited to this more inclusive approach to training.

Conclusions

The importance of developing scientifically based treatments is clearly seen in the increased emphasis at NIMH (1999) on translational research, the emergence of the clinical science movement (Baker et al., 2008), and the new RDoC framework for guiding mental health research (Cuthbert & Insel, 2013). These developments all have profound implications for mental health training. But what kind of training will be needed to produce scientists and practitioners who thrive in this new era, assume leadership positions in the field of assessment and treatment development, and help lead the charge for needed reforms in the diagnosis and treatment of mental illness?

In the broadest sense, the practical training we provide to our students should prepare them to identify treatment needs, design evidence-based treatments (EBT), market interventions, evaluate treatment efficacy, and disseminate the products and outcomes to others. This is an alternative to training that primarily prepares students to be experts in administering a set of EBT procedures, many of which will likely be supplanted by new approaches in the future. Here pedagogical models and public health finances converge, with ample evidence that EBTs can be delivered as effectively and at much lower cost by mental health specialists with associate, bachelor's, and master's degrees compared to those with doctoral training (Berman & Norton, 1985; Christensen & Jacobson, 1994).

The emergence of RDoC shows promise of being a major game-changer. Symptom-based and dimensional approaches to clinical diagnosis have certainly been proposed before (e.g., Krueger, Watson, & Barlow, 2005). However, RDoC differs in its focus on small units of behaviors that are plausibly linked to underlying neural circuits, molecules, and genes; that can be precisely measured; and that span a range of

normal to abnormal functioning. At this juncture, it is impossible to know whether RDoC will endure and flourish or just be another interesting idea that did not gain sufficient traction to survive. But the weight of the NIMH bully pulpit, the commitment of a significant portion of NIMH research funding to RDoC-based research, and the promise of having a set of mental illness-relevant constructs that are of sufficiently fine granularity to forge links with recent advances in neuroscience and molecular genetics may create the perfect storm for fomenting a revolutionary change in the understanding, assessment, and treatment of mental illness.

An RDoC-centric world would have profound implications for mental health training. The kinds of knowledge and expertise needed to navigate the RDoC framework successfully draw heavily on neuroscience and genetics, and on laboratory paradigms used to measure behavioral functioning developed in other areas of behavioral science. Students in most mental health disciplines currently do not receive a great deal of training in these areas, even in the most science-oriented training programs.

Clearly, with so much that is new, this is another excellent opportunity for problem-based learning approaches that do not give students answers (which in these domains do not yet exist) but rather give them the tools to seek those answers. Faced with the disparities between the demands of the RDoC world and current training emphases, and confronted with powerful impediments to change (e.g., accreditation requirements, existing allegiances to the DSM), mental health training may soon find itself at a crossroads. It can remain where it is now, waiting on the sidelines to see what changes actually occur, then try mightily to catch up. Or the field can begin to change now, seize the moment, figure out how to move the immovable, and set out to train a new generation of students who can help lead the way into the coming era of mental health science and practice.

Epilogue

As noted earlier, much of this chapter comes from a paper I wrote following the Delaware Conference (Levenson, 2014). In the ensuing years, significant changes have occurred in the clinical science movement, at the NIMH, and in the United States at large.

In the clinical science movement, leadership changes occurred following the deaths of Varda Shoham and Richard Bootzin and Richard McFall's retirement as Executive Director at PCSAS. In the aftermath of the revelations concerning American Psychological Association involvement in the CIA's "enhanced interrogation" of prisoners (Hoffman, et al., 2015), a summit of clinical science organizations was held in Chicago in August 2015, leading to the formation of a new clinical science umbrella organization, the Coalition for the Advancement and Application of Psychological Science (CAAPS), which is now actively involved in a range of issues including clinical science training.

At NIMH, Director Thomas Insel stepped down in 2015 and was replaced by Joshua Gordon, who, in one of his first public statements, noted the importance of brain circuits and mathematical/computational approaches in attempts to alleviate the burden of mental illness. Dr. Gordon noted that he thought RDoC was potentially very valuable and would likely be continued. Related to computation, "big data" are increasingly becoming an important part of health care decision making and research. These factors will combine to create demands for additional training that competes for our students' time and energy.

The dynamic nature of RDoC constructs and their potential for being changed as a result of new scientific discoveries was illustrated recently when the NIMH announced that the positive valence domain would be reorganized and expanded to include new constructs (e.g., probabilistic and reinforcement learning) derived from contemporary computational, human neuroimaging, and nonhuman animal research (National Institute of Mental Health, 2018). This flexibility and responsiveness to new evidence is encouraging, standing in stark contrast to the many proposed changes to the DSM that were ultimately rejected and relegated to appendices in the latest version (American Psychiatric Association, 2013).

Finally, at the national level, a new President has taken office, along with a new cabinet (there have already been two different Secretaries of Health and Human Services) and new leadership throughout the branches of government. Moreover, with ever more common and highly visible acts of public violence and continuing increases in suicide rates, the importance of mental health in the agenda of public discourse is growing. How these developments will affect mental health policy and research support remains to be seen.

Although there is much that is uncertain and many challenges lie ahead, there will also be unprecedented opportunities to move mental health training in rewarding new directions. Throughout the mental health professions, the clinical science model is likely to play a critical role in helping guide these changes.

Acknowledgments

In 2014, I wrote an article on clinical science training (Levenson, 2014) based on a presentation I made at the Delaware Project on Clinical Science Training that was held in 2011. The original article included sections on Berkeley's specialty clinics, which provide a novel model for integrating science and practice in practicum training, and on the future of clinical science training. Because I was trained as a clinical psychologist and have spent my entire career as a faculty member in university-based clinical psychology programs, I am most familiar with that role and that kind of training. Nonetheless, in this updated and expanded version of the original article, I have tried to make these issues and ideas applicable to the training of both scientists and practitioners, as well as to other mental health professions. I thank Sage Publications and the Association for Psychological Science for their permission to reproduce sections from the original article.

References

Albee, G. W. (1970). The uncertain future of clinical psychology. *American Psychologist, 25,* 1071–1080.

American Psychiatric Association. (2013). *Diagnostic and statistical manual of mental disorders* (5th ed.). Arlington, VA: Author.

American Psychological Association. (2015). *Standards of accreditation for health service psychology.* Washington, DC: Author.

Baker, T. B., McFall, R. M., & Shoham, V. (2008). Current status and future prospects of clinical psychology: Toward a scientifically principled approach to mental and behavioral health care. *Psychological Science in the Public Interest, 9,* 67–103.

Berenbaum, H., & Shoham, V. (2011). Broad and cutting-edge training in applied psychology: A clinical science perspective. *Training and Education in Professional Psychology, 5,* 22–29.

Berman, J. S., & Norton, N. C. (1985). Does professional training make a therapist more effective? *Psychological Bulletin, 98,* 401–407.

Christensen, A., & Jacobson, N. S. (1994). Who (or what) can do psychotherapy: The status and challenge of nonprofessional therapies. *Psychological Science, 5,* 8–14.

Commission on Accreditation. (2009). *Guidelines and principles for accreditation of programs in professional psychology.* Washington, DC: American Psychological Association.

Committee on Training in Clinical Psychology. (1947). Recommended graduate training program in clinical psychology. *American Psychologist, 2,* 539–558.

Cuthbert, B. N., & Insel, T. R. (2010a). The data of diagnosis: New approaches to psychiatric classification. *Psychiatry, 73,* 311–314.

Cuthbert, B. N., & Insel, T. R. (2010b). Toward new approaches to psychotic disorders: The NIMH Research Domain Criteria project. *Schizophrenia Bulletin, 36,* 1061–1062.

Cuthbert, B. N., & Insel, T. R. (2013). Toward the future of psychiatric diagnosis: The seven pillars of RDoC. *Biomed Central Medicine, 11,* 126.

Deisseroth, K., Feng, G., Majewska, A. K., Miesenbock, G., Ting, A., & Schnitzer, M. J. (2006). Next-generation optical technologies for illuminating genetically targeted brain circuits. *Journal of Neuroscience, 26,* 10380–10386.

Hoffman, D. H., Carter, D. J., Lopez, C. R. V., Benzmiller, H. L., Guo, A. X., Latifi, S. Y., et al. (2015). *Report to the special committee of the Board of Directors of the American Psychological Association.* Chicago: Sidley Austin.

Holtzheimer, P. E., Kelley, M. E., Gross, R. E., Filkowski, M. M., Garlow, S .J., Barrocas, A., et al. (2012). Subcallosal cingulate deep brain stimulation for treatment-resistant unipolar and bipolar depression. *Archives of General Psychiatry, 69,* 150–158.

Johnsen, T. J., & Friborg, O. (2015). The effects of cognitive behavioral therapy as an anti-depressive treatment is falling: A meta-analysis. *Psychological Bulletin, 141,* 747–768.

Kessler, R. C., Chiu, W. T., Demler, O., & Walters, E. E. (2005). Prevalence, severity, and comorbidity of 12-month DSM-IV disorders in the National Comorbidity Survey Replication. *Archives of General Psychiatry, 62,* 617–627.

Krueger, R. F., Watson, D., & Barlow, D. H. (2005). Introduction to the special section: Toward a dimensionally based taxonomy of psychopathology. *Journal of Abnormal Psychology, 114,* 491–493.

Levenson, R. W. (2007). The future of the clinical science movement: Challenges, issues, and opportunities. In T. A. Treat, R. R. Bootzin, & T. B. Baker (Eds.), *Psychological clinical science: Papers in honor of Richard M. McFall* (pp. 349–360). New York: Psychology Press.

Levenson, R. W. (2014). The future of clinical science training: New challenges and opportunities. *Psychological Clinical Science, 2,* 35–45.

Levenson, R. W. (2017). Clinical psychology training: Accreditation and beyond. *Annual Review of Clinical Psychology, 13,* 1–22.

Levenson, R. W., Cowan, C. P., & Cowan, P. A. (2010). A specialty clinic model for clinical science training: Translating couples research into practice in the Berkeley Couples Clinic. In M. S. Schulz, M. K. Pruett, P. K. Kerig, & R. D. Parke (Eds.), *Strengthening couple relationships for optimal child development: Lessons from research and intervention* (pp. 197–209). Washington, DC: American Psychological Association.

Levenson, R. W., & Miller, B. L. (2007). Loss of cells—loss of self: Frontotemporal lobar degeneration and human emotion. *Current Directions in Psychological Science, 16,* 289–294.

McFall, R. M. (1991). Manifesto for a science of clinical psychology. *The Clinical Psychologist, 44,* 75–88.

McFall, R. M. (2006). Doctoral training in clinical psychology. *Annual Review of Clinical Psychology, 2,* 21–49.

McHugh, R. K., & Barlow, D. H. (2010). The dissemination and implementation of evidence-based psychological treatments: A review of current efforts. *American Psychologist, 65,* 73–84.

National Institute of Mental Health. (1999). *Report of the National Advisory Mental Health Council's Behavioral Science Workgroup: Translating behavioral science into action.* Washington, DC: Author.

National Institute of Mental Health. (2018). *RDoC changes to the matrix CMAT workgroup update: Proposed positive valence domain revisions.* Washington, DC: National Institute of Mental Health.

Olney, N. T., Goodkind, M. S., Lomen-Hoerth, C., Whalen, P. K., Williamson, C. A., Holley, D. E., et al. (2011). Behaviour, physiology and experience of pathological laughing and crying in amyotrophic lateral sclerosis. *Brain, 134,* 3458–3469.

Onken, L. S., Carroll, K. M., Shoham, V., Cuthbert, B. N., & Riddle, M. (2014). Reenvisioning clinical science: Unifying the discipline to improve the public health. *Clinical Psychological Science, 2,* 22–34.

Substance Abuse and Mental Health Services Administration. (2011). *Results from the 2010 National Survey on Drug Use and Health: Summary of national findings.* Rockville, MD: Author.

Surgeon General. (1999). *Mental health: A report of the Surgeon General.* Rockville, MD: National Institute of Mental Health.

Wang, P. S., Berglund, P. A., Olfson, M., Pincus, H. A., Wells, K. B., & Kessler, R. C. (2005). Failure and delay in initial treatment contact after first onset of mental disorders in the National Comorbidity Survey Replication. *Archives of General Psychiatry, 62,* 603–613.

Weisz, J. R., Ng, M. Y., & Bearman, S. K. (2014). Odd couple?: Reenvisioning the relation between science and practice in the dissemination–implementation era. *Clinical Psychological Science, 2,* 58–74.

Weisz, J. R., Southam-Gerow, M. A., Gordis, E. B., Connor-Smith, J. K., Chu, B. C., Langer, D. A., et al. (2009). Cognitive-behavioral therapy versus usual clinical care for youth depression: An initial test of transportability to community clinics and clinicians. *Journal of Consulting and Clinical Psychology, 77,* 383–396.

Widiger, T. A., & Sankis, L. M. (2000). Adult psychopathology: Issues and controversies. *Annual Review of Psychology, 51,* 377–404.

World Health Organization. (2004). *The world health report 2004—changing history.* Geneva: Author.

Zlotlow, S. F., Nelson, P. D., & Peterson, R. L. (2011). The history of broad and general education in scientific psychology: The foundation for professional psychology education and training. *Training and Education in Professional Psychology, 5,* 1–8.

CHAPTER 24

The Role of the Consultation Team in Supporting Therapists and Preventing Burnout

CHARLES R. SWENSON

The work of psychotherapists—to alleviate suffering and transform human behavioral patterns—is extraordinarily complex. Therapists must select among a multitude of strategies, in addition to determining the timing and tact with which each one is implemented, to address targets that are influenced by a massive number of variables. Patients' responses to each intervention are difficult to predict, and early outcomes may provide few clues to eventual outcomes, even in cases that eventually succeed. The complexity of what is being attempted, including the range of intervention choices and the uncertain nature of both proximal and distal outcomes, can lead to anxiety, minimal immediate reinforcement of therapeutic choices, and low or wavering therapeutic confidence. The framework of evidence-based practice (EBP) not only supports therapists in navigating the complexities and uncertainties of clinical work but also demands that therapists learn specific protocols and apply them in ways that are sensitive to patient preferences, context, and needs.

Working so intimately with suffering individuals also often elicits intense emotions in therapists, some of which result from strong feelings of connection and attachment to one's patients. Caring deeply about one's patients may enhance patients' outcomes and therapeutic satisfaction, but it also can magnify stress on the therapist. First, there is the sense of hopeless-

ness and demoralization if this very demanding and complex work does not result in success. Moreover, since therapists commonly expose themselves to the graphic details of heartbreaking human experience of loss, neglect, mistreatment, trauma, and family dysfunction, they may internalize such experiences so thoroughly that they suffer along with their patients. They may experience what is otherwise known as *vicarious traumatization,* suffering with their own experiences of anxiety, depression, repetitive nightmares, insomnia, hypervigilance, troubling somatic sensations, and generalized fear responses. In my first job as a psychiatrist, when I treated a large number of Vietnam veterans at a Veterans Administration Medical Center, I listened carefully to many stories of experiencing near death, observing death of close friends in combat, experiencing and observing torture and suffering, and making agonizing choices regarding whether to end enemy lives, including lives of young people and families. Those stories disrupted my equilibrium at the time, and the faces of those patients remain in my memory today.

Thus, psychotherapists doing EBPs face both technical and personal challenges in their work. The technical challenge is to acquire, strengthen, and apply treatment principles and techniques correctly. The personal challenge is to maintain one's resilience as a person and motivation as a therapist in the context of close relationships with one's clients and repeated exposure to the experiences of suffering. These are interdependent tasks. Achieving technical proficiency helps the therapist to stay on track, to build confidence, and to reinforce motivation in both parties. Maintaining resiliency and motivation strengthens the therapist's capacity to achieve technical proficiency without sacrificing flexibility and spontaneity, and helps protect the therapist from burnout over time.

Often, training approaches do not include specific guidelines about how to attend to these interdependent tasks. In this chapter I initially explore how it is that therapist burnout can result from work of this kind, particularly with individuals who are severely emotionally dysregulated. In the case of one EBP, dialectical behavior therapy (DBT), a required modality, the DBT consultation team, is specifically designed to help therapists stay on track to practice the model with adherence; to continue to learn and improve as therapists; and to detect, prevent, and treat burnout in each therapist. I describe key features of the DBT consultation team, how those features support DBT therapists technically and personally, and how the team goes about detecting and dealing with burnout. It might be that other EBPs could benefit from a similar modality, adapting features from the DBT example. This may be relevant for all therapists practicing EBPs, but in particular, it may be useful for those in training.

Challenges of Doing (and Learning) EBPs

The previously mentioned stressors in the work of the psychotherapist are joined by additional stressors in the practice of EBPs.

Doing an EBP can reduce some types of stress, while increasing others. Following a manual that prescribes certain structural features, a schedule of interventions per session and per situation, and guidelines for selecting among treatment strategies can give a therapist a sense of knowing what to do under all circumstances, thereby reducing uncertainty and increasing confidence. Furthermore, knowing that the treatment has been proven to lead to positive outcomes can reassure and inspire the therapist. But when a therapist overrides "natural," spontaneous, instinctual, heartfelt relational tendencies by adhering religiously to the protocols of a manual, treatments can lose

flexibility and aliveness. The dual pressures to practice correctly and to suppress or suspend one's own spontaneous "healing" instincts can be stressful, contributing toward burnout. For some, these very pressures lead them to forgo the use of manualized treatment altogether. Yet EBPs are preferable in order to get the best outcomes. The dialectical task is to find the right balance between adhering to the treatment manual sufficiently to get the best outcomes, while at the same time remaining present, natural, spontaneous, and aligned with one's self. As an analogy, a global positioning system (the "manual") helps a driver by providing standardized directions, but even the best GPS cannot tell the driver how to drive or what the current road conditions are. The DBT consultation team is designed to help therapists align with the treatment model, align with one's self, and by doing so getting the best outcomes and preventing therapist burnout.

The strain of doing an EBP often is greater when treating individuals with severe emotional dysregulation and behavioral dyscontrol. Such patients typically present with several disorders, requiring that therapists be prepared to shift gears frequently and quickly among treatment targets. Crises are typical events in these patients' lives, including life-threatening behaviors at times, which repeatedly disrupt the therapist who is trying to stick to a treatment plan. It is often necessary to know not just one but many treatments to serve such patients well. Also, certain in-session behaviors of these patients are highly stressful for therapists: extreme noncompliance with agreed-upon practice assignments, suicidal threats which then require therapeutic focus, and intense anger directed at the therapist.

All therapists doing EBPs labor under the weight of these challenges, and many are magnified among therapists in training. They are learning a new vocabulary, learning how and when to use that vocabulary, dealing with additional relationships with teachers and supervisors, and facing the typical stresses of doing therapy as enumerated earlier. They are anxiously trying to stick to a treatment model and a treatment manual, and their work is (ideally) under scrutiny. They are even more likely than experienced therapists to sacrifice their natural response inclinations to the vocabulary and protocols that they are learning. For instance, one trainee therapist in a DBT program had learned that he was to provide skills coaching to his patients over the phone after work hours. In his first DBT case, the patient called him day and night, left messages, and when they did speak, she would devalue his efforts and almost never follow his suggestions. But because he thought he was following the protocol, he continued to take the calls in spite of his growing frustration and resentment, and his declining self-esteem. By the time he brought the problem up in the consultation team, his level of burnout was already rather advanced. The team helped him to correct course, helping him to establish a technically correct phone coaching approach, while supporting his need for personal limits, which then improved his motivation. The consultation team provides a cohesive package of technical and motivational support for the therapist in training, learning to apply EBPs effectively.

The Nature and the Toll of Therapist Burnout

The groundbreaking work of Maslach, Schaufeli, and Leiter (2001) established a field of research focused on burnout in the workplace. They defined *burnout* as "a prolonged response to chronic emotional and interpersonal stressors on the job, . . . defined by the three dimensions of exhaustion, cynicism, and inefficacy" (p. 397). The construct of burnout overlaps with others in the literature, including "compassion fatigue and secondary traumatic stress disorder" (Figley, 1995), "caregiver fatigue" (Schulz & Sherwood, 2008), "vicarious traumatization" (Bloom, 2003), and shares similarities with "combat fatigue" (shell shock) among those who have been to war (Holden, 1998). Maslach and colleagues operationalized burnout with three dimensions: *emotional exhaustion* (anxiety, depression, fatigue, poor concentration and memory, insomnia, pain, somatic complaints, and alcohol consumption); *cynicism* or *depersonalization* (increased judgment and criticism toward oneself, one's patients, and one's work context); and *inefficacy* (reduced job performance leading to reduced self-esteem). They also postulated that the causes of burnout can be categorized as (1) factors in the work context and (2) factors pertaining to the person. Of particular relevance to the work context are (1) high work demands that exceed resources, (2) low levels of personal control over work conditions and decision making, (3) insufficient social supports within the workplace, and (4) low job security. Of particular relevance to the person

are (1) conflict between pressures of work and home environments,; (2) emotional exhaustion, referring to overextension and depletion of resources; and (3) performance-based self-esteem challenges (Maslach et al., 2001).

This conceptualization of burnout and its causes are important as we consider the work of psychotherapy, including the application of EBPs. Consider, for example, the relatively new but competent DBT psychotherapist, Jeffrey, who asked his consultation team for help in his treatment of a young woman diagnosed with borderline personality disorder. His patient, who was a talented and articulate writer, complained of profound loneliness, severe anxiety, and chronic irritability. Her life had left her feeling quite bitter. In early sessions, her therapist empathized with her suffering, which she appreciated. He made behavioral suggestions that she resented, interpreting them as indicators that he did not understand her suffering. As time went on, her complaints proliferated. She communicated self-hatred, and intense resentment of those who had intimate relationships in their lives. Eventually those complaints were directed at the therapist, whom she described as "ineffectual," "removed," and "unfamiliar with suffering." The therapist, who cared about the patient, was personally hurt by her complaints. At first he felt disappointed. As he listened and validated her feelings, and as the situation persisted anyway, his feelings shifted from disappointment to shame, frustration, anxiety about provoking her criticism and anger, and even anger with her. Drawing from Maslach and colleagues' (2001) nomenclature of burnout responses, the therapist was in the early stages of *emotional exhaustion, cynicism* (judgmental reactions to the patient), and *inefficacy* (lowered self-esteem).

As the patient grew more attached to Jeffrey, she voiced resentment about his attention to others. She berated him for caring about other patients, and individuals in his family, more than he cared about her. When he was "on target" in validating her, she was generous with her gratitude, but when he was "off target," she attacked him. Essentially, on the one hand, she was punishing his change-oriented interventions and reinforcing his nurturant, empathic interventions. His balance between change-oriented and acceptance-oriented interventions shifted more toward the latter. But even though he avoided challenging her and looked for ways to validate her, her anger toward Jeffrey grew even stronger, and her behavior became more intolerant and out of control. She would not simply argue with him or dismiss his comments; she would shout at him, sometimes stomp out of the session prematurely, and slam the office door upon leaving. She left demeaning voice mail messages after sessions, wrote extensive e-mails that she expected him to read, and on two occasions she intruded upon his other patients in the waiting room, asking for details about how they were treated by the therapist.

Jeffrey's earlier training and experience as a therapist leaned heavily on patience, compassion, flexibility, and empathy, the cultivation of mutual trust, but it was not working. When she occasionally issued an apology for her "outrageous behavior" (her words), he felt a burst of hope that his approach was helping, but in fact her behavior continued to change for the worse. Because Jeffrey was embarrassed about his troubles with this, his first DBT patient, and because he feared disapproval by fellow team members, he reported any signs of a growing therapeutic alliance and omitted or minimized reports of her dysregulation. As the pressure grew, and as he continued to suppress and hide his difficulties from the team, he grew more and more isolated. Finally, Jeffrey felt that he had no choice but to ask for help.

By the time Jeffrey "came clean" with the consultation team, he was suffering mightily. His *emotional exhaustion* was unmistakable in his demoralization, resentment, shame, and anxiety; his *cynicism* was manifest in judgmental language about the patient and had spread to judgments about DBT and about himself; and his sense of *self-efficacy* was so impaired that he seriously doubted the wisdom of continuing to be a therapist. This patient pervasively occupied Jeffrey's thoughts, even during vacations. While he cared deeply about her, he dreaded each session with her. For the first time in his life, he suffered from insomnia. Seeking support, Jeffrey inappropriately shared details about this treatment with his wife, a violation from his usual practice at home, but she quickly grew tired of hearing about the case. His moods grew worse, his anxiety escalated, his sleep worsened, his confidence suffered, and he came to feel that he was a "fraud" who perhaps should leave the profession. Jeffrey suffered from a diagnosable anxiety disorder for the first time in his life, and his self-confidence was at an all-time low. By the time he revealed the extent of the trouble to his team members, his presentation was wracked with shame and anxiety. Jeffrey was convinced that all therapists on the team sat in judgment of him.

Our question here is: How can we use the consultation team to best help therapists like Jeffrey, whether in training or not? How can we help him to practice DBT in a manner that is technically aligned with the manual, that maintains his resilience and prevents burnout, and that provides effective therapy for the individual with severe and chronic emotional dysregulation?

Using the Consultation Team as Therapy for the Therapist

A core premise of DBT is that therapists need support and that "a co-supervision group, a treatment team, a consultant, or a supervisor is important for keeping therapists on track" (Linehan, 1993, p. 108). In DBT, the consultation team meeting differs distinctly from most multidisciplinary mental health team meetings in that the primary function is to support the therapist—to improve motivation and to enhance therapy skills—rather than to focus directly on how to treat the patients (Sayrs, 2019). Here, I describe the elements of the consultation team in DBT; detail how such elements are applied to the burnout syndrome experienced by Jeffrey and others in a similar situation; and consider whether and how the DBT consultation team model could be adapted in EBPs other than DBT.

The consultation process in DBT has been called *therapy of the therapist,* which is the case insofar as *therapy* refers here to one's therapeutic work life, not to one's personal life. To do so, a mutually trusting atmosphere is essential, in which each member is willing to open up to asking for help and accepting it. As was the case for Jeffrey, therapists asking for help can be as sensitive as patients asking for help. Certain basics about consultation teams serve to provide the kind of support that Jeffrey (and other therapists) need. The team comprises DBT practitioners from one, or from several, treatment contexts, who meet weekly to support each other in their practice of DBT. They do not need to come from the same treatment context or know the same patients (at first), but they do need to be engaged in the practice of DBT in some mode and in some setting, and to be willing to ask for help. Team meetings are not intended as seminars or academic discussion groups; they are more like meetings held by combat units getting ready for the next battle, or sports teams during huddles. The typical team meeting includes (1) a brief mindfulness practice; (2) a review of one of the six consultation team agreements; (3) consultation to team members regarding their cases, prioritizing cases with imminent life-threatening behaviors or cases leading to therapist burnout; and (4) a training segment to strengthen the understanding and practice of DBT. Obviously, the predicament presented to the team by Jeffrey was one in which there was already significant therapist burnout.

If we are to consider adapting features of DBT's consultation team format and function to other EBPs, we should begin by specifying the function of the meeting within that EBP, and the requirements for membership. The dual function of the team could be similar to DBT, as the effort to enhance each person's capabilities to practice the EBP adherently and effectively, and the effort to maintain or improve motivation of each therapist and to deal with burnout. Membership in consultation team meetings should be limited to those who are practicing the treatment and should not include interested onlookers who are not practicing. This creates an atmosphere in which every member is vulnerable and is therefore more willing to share genuine difficulties and to ask for help.

While a mindfulness practice to begin the meeting may or may not be appropriate in another EBP, depending on whether mindfulness plays a central role in that treatment, it may be that opening the meeting with some kind of deliberate practice that is central to the treatment is likely to help participants leave their prior mindsets at the door, and shift their attention to the functions of the meeting. Naturally, it may be helpful in any EBP to have a brief training segment each week, in which concepts are reviewed, relevant literature is discussed, therapeutic strategies are reviewed and practiced, and anything else of relevance to that treatment is included. Based on the experience in DBT consultation teams, by far the most unique and valuable feature of the team is the consultation to challenging aspects of each participant's cases and therapy sessions. There is nothing quite like presenting questions, challenges, and uncertainties to a trusted group of colleagues who are willing to give honest feedback. It provides some of the value of one-on-one supervision but has the added element of working together mutually with colleagues who have varying perspectives. Hence, it would probably be wise to make the process of consultation be the centerpiece of team meetings.

When Linehan developed the DBT consultation team, her idea was that it would be a place to practice the treatment, including the principles, strategies, and skills of DBT, with each other, for the purpose of helping each other. In other words, DBT itself was to be the vocabulary and the approach of team members to one another. For instance, team members look to balance acceptance-oriented interventions such as validation toward colleagues with change-oriented interventions, such as cognitive restructuring and exposure procedures. The effect is to strengthen the practice of DBT as the approach in therapy, as well as in teams. Whether and how to adapt this aspect of DBT consultation teams to other EBPs, whereby the underpinnings and strategies of the therapy itself are used as the underpinnings and strategies in team meetings, is an interesting question. For instance, if adapting consultation team meetings to the treatment of mindfulness-based cognitive therapy (MBCT), perhaps team members would practice mindfulness together, and in helping each other with cases, focus as well on the therapist's cognitions about treatment and the patient.

To establish the consistency, collaboration, all out engagement, and mutual trust needed to do this kind of sensitive work with each other's vulnerabilities, the team is anchored in a set of six agreements. The consultation team agreements serve the DBT team as something of a "constitution" that keeps the team on track, consistent with the principles of the treatment. When entering the consultation team, therapists are asked to study the agreements, to raise questions about them, and to commit to abide by them. These agreements pertain not so much to the content of what is discussed in team meetings; together the six agreements cultivate a multifaceted stance that DBT therapists take with respect to patients and to one another. As stated earlier, in each team meeting, members read and reflect on one of the agreements. In brief, the agreements in DBT are as follows (Linehan, 2003):

1. *Dialectical agreement.* No team member has the absolute truth. Truth is constructed, through synthesis, from the input of all team members. Team members inquired about Jef-

frey's dilemma with open minds, assessing his situation, considering the causes of it, and responding to his request for suggestions from several different vantage points that did not need to fit neatly with each other. Rather, all suggestions are welcomed and treated as having validity, and it is up to the therapist to synthesize them in practice.

2. *Consultation-to-the-patient agreement.* Team members consult with patients to help them deal with their family/social/professional networks rather than intervening directly with those networks to solve the patients' problems. Obviously, the team was trying to help Jeffrey with his own dilemmas, not directly trying to help the patient.

3. *Consistency agreement.* While consistency across members is expected in applying DBT principles, strategies, skills, and protocols, the team supports diversity (inconsistencies) in style and approach. It proved useful to Jeffrey that different team members modeled different styles themselves in the suggestions and the ways they made them. It gave him more freedom in considering what his style would be.

4. *Observing limits agreement.* Team members agree to support each therapist in determining his or her own personal limits. Different therapists are expected to have different limits. As the consultation to Jeffrey unfolded, team members supported him in identifying those personal limits that he was allowing the patient to violate.

5. *Phenomenological empathy agreement.* While remaining consistent with the facts, team members agree to interpret patient behaviors (and other team members) empathically, matching their subjective experiences. Team members looked for the validity in some of Jeffrey's approaches that were setting the stage for problems and highlighted what was valid in what he was doing prior to making change-oriented suggestions.

6. *Fallibility agreement.* Team members agree that every therapist, regardless of level of experience and expertise, is fallible. They all make mistakes in understanding and implementing DBT. The goal is to minimize defensiveness. In the course of consulting to Jeffrey, it was helpful to him that other team members shared some of their own difficult experiences managing similar situations in therapy.

In DBT, adherence to the six agreements has helped to establish a team-based approach that is in sync with DBT's underlying philosophy and principles. If the consultation team were to be adapted to a different EBP, it would begin with the elucidation of a number of agreements that are based on the underlying philosophy and principles of the treatment. Of course, one could consider whether any of the six agreements in DBT could simply be adopted, with or without modification, into that other treatment. More likely, and more creatively, agreements could be derived that are specifically based on that EBP, and that function to keep team meetings aligned with the treatment. For instance, agreements for the conduct of team meetings within acceptance and commitment therapy (ACT) should grow out of the priorities within that treatment. For instance, some might include:

1. Team members acknowledge and accept their own emotional responses and action tendencies that arise in response to patients and/or to fellow team members (acceptance of emotional responses).
2. Team members support each other, and patients, in maintaining awareness of the difference between one's thoughts/perceptions versus reality/facts (cognitive defusion).
3. Team members support each other, and one's patients, in basing action commitments on important personal values (valued committed actions).

In DBT, to ensure alignment with these agreements and to support the team structure, a clear process of commitment to the team is outlined and therapists are asked to agree to the following specific conditions:

- Attending all team meetings for the entire scheduled time, notifying the team of upcoming absences and emergencies that conflict with attendance.
- Participating actively throughout every meeting, putting other things (including cell phones) aside, consulting to one another.
- Focusing primarily on meeting each therapist's needs, as requested, rather than sharing ideas about the patient's treatment (unless that is requested).
- Assuming that each therapist shares responsibility for each patient presented and discussed by any therapist in team meetings;

this is the treatment of a group of patients by a group of therapists.

• Committing to the implementation of the six consultation team agreements.

When team members fail to adhere to these expectations, or to the team agreements, anyone on the team can place this concern on the agenda for discussion and resolution.

Not just the nature of format, agreements, and commitments made within consultation teams is drawn from the DBT treatment manual for the treatment of patients. In consulting to one another, therapists also utilize the range of DBT treatment strategies, theory, assumptions, and skills:

• DBT's *targeting strategies* for the collaborative determination of a concise treatment agenda, an agenda that includes the reduction of therapy-interfering behaviors that decrease the therapist's motivation.

• DBT's *assumptions about patients,* which provide therapists with guidelines helping them to remain compassionate and effective in the face of stress.

• DBT's *treatment strategies* that while providing a comprehensive set of tools to help patients achieve goals, also provide tools for therapists to care for themselves and to navigate burnout-promoting "traps" in treatment.

• DBT's *biosocial theory,* which while identifying causes and maintaining factors for behavioral patterns, can also be turned toward identification of causes and maintaining factors of therapist burnout.

DBT's Targeting Strategies in the Consultation Team

Patients referred to DBT typically suffer from several disorders and engage in multiple problem behaviors. This presents the therapist with the daunting, at times overwhelming, task of treating a large number of high-severity behaviors in a finite therapy session each week. The solution in DBT is to create a prioritized list of treatment targets, to be addressed one at a time, starting with those presenting the greatest severity and immediate risk, and moving down the list as high priority targets are accomplished. By focusing on one problem behavior at a time, even if several occur during the same week, therapists are less likely to be overwhelmed.

It can be demoralizing to both patient and therapist to focus one's energies entirely on problematic behaviors. Hence, problem behaviors should be seen as obstacles to articulated life-enhancing goals with which they interfere. The ultimate goal of the treatment is to build a life worth living, which is unique to each patient. Emphasizing that treatment targets are steps on the path to a life worth living is more likely to motivate the patient, as well as the therapist. This can create an upward spiral in the treatment, an antidote to the downward spiral or transaction that moves toward burnout.

For a team to consult to a therapist most effectively, a similar practice of targeting takes place in team, to ensure that the finite time for each consultation meets the highest priority needs of the therapist. While this may sound obvious on its face, in fact, in most interdisciplinary meetings in mental health settings, the usual practice is quite different. A therapist brings up a problem in the treatment of a patient, and team members begin immediately to share their experiences and suggestions in an effort to help the therapist with the treatment, without hearing first what the therapist needs from the team. This results in a "shotgun" approach that may or may not hit the target, the target being what the therapist needs most.

Therefore, each consultation begins with the therapist describing the situation with which he or she needs help, then asking the team specifically for what he or she wants. For instance, one therapist might simply ask the team to listen deeply, so that she feels less alone in a high-risk case; another might ask for input into his case conceptualization or treatment plan; a third might ask the team to brainstorm possible solutions and interventions. When Jeffrey first requested consultation on the treatment of his patient, his embarrassment and self-deprecation led him to be rather vague in defining what he needed from the team. As is the desired practice in DBT team consultations, a team member asked Jeffrey if he could tell them what he needed. Through tears, he expressed his sense of being demoralized by his failure to help the patient, feeling like a fraud given that he had been portraying things as going better than they were, and finding himself very much alone, "out on a limb" with the patient. He asked if the team members could first just listen to what was going on, and if they felt that Jeffrey should remain as the client's therapist, make suggestions about revisions that might help him conduct a more effective treatment. Having heard from him, team members then knew what to do, and what not to do.

Jeffrey described his experience and the patient's behavior. Team members inquired to get more specifics, they validated his emotional distress, and commented on how deeply he wanted to help the patient. He seemed to feel some relief as his shame dissipated, but he still expressed disappointment in himself because of how long it took for him to ask for help. Team members just listened, not offering interpretations or suggestions because he had not asked for them. Then Jeffrey asked for team members' observations and ideas about how he may have contributed to the patient's out-of-control, therapy-interfering behaviors. Team members tentatively put forward ideas for his consideration. Perhaps Jeffrey had limited experience with patients presenting with this degree of dysregulation. Perhaps he was not accustomed to taking his own personal limits seriously, directly asking patients to respect those limits in the service of their therapy. Jeffrey acknowledged that his previous therapy learning experiences emphasized therapeutic empathy, compassion, patience, and flexibility, and not interventions asking for, or insisting on, behavioral changes in the patient. He could see that in response to the patient's reinforcement of his empathic behaviors and her punishment of any slightly challenging intervention, he evolved toward using even more empathy and almost completely abandoned challenging her behaviors. Jeffrey's fear and avoidance of the patient's anger increased, which only served to prompt and reinforce her anger further, which led her, to her own dismay, to spiral further out of control.

For team members to restrain themselves from offering their best, heartfelt suggestions to their distressed colleague is not easy. It is up to the team as a whole to use discipline in providing therapists what they need rather than sharing reactions and assuming they will be helpful. This has been such a helpful approach in DBT team meetings, and so unlike usual interdisciplinary meetings in which team members share whatever they think is needed, that consultation teams created within other EBPs may want to consider defining consultation targets in a similar way.

DBT's Assumptions about Patients, as Applied within Consultation Team

In order to help DBT therapists stay on track and keep their balance between acceptance and change while treating such difficult patterns, Linehan spelled out a number of guiding assumptions to keep in mind. Some of them are acceptance-oriented, helping the therapist maintain compassion. Others are change-oriented, helping therapists continue to push for behavioral change. Acceptance-oriented assumptions include "This patient is doing the best she or he can," "This patient wants to improve," and "The lives of suicidal, borderline patients are unbearable as they are currently being lived." Acceptance-oriented assumptions can remind therapists to maintain an objective perspective and compassionate approach when frustration is generating judgments toward the patient. Change-oriented assumptions include "Patients need to do better, try harder, and be more motivated to change" and "Patients must learn new behaviors in all relevant contexts." Change-oriented assumptions remind therapists to continue to push the patient vigorously toward those changes that will accomplish their goals when feelings of defeat and hopelessness are generating therapeutic passivity and permissiveness, and when the therapist is treating the patient as fragile.

While these assumptions are meant to guide the therapist in all DBT-related contexts and work, they play a particularly salient role in the consultation team, where the difficulties that therapists bring for consultation have catalyzed drift away from maintaining the assumptions, and particularly the balance between change-oriented and acceptance-oriented assumptions. Clearly, in the work with Jeffrey, the team noticed, as did the therapist himself, that he was out of balance, relying too heavily on the side of acceptance, empathy, and compassion, while avoiding and omitting change-oriented interventions. While no one in the team needed to spell out the obvious in the consultation to Jeffrey—he already could see it—often it is important for a team member to interject something like "I wonder if the pressures in the treatment have led you to drift away from any of DBT's assumptions, especially the one that says the patient needs to be more motivated and try harder to change behaviors." Or within the team, a member might point out that there is imbalance within the team between those who see the patient as a victim needing compassion and support and those who see the patient as aggressive and destructive. The team members then can try to clarify how their various attitudes fit the assumptions and may find a better balance or synthesis between competing therapeutic tendencies.

DBT's Treatment Strategies and Skills as Used in the Consultation Team

DBT includes approximately 85 treatment strategies for therapists and 100 behavioral skills for patients, which can also be utilized by therapists. The strategies come in several "packages" from which therapists draw as needed: There are acceptance-oriented strategies to alleviate suffering and to validate, change-oriented strategies to bring about behavioral change, dialectical strategies to address therapeutic stuck-ness and irresolvable conflict, suicide crisis strategies to address patients when suicide risk is more imminent, and structural strategies to guide the therapist in the various structural elements and protocols of treatment. The mere fact that there are so many tools at his or her disposal helps the therapist to prevent his or her own burnout during sessions. When he or she gets stuck while using one strategy, he or she has many options to which to turn. The therapist can shift quickly from one change strategy to another (e.g., from exposure to skills training), pivot from a change strategy to an acceptance strategy (e.g., from exposure to validation), pivot from an acceptance strategy to a change strategy (e.g., from validation to cognitive restructuring), or pivot from either change or acceptance to a dialectical strategy (e.g., to reframe a stuck situation with a metaphor). When suicide risk seems to be heightened and more imminent, the therapist can introduce the suicide crisis protocol. Obviously, therapists need to overlearn strategies, so they can be activated automatically during sessions.

"Observing personal limits" is a crucial DBT strategy for therapists in preventing burnout. The therapist acknowledges to him- or herself that he or she has personal limits, different from other therapists, and that he or she must defend those limits in order to remain within his or her "comfort zone" while doing therapy with such severe problems. For instance, the therapist may accept too many unproductive phone calls or tolerate too many disturbing behaviors in sessions, usually motivated by wanting to bend one's usual limits to alleviate the patient's suffering. But by doing so, the therapist overestimates his or her own flexibility and endurance, and eventually finds that it is a burden to do so. Beyond that, allowing one's limits to be crossed creates conditions for strain, frustration, resentment, exhaustion of compassion, and burnout. It is deeply important for the therapist to be aware

when his or her personal limits are violated, and to have the courage and skill to communicate this to the patient without blaming, emphasizing that observing limits will actually strengthen the therapy relationship by insulating the therapist from going too far outside his or her comfort zone. As has been mentioned, one of the causes of Jeffrey's burnout, as discussed in the team, was his failure to adequately observe his personal limits.

At the core of DBT are four sets of skills. *Core mindfulness skills* help to increase awareness of reality and awareness of one's own responses; to strengthen the capacity to attend voluntarily to aspects of sensations, thoughts, emotions, and contextual factors; and to increase balance in the face of stress. *Distress tolerance skills* help one to perceive and accept realities, including unpleasant realities, to act skillfully in alignment with "the rules" of the universe, and to survive crises in life by deliberately changing the input into one's brain and body. *Emotion regulation skills* provide a set of tools for understanding and naming emotions, for increasing resiliency to negative emotions, and for reducing and transforming painful emotions once present. *Interpersonal effectiveness skills* are designed to help one to accomplish one's objectives while maintaining desired relationships and maintaining or improving self-respect.

The strategies, which are typically applied in the treatment of patients in various modes of DBT, and the skills, which are typically taught to patients to help them realize their goals, are useful for therapists in the context of consultation team.

For instance, when Jeffrey presented his predicament to the team, team members relied at first on acceptance-oriented strategies such as *warmth, responsiveness, self-disclosure,* and *validation* as they tried to understand the situation and to alleviate his shame and distress. They relied on *mindfulness skills* of *observing* and *describing* to simply observe and describe what they were hearing from Jeffrey, and to be *nonjudgmental, one-mindful,* and *effectively remain compassionate,* to stay focused, and to do what he asked for. A close relative to the mindfulness skills in DBT is a set of *reality acceptance skills,* the centerpiece of which is known as *radical acceptance.* When therapists face difficult realities in therapy, which sometimes have no immediate fix, radical acceptance can help them to see reality exactly as it is, and to accept it from deep within the self. Accepting momentarily unchangeable realities removes the therapist from fighting those realities, which can add to one's suffering. It becomes possible to "let go" of the fight against reality and to find skillful means for tolerating that reality. This can rescue the DBT therapist from unnecessary distress about any number of predicaments: the patient's lack of progress, increased risk of suicide, or relapse into addictive behaviors; or the therapist's ineffectiveness or painful emotional responses. *Radical acceptance* was a crucial skill for Jeffrey to use to accept that the patient's difficult behaviors were as they should have been given her history, and that it was not realistic for him to think that he could eliminate them by providing enough compassion.

As the consultation moved along, change-oriented strategies were brought into play. Team members helped Jeffrey *identify his personal limits* that he had not maintained, and using *role playing,* helped him to rehearse how he would ask the patient to respect his limits. The role playing relied on *exposure procedures,* which provoked Jeffrey's anxiety and helped him to approach rather than avoid the situations. Team members used *reinforcement* of his interests and capacities to establish firm limits. They helped him to *use the skill of acting opposite of his urge to avoid* situations with the patient. And they used *commitment strategies* to strengthen Jeffrey's commitment to make the changes under discussion.

Finally, dialectical strategies are added into DBT to help the therapist to navigate and transform paralyzing predicaments in therapy or in team meetings. They help the therapist to find a way to deal with intense and sustained conflict by looking for the validity on each side of the conflict, then moving toward a synthesis that incorporates the validity of both sides. They facilitate movement, speed, and flow when the situation seems stuck or irresolvable. There are nine such strategies listed in the manual. Each one helps to resolve rigid and paralyzed transactions between patient and therapist; therefore, they serve as burnout antidotes. One of them is the use of *metaphors* to represent stuck situations. In the work with Jeffrey, in trying to help him to be more willing to ask the patient to respect his personal limits, knowing that she will probably express anger forcefully, a team member suggested that he imagine he was a lion-tamer, an occupation where observing personal limits has life versus death consequences.

DBT's Biosocial Theory as Applied to the Therapist

As presented in detail in Swenson (2016), DBT's biosocial theory about the causal and maintaining factors of borderline behavioral patterns may also be applied to the identification of causal and maintaining factors of burnout behavioral patterns in therapists. This conceptualizing framework as applied to the therapist is valuable for three reasons: (1) It is parsimonious, when possible, to apply a theory that already is central to the treatment; (2) it provides a nonpejorative explanation of therapist burnout; and (3) it generates practical suggestions for preventing and treating burnout. Consultants, supervisors, and DBT's consultation teams (see below) can use the theory to assess the factors causing and maintaining burnout in fellow therapists, guiding them toward specific solutions that come from the DBT lexicon. Space prohibits a detailed account of the biosocial theory here (see Linehan, 1993), but a brief overview indicates how this can be helpful in supporting therapists.

The theory posits a transaction between a person and that person's environment or, more particularly, between a person's biologically based emotional vulnerabilities and impulsive tendencies, and that person's pervasively invalidating environment. The emotionally vulnerable person remains in transaction over time with an environment that invalidates valid behaviors. A transaction refers to a bidirectional interaction. Invalidated, the emotionally vulnerable person becomes more reactive or impulsive, lacking other means to self-regulate. In response to heightened reactivity and impulsivity, those in the invalidating environment become even more invalidating, a sign of intolerance, a lack of understanding, and an effort to control. This transaction goes back and forth until the individual is stuck in a pattern of severe and chronic emotional dysregulation. The individual completes the genesis of borderline personality disorder by adopting problematic behaviors that provide short-term relief, such as suicide attempts, self-injury, substance use, dissociative episodes, eating disorders, and so on. As consequences of the transaction, the individual fails to learn to observe and label specific emotions, fails to acquire skillful means for modulating emotions, learns to invalidate him- or herself much as the environment did, tends to alternate between emotional suppression and escalation, and searches the interpersonal environment to figure out how to behave. Broadly, DBT's treatment approach addresses the two sides of the theory, providing a relatively validating environment in which patients are taught emotion regulation strategies to use instead of the problematic patterns.

How can this theory, which helps to conceptualize the path to borderline personality disorder in patients, be used to conceptualize the path to burnout among DBT therapists, and in so doing provide a framework for the consultation team's work to prevent and treat burnout in each therapist? The key is to realize that while quite different in scope, the two problems (borderline personality disorder and therapist burnout) are actually similar in nature. In some cases, one could fairly say that the syndrome of therapist burnout is a circumscribed version of borderline personality disorder, revolving around the treatment of a particular patient or clinical situation. In applying the theory, the emotionally vulnerable person in the case of burnout is the psychotherapist. The relevant environment for that person includes those individuals and those interactions associated with the treatment of that patient, including interactions with the patient him- or herself. This may include interactions with the patient, collateral contacts regarding the patient, payors and administrators relevant to the patient's treatment, the patient's social–professional network, including family members, colleagues, and supervisors with whom the therapist interacts regarding the patient, and the context of the consultation team. Let's outline how the process toward burnout unfolds step by step, aligned with the biosocial theory. Every step in the sequence matches the steps in the evolution of Jeffrey's burnout.

1. Prior to the beginning of treatment with the patient, the therapist has a certain level of biologically based emotional vulnerability as a result of his or her biology and life history, and certain impulsive tendencies.
2. From the beginning of therapy with the index patient, the therapist is exposed repetitively to a large number of patient-associated cues, some of which are emotionally evocative, including in-session and out-of-session contacts with the patient, and contacts with other associated parties as mentioned earlier.
3. Many of these cues trigger aversive emotional responses in the therapist (e.g., sad-

ness, shame, fear, anger, or frustration), adding to preexisting vulnerabilities.
4. Following norms in mental health environments, in combination with lifelong values of the therapist, the therapist tries to handle the emotions by him- or herself.
5. As his or her emotions intensify and proliferate "underground," the therapist's efforts to suppress them grow stronger.
6. Avoidance of cues and suppression of emotions affect therapist behaviors in treatment, such as an increase in disrespect, a lack of balance between poles such as acceptance and change, and departure from standard practices of DBT. Toward the patient or team, the therapist might show detachment or excessive closeness, forgetfulness or neglect, decreased tolerance, decreased compassion and validation, or increased judgment.
7. The patient is likely to feel invalidated by these changes in the therapist, leading to escalated emotion dysregulation and problem behaviors.
8. The escalation of emotions in the transaction between therapist and patient, while the therapist has not yet confronted the reality of his or her own emotional dysregulation leads him or her to "fall out" of adherence to the treatment, and to feel a sense of entrapment or loss of control.
9. By this point, it is a transactional burnout spiral, with the patient falling into borderline behavioral patterns and the therapist falling into burnout.
10. The therapist, feeling demoralized and drained, may become convinced that he or she cannot treat that patient, may come to deeply doubt his or her capacities as a therapist, may develop signs of burnout more broadly, and may want to change his or her career.

Sometimes therapy is actually dead long before either party is aware of it, and it has damaging effects for both. At this point, the therapist is suffering from a full-blown case of therapist burnout.

In this account, it is usually rather easy to see signs of emotional vulnerability in the therapist, but not so easy to see the nature of the therapist's invalidating environment. It may not look like the sometimes grossly invalidating environment our patients have experienced. It may not look invalidating from the outside, but it still can be highly invalidating to the therapist. The therapist may find that those around him or her subtly but pervasively react to his or her as if he or she is doing something wrong in the treatment of the patient: "overinvolved," "hyperreactive," "hypersensitive," "obsessed," "overidentified," and so on. These communications might not be stated plainly or directly, but they may be communicated through what is not said or how something is said, through tones of voice and nonverbal communications. Perfectly valid responses of therapists in difficult treatments can be quietly invalidated in environments in which it is a prevailing norm that professionals are expected to regulate themselves without much complaint, especially if it is an environment where the demands exceed the resources. More obvious is the invalidation that comes to the therapist from the detached or angry patient, the disgruntled family, and the third-party payors that audit treatments and require documentation justifying ongoing treatment

The evolution of Jeffrey's burnout syndrome follows the sequence just outlined, in which the biosocial theory is used as a framework for understanding the development of therapist burnout. First, we can assume that he entered into the case already having his own emotional vulnerabilities, as is the case with all of us, and with the additional vulnerability of being relatively new to the treatment. Second, as therapy progressed, Jeffrey encountered cues, as the patient more and more directly, and more and more frequently, berated and verbally attacked him in and outside of sessions, eliciting increasingly negative emotions in him. Following norms that he had learned in prior environments in his life, including prior psychotherapy training environments, Jeffrey assumed that he should be able to handle the situation on his own, without help. He proceeded to try to suppress the growing intensity of his emotions. These efforts contributed to a growing imbalance between acceptance and change in the therapy, where Jeffrey allowed his own limits to be violated, where he did not confront the patient but instead looked for opportunities to empathize with her. As a result, the patient's needs for natural consequences were not met; she ran into no barriers despite her increasing loss of control, and her clinical presentation grew worse, as did her level of distress. In this respect, she was invalidated and increasingly evidenced borderline behavioral patterns. Meanwhile, the therapist grew more despairing,

suffered from burnout, was losing hope, and the therapy was dying. The transactional burnout spiral was well under way, and had Jeffrey continued to conceal it from the team, it would likely have led to the end of therapy, with a bad outcome for both parties. Instead, it was turned around with the institution of more appropriate personal limits and a better balance between acceptance and change.

Jeffrey was relatively new to the treatment of borderline personality disorder, new to DBT, and new to the consultation team. He was still working under the norms he learned in prior training and treatment environments, which could be considered invalidating in that they encouraged him to suppress any negative emotional responses. Once Jeffrey got to the point of sharing his increasingly desperate situation with this consultation team, and once he experienced that the team was respectful, supportive, and validating, he began to appreciate the value of a DBT-oriented consultation team that helped him to become remoralized and remotivated, but also offered concrete suggestions to get the therapy back on track.

Assessing and Treating Burnout in the Team

Certain features of consultation team are especially helpful in buernout prevention and treatment. The team accepts burnout in therapists as a natural consequence of being therapists, not as something that indicates weakness, lack of skill, or something of which to be ashamed. Hence, team members routinely "scan" one another for signs of burnout, which are sometimes identifiable before the therapist him- or herself is aware of them. Some typical suggestive signs of burnout include:

- The therapist directly complains of burnout, or shows signs of increased emotional exhaustion or sensitivity.
- The therapist becomes more detached from the patient and/or the team.
- The therapist (prematurely) suggests termination with the patient.
- The therapist becomes more judgmental regarding him- or herself, the patient, and/or his or her team.
- The therapist falls out of compliance with the usual agreements, commitments in team, assumptions, and theory that are central to DBT.

- The therapist becomes more defensive in team meetings.
- The patient is complaining that the therapist has changed, either providing less validation than before, becoming more pushy, or becoming more passive.

Once aware of the presence of burnout in a therapist, team members can refer to the following list of factors that are known to promote burnout in therapists:

- Factors in the work environment
  - Work demands exceed personal resources.
  - Compensation is lower than in other possible work settings.
  - The therapist has little control over work conditions.
  - The therapist receives insufficient social support.
  - The therapist experiences minimal job security.
  - Emotional suppression is a norm in the work setting.
- Factors in the therapist's personal life
  - Stress, illness, personal, and family problems.
  - Insufficient attention to sleep, exercise, nutrition, leisure interests.
  - Life imbalance, with attention to work seriously outweighing attention to home and personal life.
- Factors arising in the treatment of a particular patient
  - Pathology is severe, complex, and chronic.
  - Patient repeatedly shows poor response to interventions.
  - Patient has a number of factors indicating high risk, including risk of suicide.
  - The therapist cares deeply about the patient, and extends personal limits, for an extended period, beyond his or her comfort zone.
  - The therapist takes on a sense of "omnipotence," assuming the job of "rescuing" the patient him- or herself.
  - The therapist is repeatedly exposed to disturbing details of the patient's history and current life.
  - The therapist becomes the object of the patient's anger and disappointment.

Having detected signs of burnout in a fellow therapist, and having helped to assess the causes and conditions leading to burnout, the consulta-

tion team has certain practices that are antidotes to the further progression of burnout. The team encourages each member to be open and transparent about what is happening in treatment, including uncertainty, doubts, and "mistakes." Team members assess, rather than assume, the causes of burnout. In so doing, the team helps the therapist recognize his or her own burnout-promoting cognitions and judgments that may be fueling unrealistic expectations or damagingly excessive self-criticism. Therapists are regularly encouraged to observe their own personal limits. The team helps each therapist find the optimal "distance" from the patient and to shift as needed, to move in closer when becoming more detached, and to move back from the patient when becoming overinvolved and overly responsible. At times when a team member is feeling overwhelmed in a treatment, or in general, and is therefore more vulnerable to burnout, team members may offer concrete help (e.g., make phone calls for the therapist). Finally, the team establishes an atmosphere of warmth and spontaneity that generates positive emotions and promotes bonding among members.

Concluding Comments

Having presented and discussed the elements of the DBT consultation team, having considered whether other EBPs may benefit from such a modality, and having illustrated the working of the consultation team with a therapist having difficulties in a treatment, I have focused on the issue of therapist burnout: how it arises, how it manifests, and how it can be addressed in a consultation team format. Preventing and treating burnout, as stated earlier, is one of the two primary functions of the consultation team. The other is to enhance each therapist's capacities to practice DBT with adherence to the manual. In this respect, the team takes on functions of supervision and training. In both content and process of team functioning, expertise in the practice of DBT is both discussed and modeled. In training segments in team meetings, every therapist's understanding and practice of DBT is improved. In consulting to one another's treatments, therapists in training and experienced therapists take part together, and all are repeatedly exposed to the vocabulary, the concepts, the treatment strategies, and the skills that are central to the treatment. This is a "hands-on" format for training. Cases are formulated again and again within the DBT model. In presenting his or her own cases, each therapist articulates what he or she is doing, formulates cases, assesses progress, and receives feedback from other therapists within the DBT framework. In role plays, therapists engage in deliberate practices of therapeutic strategies. Reviewing one's own therapies on videotape with team members is a uniquely valuable opportunity to get specific feedback on practice. On occasion, team members take advantage of training opportunities and bring their learning back to the team. The entire treatment, again and again, is discussed, applied, modeled, and assessed in team meetings.

Well-conducted consultation team meetings represent a superb example of on-the-job training that enhances capabilities and improves motivation. A good team leads to an engaged, motivated therapist, with reduced likelihood of burnout, who acquires the sense of being an integral part of a team rather than "going it alone." Team members validate each other, challenge each other, and learn from each other. A well-functioning team leads everyone to feel more positive about the work, leads everyone at all levels of experience to receive help and to improve, and ultimately leads patients to get better. To repeat the central concept, DBT is the treatment of a group of people (patients) by a group of people (therapists).

References

Bloom, S. (2003). Caring for the caregiver: Avoiding and treating vicarious traumatization. In A. P. Giardino, E. M. Datner, & J. B. Asher (Eds.), *Sexual assault: Victimization across the lifespan—a clinical guide* (pp. 459–470). Maryland Heights, MO: G. W. Medical Publishing.

Figley, C. R. (Ed.). (1995). *Compassion fatigue.* New York: Brunner/Mazel.

Holden, W. (1998). *Shell shock.* London: Channel 4 Books.

Linehan, M. M. (1993). *Cognitive-behavioral treatment for borderline personality disorder.* New York: Guilford Press.

Maslach, C., Schaufell, W. B., & Leiter, M. P. (2001). Job burnout. *Annual Review of Psychology, 52*(1), 397–422.

Sayrs, J. (2019). Running an effective DBT consultation team: Principles and challenges. In M. Swales (Ed.), *The Oxford handbook of dialectical behavior therapy* (pp. 147–166). Oxford, UK: Oxford University Press.

Schulz, R., & Sherwood, P. R. (2008). Physical and mental health effects of family caregiving. *American Journal of Nursing, 108*(9), 23–27.

Swenson, C. R. (2016). *DBT principles in action: Acceptance, change, and dialectics.* New York: Guilford Press.

CHAPTER 25

Why Therapists Need to
Take a Good Look at Themselves

*Self-Practice/Self-Reflection as an Integrative
Training Strategy for Evidence-Based Practices*

JAMES BENNETT-LEVY
BEVERLY HAARHOFF

The "long, textured path" of the therapist's journey toward evidence-based practice (EBP) in action has many ups and downs (Skovholt & Rønnestad, 2001); for instance, there are times when we consider ourselves incredibly fortunate to be doing such interesting and important work, and times when we may doubt ourselves and wonder what we are doing, and whether we are the best people to be doing it. This is true for therapists at all levels of experience.

Experienced therapists may go through periods in which their practice has gone stale. They may look for inspiration by going to conferences or attending lectures by experts. Sometimes they may get excited by a workshop presenting new ideas. But 10 weeks later, often not much has changed. Without follow-up consultation, supervision, or structured self-reflection, one-off training tends not to "work" (Bennett-Levy & Padesky, 2014; Lyon, Stirman, Kerns, & Bruns, 2011; Nadeem, Gleacher, & Beidas, 2013).

Novice therapists and trainees may struggle with learning the many components of empirically supported treatment and integrating basic theory with technique. Moreover, they may find that core empathy and relationship skills get left inadvertently outside the therapy room as their attention is dominated by what tech-

nique to use next (Bennett-Levy & Thwaites, 2007; Thwaites & Bennett-Levy, 2007). Depression and anxiety appear to be rife among therapy trainees (Cushway, 1992; Pakenham & Stafford-Brown, 2012), and frequently trainees (and the educators and supervisors who support them) may find themselves doubting their capabilities and the path that they have chosen (Bennett-Levy & Beedie, 2007; Pakenham & Stafford-Brown, 2012).

All therapists, regardless of level of training and expertise, may have particular difficulty with certain clients or types of clients. Some irritate you or make you feel inadequate. You realize that you need to address your personal reactions if you are to make headway. At other times, you may struggle with work overload, burnout, organizational hassles, or personal issues. Your therapy has become very ordinary. It has lost its coherence. Your work does not satisfy you. You suspect client outcomes are not as good as they should be. You feel guilty that perhaps clients are not getting much bang for their buck.

Are any of these scenarios familiar? Is more knowledge the answer? More reading? More workshops? More practice? Lifestyle adjustments? Personal therapy? More supervision? Any of these strategies might be useful for particular purposes, but most are only available infrequently—for an hour every couple of weeks, or a day every so often. Your supervisor is not there beside you in the therapy room.

A key focus of this book is the integration of science and practice in the delivery of clinical interventions. However, although a useful evidence base for therapist training has developed in recent years (Beidas & Kendall, 2010; Edmunds, Beidas & Kendall, 2013; Gale & Schröder, 2014; Nadeem et al., 2013), too often training is delivered with little regard to theories of therapist skill development (Bennett-Levy, 2006; Skovholt & Rønnestad, 2001) or evidence-based training practices.

So what to do on a day-to-day basis? As novice therapists, how can we acquire new skills and address crises of confidence at those times when, almost inevitably, we feel out of our depth (Bennett-Levy & Beedie, 2007)? As experienced therapists, how can we enhance our practice and well-being—and that of our clients—when we are seeing many clients a day? As supervisors or educators, how can we design training programs that help trainees integrate conceptual and technical skills, that ensure that trainees' interpersonal skills do not drop through the floor, and that give them some tools to address crippling self-doubt and lack of confidence?

Self-practice/self-reflection (SP/SR) is an evidence-based training approach that has the capacity to address many of these issues. Central to SP/SR is the self-practice of the core therapy skills that we are teaching others and self-reflection, a metacognitive skill that the adult learning, social psychology, and psychotherapy literatures have consistently identified as a core component of clinical and personal wisdom (Bennett-Levy, Thwaites, Chaddock, & Davis, 2009; Haarhoff & Thwaites, 2016; Levitt & Piazza-Bonin, 2016; Schön, 1983; Staudinger & Gluck, 2011). A significant benefit of SP/SR practices is that they can be available to therapists at any time on a day-to-day basis.

In this chapter, we suggest that it is important for therapists to take a good look at themselves for two reasons: to enhance their therapy skills and to attend to caring for themselves as people, which can impact on their therapeutic effectiveness. SP/SR is an integrative training strategy for achieving these aims, derived from a theoretical model of therapist skill development (Bennett-Levy, 2006), and supported by empirical research (Davis, Thwaites, Freeston, &

Bennett-Levy, 2015; Thwaites, Bennett-Levy, Davis, & Chaddock, 2014), as demonstrated by a recent metasynthesis of SP/SR studies (Gale & Schröder, 2014). Our aims for the chapter are to:

- Define and describe SP/SR.
- Provide a theoretical framework to understand the process and impact of SP/SR.
- Identify the differences between SP/SR and traditional forms of training.
- Review the evidence base for SP/SR.
- Provide guidelines for the introduction and use of SP/SR in one's practice or in training programs.

In addition, in the last part of the chapter, readers have the opportunity to experience several SP/SR exercises for themselves. One of the guiding philosophies of SP/SR is that "just reading" about therapy techniques or "just listening" to lecture or workshop material is of limited benefit. Therapists need to experience therapeutic practices from the "inside out," and reflect on that experience, to enhance their capacities to implement EBP in action. A similar philosophy has underpinned the practice of personal therapy for therapists since the birth of psychoanalysis (Freud, 1937/1957).

Although the main body of SP/SR research to date has focused on Beckian cognitive-behavioral therapy (CBT), it should be noted that self-experiential and self-reflective approaches have also been advocated for practitioners from other evidence-based therapeutic approaches such as acceptance and commitment therapy (Pakenham, 2015), dialectical behavior therapy (Linehan & McGhee, 1994), schema therapy (Farrell & Shaw, 2018) and compassion-focused therapy (Gale, Schröder, & Gilbert, 2017; Kolts, Bell, Bennett-Levy, & Irons, 2018).

What Is SP/SR?

SP/SR is a self-experiential training strategy in which participants practice therapy strategies on themselves (e.g., self-formulation, behavioral activation, imagery), then reflect on the experience, first from a personal, then from a professional, perspective. Key formative influences on the development of SP/SR were seminal texts in the 1980s adult education literature (Kolb, 1984; Schön, 1983) highlighting the value of experiential learning (Kolb, 1984) and self-reflection for adult learning. In particular,

Schön (1983, p. 42) distinguished between the "the high ground where practitioners can make effective use of theory and technique" (e.g., highly selected clients with defined disorders in clinical trials) and "the low swampy ground where situations are confused messes" (e.g., complex multifaceted clinical issues, typical of clinical practice). Schön suggested that practitioner reflection is a core skill for navigating "confused messes." A further impetus to the development of SP/SR was suggestions in the 1990s by leading CBT therapists that practicing therapy techniques on oneself is one of the best ways to learn CBT skills and develop self-awareness (A. T. Beck, Freeman, & Associates, 1990; J. S. Beck, 1995; Padesky, 1996).

To date, the primary focus of SP/SR has been to develop and/or refine therapist skills (Thwaites et al., 2014). However, SP/SR participants often report personal as well as professional benefits (Bennett-Levy et al., 2001), and increasingly, educators are realizing that SP/SR and other personal practices (e.g., meditation or compassion programs) can be used for personal development and well-being purposes such as enhancing therapist self-care (Bennett-Levy, 2019; Bennett-Levy & Finlay-Jones, 2018; Boellinghaus, Jones, & Hutton, 2013; Haarhoff & Thwaites, 2016; Pakenham, 2015; Shapiro, Brown, & Biegel, 2007), a theme that we revisit in the exercises at the end of the chapter.

The key principles of SP/SR, self-experiential learning and self-reflection, may be implemented by a variety of methods (e.g., personal therapy, therapeutic writing, mindfulness) in a variety of contexts (supervision, consultation, personal reflective practice, group programs). Our research on SP/SR has taken two forms: "limited co-therapy pairs," in which practitioners take turns being therapist and client, and reflect on their experience in both roles (Bennett-Levy, Lee, Travers, Pohlman, & Hamernik, 2003), and SP/SR workbooks, which are rather more frequently offered and researched.

The workbook form of SP/SR involves working through a structured workbook (e.g., Bennett-Levy, Thwaites, et al., 2015; Kolts et al., 2018), in which the exercises are particular therapeutic interventions presented as modules guiding the therapist toward first understanding, then modifying or changing an identified personal or professional problem. In the CBT workbook (Bennett-Levy, Thwaites, et al., 2015), we offer 12 modules with about 1-hour of self-practice each. Each module systematically guides and supports therapists through a series of SP exercises and structured SR questions. SP can focus on personal or professional problems. Personal problems are the problems in living that we all experience. Professional problems can be difficulties with colleagues or supervisors, the stress of training, unreasonably high expectations for oneself, difficult or complex clients, and so forth. SP/SR participants are advised to choose problems that can be subjectively rated as having a 50–80% negative emotional impact (choosing something with very little emotional impact does not generally generate enough content to be helpful). Participants, however, are cautioned against choosing personal problems that are acute, related to trauma and loss, or chronic and enduring. Personal and professional problems can (and often do) overlap, and this can be accommodated as the workbook progresses.

The next step is to apply selected therapeutic interventions to manage or make changes to the identified problem. The SP exercises incrementally build up the participant's understanding and ability to modify or change an identified problem in much the same way that clients would progress in therapy. In this way, they experience therapy processes "from the inside out."

Each set of SP interventions is followed by SR questions. These usually start with personal SRs (e.g., "What was my experience?"; "How do I understand my experience?") before bridging to therapist SRs (e.g., "What are the implications of my own—and others—experience for my clinical practice?"; "What are the implications for my understanding of CBT theory?"). The "reflective bridge" from personal experience to implications for therapeutic practice is one of the defining features of SP/SR (Bennett-Levy, 2019; Bennett-Levy & Finlay-Jones, 2018). Personal SR is not an end in itself, but rather is the vehicle for skill development of the therapist self.

Writing the self-reflections down is an important part of the process (Bolton, 2010). SP/SR participants report, often to their surprise, that the process of writing is a deeper, more effective way of reflecting than simply "thinking about" their experience. Additionally, when SP/SR is delivered to groups of trainees, it is recommended that members of the group share their SRs, using online discussion forums or SR blogs (Farrand, Perry, & Linsley, 2010; Spafford & Haarhoff, 2015). Sharing SRs achieves a number of goals (e.g., normalizing unexpected emotional or behavioral reactions, overcoming difficulties in executing the SP, and learning from the experience of others).

Finally, we note that brief forms of SP exercises and SR processes are often included in training workshops and supervision, and may play a useful role (Haarhoff & Thwaites, 2016). However, when we use the term *SP/SR* in this chapter and elsewhere, we are not referring to "one-off" SP exercises. *SP/SR* refers to a formal self-experiential training process over an extended period of time, following through on real-life issues and developing reflective skills as a bridge between personal impact of the therapeutic techniques and implications for the therapist role.

Framing SP/SR: The Declarative–Procedural–Reflective Model of Therapist Skills Development

Hand-in-hand with the development of SP/SR has been the development of a theoretical framework, the declarative–procedural–reflective (DPR) model, to conceptualize therapist skills development and understand the impact of SP/SR and other training strategies. Lately, the DPR model has been supplemented by the Personal Practice model to conceptualize the specific impact of personal practices, including SP/SR, on therapist skills (Bennett-Levy, 2019; Bennett-Levy & Finlay-Jones, 2018).

The DPR model has been widely adopted since it was first published (Kuyken, Padesky, & Dudley, 2009; Ludgate, 2016; Whittington & Grey, 2014), and has been presented in a number of different ways to emphasize different aspects of the model (Bennett-Levy, 2006; Bennett-Levy & Thwaites, 2007; Bennett-Levy et al., 2009a). A key distinction in the model is between declarative knowledge (e.g., facts and information about therapy) and procedural skills in action. For instance, a theorist with no clinical involvement may have excellent declarative knowledge but poor procedural skills, while the reverse might be the case for a clinician who has not kept abreast of the literature. The third DPR element, reflection, is seen as "the engine of lifelong learning" (Bennett-Levy, Thwaites, et al., 2009). Drawing on Schön's (1983) work, reflection helps therapists navigate the "low swampy ground" to determine which problem to address with which person, in which particular situation at which time in therapy, drawing

on which kind of conceptualization for selecting which therapeutic skill.

In the context of this chapter, a key DPR distinction is between the personal self and the therapist self (Bennett-Levy, 2019; Bennett-Levy & Finlay-Jones, 2018; Bennett-Levy, Thwaites, et al., 2009). As illustrated in Figure 25.1, these two selves are seen as overlapping but partially distinct. Necessarily, the personal self predates the development of the therapist self. We start the therapist journey with a pre-formed set of attitudes and beliefs (personal self), which are likely to translate into some of the skills, attitudes, and beliefs that we bring to therapy (therapist self). For instance, an empathic attitude toward those in distress would, we hope, characterize those who decide to train as therapists.

However, when we become therapists, we acquire a new set of conceptual and technical skills specific to therapy (e.g., behavioral activation, imagery rescripting, defusion techniques; see Figure 25.1. We may also to some extent add to or modify our interpersonal skills through training; for instance, learning how to repair therapeutic ruptures (see Kraus, Safran, & Muran, Chapter 26, this volume). Hence, we have a therapist self identity and set of behaviors, which is at least partially distinct from the personal self of our day-to-day life. As Figure 25.1 illustrates, we also have a set of personal self beliefs, attitudes, and behaviors (e.g., our cultural or sporting interests) that may play a prominent part in our personal lives but little part in the therapy room. However, there are large degrees of intersection between the personal self and the therapist self, particularly when it comes to interpersonal skills and self-awareness, which are central to both personal and therapeutic relationships. And as we become more experienced as therapists, it seems that we bring more and more of our "personality" or "authentic self" into the therapeutic relationship (Bennett-Levy, 2006).

The overlap between the personal self and therapist self also extends to the impact that personal self beliefs and attitudes may have on therapist self-care, resilience, and burnout (Bennett-Levy & Finlay-Jones, 2018). For instance, patterns of striving to meet unrelenting or perfectionist standards and excessive self-sacrifice, which may often predate therapy training, can make therapists particularly prone to burnout (Haarhoff, 2006; Kaeding et al., 2017). Other beliefs and attitudes may develop

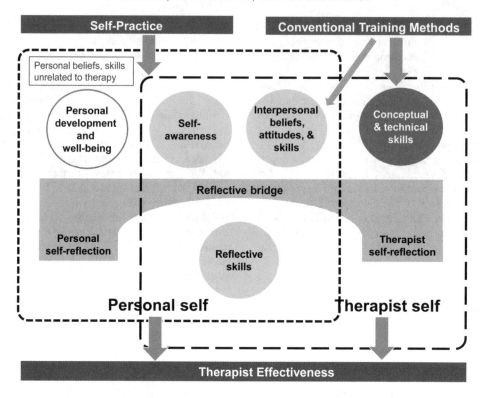

FIGURE 25.1. The personal practice model. From Bennett-Levy and Finlay-Jones (2018) and Bennett-Levy (2019).

specifically within the context of the therapist role (e.g., the belief that we may enjoy working with some clients more than others, or that we have failed if we don't get everyone better).

Many of our interpersonal skills predate the development of the therapist self (Bennett-Levy, 2006), and are brought into our therapist role. Therapists vary in the degree to which they already have strong empathic skills or struggle to make warm, empathic connections. Some authors have suggested that interpersonal skills are relatively immutable through training (Dobson & Shaw, 1993). However, this probably overstates the case, since certain interpersonal skills may be learned through training (e.g., repairing therapeutic ruptures), and as the empirical research on SP/SR demonstrates (see below), one of the chief impacts of SP/SR appears to be an enhancement of interpersonal skills.

This distinction between the personal self and the therapist self becomes important when considering the specific impact of SP/SR and its differentiation from more conventional training methods (see Table 25.1). Typically,

workshops and training programs in most evidence-based therapies tend to be heavily—often exclusively—focused on the therapist self. Conventional training methods such as reading, lectures, modeling, and role play are conceptually driven, with the focus of training on conceptual and technical skills (see Figure 25.1). In the initial stages of training in particular, the pedagogical approaches are often highly didactic, learning can easily become intellectualized, and trainees may require considerable practice to translate declarative knowledge into procedural skills (Bennett-Levy, 2006). In the absence of self-experience, therapy can be "clunky" and overly mechanistic, with therapists sometimes not fully grasping the "nuts and bolts" of applying EBP "in action," or lacking the confidence to translate conceptual understandings into new practices.

In contrast, SP/SR is a self-experiential training strategy focused on both the personal self and therapist self. Learning is experienced through an inductive–reflective process from the "inside out" rather than the "outside in." In

TABLE 25.1. Comparison of SP/SR with Conventional Training Methods

	SP/SR	Conventional training methods
Perspective of training	First-person process—"self-experience"	Third person process – how to deliver therapy to others
Focus of training—which "Self"?	Personal self ("experiencer") and therapist self	Therapist self only
Focus of training—which elements?	• Personal experience of therapy techniques • Experience of problematic feelings, thoughts, and habits • The struggle of achieving personal change	• Conceptual and technical understanding of empirical literature (declarative) • Putting understandings into practice (procedural)
Key learning processes	• Experiential learning of the therapy • Self-reflection as experiencer and therapist: in particular, making the Reflective bridge from "personal self" to "therapist self"	• Reading about therapy and didactic learning from lectures or workshops (declarative) • Modeling, role playing, and feedback (procedural)
Role of educator	Process facilitator	Teacher

the terms of Epstein's (1994, 2014) cognitive–experiential theory, both the experiential system and the rational system are engaged: the experiential system as the "experiencer" of therapeutic techniques; the rational system in reflecting first for the personal self, then for the therapist self. Hence, the SP/SR model (Figure 25.1) predicts that whereas conventional therapist self-oriented training strategies should impact primarily on conceptual and technical knowledge and skills, the self-experiential nature of SP/SR should additionally impact on self-awareness and interpersonal beliefs, attitudes and skills that lie at the interface of the personal self and therapist self (Bennett-Levy, 2019). Consistent with these predictions, in a study of 120 experienced CBT therapists, Bennett-Levy, McManus, Westling, and Fennell (2009) reported that while conventional training methods such as reading, lectures, modeling, and role play were rated as effective in enhancing conceptual and technical skills, self-experiential work and reflective practice were rated as the methods of choice for enhancing interpersonal skills and reflective skills. As we see in the next section, the findings from this study are supported and reinforced by studies of SP/SR across a range of practitioners from different countries with different levels of experience.

SP/SR may also be differentiated from per-

sonal therapy. Large-scale surveys of therapists' personal therapy indicate that the prime reasons that therapists seek therapy is for personal problems and personal growth (Orlinsky, Schofield, Schroder, & Kazantzis, 2011). In other words, the data suggests that, for most therapists, personal therapy is focused largely or exclusively on the personal self. In contrast, SP/SR has been specifically developed to enhance therapist skills. In SP/SR the focus on the personal self is primarily to develop and enhance the therapist self. Consequently, we argue that in many contexts, SP/SR may be a more targeted therapist training strategy than personal therapy, since the reflective process in SP/SR is specifically geared to creating a reflective bridge between the personal self and the therapist self (Bennett-Levy & Finlay-Jones, 2018).

Empirical Research on SP/SR

Since 2001, SP/SR publications have featured researchers from a number of different countries (e.g., Australia, New Zealand, United Kingdom, Austria, Germany) and therapists with different levels of experience and specialities, including experienced CBT therapists and supervisors (Bennett-Levy et al., 2003; Davis et al., 2015), clinical psychology trainees (Bennett-Levy et al., 2001; Schneider & Rees, 2012; Spendelow & Butler, 2016), diploma CBT students (Chaddock, Thwaites, Bennett-Levy, & Freeston, 2014; Haarhoff, Gibson, & Flett, 2011; Spafford & Haarhoff, 2015), experienced low-intensity CBT practitioners (Thwaites, Cairns, et al., 2015), and allied health professionals (Farrand et al., 2010).

Although much work is needed to determine similarities and differences in SP/SR impact in practitioners with different experience levels (McGinn, 2015; Thwaites, Bennett-Levy, & Haarhoff, 2015), there are some clear consistencies across groups and countries. A meta-synthesis of existing studies concluded that SP/SR increases understanding of the model and techniques (declarative system), improves application of the techniques (procedural system), and increases reflective skills and ongoing refinement of therapeutic understanding and skills (reflective system) (Gale & Schröder, 2014).

The impact of SP/SR appears to vary according to the stage of development of the therapist. SP/SR seems to have the most impact on declarative understandings in novice therapists by reinforcing and internalizing learning from books or workshops (Bennett-Levy et al., 2001); SP/SR also assists their translation from declarative information to procedural skills, since therapeutic techniques become "lived experience" rather than words on a page (Thwaites et al., 2014). For more experienced therapists who have already internalized their declarative understanding and basic techniques, the impact of SP/SR is more nuanced. For instance, Bennett-Levy and colleagues (2003) reported that in a group of experienced therapists, SP/SR enabled therapists to refine CBT techniques and enhance their interpersonal skills and metacognitive skills (e.g., enhanced self-reflection and therapist flexibility).

The consistent finding across all SP/SR studies is the impact of SP/SR on interpersonal skills and self-awareness (Bennett-Levy, 2019; Laireiter & Willutzki, 2003; Thwaites et al., 2014). Being "in the client's chair" and experiencing the difficulties in facing rather than avoiding emotional issues, and the difficulties in making changes to existing ways of feeling and behaving, creates empathy and respect for the struggles that clients face. For experienced therapists, this might be a "tap on the shoulder" reminder; for all therapists, SP/SR helps to at-

tune them to what their clients are expressing verbally and nonverbally. They report that they are more perceptually attuned, more empathic and compassionate. There is always a danger in more conceptual/technical therapies that therapists place too much attention on ensuring they are delivering an evidence-based intervention "correctly," and in doing so, lose connection with the client (Bennett-Levy, 2006). SP/SR appears to serve as an experiential reminder of the centrality of the therapeutic relationship.

Enhanced self-awareness is also a consistent effect of SP/SR (Bennett-Levy & Finlay-Jones, 2018). It is the nature of SP/SR that participants become more aware of their negative automatic thoughts, internal reactions, and underlying patterns of behavior and feelings that serve as barriers to change. This can be challenging. However, when SP/SR participants experience firsthand the impact of therapeutic strategies such as imagery and behavioral experiments, it can renew or enhance their belief in the therapy and give added impetus to their delivery of EBPs.

Finally, although the purpose of SP/SR has not primarily been to solve personal problems or create personal growth, recent studies have suggested the potential to use SP/SR processes to enhance therapist self-care (Bennett-Levy, Wilson, et al., 2015; Pakenham, 2015), a major issue for trainees and therapists alike (Haarhoff & Thwaites, 2016; Haarhoff, Thwaites, & Bennett-Levy, 2015; Pakenham, 2015). We anticipate that future SP/SR studies will be increasingly oriented toward therapist self-care. In the latter part of this chapter, we introduce some SP/SR exercises focused on self-care, so that readers can experiment with some CBT-based SP/SR for themselves.

A caveat about SP/SR research to date is that it is largely based on self-report, and most have been qualitative studies. Qualitative research methods are valuable and fitting for descriptive questions and efforts to map the territory of interest. Now that research is clearer about potential impacts of SP/SR, quantitative studies are starting to emerge (Davis et al., 2015; Pakenham, 2015; Spendelow & Butler, 2016). There is clearly a need at this stage to progress with more refined studies, ideally conducting randomized trials that compare clinicians and trainees who receive SP/SR with those who receive other types of training to determine whether the predicted impacts of SP/SR hold up under these conditions. The prior work on developing the SP/SR approach, qualitatively mapping the self-reported outcomes of SP/SR across many settings and clinician groups, and the guiding DPR theoretical model inform clear predictions and measurement strategies that are ripe for empirical investigation (Bennett-Levy & Finlay-Jones, 2018).

In summary, we see SP/SR as an integrative training strategy. It is designed to integrate the personal self with the therapist self; the declarative with the procedural; the interpersonal with the technical and conceptual; and the experiential with the rational. Self-awareness and self-reflection provide the glue that enables the personal self to inform and influence the therapist self and the different therapy skills to blend effectively with one another. Those who engage effectively with SP/SR tend to report major shifts in their appreciation of the therapeutic process, and in the ways that they engage with clients.

Guidelines for Using SP/SR

To date, studies of SP/SR have all been undertaken in the context of group training programs. However, there is no reason why SP/SR cannot be undertaken by individuals, or within the context of a supervisory relationship or consultation team, and guidelines are available for this purpose (Thwaites & Haarhoff, 2016). Most therapists believe that SP/SR may be of benefit, but not all SP/SR participants engage well enough with SP/SR to derive benefit, and many are stopped by issues such as lack of time from engaging with SP/SR in the first place (Bennett-Levy & Lee, 2014; Haarhoff et al., 2015). Furthermore, a small minority of therapists may have difficult experiences from SP/SR, when the process triggers an unexpectedly strong reaction.

Awareness of these issues has meant that it has taken 15 years to create guidelines and scaffolding materials for self-guided SP/SR in publicly

Sources of therapist stress	What are the factors contributing to my work-related stress?
Client factors: difficult interpersonal styles, emotional dysregulation, therapy-interfering behaviors such as avoidance, unrealistic expectations of therapy, paranoid or litigious behavior, self-harm, suicide attempts, or completions.	
Work-related factors: unmanageable caseloads, staff shortages, restructuring, poor supervision or lack of supervision, unrealistic goals and expectations, competency requirements, workplace bullying, difficult relationships with other staff members.	
Event-related factors: life crises such as bereavement, divorce, moving home, loss of employment, poor health, and money problems.	
Self-evaluative factors: negative beliefs about ability and competence, self-doubt, fear of being judged, perfectionism and negative self-schemas, such as beliefs concerning failure or not being good enough.	
Educational or training factors: high expectations, difficult-to-meet academic standards, being required to take on complex cases too soon, increasing self-awareness regarding "what I don't know," and continual evaluation.	

FIGURE 25.2. Sources of Therapist Stress Questionnaire. Copyright © 2019 B. A. Haarhoff and J. Bennett-Levy.

available forms. We wanted to be confident that we had addressed engagement and safety issues with SP/SR as effectively as possible. Guidelines for SP/SR are now readily available (Bennett-Levy & Lee, 2014; Farrell & Shaw, 2018; Freeston, Thwaites, & Bennett-Levy, 2019; Kolts et al., 2018; Thwaites & Haarhoff, 2016). Specific chapters for SP/SR participants and trainers are included in the SP/SR CBT workbook (Bennett-Levy, Thwaites, et al., 2015), which was written to reflect contemporary understandings of CBT and promote the processes of value for both therapists' personal selves and their therapist selves. The specific features built into the workbook were that it should be transdiagnostic, strengths-based, experiential (e.g., featuring behavioral experiments and imagery), process oriented (as well as content oriented), and include body-oriented interventions.

While a detailed discussion of all SP/SR guidelines is beyond the scope of this chapter, clinicians, trainers, and supervisors should note that it is important to spend time addressing all issues of concern to SP/SR participants (e.g., safety, confidentiality, course expectations, the difference between private reflections and shared reflections, addressing the potential for dual relationship). SP/SR processes should be negotiated and agreed upon with individuals and groups prior to the commencement of a program. Creating a context of safety and anticipating that SP/SR will be beneficial and worthwhile are both central to promoting engagement and benefit from programs (Bennett-Levy & Lee, 2014; Freeston et al., 2019). Other important issues include being clear about where and how SP/SR fits into training or course requirements; creating a supportive group environment; ensuring that participants have a personal safeguard strategy in place (e.g., reducing involvement with SP/SR if they are feeling unduly stressed); and providing guidance for the how-tos of SR (e.g., written examples of "good" SR, scheduling regular uninterrupted time).

Experiencing SP/SR Exercises

As we have emphasized, there is a difference between reading about a technique and experiencing it from the inside out, so this last part of the chapter is devoted to experiencing. Since therapist self-care is an issue that affects many health professionals, and in particular students (Pakenham, 2015) (e.g., more than 50% of clinical psychology students report levels of psychological distress), we have focused the following SP/SR exercises on self-care issues to bridge both the personal self and therapist self.

Exercise 1: How Is My Self-Care Being Compromised?

Identify which sources of therapist or trainee stress listed in the Sources of Therapist Stress Questionnaire (page 387) may be compromising your self-care. Bring to mind some specific situations and, in the space provided, note what factors may have contributed to the stress. Some of these factors may be more external pressures (e.g., academic demands, organizational problems, adverse events), others may be more internal (e.g., negative self-evaluation, perfectionistic standards). Select one of these factors for Exercises 2 and 3.

Self-Reflective Questions

1. How was it to do this questionnaire? Did your answers surprise you in any way? If so, how?
2. Reflecting on your feelings as you completed and reviewed the questionnaire: Do you have any thoughts about how it might be for clients who are asked to complete similar questionnaires? Would this change in any way the ways in which you present questionnaires to clients? Or the ways in which you debrief their experience of questionnaires?

Exercise 2: Identifying Your Old/Unhelpful Ways of Being

Referring to Exercise 1, bring to mind a specific recent situation in which your self-care was compromised by the issue that you identified. What were your . . .

Emotions	
Bodily sensations	
Thoughts/images (complete phrases)	
Behaviors/actions	

Now, do the same with a second situation in which your self-care was compromised by the issue that you identified, and complete the chart below:

Emotions	
Bodily sensations	
Thoughts/images (complete phrases)	
Behaviors/actions	

If a third or fourth situation come to mind, you can complete the same chart again.

Now transfer items from these charts into the Old/Unhelpful Ways of Being disk model (Figure 25.3). The Ways of Being disk model is a holistic framework within which to formulate and contrast Old/Unhelpful Ways of Being with New/Desired Ways of Being (Bennett-Levy, Thwaites, et al., 2015). While a detailed explanation of the Ways of Being (WoB) model is beyond the scope of this chapter, here, we guide you in two exercises featuring the model to give you a "taste" of the process (see Chapter 2 and Modules 9–11 of Bennett-Levy, Thwaites, et al., 2015, for further information). The more situations in which you can add to the Old/Unhelpful Ways of Being disk, the fuller the picture. If you detect consistent behavioral or emotional patterns from your charts (e.g., avoidance, rumination, safety behaviors), add these to the Old Underlying Patterns section (for an example, see Bennett-Levy, Thwaites, et al., 2015, Module 9).

Self-Reflective Questions

1. What was my experience of completing the charts? And then framing these elements within the Old/Unhelpful Ways of Being disk model?
2. Does the disk model help me to understand my experience?
3. How much might my emotional and/ or cognitive experience of doing this exercise be reflected in the experiences of clients who are focusing on "how things go wrong"? What are the implications for the way I work with clients on such issues?

Exercise 3: Creating New/Desired Ways of Being

If you are following on immediately from the previous exercise, we would suggest a break, a cup of tea, and some simple mind-changing exercises (e.g., recall past successes, imagine yourself engaging in a favorite pleasurable activity) to change your mindset from a problem-oriented approach to one of creative possibility. With clients, we would leave the New Ways of Being exercise for a new session rather than mix it with the Old Ways of Being.

The foundation for creating New/Desired Ways of Being is an imagery exercise that should be repeated on several occasions in order to strengthen and enrich the New Ways. First, notice your strengths, talents, interests, and abilities that show themselves in contexts not necessarily related to the present problem. Experience the feeling of these strengths in your body, perhaps accompanied by memories of times that you have used them. Write down your strengths in the Personal Strengths section of the New Ways disk (see Figure 25.4).

Next, ask yourself, in relation to the problem area: "How would I like to be in these types of situations?" Imagine yourself being exactly as you would like to be in the situations that have been a problem, even if right now it is hard to believe that you could feel or act in this way. Bring your Personal Strengths into focus. How might these help you? See yourself clearly in one of the problem situations, but feeling exactly as you would like to feel, behaving in exactly the way that you would like to be behaving, thinking in exactly the way that you would like to be thinking about yourself and the situation. How do you want to be feeling? Do you notice any particular place in your body that you feel this? What do you see yourself doing? How does that feel? How does it feel to feel this way in your body? What personal strengths are you drawing on? What thoughts and images are you having: about you and about the situation? How is what you see yourself doing different from before? Note your thoughts, images, behaviors, bodily sensations, strengths, underlying patterns, and motives on the New/Desired Ways of Being disk.

Although there is not the space to go further with developing the New Ways in this chapter, the next steps would be to strengthen and embed the New Ways, using experiential strategies such as imaging past experiences of similar successes, undertaking behavioral experi-

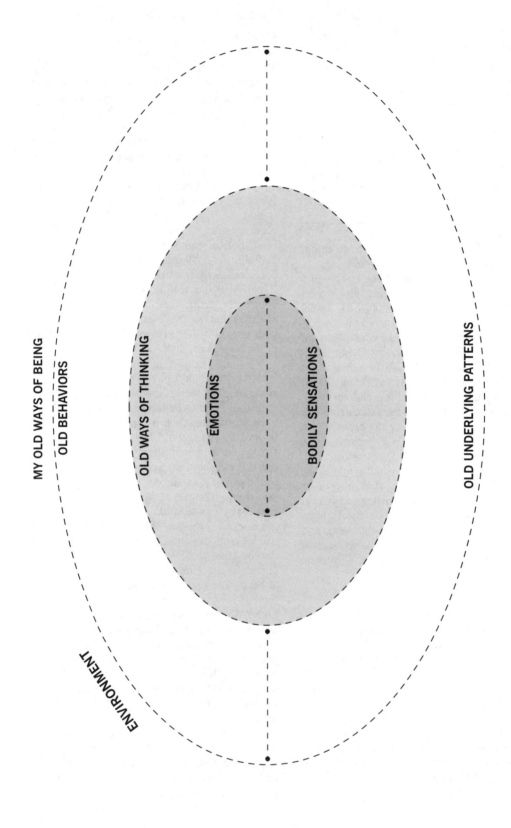

MY OLD WAYS OF BEING

OLD BEHAVIORS

OLD WAYS OF THINKING

EMOTIONS

BODILY SENSATIONS

OLD UNDERLYING PATTERNS

ENVIRONMENT

FIGURE 25.3. My Old/Unhelpful Ways of Being. From Bennett-Levy, Thwaites, Haarhoff, and Perry. Copyright © 2015 from The Guilford Press. Reprinted with permission.

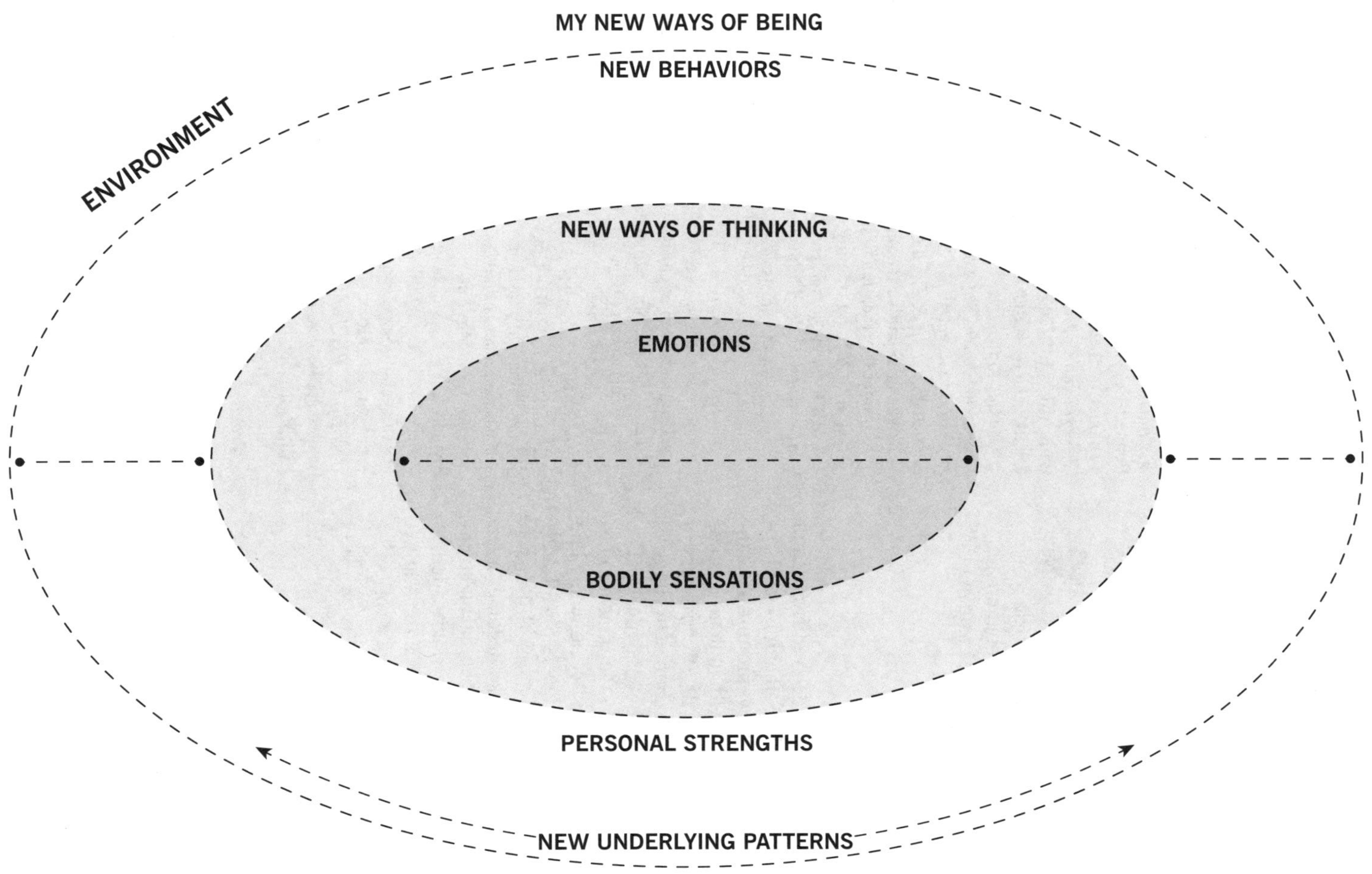

FIGURE 25.4. My New/Desired Ways of Being. From Bennett-Levy, Thwaites, Haarhoff, and Perry. Copyright © 2015 from The Guilford Press. Reprinted with permission.

ments, experimenting with empowering body movements, and playing evocative music (see Bennett-Levy, Thwaites, et al., 2015, Modules 10 and 11).

Self-Reflective Questions

1. What was your experience with accessing your strengths? How easy or difficult was it to do the imagery exercise? Were you able to form a strong image of your New Ways? Anything get in the way? What?
2. How do you understand your experience?
3. If you were to introduce the Old Ways/New Ways ideas to clients, what rationale would you give? How would you go about creating the experiential exercise? And ensuring that they embed the learning?

Conclusion

SP/SR is a training strategy derived from adult education theory and the DPR therapist skill development model, which shows promise as an integrative training strategy. Although more studies are required to establish its effectiveness in different settings, our research to date suggests that SP/SR puts flesh on the bones of declarative understandings and assists in the translation to procedural skills for novice practitioners, while for more experienced practitioners SP/SR adds nuance and quality to procedural skills. Additionally, interpersonal skills become more seamlessly integrated with conceptual and technical skills, practitioners become more adept at self-reflection, and SP/SR provides tools to explore the personal self and to create a reflective bridge to the therapist self.

Ultimately, SP/SR should not be seen as a once-off training program. The aim of SP/SR should be for therapists to create new ways of being that enhance their personal and professional wisdom and skills. In this sense, SP represents an ongoing commitment to growth of the personal self and a deepened understanding of the therapist self, while SR is a metacognitive skill, which both the therapy and social psychological literatures consistently identify as central to personal and therapeutic wisdom. The challenge for future clinicians and researchers is to create and research SP/SR programs that embed these practices in the long term, with demonstrated effectiveness for the well-being of clients and therapists alike.

References

Beck, A. T., Freeman, A., & Associates. (1990). *Cognitive therapy of personality disorders*. New York: Guilford Press.

Beck, J. S. (1995). *Cognitive therapy: Basics and beyond*. New York: Guilford Press.

Beidas, R. S., & Kendall, P. C. (2010). Training therapists in evidence-based practice: A critical review of studies from a systems-contextual perspective. *Clinical Psychology: Science and Practice, 17*, 1–30.

Bennett-Levy, J. (2006). Therapist skills: A cognitive model of their acquisition and refinement. *Behavioural and Cognitive Psychotherapy, 34*, 57–78.

Bennett-Levy, J. (2019). Why therapists should walk the talk: The theoretical and empirical case for personal practice in therapist training and professional development. *Journal of Behavior Therapy and Experimental Psychiatry, 62*, 133–145.

Bennett-Levy, J., & Beedie, A. (2007). The ups and downs of cognitive therapy training: What happens to trainees' perception of their competence during a cognitive therapy training course? *Behavioural and Cognitive Psychotherapy, 35*, 61–75.

Bennett-Levy, J., & Finlay-Jones, A. (2018). Personal practice for therapists: A model to guided therapists, educators, supervisors and researchers. *Cognitive Behaviour Therapy, 47*, 185–205.

Bennett-Levy, J., & Lee, N. (2014). Self-practice and self-reflection in cognitive behaviour therapy training: What factors influence trainees' engagement and experience of benefit? *Behavioural and Cognitive Psychotherapy, 42*, 48–64.

Bennett-Levy, J., Lee, N., Travers, K., Pohlman, S., & Hamernik, E. (2003). Cognitive therapy from the inside: Enhancing therapist skills through practising what we preach. *Behavioural and Cognitive Psychotherapy, 31*, 145–163.

Bennett-Levy, J., McManus, F., Westling, B., & Fennell, M. J. V. (2009). Acquiring and refining CBT skills and competencies: Which training methods are perceived to be most effective? *Behavioural and Cognitive Psychotherapy, 37*, 571–583.

Bennett-Levy, J., & Padesky, C. A. (2014). Use it or lose it: Post-workshop reflection enhances learning and utilization of CBT skills. *Cognitive and Behavioral Practice, 21*, 12–19.

Bennett-Levy, J., & Thwaites, R. (2007). Self and self-reflection in the therapeutic relationship: A conceptual map and practical strategies for the training, supervision and self-supervision of interpersonal skills. In P. Gilbert & R. Leahy (Eds.), *The therapeutic relationship in the cognitive behavioural psychotherapies* (pp. 255–281). London: Routledge.

Bennett-Levy, J., Thwaites, R., Chaddock, A., & Davis, M. (2009). Reflective practice in cognitive behavioural therapy. In J. Stedmon & R. Dallos (Eds.), *Reflective practice in psychotherapy and counselling* (pp. 115–135). Maidenhead, UK: Open University Press.

Bennett-Levy, J., Thwaites, R., Haarhoff, B., & Perry, H. (2015). *Experiencing CBT from the inside out: A self-practice/self-reflection workbook for therapists.* New York: Guilford Press.

Bennett-Levy, J., Turner, F., Beaty, T., Smith, M., Paterson, B., & Farmer, S. (2001). The value of self-practice of cognitive therapy techniques and self-reflection in the training of cognitive therapists. *Behavioural and Cognitive Psychotherapy, 29,* 203–220.

Bennett-Levy, J., Wilson, S., Nelson, J., Rotumah, D., Ryan, K., Budden, W., et al. (2015). Spontaneous self-practice of CBT by Aboriginal counsellors during and following CBT training: A retrospective analysis of facilitating conditions and impact. *Australian Psychologist, 50,* 329–334.

Boellinghaus, I., Jones, F. W., & Hutton, J. (2013). Cultivating self-care and compassion in psychological therapists in training: The experience of practicing loving-kindness meditation. *Training and Education in Professional Psychology, 7,* 267–277.

Bolton, G. (2010). *Reflective practice: Writing and professional development.* London: SAGE.

Chaddock, A., Thwaites, R., Bennett-Levy, J., & Freeston, M. (2014). Understanding individual differences in response to self-practice and self-reflection (SP/SR) during CBT training. *The Cognitive Behaviour Therapist, 7,* e14.

Cushway, D. (1992). Stress in clinical psychology trainees. *British Journal of Clinical Psychology, 31,* 169–179.

Davis, M. L., Thwaites, R., Freeston, M. H., & Bennett-Levy, J. (2015). A measurable impact of a self-practice/self-reflection programme on the therapeutic skills of experienced cognitive-behavioural therapists. *Clinical Psychology and Psychotherapy, 22,* 176–184.

Dobson, K. S., & Shaw, B. F. (1993). The training of cognitive therapists: What have we learned from treatment manuals? *Psychotherapy, 30,* 573–577.

Edmunds, J. M., Beidas, R. S., & Kendall, P. C. (2013). Dissemination and implementation of evidence–based practices: Training and consultation as implementation strategies. *Clinical Psychology: Science and Practice, 20,* 152–165.

Epstein, S. (1994). Integration of the cognitive and the psychodynamic unconscious. *American Psychologist, 49,* 709–724.

Epstein, S. (2014). *Cognitive-experiential theory: An integrative theory of personality.* New York: Oxford University Press.

Farrand, P., Perry, J., & Linsley, S. (2010). Enhancing Self-Practice/Self-Reflection (SP/SR) approach to cognitive behaviour training through the use of reflective blogs. *Behavioural and Cognitive Psychotherapy, 38,* 473–477.

Farrell, J. M., & Shaw, I. A. (2018). *Experiencing schema therapy from the inside out: A self-practice/self-reflection workbook for therapists.* New York: Guilford Press.

Freeston, M. H., Thwaites, R., & Bennett-Levy, J. (2019). "Courses for Horses": Designing, adapting and implementing self-practice/self-reflection programmes. *The Cognitive Behaviour Therapist, 12,* e28.

Freud, S. (1957). Analysis terminable and interminable. In J. S. Strachey (Ed.), *Complete psychological works of Sigmund Freud.* London: Hogarth Press. (Original work published 1937)

Gale, C., & Schröder, T. (2014). Experiences of self-practice/self-reflection in cognitive behavioural therapy: A meta-synthesis of qualitative studies. *Psychology and Psychotherapy: Theory, Research and Practice, 87,* 373–392.

Gale, C., Schröder, T., & Gilbert, P. (2017). Do you practice what you preach?: A qualitative exploration of therapists' personal practice of compassion focused therapy. *Clinical Psychology and Psychotherapy, 24,* 171–185.

Haarhoff, B. (2006). The importance of identifying and understanding therapist schema in cognitive therapy training and supervision. *New Zealand Journal of Psychology, 35,* 126–131.

Haarhoff, B., Gibson, K., & Flett, R. (2011). Improving the quality of cognitive behaviour therapy case conceptualization: The role of self-practice/self-reflection. *Behavioural and Cognitive Psychotherapy, 39,* 323–339.

Haarhoff, B., & Thwaites, R. (2016). *Reflection in CBT.* London: SAGE.

Haarhoff, B., Thwaites, R., & Bennett-Levy, J. (2015). Engagement with self-practice/self-reflection as professional development: The role of therapist beliefs. *Australian Psychologist, 50,* 322–328.

Kaeding, A., Sougleris, C., Reid, C., van Vreeswijk, M. F., Hayes, C., Dorrian, J., et al. (2017). Professional burnout, early maladaptive schemas, and physical health in clinical and counselling psychology trainees. *Journal of Clinical Psychology, 73,* 1782–1796.

Kolb, D. (1984). *Experiential learning: Experience as the source of learning and development.* Englewood Cliffs, NJ: Prentice Hall.

Kolts, R. L., Bell, T., Bennett-Levy, J., & Irons, C. (2018). *Experiencing compassion-focused therapy from the inside out: A self-practice/self-reflection workbook for therapists.* New York: Guilford Press.

Kuyken, W., Padesky, C. A., & Dudley, R. (2009). *Collaborative case conceptualization: Working effectively with clients in cognitive-behavioral therapy.* New York: Guilford Press.

Laireiter, A.-R., & Willutzki, U. (2003). Self-reflection and self-practice in training of cognitive behaviour therapy: An overview. *Clinical Psychology and Psychotherapy, 10,* 19–30.

Levitt, H. M., & Piazza-Bonin, E. (2016). Wisdom and psychotherapy: Studying expert therapists' clinical wisdom to explicate common processes. *Psychotherapy Research, 26,* 31–47.

Linehan, M. M., & McGhee, D. E. (1994). A cognitive-behavioural model of supervision with individual and group components. In S. E. Greben (Ed.), *Clini-*

cal perspectives on psychotherapy supervision (pp. 165–188). Washington, DC: American Psychiatric Press.

Ludgate, J. (2016). Self-management in CBT training and supervision. In D. M. Sudak, R. T. Codd, III, J. W. Ludgate, L. Sokol, M. G. Fox, R. P. Reiser, et al. (Eds.), Teaching and supervising cognitive behavioral therapy (pp. 243–264). Hoboken, NJ: Wiley.

Lyon, A. R., Stirman, S. W., Kerns, S. E. U., & Bruns, E. J. (2011). Developing the mental health workforce: Review and application of training approaches from multiple disciplines. Administration and Policy in Mental Health and Mental Health Services Research, 38, 238–253.

McGinn, L. (2015). Enhancing cognitive-behavioural therapy (CBT) skill acquisition through experiential and reflective learning: A commentary on studies examining the impact of self-practice and self-reflection in CBT. Australian Psychologist, 50, 340–343.

Nadeem, E., Gleacher, A., & Beidas, R. S. (2013). Consultation as an implementation strategy for evidence-based practices across multiple contexts: Unpacking the black box. Administration and Policy in Mental Health and Mental Health Services Research, 40, 439–450.

Orlinsky, D. E., Schofield, M. J., Schroder, T., & Kazantzis, N. (2011). Utilization of personal therapy by psychotherapists: A practice-friendly review and a new study. Journal of Clinical Psychology: In Session, 67, 828–842.

Padesky, C. A. (1996). Developing cognitive therapist competency: Teaching and supervision models. In P. M. Salkovskis (Ed.), Frontiers of cognitive therapy (pp. 266–292). New York: Guilford Press.

Pakenham, K. I. (2015). Effects of acceptance and commitment therapy (ACT) training on clinical psychology trainee stress, therapist skills and attributes, and ACT processes. Clinical Psychology and Psychotherapy, 22, 647–655.

Pakenham, K. I., & Stafford-Brown, J. (2012). Stress in clinical psychology trainees: Current research status and future directions. Australian Psychologist, 47, 147–155.

Schneider, K., & Rees, C. (2012). Evaluation of a combined cognitive behavioural therapy and interpersonal process group in the psychotherapy training of clinical psychologists. Australian Psychologist, 47, 137–146.

Schön, D. A. (1983). The reflective practitioner. New York: Basic Books.

Shapiro, S. L., Brown, K. W., & Biegel, G. M. (2007). Teaching self-care to caregivers: Effects of mindfulness-based stress reduction on the mental health of therapists in training. Training and Education in Professional Psychology, 1, 105–115.

Skovholt, T. M., & Rønnestad, M. H. (2001). The long, textured path from novice to senior practitioner. In T. M. Skovholt (Ed.), The resilient practitioner: Burnout prevention and self-care strategies for counselors, therapists, teachers, and health professionals (pp. 25–54). Boston: Allyn & Bacon.

Spafford, S., & Haarhoff, B. (2015). What are the conditions needed to facilitate online self-reflection for CBT trainees? Australian Psychologist, 50, 232–240.

Spendelow, J. S., & Butler, L. J. (2016). Reported positive and negative outcomes associated with a self-practice/self-reflection cognitive-behavioural therapy exercise for CBT trainees. Psychotherapy Research, 26, 602–611.

Staudinger, U. M., & Gluck, J. (2011). Psychological wisdom research: Commonalities and differences in a growing field. Annual Review of Psychology, 62, 215–241.

Thwaites, R., & Bennett-Levy, J. (2007). Conceptualizing empathy in cognitive therapy: Making the implicit explicit. Behavioural and Cognitive Psychotherapy, 35, 591–612.

Thwaites, R., Bennett-Levy, J., Davis, M., & Chaddock, A. (2014). Using self-practice and self-reflection (SP/SR) to enhance CBT competence and meta-competence. In A. Whittington & N. Grey (Eds.), How to become a more effective CBT therapist: Mastering metacompetence in clinical practice (pp. 241–254). Chichester, UK: Wiley-Blackwell.

Thwaites, R., Bennett-Levy, J., & Haarhoff, B. (2015). Invited response to commentaries: Self-practice/self-reflection (SP/SR): Contexts, challenges and ways forward. Australian Psychologist, 50, 344–349.

Thwaites, R., Cairns, L., Bennett-Levy, J., Johnston, L., Lowrie, R., Robinson, A., et al. (2015). Developing metacompetence in low intensity CBT interventions: Evaluating a self-practice/self-reflection program for experienced low intensity CBT practitioners. Australian Psychologist, 50, 311–321.

Thwaites, R., & Haarhoff, B. (2016). Experiencing CBT for yourself: Using self-practice and self-reflection (SP/SR) to develop therapeutic competence and metacompetence. In B. Haarhoff & R. Thwaites (Eds.), Reflection in CBT (pp. 127–140). London: SAGE.

Whittington, A., & Grey, N. (2014). How to become a more effective therapist: Mastering metacompetence in clinical practice. Chichester, UK: Wiley.

CHAPTER 26

Augmenting Cognitive-Behavioral Therapy with Alliance-Focused Training

A Research-Informed Case Study

JESSICA KRAUS
JEREMY D. SAFRAN
J. CHRISTOPHER MURAN

Like any relationship, the relationship between patient and therapist is subject to occasional misunderstandings, tensions, and disagreements. But what happens to the therapeutic relationship if these types of strains become ongoing events? Perhaps your patient chronically arrives late, is not following through with out-of-session assignments, is overly deferential, or is given to long silences. Perhaps you feel detached or disconnected from your patient, and the vital connection that you expect to have is instead pervaded by a sense of dullness or irritation. Whether you regard a collaborative relationship with your patient to be a necessary condition of treatment, an epiphenomenon, or the vehicle of change, these signs of relational breakdowns can be challenging. Even the most experienced of practitioners is put to the test when working to effectively address deterioration in the therapeutic alliance.

The therapeutic alliance—the bond or relationship between patient and therapist as they engage in the collaborative work of treatment—is perhaps the most exhaustively studied construct within the field of psychotherapy research. For more than three decades, research findings have consistently shown that the quality of the alliance predicts treatment outcome (Horvath, Del Re, Flückiger, & Symonds, 2011).

Although the concept of alliance arose out of developments in the psychoanalytic field, the importance of establishing and maintaining a positive connection between patient and therapist emerges as an important factor across diverse schools of treatment, from humanistic to behavioral (Flückiger, Del Re, Wampold, Symonds, & Horvath, 2012). Increasingly, researchers are turning their attention to defining alliance-fostering skills and developing effective ways of training clinicians from diverse orientations and developmental stages of professional development to incorporate these skills into practice.

Among the most important skills are those that support clinicians in successfully managing negative interpersonal process, which describes the tendency for therapists to respond to patient hostility with counterhostility (Binder & Strupp, 1997). When unaddressed, negative process often results in premature termination or poor outcome (Anderson, Knobloch-Fedders, Stiles, Ordoñez, & Heckman, 2012; Binder & Strupp, 1997; Martin, Garske, & Davis, 2000). These findings may seem self-evident; however, negative process in most cases does not present as open conflict or dramatic confrontation but arises within the treatment in a more subtle fashion and is frequently not easy to detect. For example, the therapist who pursues a task for which the patient shows little enthusiasm, or the overly compliant or deferential patient may indicate the presence of negative process which, along with more obvious shows of hostility, suggest a strain or rupture in the alliance. Although ruptures signal a breakdown in the therapeutic alliance, they also offer opportunities to explore and challenge the maladaptive beliefs and interpersonal patterns that are often central to the difficulties that bring patients into treatment (Safran & Segal, 1990). Because ruptures in the alliance are both inevitable and ubiquitous within clinical practice, learning the skills to successfully detect and manage these tensions are essential to the novice and the seasoned clinician alike (Safran & Muran, 2000).

Surprisingly few approaches have focused directly on training clinicians to attend to strains in the alliance or to address ruptures when they occur. In fact, in a meta-analysis of the impact of rupture resolution training and/or supervision on outcome, only eight studies were identified for inclusion (Safran, Muran, & Eubanks-Carter, 2011). In the course of an ongoing initiative to extend research on the therapeutic alliance and to translate study findings into clinical practice, Safran, Muran, and colleagues developed a protocol known as alliance-focused training (AFT; Muran, Safran, & Eubanks-Carter, 2011; Muran, Safran, Samstag, & Winston, 2005; Safran & Muran, 2000; Safran, Muran, Samstag, & Winston, 2005). AFT assumes that a strong therapeutic alliance is a precondition for success in all forms of therapy. The training emphasizes experiential learning and self-exploration, and employs a set of core principles and strategies drawn from research and contemporary relational theory that can be taught to therapists of any orientation as an adjunctive form of training. AFT is intended to elucidate the rupture and repair process, and to provide a framework for cultivating the therapeutic alliance. AFT also helps therapists develop and refine their abilities to engage "hard to reach" clients, and it revitalizes and deepens the everyday clinical work of even the most experienced practitioners (Eubanks-Carter, Muran, Safran, 2010; Safran et al., 2011; Safran, Muran, Samstag, & Stevens, 2002).

AFT is based on the foundational belief that all interventions are relational acts. The content or activity of the session—constructing a thought record, identifying and challenging core beliefs, offering an interpretation—are in-

separable from and determined by the quality of the interpersonal relationship within which they occur (Safran & Muran, 2000; Safran & Segal, 1990). Therapists are taught to monitor what is taking place in the alliance on an ongoing basis and to explore the patient's emerging feelings in the context of the relationship. They are sensitized to how the patient's verbal and nonverbal expressions may serve as a source of information about the patient's thoughts and feelings. The therapist is guided to identify subtle indicators—such as sighs, gestures, and glances—and to draw the patient's attention to his or her emotions and the information these emotional responses provide about the patient's goals and needs (Greenberg & Safran, 1989).

In AFT, therapists are also encouraged to attend to their own internal experience in session as important data regarding what may be occurring in the context of the interaction with the patient. Therapists come to recognize that they may be unaware of how they may contribute to tension in the relationship. Mindfulness training is used in this context to help therapists develop a nonjudgmental awareness of their internal experiences on a moment-to-moment basis in order to become more fully attuned to the unfolding relational dynamic. By attending in this way, the therapist can also begin to recognize *enactments*—the subtle tug and pull of transference–countertransference interactions—that may be playing out across the treatment. AFT is predicated on the assumption that alliance ruptures and enactments result from patients' and therapists' contributions and are resolved through collaborative investigation (Safran & Muran, 2000).

A central strategy in AFT for resolving ruptures is metacommunication, which refers to the therapist actively engaging the patient in a mutual exploration of the implicit relational process occurring within the treatment (Kiesler, 1996; Safran et al., 2002; Safran & Muran, 2000). Metacommunication strategies keep the focus on in-session events that arise within the context of therapeutic relationship and include judicious self-disclosure and facilitation of a collaborative exchange about underlying anxiety or unspoken tension. One way of conceptualizing metacommunication is *mindfulness in action*—the therapist, using his or her awareness of emerging feelings and impressions, explicitly engages the patient in a *here-and-now* exploration of subtle shifts in the unfolding interpersonal process.

Recently, a study that investigated incorporating AFT into standard cognitive-behavioral therapy (CBT) training revealed resulting improvements in the quality of interactions between therapists and their patients (Safran et al., 2014). Preliminary findings also suggest that the improvement in interpersonal process between patient and therapist has implications for better outcome and that AFT enhances therapists' abilities to reflect on their emotional engagement with their patients (Muran, Gorman, Safran, Eubanks-Carter, & Winston, 2014). An earlier study found that AFT practices are more effective for patients with whom it is difficult to establish a therapeutic alliance than either CBT or short-term dynamic therapy (Safran et al., 2005). A number of independent research teams have also found evidence regarding the positive impact of augmenting cognitive therapy and other treatment modalities with AFT principles derived from our research program (e.g., Castonguay et al., 2004; Constantino et al., 2008; Crits-Christoph et al., 2006; Harmon et al., 2007; Newman, Castonguay, Borkovec, Fisher, & Nordberg, 2008).

In this chapter, we describe the core elements of the AFT approach, then illustrate the application of these through the case of Ellen, whose therapist Rob introduced AFT following 16 sessions of standard CBT. The case, which is drawn from the study previously described (Safran et al., 2014), illustrates the nature of learning for the therapist and the shift in interpersonal process following the initiation of AFT training and supervision. The case focuses on the evolution and transformation of the therapeutic relationship as the therapist becomes more attuned to and adept at managing negative process following AFT training. The case illustrates the way in which the therapist's ability to work more collaboratively with the patient increases with training and coincides with subtle but meaningful changes in the treatment process and patient outcomes over the course of 30 weeks of therapy.

AFT and Supervision

AFT (Muran et al., 2010; Safran & Muran, 2000) was derived from ongoing research on resolving therapeutic alliance ruptures (see Safran, Muran, & Eubanks-Carter, 2011) as well as contemporary developments in relational psychoanalysis (e.g., Aron, 1996; Benjamin, 2004; Mitchell, 1988). *Negotiating the Therapeutic Alliance: A Relational Treatment Guide* (Safran & Muran, 2000) serves as the training manual for AFT, and trainees are provided with readings that review the theoretical evolution of the therapeutic alliance and detail core principles that guide the process of rupture resolution strategies.

In our clinic, AFT is conducted in a weekly 90-minute group supervision format that consists of video-recorded sessions, experiential exercises, and modeling by the supervisor. The recorded sessions are reviewed with an eye toward identifying possible moments of strain or tension in the alliance, in order to explore the therapist's in-session subjective experience. Role-playing exercises also provide therapists with the opportunity to simulate working through difficult moments in treatment and to experiment with metacommunication strategies. Exercises give therapists the opportunity not only to practice technical skills but also to develop awareness of their own feelings and internal conflicts as they emerge during alliance ruptures (countertransference responses). Supervision sessions also employ mindfulness training in order to help therapists cultivate the capacity to observe their inner experiences and begin to develop a nonjudgmental stance toward their possible contributions to moments of deterioration within the alliance (Safran & Reading, 2008).

As part of our research AFT program, we administer a series of outcome and process measures to assess the impact of AFT on therapeutic process and outcome. Patient-focused measures include the Symptom Checklist–90—Revised (SCL-90-R; Derogatis, 1994), the Inventory of Interpersonal Problems (IIP; Horowitz, Alden, Wiggins, & Pincus, 2000), and the Target Complaints Instrument (TC; Battle et al., 1966). Postsession questionnaires are administered to both patient and therapist, and include the Working Alliance Inventory (WAI; Tracey & Kokotovic, 1989) along with specific questions that are designed to evoke information about any ruptures or tension that might have occurred in the course of that session. While the data collected in the postsession questionnaires (PSQs) are utilized for research, they also allow the therapist to reflect more fully on relational dynamics of each session. In addition to these self-report measures, both patients and therapists participate in extensive interviews that probe for relational factors and experiences of ruptures. Therapists are interviewed during the midphase of treatment and again at termination, while patients are interviewed at termination and again at 6-month follow up. Although a full summary of the specific assessments for the case of Ellen and her therapist Rob is beyond the scope of this chapter, we discuss the results from the PSQs and termination and follow-up interviews with both Ellen and Rob.

A Case of CBT Integrating AFT Principles

Ellen, a 38-year-old, single, white female, sought time-limited CBT treatment to address recurrent depression and low self-esteem. She reported feeling isolated, stuck, and hopeless about her future prospects. At intake, following a Structured Clinical Interview for DSM-IV Axis I and Axis II (SCID; First, Spitzer, Gibbon, & Williams, 1995), Ellen met criteria for Axis I diagnoses of major depressive disorder and dysthymic disorder, early onset and an Axis II diagnosis of avoidant personality disorder (American Psychiatric Association, 2000).

Ellen's therapist, Rob, was a 29-year-old, white, male doctoral candidate in clinical psychology. When treatment began, he had 3 years of training, including 9 months of CBT supervision, and this was his second CBT case assignment. During the first half of the 30-session treatment, Rob continued to receive CBT supervision, then, in keeping with study protocol, switched to AFT training and supervision for the remainder of the case.

Ellen was attractive in an understated way that was easy to miss. She seemed almost to retreat into herself, as if attempting to hide in plain view of the therapist. She lived alone and worked as a clerk in the permissions department of a large publishing house, while, with waning interest, she pursued a career as an actress. Two years earlier, Ellen and her long-term boyfriend had broken up by mutual consent. Although she was lonely and had few close friends, Ellen was disinclined to seek new relationships. She usually wore jeans, sneakers and T-shirts and these, along with her hesitant manner, gave the impression of someone much younger than her actual age. Ellen's speech often faltered as she struggled to put her experiences into words, and her anxiety would culminate in a tight smile and a nervous laugh that signaled the onset of tears.

In contrast, Rob projected an air of easy confidence. He had a quick and lively mind and was articulate and engaging. Both his thoughts and speech tended to move rapidly. Dressed in shirt and tie, Rob presented a polished and professional demeanor. While he initially accommodated to Ellen's measured pace, he soon betrayed difficulty in remaining silent in the face of her halting self-expression. As Ellen strained to communicate, Rob would often jump in to complete her sentences or elaborate on her behalf. He tended to counter her anxiety with uplifting stories and exhortatory remarks—words to motivate and encourage ("You're doing a great job!"; "You're making real progress!")—and he often talked more than Ellen in their sessions.

The Initiation of CBT

During the first weeks, as Rob began to socialize Ellen to the structure of CBT sessions and cognitive principles and strategies, details about her life began to emerge and her schema-level beliefs began to emerge. She was the third of five siblings in a devoutly religious family with limited resources. Ellen conveyed how she learned early on to keep her thoughts and feelings to herself and, in the course of treatment, she came to associate this strategy with the belief, "It's not OK to say what I want to say or feel what I feel." In order "to keep the peace," she often submitted to her parents or "sacrificed" her needs in favor of the demands of her siblings. Growing up, Ellen felt reluctant to make requests, believing, "If I get what I want, someone else loses." Early in the course of treatment, she wrestled with whether she should return to the Midwestern state where her family still lived or commit to cultivating a potentially more satisfying life for herself in New York. This indecision about moving "home" deferred Ellen's investment in her future and prevented her from seeking more fulfilling work or cultivating new relationships.

Ellen quickly took to the structured approach of CBT and appeared to draw comfort from the predictability of the sessions, with their agendas, mood checks, and homework assignments, which she diligently completed. She seemed grateful for the Rob's guidance and the skills he was teaching her. In turn, he was gratified by her responsiveness to his instruction and obvious commitment to treatment. However, as the weeks wore on during the first phase of treatment, a distinct relational pattern between the two began to take shape. Ellen, in a submissive and childlike fashion, would seek direction, reassurance, and approval from Rob. She questioned whether she was doing the assignments "right" and, when uncertain with how to proceed in a session, would ask, "What do people usually do?" Frequently, as if trying to gauge his reactions to her, Ellen would cautiously study him, then quickly look away. For his part, Rob seemed to be caught between taking a more directive approach to the interaction and encouraging Ellen's independence. At times, this resulted in his intervening while she was still struggling to clarify her thoughts. In Session 6, as Ellen tentatively produced reasons why her parents might not be calling her, Rob preempted her exploration to impose a conclusion:

THERAPIST: I can think of a couple of others. Maybe they're respecting your privacy.

ELLEN: (*Laughs.*) Really? (*Reaches for tissue.*)

THERAPIST: Is it possible?

ELLEN: I don't know.

THERAPIST: Well think about it (*After a few moments of silence, he pushes on.*) Or maybe we can rephrase it as "respecting your autonomy or your life in New York."

ELLEN: Yeah, maybe. . . .

THERAPIST: Write that down.

At times, the clash between Rob's swift pace and Ellen's slower tempo led to misunderstandings and disturbances in the otherwise positive alliance. A notable instance of this occurred in Session 7. Rob asked Ellen to start paying attention to whether there was a discrepancy between what she was thinking and feeling, and what she was saying in conversations. He quickly devised a homework assignment (a thought record on an interpersonal situation in which she would track what she said, felt, and thought) and, in his eagerness, he overwhelmed Ellen and missed her mounting distress:

THERAPIST: So this is an experiment, we're going to be good social scientists. We're going come up with an experiment, which we just did, and then we're going come up with data.

ELLEN: Mmhmm.

THERAPIST: This is the data collecting. And then next week we'll look at the data and see if there are some interesting patterns.

ELLEN: OK.

THERAPIST: Because you remembered what . . .

ELLEN: My parents . . .

THERAPIST: . . . What your folks said but not . . .

ELLEN: What I said.

THERAPIST: Not that that's right or wrong or anything in between, but it's interesting. And I think that if there are things we're not aware of and we bring awareness to them, it'll give us more information and it'll help us understand what's going on. OK?

ELLEN: All right.

THERAPIST: (*Gives a thumbs-up as if an agreement has been reached and he's ready to move on, then almost as an afterthought*) Anything else about the parents?

ELLEN: No (*Smiles, laughs, and looks down.*)

THERAPIST: Why are you smiling?

ELLEN: No, I'm not smiling (*Flips through notebook, smiling.*)

THERAPIST: No, I'm curious . . .

ELLEN: No, I just, uh . . .

THERAPIST: Is that a discomfort? Is that an uncomfortable smile?

ELLEN: Um, no uh, just I thought that you want me to do this because something's wrong with me. (*Wipes eyes.*)

THERAPIST: That something's wrong—oh, so just now, a thought came up that the reason I want you to do this is that I think that there's something wrong with you.

ELLEN: Yeah. (*Laughs, wiping eyes.*)

Rob, in his haste to keep things moving along, seemed blindsided by Ellen's response and quickly backtracked to address her concerns. So intent was he on the task at hand that he seemed to have lost sight of Ellen. At other times, in order to soothe her and to alleviate his own uneasiness in the face of her obvious distress, he was given to extended analogies with uplifting messages, as occurred at the end of Session 9:

THERAPIST: . . . The avoidance of the pain doesn't work. And it's sort of, sort like the same theory behind homeopathic medicine.

ELLEN: (*Nods.*)

THERAPIST: . . . Where they take a very tiny dose of something that's poisonous and they distill it in a huge amount of like, sugar water and then you take it and it's actually, actually palliative . . .

ELLEN: Oh, really?

THERAPIST: It actually, like, reduces pain.

ELLEN: Hmm.

THERAPIST: Yeah, or like vaccines, they take a little bit of the disease and they inject it into you and your body builds antibodies against it.

ELLEN: Oh yeah, right.

THERAPIST: It's kind of like the same thing; taking too much is not a healthy thing, right. So we don't want you to do something that feels overwhelming, which is why I was asking about, you know, how anxiety inducing this is. But a little bit is good because that's what builds your emotional immune system. (*Smiles and nods.*)

ELLEN: Right. (*Closes her notebook and looks ready to leave.*)

While there were instances when Ellen seemed to draw solace from Rob's words, on this occasion she silently acquiesced. His remarks were meant to hearten her, but her rigid body language conveyed distress.

Within the first 3 months, the content and themes that would recur across the balance of the treatment were well established. Among them were Ellen's ambivalence about moving "home," her conviction of her sense of inadequacy ("There's something wrong with me"), her apprehension concerning interpersonal relationship, and her small smile and nervous laugh that served as a defense against the expression of confusion and pain.

Introducing AFT training and Supervision

Midway through Ellen's treatment, Rob began AFT training and supervision. Therapists transitioning from CBT supervision into AFT are instructed to begin incorporating AFT principles into treatment by bringing greater awareness to their own experience and paying attention to the relational patterns within the therapeutic alliance. Therapists in this study did not directly address with their patients the shift initiated by AFT; however, they were instructed to provide patients with rationales for employing interventions they had not previously used. For Rob, the initial focus of supervision was on

cultivating a greater capacity for self-reflection and beginning to observe the impact that his interventions had on Ellen. Although the training protocol encourages therapists to introduce aspects of AFT gradually and in a fashion that feels appropriate for their particular case, Rob transitioned abruptly and, in so doing, unwittingly initiating a rupture. As Session 16 began, Ellen looked to Rob to set the agenda, but in a break from their accustomed routine, he cedes the responsibility to her, stating, "The floor is all yours." Ellen seems caught off guard and tentatively begins going through the established protocol:

ELLEN: OK, so, I think this is number 16 . . .

THERAPIST: Uh, huh. How are you feeling today?

ELLEN: I'd say seven and a half.

THERAPIST: (*Notes Ellen's mood in the chart.*)

ELLEN: (*Waits.*)

THERAPIST: (*pause*) And, uh. . . . (*pause*)

ELLEN: And what do I attribute that to?

THERAPIST: (*Smiles.*) or, sure . . .

ELLEN: Agenda?

THERAPIST: (*Smiling, regards Ellen for a moment and gestures with open hands toward her.*)

ELLEN: What were you going to say?

THERAPIST: As you like it.

ELLEN: (*Laughs and for a moment covers her eyes with a hand. After a moment, she gathers herself and forges on.*) Um . . . yeah. I think the work that I'm doing is helping.

THERAPIST: Uh huh.

ELLEN: Um . . . so. . . .

Ellen looks expectantly at Rob, laughs, and looks down. Rob looks to Ellen and a moment of silence ensued in which both nod and smile at each other. She then breaks the silence with a nervous laugh and covers both eyes with a hand.

THERAPIST: (*Laughs.*) You look like you want me to. . . .

ELLEN: I want you to be the leader.

THERAPIST: Be the leader. (*Both smile and nod.*)
So it seems like you're aware of that thought.

ELLEN: That thought?

THERAPIST: The one that you just said, that you want me to be the leader.

ELLEN: (*Laughs uncomfortably.*) Yeah, I'm aware of that thought.

THERAPIST: Uh-huh. (*Remains silent, waiting.*)

ELLEN: Homework review?

THERAPIST: Sure, OK. What else should we put on the agenda?

ELLEN: I think that's it.

It is here that Rob begins to employ a variety of metacommunication strategies. He explicitly calls Ellen's attention to her immediate experience, then discloses his impression of what he observes in order to facilitate an exploration of her thoughts and feelings.

THERAPIST: OK. Before we jump into the homework review, any sense of why that thought just popped into your head?

ELLEN: Maybe because it's easier for me if you do the work. (*Laughs.*)

THERAPIST: (*Laughs.*) If I do the work. And I've been doing the work?

ELLEN: (*Laughs nervously, suddenly looks up in confusion.*) What?

THERAPIST: It's easier, you said, if I do the work. And what work specifically?

Ellen begins to talk about the recommended assignments in the CBT book that she's reading, but Rob brings her back to what just transpired between them.

THERAPIST: But specifically what just happened here, where I was. (*Pauses and gestures with open hands toward Ellen.*) Well, what did you experience?

ELLEN: Well, I said that I wanted you to lead.

Ellen tries to identify what she was thinking and feeling about their exchange, and Rob finally offers his impressions:

THERAPIST: The emotion that I saw was a little bit of anxiety.

ELLEN: Hmm.

THERAPIST: It seemed like you were uncomfortable.

ELLEN: (*Laughs.*) Well, yeah.

THERAPIST: And, all fairness, silence can be anxiety provoking.

ELLEN: Right, right.

THERAPIST: Is that what you . . . is that close to what you were feeling, or was it just, I'm not up to this?

ELLEN: Yeah I feel a little anxious. I think it's pretty regular.

THERAPIST: Pretty regular? Say more.

ELLEN: Like, uh, like coming here (*Leans forward and looks directly at Rob.*) I feel anxious about coming here.

THERAPIST: Do you have some sense of why you feel anxious?

ELLEN: (*Laugh and tears up.*)

THERAPIST: Do you, uh, let me ask, do you feel anxious because you've chosen to come here, or anxious becomes of what coming here entails?

ELLEN: That one. (*Begins to wipe away tears.*) I feel anxious that I might feel more pain.

THERAPIST: Hum, and it's less painful if . . .

ELLEN: I do nothing. If I don't come here. (*Wipes eyes and laughs.*)

THERAPIST: But also in the session, um, uh, perhaps, letting me do the work, or however you phrased it, minimizes the chances that you'll say, you'll go somewhere that feels painful or say something that feels painful.

By not acting on his usual impulse to end the silence, Rob forced them both to endure and explore the discomfort. By yielding the floor, he drew Ellen out into the open and encouraged her to take the lead. By asking her to bring her awareness to what was transpiring in the here and now of the session, she started to address the anxiety that flooded her and impinged on her capacity to directly express her needs. Throughout much of the session Ellen laughed and covered her face with her hands like a bashful child trying to find a place to hide. Only when Rob communicated (metacommunicated) his observation to her did she display an uncharacteristic moment of frankness by leaning forward and, looking directly at Rob, stating, "I feel anxious about coming here."

The change into AFT disrupted what had become the predictable form of the treatment and the conventional pattern of their interaction. Over the course of the following weeks, changes in their interpersonal process were perceptible. Rob began to moderate his pace and made a concerted effort to listen more and speak less. He tempered his upbeat and jaunty demeanor, and let Ellen set the tone. At times, he visibly compressed his lips or covered his mouth with his hand as if in an effort to keep from interrupting Ellen or intervening to forestall her suffering. In a posttreatment interview, Rob reflected on the phase of treatment following the change in AFT:

"Once I made the switch to relational work and I was paying attention to my own internal emotional experiences on a much more fine-grain level, it was not always comfortable. . . . [I] got comfortable with saying less, more comfortable introspecting more, got very interested in finding ways of using that data in treatment."

Shifts began to occur in Ellen's behavior as well. Though reluctantly at first, she hesitantly tried to "take the lead" and assumed a more active role in the treatment. When a misunderstanding occurred during a discussion of her brother's illness in Session 17, Ellen, without prompting, confronted Rob in the next session with what she regarded as his negative judgment of her. Over the course of the next two sessions, Ellen, together with Rob, was able to closely examine and work through their interaction, connecting it to her maladaptive belief that she's a flawed or "terrible person." In the postsession questionnaire, she recorded that what transpired in session was neither "conflict" nor "misunderstanding" but rather a "misinterpretation" that was clarified by "talk[ing] about it" with Rob.

As treatment progressed Rob seemed more attuned to Ellen. His voice, like hers, became lower, and his manner gentler and more ruminative. During Session 19, as Ellen related a conversation she had with a distant cousin, Rob, noting a shift in her emotions, asked her to explore what occurred:

ELLEN: It's hard to talk about. (*Reaches for a tissue*) Like I'm not really. . . . No, I think it's just that, I'm not even that close to him. I've seen him maybe once in the past 5 years. (*Dabs at her eyes.*) I think it's. . . . It's just that like . . . (*Sobs, looks stricken.*)

THERAPIST: It's OK.

ELLEN: I . . . (*Blots face, pauses.*) I think I just,

uh, like when he called me I was surprised but it was also like . . . (*Sobs again and reaches for another tissue.*) God, I don't know why this is so hard. It's more just finally somebody saw me. (*Reaches for another tissue.*) Somebody saw through, like, my charade, or what I was trying to put out and hide, you know?

THERAPIST: Hmm.

ELLEN: Like somebody finally . . . noticed . . . (*Spreads her hands in front of her.*)

THERAPIST: You. (*Both nod.*)

ELLEN: Um, why do you think that's such a . . . hard thing to talk about?

THERAPIST: Any ideas?

ELLEN: (*Laughs, blots eyes.*) Like I've tried so long, like to hide. I hide everything. And I don't know exactly what I'm trying to hide or even how I do it. (*Laughs and puts her notebook away, getting ready to go.*)

THERAPIST: Before we stop, I just want to acknowledge your willingness to stay open and um, your courage at being able to look at this stuff. It's not always easy, so my hat is off to you.

ELLEN: Thanks.

ELLEN: And uh, and sometimes when people see us as we see ourselves down deep, it can be a bit of a shock, it can feel like someone can see that, oh, oh, what does that mean? That can be a little unnerving . . .

ELLEN: Yeah, yeah.

THERAPIST: And simultaneously relieving.

In the ensuing weeks, Ellen became increasingly forthcoming, disclosing more about her past relationships and her need for love, confusion about her sexual orientation, and ambivalence about intimacy. During Session 21, following an extended trip to see her family for the holidays, Ellen discussed how returning gave her a new appreciation for her independence:

ELLEN: I feel like a child when I'm back in their house. I feel like I'm smothered. (*Begins to explore the burden of her parents' silent demands to feel and behave in a prescribed fashion and Rob pursued this point.*)

THERAPIST: I wonder if there's something about being close that's disquieting somehow?

ELLEN: (*Laughs.*) I think so. I don't really like it. When you grow up with four other siblings

. . . even then I tried to distance myself, get my own space, it didn't always feel like I had the same ideas. Wow. (*Reaches for tissue and begins to cry.*) I, most of the time I prefer to be alone and, like, my life here is like pretty solitary. Like, my job doesn't require me to interact with a ton of people. And I go home, and I live alone, I don't have a boyfriend or a huge social life. And at my parents' house, it's sort of the opposite, where it's constant, with people. So I mean I think I'd prefer a balance between the two.

This seems to be a new insight for Ellen and, Rob reflects on her ambivalence regarding interpersonal relations and remarks:

"If in some relationships, like with your parents, intimacy comes with strings attached . . . then I can understand why having your own space to tend to your needs is a really smart choice. But I also hear that you want some more connection with friends and in some cases with family but in a different sort of way that allows you to feel what you're feeling, think what you're thinking, and have that be sort of acknowledged and validated."

Ellen's interpersonal relationships—friends, family, and romantic partners—occupied a good deal of the remainder of treatment as she explored what it meant to have intimate relationships and yet not give up her autonomy or sense of self. Although a struggle for both of them, Ellen and Rob continued to navigate the difficulties of managing issues of interpersonal control across the remainder of treatment—he to relinquish it and she to claim it. Rather than respond to her pull for guidance, Rob tried to create an environment in which Ellen could safely explore her more disturbing thoughts and feelings without his active intervention. Ellen, rather than abdicating her independence to Rob's authority, challenged herself to look for answers within.

Approaching Termination

In Session 27, the two began to discuss the impending termination of their treatment. Ellen revealed feeling both apprehensive and excited. When Rob asks her about her apprehension, she cries and expresses uncertainty over whether she's done therapy the "right way." El-len's distress becomes the focus of Rob's ensuing metacommunication about their relational dynamic:

THERAPIST: So as you're talking about this I'm also really aware, in relation to you, wanting to offer some certainty.

ELLEN: Right.

THERAPIST: What's it like to hear me say that?

ELLEN: (*Silently considers for a few moments.*) Um, well. Like I think I want you to know all the answers.

THERAPIST: Right, right.

ELLEN: I think I also know that you don't and you can't.

THERAPIST: And I feel you asking for certainty.

ELLEN: Right.

THERAPIST: On the one hand, I would like to offer it, and on the other hand, uh, not only are individual people's certainties different. . . .

ELLEN: Yeah, right.

THERAPIST: But I don't know that offering it would actually be helpful.

The issue of uncertainty—of not knowing the answers—became a dominant theme for both Ellen and her therapist as the treatment reached termination. She sought the security of ready answers as a way of avoiding the process of examining her painful thoughts and feelings. For his part, Rob was avid to know. He wanted to know in order to offer Ellen the solace she so desperately longed for, but he also derived comfort from the role of being the *knowing one* with the ready answers. In looking back 2 years after the case, Rob would speak lucidly on this topic:

"Mind always wants to know, that's what mind does. Mind's function is to know. . . . The only other thing I can say in retrospect is, uh, um, I think I'm a little more balanced like in my interest in knowing what it's like to not know in the presence of someone that's there for help and implicitly saying like, 'Help me know the right way'. . . . Sometimes what's actually more mutative is not knowing."

This point is well illustrated in Session 29 as Rob and Ellen together grapple with the difficulty of "not knowing":

ELLEN: Well I'm not sure I ever really understood feelings, like I always felt kind of beholden to them.

THERAPIST: Uh-huh. In what regard?

ELLEN: Sort of as if they were factual.

THERAPIST: Ummm.

ELLEN: Like I feel this way, therefore

THERAPIST: I must be deformed.

ELLEN: Yeah, right.

THERAPIST: And now?

ELLEN: Hmm, I'm starting to change how I think of them.

THERAPIST: In what ways?

ELLEN: (*pause*) Well, (*pause*) well, just in some work that I've done . . . here, uh. Noticing that they come and go and they are not constant.

THERAPIST: Um, hum. (*pause*) That you're not your feelings.

ELLEN: Yeah.

THERAPIST: They affect how we think and function but we are not them.

ELLEN: I always thought I was. (*Laughs.*)

THERAPIST: (*nodding*) Yeah.

ELLEN: So . . .

THERAPIST: I know.

ELLEN: (*Laughs.*).

THERAPIST: Well that's huge. It's like the chains coming off.

ELLEN: Um. (*Laughs.*) So then what am I, if I'm not my feelings what determines who I am? Do you know? (*Laughs.*)

THERAPIST: (*Tightly crosses his arms and legs.*) Do I know who you are?

Rob seems uncomfortable with not knowing and remaining silent in the face of Ellen's importuning. He begins to speak, sputters and then falls silent. Finally, he uncrosses his arms.

THERAPIST: The challenge is for each of us to find that out ourselves. I think it would be counterproductive at best if I . . .

ELLEN: Well, I mean in general, like as people. (*Sighs, pauses, looks at Rob.*) What are we? (*Laughs, covers her face with her hand.*)

THERAPIST: (*Laughs.*) You're asking some big questions. If you're willing to close your eyes a moment. . . .

Ellen does so and Rob initiates a mindfulness exercise, inviting her to bring her attention to what she's experiencing. Rob closes his eyes as well. After a minute, he asks Ellen what she discovered.

ELLEN: Well, at the beginning of the exercise I felt like I was standing on a river bank throwing a fishing line in, trying to catch a fish (*laughs*), desperate for some answer.

THERAPIST: Uh-huh.

ELLEN: And then the thought came that it's OK not to know the answers.

THERAPIST: Uh-huh.

ELLEN: Then I thought that, uh, then I thought that (*laughs*) . . . I had this thought that I'm a loving and giving person, that, that . . . (*Throws up hands and laughs.*) That's it.

THERAPIST: And were there any shifts in what it felt like between those different things?

ELLEN: Yeah. At first I felt panicked and desperate.

THERAPIST: Have to find something . . .

ELLEN: (*Nods.*) Searching.

THERAPIST: Uh-huh.

ELLEN: I'm not even a fisher; I don't know how to fish. (*Both therapist and Ellen laugh.*) And then, uh, I just felt really calm (*pause*), uh, peaceful about it.

During the final session, Ellen and Rob together review the course of treatment: her efforts to acknowledge her feelings; her growing self-acceptance and self-awareness; and her disappointment that he did not have "the answers." Rob commented that he noticed changes in Ellen and felt a greater sense of connection to her. Before the session ended, Ellen asked Rob to review the mindfulness exercise that he had led her through the week before, adding that she wants to know, "How I can do it myself." He slowly goes through the steps with her while she intently takes notes. As she gathers her bag and notebook, Ellen smiles tearfully at Rob.

ELLEN: Thanks. I couldn't have done it without you.

THERAPIST: I couldn't have done it without you.

Postscript: Evaluating the Impact of AFT

During her termination interview, Ellen was noticeably anxious and uncomfortable. She described her relationship with Rob in positive terms and remarked that she felt that she had grown as a result of the treatment. More informative than the content of the interview were her interactions with the interviewer. Mostly, Ellen offered terse responses to the questions and seemed guarded and wary, stating that she had not expected to be "delving into all of this." As the interview progressed, she became tearful and expressed her dismay at what seemed to her to be the invasive nature of the questions and finally remarked, "I'm sorry, I really don't want to do this. Is there a lot more that you have?" For someone who entered treatment believing "It's not OK to say what I want to say or feel what I feel," the moment of self-assertion, albeit awkwardly executed, was striking.

At her 6-month follow-up interview, Ellen appeared far more relaxed and assured. While she credited working with Rob as having helped her to change and expressed feelings of gratitude toward him, she also noted: "I've done some other things that have helped me have a better outlook, have a more positive outlook, and take better care of myself, so I can't say that it was just the therapy." Ellen seemed to have moved from her stance of dependence toward acknowledging and appreciating a greater sense of autonomy.

During both his midterm and termination interviews, Rob recognized that Ellen derived obvious benefits from the cognitive therapy aspect of the treatment. However, he conceded, "There was a way in which the structure that I was imposing prevented her from having agency," adding that the addition of the AFT interventions "allowed for a certain different range of exploration." For his part, Rob related how the training had resulted in a growing receptiveness to his own internal experience within session:

"I'm very aware of enactments now. . . . She pulled for a lot of soothing, and those were enactments and it didn't, after a while it didn't really help things very much, um, to soothe . . . as opposed to perhaps you know conveying my awareness that in that moment I felt like I wanted to help make her feel better, but feeling like perhaps that's not what would be helpful and, uh, leaving

space for her to join me in that inquiry to sort of like figure out what would actually be therapeutic."

Rob also observed that there were changes in Ellen across the course of treatment:

"I think she felt more comfortable to experience what she was feeling, she was much more aware of the cognitions they engendered, or that preceded them. Um, she was aware of a new sense, like a fledgling sense, of self-efficacy. . . . I think she was surprised initially by her ability to change what she was feeling, or to augment it. . . . She developed a lot of insight into her long-standing schemas and was able to sort of deploy some of the coping strategies. . . . Um, I think she developed a little more of a compassionate self-stance."

Two years after the termination of the case, Rob reflected on the treatment, his assessment of himself as a therapist at the time, and the benefits he derived from the AFT training:

"[My supervisor] had been sort of very gently orienting me toward seeing how some of my own sort of strengths as a therapist and tendency to pull for positive, uh, future-oriented stuff precluded [Ellen] from actually being able to uh, express some degree of discomfort in sessions. . . . I learned a lot about sort of how I organize and sort of protrude into interpersonal space in different ways. . . . There is nothing that we do in session that is neutral. . . . It's like, you know, walk into a pond and it creates ripples. . . . He helped me become aware of the kind of ripples I was making at different times and invited me to become very curious about what was going on inside of me in those moments when I felt compelled to do, say those types of things, which in turn over the past few years has really led me to . . . develop quite a sensitive internal instrument for becoming quite aware when I'm in the midst of enactments, when I'm sort of defending against my own discomfort."

Turning his attention to Ellen, Rob was pensive:

"I hope I was helpful. I sort of feel bad in retrospect that she had a therapist that was just figuring out what he was doing because she really needed help. I just hope that the time was of use to her and her life is a little bit, feels a little bit, more easy."

Summary

In a sense, the dyad at the outset of treatment was a perfect match: The patient looked to Rob to care for her and provide guidance, and Rob responded in a way that was in keeping with his own natural tendencies to step in, take charge, and comfort the patient. While his encouragements and steady flow of soothing inspirations were what the patient wanted, they were not ultimately what she most needed. Although Ellen and Rob reported and evidenced a positive alliance across all sessions (as confirmed by the PSQs, observation-based measures, and the interviews), during the first half of treatment, the ways in which Rob was delivering the CBT model seemed to have kept both participants in the dyad locked into an interpersonal pattern that precluded the type of growth and development that Ellen needed to begin to step out of the shadow of dependency.

As Safran (1984, p. 260) warns, the cognitive-behavioral therapist who does not pay sufficient attention to the relational dimensions of the treatment is in "danger of helping clients maintain their maladaptive behaviors . . . by virtue of inattention to his or her own behaviors." With the initiation of AFT training, Rob started to attend to his experience within session and assumed a new relational stance toward the patient. The core elements of AFT that helped him make this shift included attending more to his internal experience, an expanding awareness of his impact on Ellen, and utilizing metacommunication strategies to initiate a dialogue with Ellen about the interpersonal dynamic between them. The impact of these changes within Rob was clear in the sessions with Ellen. He began taking a less dominant or controlling position, which in turn led Ellen to assume greater agency in the exploration and articulation of her feelings. After the change into the more relationally focused AFT process, Rob exerted less paternal control and instead offered Ellen understanding and support without protecting her from encountering her painful affect. In exploring the relational underpinnings of AFT, Muran (2002) asserts that in any treatment, change is a mutual process:

The relational formulation . . . suggests that change should also include the therapist. In other words, the clarification of the patient's self-definition invariably involves the clarification of the therapist's self-definition. . . . Thus, with every therapeutic encounter, therapists must confront themselves and expand their awareness of themselves. (p. 132)

Corresponding changes were observed in Ellen's interactions as she became less submissive and more autonomous. The language that she used in the PSQs suggested subtle changes in her self-conception. Specifically, after the switch into AFT, the language Ellen uses emphasizes herself as an active and mutual participant in the interaction: "We talked about it/we addressed it"; "I wanted to clear up something I said last session"; "I think the resolution will need to come from me." Her remarks hint at a nascent sense of independence. The TC that she filled out before and immediately after treatment and again at follow-up documented a notable decrease in symptom severity. In describing the alteration of the depression that led her to seek therapy, Ellen noted at termination, "Seeing the growth I've made in treatment over the past 8 months has inspired me to have hope and to keep striving for greater self-awareness and health." In her self-assessment can be heard an echo of the therapist's observation at termination: "She was aware of a new sense, like a fledgling sense, of self-efficacy."

Conclusion

AFT was developed as an approach to teaching fundamental clinical skills to therapists of all orientations. It may well be the case that experienced clinicians of all orientations already incorporate some, if not all, of these skills into their everyday clinical work. The growing emphasis on integrating science and practice in our field has many virtues. One of the potential limitations to this emphasis, however, is that it can sometimes lead to a skewed interpretation of what the evidence actually demonstrates. It is unfortunate when clinicians become locked into turf wars about which therapeutic approaches have the best supporting evidence. While meta-analyses abound demonstrating the efficacy of both CBT and other approaches, there are also abundant meta-analyses supporting the conclusion that the therapy brand accounts for a relatively small proportion of the outcome variance and that so-called *nonspecific factors* (including the alliance, empathy, therapist facilitative interpersonal skills) account for a considerably larger proportion of the outcome variance than treatment modality (Wampold & Imel, 2015). Our goal in AFT is to continue to refine our ability to facilitate therapists' acquisition of these *nonspecific therapeutic skills*—skills that are indispensable when it comes to treating patients in the real world.

Acknowledgment

The research described in this chapter was supported by Grant No. MH071768 from the National Institute of Mental Health (Principal Investigator: J. Christopher Muran).

References

American Psychiatric Association. (2000). *Diagnostic and statistical manual of mental disorders* (4th ed., text rev.). Washington, DC: Author.

Anderson, T., Knobloch-Fedders, L. M., Stiles, W. B., Ordoñez, T., & Heckman, B. D. (2012). The power of subtle interpersonal hostility in psychodynamic psychotherapy: A speech acts analysis. *Psychotherapy Research, 22,* 348–362.

Aron, L. (1996). *A meeting of minds: Mutuality in psychoanalysis.* Hillsdale, NJ: Analytic Press.

Battle, C. C., Imber, S. D., Hoehn-Saric, R., Stone, A. R., Nash, E. R., & Frank, J. D. (1966). Target complaints as criteria of improvement. *American Journal of Psychotherapy, 20,* 184–192.

Benjamin, J. (2004). Beyond doer and done to: An intersubjective view of thirdness. *Psychoanalytic Quarterly, 73,* 5–46.

Binder, J. L., & Strupp, H. H. (1997). "Negative process": A recurrently discovered and underestimated facet of therapeutic process and outcome in the individual psychotherapy of adults. *Clinical Psychology: Science and Practice, 4,* 121–139.

Castonguay, L. G., Schut, A. J., Aikins, D., Constantino, M. J., Lawrenceau, J. P., Bologh, L., et al. (2004). Repairing alliance ruptures in cognitive therapy: A preliminary investigation of an integrative therapy for depression. *Journal of Psychotherapy Integration, 14,* 4–20.

Constantino, M. J., Marnell, M. E., Haile, A. J., Kanther-Sista, S. N., Wolman, K., Zappert, L., et al. (2008). Integrative cognitive therapy for depression: A randomized pilot comparison. *Psychotherapy: Theory, Research, Practice, Training, 45,* 122–134.

Crits-Christoph, P., Gibbons, M. B. C., Crits-Christoph, K., Narducci, J., Schamberger, M., & Gallop, R. (2006). Can therapists be trained to improve their alliances?: A preliminary study of alliance-fostering psychotherapy. *Psychotherapy Research, 16,* 268–281.

Derogatis, L. R. (1994). *Symptom Checklist–90—Revised.* Bloomington, MN: Pearson.

Eubanks-Carter, C., Muran, J. C., & Safran, J. D. (2010). Alliance ruptures and resolution. In J. C. Muran & J. P. Barber (Eds.), *The therapeutic alliance: An evidence-based guide to practice* (pp. 74–94). New York: Guilford Press.

First, M. B., Spitzer, R. L., Gibbon, M., & Williams, J. B. W. (1995). *Structured Clinical Interview for DSM–IV.* New York: Biometrics Research Department, New York Psychiatric Institute.

Flückiger, C., Del Re, A. C., Wampold, B. E., Symonds, D., & Horvath, A. O. (2012). How central is the alliance in psychotherapy?: A multilevel longitudinal meta-analysis. *Journal of Counseling Psychology, 59,* 10–17.

Greenberg, L. S., & Safran, J. D. (1989). Emotion in psychotherapy. *American Psychologist, 44,* 19–29.

Harmon, S. C., Lambert, M. J., Smart, D. M., Hawkins, E., Nielsen, S. L., Slade, K., et al. (2007). Enhancing outcome for potential treatment failures: Therapist–client feedback and clinical support tools. *Psychotherapy Research, 17,* 379–392.

Horowitz, L. M., Alden, L. E., Wiggins, J. S., & Pincus, A. L. (2000). *Inventory of Interpersonal Problems manual.* San Antonio, TX: Psychological Corporation.

Horvath, A. O., Del Re, A. C., Flückiger, C., & Symonds, D. (2011). Alliance in individual psychotherapy. *Psychotherapy, 48,* 9–16.

Kiesler, D. J. (1996). *Contemporary interpersonal theory and research: Personality, psychopathology, and psychotherapy.* New York: Wiley.

Martin, D. J., Garske, J. P., & Davis, M. K. (2000). Relation of the therapeutic alliance with outcome and other variables: A meta-analytic review. *Journal of Consulting and Clinical Psychology, 68,* 438–450.

Mitchell, S. A. (1988). *Relational concepts in psychoanalysis: An integration.* Cambridge, MA: Harvard University Press.

Muran, J. C. (2002). A relational approach to understanding change: Plurality and contextualism in a psychotherapy research program. *Psychotherapy Research, 12,* 113–138.

Muran, J. C., Gorman, B. S., Safran, J. D., Eubanks-Carter, C., & Winston, A. (2014, June). *Exploring changes in interpersonal process, intermediate, and ultimate outcome in a within-subject experimental study of an alliance-focused training.* Paper presented at the annual meeting of the Society for Psychotherapy Research, Copenhagen, Denmark.

Muran, J. C., Safran, J. D., & Eubanks-Carter, C. (2010). Developing therapist abilities to negotiate alliance rupture. In J. C. Muran & J. P. Barber (Eds.), *The therapeutic alliance: An evidence-based guide to practice* (pp. 320–340). New York: Guilford Press.

Muran, J. C., Safran, J. D., Samstag, L. W., & Winston,

A. (2005). Evaluating an alliance-focused treatment for personality disorders. *Psychotherapy: Theory, Research, Practice, Training, 42,* 532–545.

Newman, M. G., Castonguay, L. G., Borkovec, T. D., Fisher, A. J., & Nordberg, S. S. (2008). An open trial of integrative therapy for generalized anxiety disorder. *Psychotherapy: Theory, Research, Practice, Training, 45,* 137–147.

Safran, J. D. (1984). Some implications of Sullivan's interpersonal theory for cognitive therapy. In M. A. Reda & M. J. Mahoney (Eds.), *Cognitive psychotherapies: Recent developments in theory, research and practice* (pp. 251–272). Cambridge, MA: Ballinger.

Safran, J. D., & Muran, J. C. (2000). *Negotiating the therapeutic alliance: A relational treatment guide.* New York: Guilford Press.

Safran, J. D., Muran, J. C., Demaria, A., Boutwell, C., Eubanks-Carter, C., & Winston, A. (2014). Investigating the impact of alliance-focused training on interpersonal process and therapists' capacity for experiential reflection. *Psychotherapy Research, 24*(3), 269–285.

Safran, J. D., Muran, J. C., & Eubanks-Carter, C. (2011). Repairing alliance ruptures. In J. C. Norcross (Ed.),

Psychotherapy relationships that work (2nd ed., pp. 224–238). New York: Oxford University Press.

Safran, J. D., Muran, J. C., Samstag, L. W., & Stevens, C. (2002). Repairing alliance ruptures. In J. C. Norcross (Ed.), *Psychotherapy relationships that work: Therapist contributions and responsiveness to patients* (pp. 235–254). New York: Oxford University Press.

Safran, J. D., Muran, J. C., Samstag, L. W., & Winston, A. (2005). Evaluating an alliance-focused treatment for potential treatment failures. *Psychotherapy, 42,* 512–531.

Safran, J. D., & Reading, R. (2008). Mindfulness, metacommunication, and affect regulation in psychoanalytic treatment. In S. Hick & T. Bien (Eds.), *Mindfulness and the therapeutic relationship* (pp. 122–140). New York: Guilford Press.

Safran, J. D., & Segal, Z. V. (1990). *Interpersonal process in cognitive therapy.* New York: Basic Books.

Tracey, T. J., & Kokotovic, A. M. (1989). Factor structure of the Working Alliance Inventory. *Psychological Assessment, 1,* 207–210.

Wampold, B. E., & Imel, Z. E. (2015). *The great psychotherapy debate: The evidence for what makes psychotherapy work* (2nd ed.). New York: Routledge.

CHAPTER 27

Training Evidence-Based Practitioners

Recommendations for the Improvement
of Instructional Design and Delivery

DONNA M. SUDAK
RICHARD TRENT CODD III

There is a lack of adequate treatment provided worldwide for mental health disorders. Treatment is insufficient both in quality and quantity. The global median treatment gap, or the percentage of individuals who require care yet do not receive it, for mental health disorders, ranges from 78.1% for alcohol abuse and dependence to 32.2% for schizophrenia (Kohn, Saxena, Levav, Saraceno, 2004). Mental health treatment is similarly lacking when considering high-income countries such as the United States. The size of the population in need of treatment in the United States relative to the numbers treated is shocking. For example, 8.4% of adults in the United States screen positive for depression and only 28.7% of these individuals report receiving treatment; of those treated, only 23% receive psychotherapy of any type (Olfson, Blanco, & Marcus, 2016). Of the severely depressed patients receiving treatment in this study, fewer than half reported seeing a psychiatrist or mental health professional, and one-third obtained treatment with only antidepressant medication. When considering lifetime history of depression, only about 50% of adults in the United States receive treatment. Moreover, as troubling as these statistics are, rates of psychotherapy provided to individuals in the United States are continually declining. Only 3.18% of a large sample of people surveyed in 2007 in the United States reported receiving psychotherapy as outpatients (Olfson & Marcus, 2010). In outpatient mental health care, the percentage of patients receiving medications alone went from 44.1 to 57.4%, and those receiving psychotherapy alone went from 15.9 to 10.5% between 1998 and 2007 (Olfson & Marcus, 2010). In addition to the overwhelming lack of services, it is difficult to evaluate the type and quality of therapy that is delivered.

Insufficient access and affordability are factors contributing to this problem, as are indirect barriers such as stigma and perceived ineffectiveness of treatment (Kohn et al., 2004). Attitudinal barriers are more pervasive in severe psychiatric disorders; studies indicate that persons with more severe illness more often cite having a negative reaction to a provider, or thoughts that psychotherapy is ineffective, as reasons not to seek care or to drop out of care (Mojtabai et al., 2011). The World Health Organization recommends increasing and improving the training of mental health professionals as one way to address the enormous treatment gap (Kohn et al., 2004).

The chapters that precede this one have presented a state-of-the-art depiction of the progress in the conceptualization and application of evidence-based treatment for mental health problems. Although they showcase innovations in our field, the remarkable advances described in this book are infrequently available and rarely taught. There exist but a few models for how to disseminate evidence-based treatments in a way that impacts the needs of patients (Improving Access to Psychological Therapies, 2008; Karlin et al., 2012). The irony is that we have the greatest number of effective treatments for mental health disorders at any time in history, but they remain underused and often incompletely and/or incorrectly implemented. Our goal in writing this chapter is to present some ideas about how training and supervision can be improved in order to produce therapists who provide care that aligns with the aspirations of chapter authors within this book.

Challenges in Evidence-Based Practice Training

Training in mental health professions is variable and scarce regardless of the discipline (Weissman et al., 2006). There is no national standard for training in evidence-based practice (EBP). No national certification body ensures that practitioners adhere to particular forms of treatment or remain competent to deliver treatment over time. In fact, there is widespread confusion among mental health professionals regarding what constitutes EBP, primarily the notion that EBP solely refers to a list of treatments (Codd, 2017). However, EBP refers to three equally weighted[1] components: "the integration of the best available research with clinical expertise in the context of patient characteristics, culture, and preferences" (American Psychological Association, 2005, p. 5; see Table 27.1 for steps in EBP). Spring, Marchese, and Steglitz (Chapter 1, this volume) detail the basic knowledge and skills that clinicians must learn to adhere to EBP. Unfortunately, there has been insufficient attention to how best to train clinicians to achieve competency in EBP.

Even in the contexts in which standards for EBP training exist, such as requiring psychiatry residents to be competent in cognitive-behavioral therapy (CBT), there is no precise specification of what is to be taught, and no required assessment of competence. Requirements for training often simply specify the

amount of training that must be completed (e.g., number of courses or training hours), but no other outcomes. This is problematic for several reasons. First, this method assumes that competence is produced at the completion of the specified amount of training, despite a lack of evidence to support this conclusion. Trainees may or may not develop competent repertoires solely due to the dose of instruction, and if they do acquire competence, they may do so at substantially different rates. Some trainees are likely to require more than the minimum hours required to reach criterion, whereas others will reach acquisition more quickly. Both are undesirable outcomes.

In the first case, the instruction failed to produce a competent clinician, and because the requirements were "met" by that clinician, he or she is generally unlikely to pursue additional training, and, if measures of competence are not employed, may assume that he or she is competent (and tell patients this as well). In the latter case, there is an opportunity cost. The clinician acquired the desired repertoire but did so over a shorter time horizon and could have progressed to other important instructional areas or the training resources deployed elsewhere. To put it colloquially: The time was wasted. Clinicians are likely to achieve competence at different rates, so "cookie cutter" blocks of training time are not economical; this is particularly critical, since the time and money involved represents a major barrier to agency support. Mental health agencies bear the direct cost of training and a simultaneous reduction in clinician billable hours during training (private practitioners incur these costs as well). Furthermore, competence in the desired model of therapy, the presumed goal of required training, is rarely measured directly. Generally, in postgraduate training opportunities, trainees complete a paper-and-pencil measure, most commonly a true–false and/or multiple-choice assessment of knowledge to assess educational outcomes. In graduate coursework, students are typically assessed with similar methods (i.e., exams) along with papers and presentations. Actual clinical acumen, the desired training result, is rarely directly assessed. Skills-based measures of therapist competence are few and have multiple disadvantages (e.g., cost, limited generalizability). More recent efforts to develop Internet-based measures that assess therapist performance are promising and may provide a more scalable means of assessment (Cooper et al., 2017).

---

[1] Although some authors argue for increasing the relative weight afforded to the empirically supported treatment component. See Lilienfeld, Ritschel, Lynn, and Latzman (Chapter 3, this volume).

TABLE 27.1. Sample Training Hierarchy for FiLCHeRS

Training step	Training focus
1	Basic definitional awareness of acronym elements
2	Discrimination training involving examples and nonexamples of each element of the acronym
3	Application—identifying violations of acronym in clinically relevant written scenarios
4	Application—specification regarding remediation of violations of acronym (e.g., how they would turn a nonfalsifiable claim into a falsifiable one, and how they might test out the claim)
5	Application—use trainee-specific examples to identify violations of the acronym
6	Application—use trainee-specific examples to specify remediation methods for acronym violations

A greater focus on clinician training is an integral part of addressing the global treatment gap and the multitude of barriers to effective treatment implementation. Often, when instruction in EBP exists, it presumes that remediation of knowledge deficits is all that is necessary. However, cognitive and emotional factors may produce capability deficits. Administrators who maintain the mantra "we need more training" whenever they identify behavioral deficits are not considering this possibility. Agencies would be more effective by considering "Is this a can't-do or a won't-do problem, or both?" to implement the most appropriate training interventions. Finally, existing training generally does not isolate the most crucial repertoires for training, nor does it seek to bring relevant repertoires to fluent levels or program for generalization. The following sections offer some general solutions that target these deficiencies in training, introduce an empirically supported instructional method, and provide an example of the application of that method to relevant training targets.

Intervention 1: Target Cognitive Biases in Training

Several cognitive biases (e.g., confirmation bias, fundamental attribution error) can negatively impact patient care through their impact on clinician decision making, unhelpful belief development, and openness to adopting or maintaining EBP. These biases are well known and fully detailed in several publications (e.g., Gilovich, 2008; Kahneman, 2011), including chapters in this volume (e.g., Lilienfeld et al., Chapter 3). Because cognitive biases impede the initial pursuit as well as the maintenance of

EBP, they should be directly targeted in training. Empirical studies have not yet identified the most efficacious mechanism for targeting such biases in training clinicians; however, we provide some recommendations by generalizing from empirical findings in related areas, with the caveat that these recommendations should be evaluated empirically.

Introducing trainees to the existence and nature of cognitive biases is unlikely to be sufficient to produce therapists who incorporate ways to guard against their interference. In fact, when cognitive biases are incorporated into training, such training is likely to be in the form of a lecture introducing trainees to one or more biases, with a focus on their definition and perhaps some examples of how they relate to clinical practice. Biases may also be highlighted because of their impact on clinical and diagnostic judgment (certainly a worthy goal) rather than their relation to EBP more broadly. This educational effort, however, is likely to be insufficient. First, it is unlikely that fluent acquisition and change are achieved by lectures. Second, even if a fluent repertoire is developed, this does not imply sufficient environmental support to reinforce its continued use. Third, trainees are unlikely to generalize from examples provided during training to individual practice behaviors and practice environments. Knowing about the existence of cognitive biases is not the same as recognizing and evaluating their effect on clinical work. Largely absent from the literature is an emphasis on inculcating protective factors with respect to these biases into clinician training.

Clinical strategies for patients who have deficits with receptivity to feedback have been developed and are effective in producing a "healthy sense of self-doubt" (see Lynch, 2018), which is an important prerequisite to recognizing biases and seeking disconfirmation of one's beliefs. These skills might also be useful to transport to training. For example, developing a healthy sense of self-doubt about the effectiveness of therapy efforts and the ability to assess patient improvement without measurement could significantly improve care. Trainees should be measuring outcomes regularly and encouraged to predict how well the patient is doing prior to obtaining ratings. There should be a requirement to bring patient ratings to supervision, and the rating should be discussed at every supervision session. Wampold, Lichtenberg, Goodyear, and Tracey (Chapter 10, this volume) describe in detail the value of professional self-doubt.

Also, some trainees may have difficulty with fully examining cognitive biases in themselves and their clinical effectiveness because doing so produces discomfort that is difficult to tolerate. In this instance, the barrier is an emotional one (i.e., poor distress tolerance with respect to personal fallibility) rather than a knowledge deficit. Instruction alone cannot remedy this problem. One key skills set should involve values identification and values expression in the context of these emotional barriers. *Values identification* entails guiding trainees in pinpointing and verbally describing "life directions" of central importance to them. These descriptions operationalize what a life lived well means to them in terms of large patterns of behavior. For example, a trainee might specify "taking care of others" or "learning new things" as important life directions. There exists a sizable literature indicating that expansion of attention to valued directions in the context of aversives (e.g., emotional discomfort) reduces attempts at escape and avoidance of those aversives (e.g., Cresswell et al., 2005; Crocker, Niiya, & Mischkowski, 2008; Dahl, Lundgren, Plumb, & Stewart, 2009; McQueen & Klein, 2006; Sherman & Cohen, 2006; Tesser, Martin, & Cornell, 1996; Wilson & Sandoz, 2008). For example, attention to values has been shown to increase smokers' willingness to acknowledge health risks associated with smoking (Crocker et al., 2008) and similarly to increase acceptance of risks of sexual behavior among those who are sexually active (Sherman, Nelson, & Steele, 2000). It seems reasonable, therefore, that impacting trainee attention to values may also be useful in this context—the context only differs in content, not in the central feature of aversive private experiences. For example, a therapist

who values being effective at providing durable relief from suffering may be impacted by information about the relief provided by exposure when implementing it with a patient.

Therapists who are anxious about using particular interventions are less likely to execute them in treatment and may avoid behavioral interventions that are key to positive outcomes (Scherr, Herbert, & Forman, 2015). This suggests that identifying and intervening upon clinician anxiety is likely an important part of training and dissemination efforts. Beliefs about the therapy may interfere with effective interventions by the therapist. Validated instruments have been developed that can identify therapists who have negative beliefs about exposure; this is often cited as a potential reason for its underutilization (Deacon et al., 2013). Therapists with such beliefs may avoid the use of exposure and/or interfere with its effectiveness by providing patients reassurance or otherwise attenuate a patient's experience of anxiety (Deacon et al., 2013). Farrell, Deacon, Kemp, Dixon, and Sy (2013) demonstrated that uncorrected negative beliefs about exposure influence clinicians to recommend suboptimal delivery of the treatment. This could lead to poor outcomes that confirm the therapist's belief about the ineffectiveness of the treatment, or its association with dropout and poor outcome. Several empirically supported methods of managing such clinician beliefs about exposure serve as an example of what might be done to influence interfering belief systems in training and supervision. Didactic training has been shown to improve attitudes and impact clinical decision making when it directly addresses common misconceptions about exposure (Deacon et al., 2013). Managing therapist anxiety by role-playing "worst-case" scenarios may be useful—for example, role-playing how to manage the patient having a panic attack in the session. Negative beliefs may also be reinforced by a therapist's practice environment. For example, many clinical settings forbid therapists from conducting exposure outside the clinic because of malpractice insurance constraints, which then may be misconstrued as evidence that such practices are truly risky.

Finally, a common pernicious bias in therapists involves the perception of their own therapeutic efficacy. Studies have shown that the less experience therapists have, the higher they rate their skills level (Kavanaugh, 1994). Most therapists in practice believe that their skill level is well above average and that what they are doing is effective (Walfish, McAlister, O'Donnell, & Lambert, 2012). In fact, "25% of mental health professionals viewed their skill to be at the 90th percentile when compared to their peers, and none viewed themselves as below average." In this study, a group of 129 therapists responded to an online survey asking about their abilities, and their patients' improvement. The self-assessment bias extended to the progress the therapists perceived in their patients, with nearly two-thirds of respondents indicating that 80% or more of their clients improved in therapy (Walfish et al., 2012). Similar to many other professions, therapists become gradually less effective with time following initial training (Goldberg et al., 2016; Waller & Turner, 2016) in the absence of continual work to maintain their skills level. Training must include at least two core processes to manage this self-assessment bias and erosion of skills level: monitoring patient progress with validated rating scales and regularly assessing one's own skill at employing therapy faithfully.

A novel solution to this dilemma is via computer software that can provide "just in time" training to be responsive to clinicians' needs. For example, Willow (K. Koerner & L. Dimeff, personal communication, January 25, 2016) is a platform that helps providers learn and deliver empirically supported treatments (ESTs) by giving clinicians progress monitoring tools, training on the spot in key competencies with computerized videos and scripts, and access to immediate indicators of suicide risk and lack of progress. Such innovations may make it easier for systems of care to facilitate the implementation of EBP by making available training that supports ongoing commitment to EBP among clinicians.

Therapists frequently make errors in estimating the degree of patient improvement without validated scales (Hannan et al., 2005; Lambert, Harmon, Slade, Whipple, & Hawkins, 2005). Toward this end, we recommend measurement-guided care as a part of continuing education events. Most professional boards require that a minimum number of continuing education (CE) hours for continual licensure include ethics-specific content. Our view is that a minimum number of hours each renewal period should similarly be specific to undermining cognitive biases and to providing therapists with concrete tools to evaluate their work and the progress of their patients more accurately. Regular rating of therapy performance might be a more benefi-cial licensure renewal requirement relative to attending a CE or continuing medical education seminar and taking a multiple-choice quiz.

Also, when a patient is not improving, there is a natural tendency to make a fundamental attribution error and attribute lack of progress to the patient (or consumer) (Gambrill, 2006). An example of such an error is when students are learning less well, teachers often attribute this to a lack of motivation (e.g., "Residents don't read") rather than to the instructional method and environment. Similarly, when patients do not improve, therapists often erroneously attribute lack of success to patient character-istics, such as diagnosis, lack of motivation, comorbidity, or external circumstances, rather than to the adequacy of the treatment delivery or the limited efficacy of the treatment itself (Kendall, Kipnis, & Otto-Salaj, 1992). A well-known mantra in the behavioral litera-ture, first attributed to Skinner, is "The rat is always right." This mantra was applied to the educational environment by Ogden Lindsley, who said, "The child is always right" (Linds-ley, 1971). Skinner and Lindsley both taught us that the organism always behaves as it should given the environmental conditions and the his-tory of prior learning. This mantra has served many behavior analysts in protecting against fundamental *attribution errors* (e.g., interpreta-tion of client problem behavior with objectify-ing and demeaning statements such as "That's what Borderlines do!"). It is important because it not only protects against the natural tendency for pejorative responding, but it also focuses the instructor/clinician on areas where he or she can be more effective at assisting the individual to change (i.e., alter the environment rather than blame the individual).

Intervention 2: Train Clinicians in Critical Thinking

Training clinicians in critical thinking for the purposes of countering misinformation, which frequently comes close to propaganda regard-ing non-scientifically supported approaches, is another way to support therapists in implement-ing EBP. There are several approaches to train-ing critical thinking. One such approach in-volves the acronym FiLCHeRS (Ruscio, 2006). The acronym stands for (the *i* and *e* are "silent" and only used to assist recall of the acronym): F̲alsifiable, L̲ogic, C̲omprehensive, H̲onesty,

Replicable, and Sufficient. Trainees can be taught to think of each element of the acronym as a test to assess the validity of claims about a treatment approach, as the following summary indicates.

1. *Falsifiable* refers to the importance of claims being framed in such a manner that they can, in principle, be demonstrated false; that is, falsifiable claims are framed in a way that affords empirical testing, whereas nonfalsifiable claims are sheltered from disconfirming evidence.

2. *Logic* prompts us to consider whether arguments are logically sound. We can evaluate this by examining whether the premises used to arrive at a conclusion are accurate, and whether deriving the conclusion from the premises offered is valid.

3. When we consider the *comprehensive* component, we ask whether the claim can account for all available information instead of a subset of information.

4. *Honesty* is included in the acronym to remind us to check for the influence of our own, or other researchers', cognitive biases, conflicts of interest, and preexisting beliefs. We discussed examples of such biases and beliefs earlier (e.g., fundamental attribution error).

5. *Replicability* represents an important test of claims. It concerns the repeatability of effects with subsequent experiments, and by differing researchers, in differing locations, and with different stimuli. The more repeatable an effect, especially with the noted variations, the more replicable the claim.

6. *Sufficiency* primarily refers to the amount of available evidence; that is, is the amount of available evidence sufficient to be confident in the claim? Ruscio (2006) also suggests that the burden of proof belongs to the person making the claim, that argument from authority does not satisfy sufficiency, and that extraordinary claims require extraordinary evidence.

Trainees must learn that the satisfaction of all six tests does not guarantee the accuracy of a claim, but it does provide the conditions by which one can be most confident and less susceptible to incorrect conclusions. Training should involve practice in the application of these criteria to clinically relevant matters, and

should do so with many practice trials. Practice trials should involve a hierarchical progression, an example of which appears in Table 27.2.

This exercise may be inculcated into training in several ways. For example, in a graduate course, this may form the basis of a written assignment in which students evaluate one or more interventions or claims (e.g., astrological counseling, the suggestion that vaccines cause autism) in terms of each element of the acronym. Another strategy involves taking advantage of the natural emergence of claims in a course or supervision, as this provides an opportunity to assist the trainee in evaluating the claim(s) via FiLCHeRS.

Another important strategy is to train practitioners to routinely ask themselves the following questions: Is the treatment I'm delivering the same I'd want for myself? Are the methods in support of this method the same kind of support I'd feel comfortable with my care providers using? Is this treatment in line with my profession's code of ethics? Is my choice of interventions based on my personal preference, comfort, or ability level or is it based on what's in the best interest of my patient(s)? Guided self-reflection transforms "routine" management of patients and helps clinicians more frequently consider alternative approaches.

Intervention 3: Train for "Flexibility" with Precision

Practitioners are routinely confronted with novel clinical presentations and idiosyncratic expressions of clinical phenomena. This text vividly illustrates how frequently in complex, real-world situations, standard treatment protocols do not adequately produce relief. Adapting and modifying treatments with creativity and careful attention to the patient's symptoms and case conceptualization is often required to provide care and relief. Unfortunately, the education provided to therapists in training often is unable to produce such skills (Sudak & Goldberg, 2012; Weissman et al., 2006). It generally results in only minimal competence in the skills to treat patients with uncomplicated severity, let alone to adapt to those patients with substantial complexity. Training should provide experiences that enable the clinician to be flexible; that is, clinicians need to be able to adapt to a dynamic clinical environment, while remaining faithful to the overall framework of EBP. Teaching re-

TABLE 27.2. Steps in EBP

1. Convert the need for information into an answerable question.

2. Track down the best clinical evidence to answer that question.

3. Critically appraise that evidence in terms of its validity, clinical significance, and usefulness.

4. Integrate this critical appraisal of research evidence with the available clinical expertise and the patients values and circumstances.

5. Evaluate the effectiveness and efficiency in undertaking the four previous steps, and strive for self-improvement.

Note. From Thyer (2004, p. 168). Copyright © 2004 Oxford University Press. Reprinted by permission.

flective practices is an invaluable part of what allows for flexibility. The conditions of therapy are constantly changing, so that the therapist must be similarly adapting to the present reality. This is akin to the concept of "open skill" training in sports, where varied practice is superior in sports that require a nimble and reflective participant. Incorporating variety and depth in role plays and reflective practice in supervision may increase such capacities in therapists. For example, role plays should be stratified across levels of complexity, so that trainees first master the skill and are then required to make modifications of the skill "on the fly" with a more complicated clinical situation. In supervision, supervisees should have ample time to struggle with a clinical matter on their own, with the supervisor playing a supportive role but not necessarily telling the supervisee how to proceed unless a skill is absent or the clinical situation is urgent.

Flexibility, of course, is a colloquial term that we use here because it affords an economical means of communicating about a phenomenon. However, the method for producing such a complex behavioral repertoire rests on highly specified scientific concepts and empirically derived instructional procedures. We introduce this body of empirical instruction, known as *precision teaching* (PT; Kubina & Yurich, 2012). PT produces complex repertoires by carefully identifying their key components and focusing instructional and extensive practice efforts on such components. A large body of research indicates that complex repertories can emerge without explicit training (e.g., Alessi, 1987; Andronis, Layng, & Goldiamond, 1997; Johnson & Layng, 1992) as individuals successfully recruit necessary components as the context requires. Originally, the phenomenon of emergent complex behavior, based on isolated component training, was known as gen-

erativity and emerged from early experimental work on insight (Epstein, 1991; Epstein, Kirshnit, Lanza, & Rubin, 1984). This experimental work, initially with animal subjects and later with human participants, involved training isolated behaviors and subsequently confronting participants with a novel problem. Subjects had not been specifically trained to solve the new problem but were nevertheless able to effectively recruit the separately trained behaviors into a new behavioral pattern. In the late 1990s, Andronis and colleagues (1997) advanced this work. They demonstrated that the implementation of new contingencies can recruit behavioral patterns previously learned under different performance requirements, a phenomenon they labeled *contingency adduction*; that is, contingencies can adduce novel behavioral patterns, one of several empirically derived outcomes of behavioral fluency.

PT is designed to bring performance to fluent levels. Fluency is used in two ways in PT: (1) metaphorically and (2) to refer to several empirically derived outcomes. Its metaphorical use references several topographical characteristics of expert performance, such as its smooth, flowing, and nonhesitant nature. The empirically derived outcomes of fluent behavior are captured by the acronym *MESAG*: Maintenance, Endurance, Stability, Application, and Generativity (Johnson & Street, 2004). Fluent repertoires are maintained when they persist over long time frames without additional training (i.e., they do not drift), demonstrating endurance when the performance persists without fatigue, when they are stable and continue despite environmental distractions, demonstrating applicability when executed in functional ways, and when they exemplify generativity as differing component repertoires combine in ways to produce novel composite behaviors. Generativity is the primary outcome of interest

TABLE 27.3. Examples of Tool Skills and Component and Composite Repertoires—EBP

Tool skills	Components	Composites
• Identifying databases	• Literature search	• EBP
• Saying EBP steps	• Critical evaluation of research	
• Identifying outcome measures	• Measure treatment outcomes and process	
• Specifying needed information	• Formulate effective questions	
• Defining important terms	• Integrate evidence, expertise, and patient values	

in this section because it is impossible to train clinicians for all possible required behavioral repertoires, and because the focus on training key component repertoires affords a more economical training time frame.

Determining the key component repertoires that must be the targets of intervention, known as *pinpointing* in PT, is a crucial step. Component skills can, in turn, be broken down further into tool skills, the most basic elements of performance. Examples of component and tool skills for the composite repertoire "psychotherapy practice" are "active listening skills" and "reflective statements," respectively. Additional examples of relevant tool skills, as well as component and composite repertoires, can be found in Tables 27.3, 27.4, and 27.5.

Precision teachers describe performance in terms of learning channels. Such descriptions refer to the specification of the stimulus and response characteristics of repertoires. Examples of learning channels include *see–say, hear–say, free–say, hear–write,* and so forth. The channels describe the sensory organ receiving the stimuli and the characteristics of the response. The one exception is the designation *free*, as in *free–write* or *free–say*. In this context, *free* means there is no external stimulus; rather, there is an internal one, such as thinking. For example, we might be in interested in *free–say*

steps in EBP or *hear* treatment claim–*say* logical errors. When pinpointing, one identifies the tool skills, component and composite repertoires of interest, as well as the relevant learning channel. Specifying performance in terms of learning channels is an essential element of pinpointing because it ensures that all aspects of performance are adequately trained and because fluent performance in one channel does not always generalize to other channels.

A key procedure in PT is known as a *timing*. Timings are brief but intense periods of practice in which the performer emits component skills as rapidly and accurately as possible. For example, a timing might involve a 30-second timed period in which the trainee lists cognitive biases, or as many steps in a particular sequence as possible. At the end of the timing period, the trainee counts how many correct and incorrect responses were provided and expresses these data in terms of correct–incorrect responses per minute (count per minute is a standard unit in PT). These practice periods occur frequently within each instructional period (and preferably between them).

Another important step is to set an *aim* for performance, a description of the desired performance level in terms of speed and accuracy. Importantly, aims do not make use of targets involving percent correct measures because per-

TABLE 27.4. Examples of Tool Skills and Component and Composite Repertoires—Claim Appraisal

Tool skills	Components	Composites
• Saying/defining elements of FiLCHeRS	• Discriminate falsifiable from nonfalsifiable claims	• Critically appraise claims
	• Restate nonfalsifiable claims in testable terms	
	• Determine whether conclusions follow from premises	

TABLE 27.5. Examples of Tool Skills and Component and Composite Repertoires—Remediating Cognitive Biases

Tool skills	Components	Composites
• Listing/defining cognitive biases	• Identifying cognitive biases	• Remediating cognitive biases
• Listing remediation steps	• Emitting remediation steps	
• Listing protective measures	• Executing cognitive biases prevention strategies	

cent correct only contains an accuracy dimension, and because such benchmarks provide a ceiling that suppresses performance. Consider, for example, two students enrolled in a graduate psychopathology course, who must master DSM-5 criteria sets. Their instructor seeks to evaluate their knowledge with a written exam that requires them to list criteria for several diagnostic categories. Both students are perfectly accurate in listing the requested criteria, but whereas one can do so in 10 minutes, the other requires a full hour. Their respective performances indicate different levels of competence. If the requirements are fully satisfied when both students reach a 100% accuracy criterion, then the slower student will not be trained to the same level of competence. In addition, a 1-hour latency would not meet real-world diagnostic interview performance requirements. Rather, PT sets

aims in terms of rate of response that involves both an accuracy and a time dimension, such as 30 corrects per minute with zero errors. Aims can be determined in several ways, but a useful guide is to determine what expert performers can achieve. For example, how quickly and accurately do experts say the steps in a clinical procedure sequence? The goal is for each trainee to reach the aim on all trained repertoires.

After each timing exercise, trainees immediately plot their data to contact the frequent reinforcing properties of graphically displayed feedback and to inform subsequent instruction. To understand the latter use, imagine a graphical display showing the number of correct responses increasing, while also showing incorrect responses decreasing (a desirable pattern known as "jaws"). See Figure 27.1 for an example.

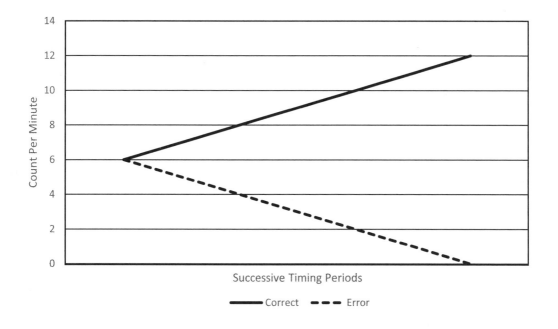

FIGURE 27.1. Example of the "jaws" pattern.

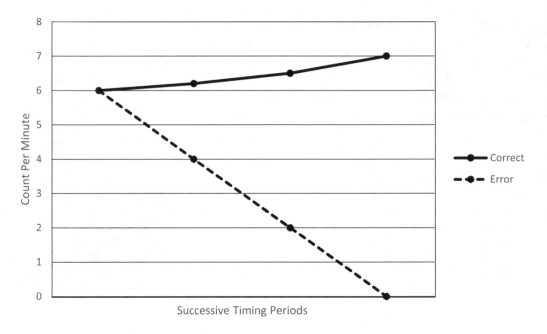

FIGURE 27.2. Example of an undesirable rate of increase in correct responding.

Instructional procedures would remain the same because the performance levels are progressing toward the specified aim. In contrast, imagine that correct responses are not increasing or they are increasing, but not at a favorable rate, as seen in Figure 27.2. In this circumstance, the instructional procedures should be altered in the interest of producing a more desirable performance pattern. Many other performance pictures are possible (e.g., both correct and incorrect responses increasing, no change in correct or error responding), with each suggesting a different course of action. Frequent and sensitive measurement of this kind allows the instructor to make real-time changes in instruction, thus maximizing effectiveness. This approach contrasts substantially with the all-too-common approach of infrequent, insensitive measurement procedures, such as tests at the end of a semester, which disallow real-time alteration in instruction.

In summary, PT involves several components: (1) pinpointing component repertoires and their sequence for training; (2) frequent, brief timed practice periods that emphasize speed and accuracy; (3) setting an aim; (4) frequent, sensitive measurement methods; and (5) altering instructional intervention based on measurement previously obtained. Here, we provide a brief example of the application of PT when targeting the cognitive biases. The first step is to select a specific cognitive bias to target; we'll use the fundamental attribution error (FAE). First, definitional awareness of the FAE is trained, which involves direct instruction and discrimination training using many examples and non-examples of the FAE. For example, we might provide a didactic overview of the FAE. Then the discrimination training would include timing periods in which the trainee will *see* written examples/non-examples and *write* "example" or "non-example." These visual stimuli must be contained in a document with items so numerous that the trainee could not possibly exhaust the list in the time afforded. Sample visual stimuli representing examples of the FAE might include "This patient is . . . 'not motivated,' 'resistant,' or 'an Axis II.'" We would provide the trainee with many brief, sprint-type trials, in which he or she notes "example," and "non-example," as he or she progresses through the sheet, and we would be sure to vary the stimuli considerably, such that there are "close in" and "far out" examples. This is an example of training along a *see–write* learning channel in which the learner is asked to "*see* written example" and then to "*write*" either FAE or not FAE. After each timing, we would calculate the number of responses that were correct and incorrect, then immediately plot these data, produce a graphical display of the data, and determine whether to continue with the current instructional procedures or change direction based on the observed trend.[2] Between timings, instruction would occur specifically about noted incorrect responding. Then instruction would alternate between timing trials, and instructional intervention, until the trainee(s) reached the *specified aim*, which, by definition, means they achieved fluency with that component repertoire. Next, the FAE training would continue with different stimuli, such as video examples of clinicians demonstrating and not demonstrating the FAE in clinically relevant contexts, a *see* video example—WRITE FAE or Not FAE learning channel. The same previously described methodology would continue until the group met the specified aim. Our use of cognitive biases when introducing PT is only by way of example. PT is applicable to any content area, limited only by the creativity of the trainer.

Intervention 4: Leverage Supervision to Improve the Dissemination of EBP and ESTs

There is evidence that supervision increases skills and confidence in therapists (Bambling, King, Raue, Schweitzer, & Lambert, 2006; Sholomskas et al., 2005; Simons, Rozek, & Serrano, 2013). Supervisors must adhere to a model to maintain fidelity in their supervisees and must also be aware of their own cognitive biases and faulty beliefs. For example, it is easy to assume that a "good" trainee will behave in ways that are always in the patient's best interests and have good patient outcomes. Supervisors may develop a confirmatory bias about a trainee who has excellent interpersonal skills

and a good work ethic regarding that trainee's patient care. Beliefs may influence a supervisor's adherence to treatment protocols, assessment of the supervisee ("the halo effect"), and estimations of the benefits of supervision. An example of such influential beliefs is a study that indicated that high supervisee anxiety in female supervisees resulted in supervisors of both genders being less likely to focus the female supervisee's work on therapeutic technique, compared to when a male supervisee was anxious (Simpson-Southward, Waller, & Hardy, 2016). Supervisors must directly assess patient care with a fidelity instrument for the trainee's behavior, and monitor patient outcomes and their own supervisory practices routinely.

Another intervention target during supervision that may enhance trainees' future pursuit of EBP relates to their values, as we indicated in a prior section. Values are what a person holds most dear and have been described in terms of directions rather than concrete ends. For example, being a compassionate therapist is a value because one can always be more compassionate, whereas taking on one pro bono therapy case per year is a goal because it has a concrete outcome. The two are related because setting goals, which contain concrete outcomes, indicates to an individual that he or she is moving in a valued direction. Most commonly, trainers attempt to persuade trainees to pursue EBP through the provision of data and rational argument. This may not be persuasive to many trainees and is unlikely to be salient for trainees after training. Assisting trainees in values identification, then connecting their identified values to the provision of care with EBP may function to enhance motivation, especially in the context of the supervisory relationship. For example, enhanced training in exposure-based treatments that included influencing clinicians by appealing to their emotions regarding exposure's safety and tolerability, as well as providing data about its effectiveness, was more effective at changing attitudes (Farrell, Kemp, Blakey, Meyer, & Deacon, 2016). Socratic questions that facilitate reflection regarding the trainee's prior experiences with an intervention and how he or she might want to improve may facilitate goal setting. Asking trainees to assess their confidence in executing certain therapeutic procedures amplifies goals about therapeutic confidence and enhances motivation. A trainee who believes EBP is the compassionate

---

[2]Precision Teachers make use of a sophisticated semilogarithmic chart known as a *standard celeration chart* (SCC) for measurement purposes. The SCC requires substantial training to use and is beyond the scope of this chapter. However, a highly useful service for this purpose is an Internet-based platform known as Chartlytics (*www.chartlytics.com*), which is particularly useful because it is specifically designed for the PT approach and is constructed in such a way that the user does not need to be intensively trained in PT or the SCC; it is also inexpensive and easy to use.

or most effective thing to do, and values being a compassionate or highly effective, confident therapist, is more likely to pursue EBP than one who simply received a logical argument for doing so.

Developing a cooperative climate with defined objectives is a central feature of effective supervisory relationships (Milne & Reiser, 2017). Like therapy, learning in supervision occurs in the context of a relationship. The supervisory working alliance, first described by Bordin (1983), mirrors that of therapy, with bonds, tasks, and goals at its core. Genuine interest in the supervisee as a growing professional is essential. As with therapy, a clearly defined framework reduces anxiety and sets out the tasks at hand. A written supervision contract, describing time frame, tasks to be performed, and methods of evaluation provides clarity and solidifies commitment. Supervisors must be mindful of the tremendous anxiety inherent in the process of therapist development and normalize struggles, praise courage, and highlight effective interventions. Decreasing anxiety is essential for honest disclosure, known to be a problem in supervision (Ladany, Hill, Corbett, & Nutt, 1996). A challenge for the supervisor is to balance support, while not interfering with supervisee self-reflection, to encourage the capabilities necessary for independent practice. Because supervision frequently has an evaluative function, which increases anxiety, the supervisor must very carefully review with the supervisee the required methods of evaluation.

Setting learning goals is a critical initial step in CBT supervision. Goal setting is facilitated by assessing the supervisee's baseline skills. This may be accomplished by listening to a therapy recording and rating it with fidelity instruments. Supervisors must assess supervisees' prior training in basic psychotherapy and CBT-specific skills, with special attention to actual skills practiced and evaluated during training. The supervisee's working and learning environment also influences the goals for supervision. Clear, collaborative, and explicit learning objectives distinguish supervision from case management.

Early literature regarding CBT supervision recommended a structure similar to that of therapy (Liese & Beck, 1997; Padesky, 1996) to enhance learning and efficiency. Agenda setting targets the most important concerns of the supervisee and most central issues regarding

patient safety. Deliberate selection of varyious teaching strategies is often neglected by supervisors. "Gold standard" but underused methods for CBT supervision, as defined by Dorsey and colleagues (2018), include experiential and interactive methods such as direct observation, modeling, and behavioral rehearsal. Skills must be trained as needed, and sufficient time must be provided for the supervisee to struggle to determine the best course of action independently.

Summaries and feedback are some of the most essential supervisory behaviors. Clear and specific observation of supervisees is necessary to provide formative feedback. Supervisors must give details about effective supervisee behaviors prior to addressing what must be modified or changed. Measures of treatment fidelity and patient outcome assist the supervisor in providing feedback. Recordings of sessions or direct observation of patient care should be evaluated with fidelity instruments. Patient outcome rating scales are essential to monitor patient progress and improve outcomes (Lambert et al., 2005). Regular feedback from the supervisee regarding the supervisory relationship and progress toward supervision goals ensures continual progress.

Intervention 5: Develop Systems That Reinforce Training

A final barrier to EBP is the absence of reinforcing consequences that sustain behavior over time. Simply put, systems of care often are not designed to reinforce EBP. For example, compensation for reflection and research about a patient's lack of progress is not generally provided. Such a lack of reinforcement is important because clinicians will not continue to engage in EBP unless such behavior contacts reinforcing consequences. Training is merely an antecedent condition; thus, it cannot impact the subsequent probability of this behavior. The purpose of an antecedent is to provide an occasion for behavior; it is designed to get a behavior to occur once. Consequent events determine the subsequent probability of behavior. By way of illustration, consider the parents of an oppositional child. One is likely to observe endless prompts (antecedents) for desired behavior, such as "Johnny, quit standing on the couch," "Johnny, I said sit down," "Johnny, you better sit down right now!" The behavioral clinician would teach these parents (among other things) to provide only one prompt, if necessary, and to instead look for ways to rearrange the environment so that opportunities for reinforcing (consequent event) sitting behavior are more likely. Similarly, little attention is paid to the need for reinforcement for EBP in systems of care or in the training of private practitioners who would need to set up facilitating conditions for themselves.

One solution is to train clinicians and administrators to rearrange their practice environments so that they maintain consequences for EBP behavior. A recent training effort by the Academy of Cognitive Therapy, in conjunction with the Texas Department of Health and Human Services (DHHS), implemented a successful alternative strategy. In brief, DHHS established CBT competence requirements, tied to reimbursement, for all clinicians employed in community mental health agencies that maintain contracts with the state of Texas to provide mental health services. Agencies, in turn, satisfied this requirement by stipulating demonstrated competence as a condition of employment. Competence was assessed through the independent evaluation of work samples (by calibrated raters available through the Academy of Cognitive Therapy) and was defined as a score of 40 or higher on the Cognitive Therapy Rating Scale (CTRS; Young & Beck, 1980). Agencies were motivated to apply this measure because they were unable to bill for CBT unless their employees met this criterion. The number of training and/or supervision hours in CBT were intentionally not specified as requirements by the state. Clinicians could pursue whatever level or duration of training was required to demonstrate a competent repertoire. This strategy solved several problems. First, it removed uncertainty regarding competence because it was measured directly rather than presumed to result from a prescribed amount of training. Second, mental health agencies were no longer burdened with pursuing arbitrary training hour requirements. Third, it motivated agency administrators to value and thus seek competent CBT instruction. This protects against the pursuit of inexpensive, but incompetent instruction. This effort, initiated in 2013, has been successful, as evidenced by the submission and subsequent evaluation of 715 work samples. The training model of the Academy of Cognitive Therapy and the Texas DHHS may serve as a useful paradigm for similar programs. We would suggest one modification, namely, we recommend that demonstration of competence occur more than once. Currently, satisfying the Texas requirements only requires a single demonstration, which does not attenuate competence drift. Nevertheless, we believe this program is a substantial step forward in disseminating and measuring clinician competence and sustaining EBP over time.

Training administrative staff—those with the power to arrange organizational environments—in how to support fidelity monitoring is critical. However, it is also possible to teach frontline clinicians about the importance of fidelity monitoring and how to achieve it in individual practice. Therapists should be taught the literature regarding deterioration of skills levels and fidelity over time, and instructed in the application of rating scales such as the CTRS. Individuals can be trained to identify others within their organizations who share a similar commitment to EBP and self-examination, to approach those persons effectively, and to establish a means to continually monitor treatment fidelity. Such a practice can take a variety of forms, but may include reviewing, rating, and discussing recordings of therapy sessions for fidelity, reinforcing each other's EBP behavior, and regular peer meetings. Other options involve rating and engaging in role plays with direct observation. Such role plays can be constructed to highlight key clinical skills and can vary by difficulty (e.g., cooperative and noncooperative patients). This practice allows for immediate feedback and shaping if recording and scoring of therapy sessions are not easily available. Individual therapists can also be trained to advocate for the arrangement of EBP-supporting contingencies within their organization. Examples of such contingencies include the provision of reinforcement for key EBP behaviors. For example, administrators can deliver reinforcement such as time off, or other desirable consequences. Training therapists to advocate for these changes may involve instruction in specific persuasion and negotiation skills and may also include distress tolerance training to increase clinicians' endurance in the face of likely slow change. Marsha Linehan very effectively incorporates such skills training in teaching therapists to advocate for instituting DBT programs (*http://behavioraltech.org/training/implementation.cfm*).

Conclusion

Several barriers to EBP exist. We have a paucity of evidence regarding effective means to address these barriers. In this chapter, we have discussed a specific subset of barriers that, we believe, have not been adequately leveraged, including cognitive biases, beliefs, emotional barriers, and critical thinking deficits. We also addressed what we perceive as inadequacies in instructional design and delivery, training efforts that fail to target these content areas, and those that do not focus on bringing performance to fluent levels. We hope our recommendations will inspire research in training to determine whether these suggestions improve delivery of care.

References

Alessi, G. (1987). Generative strategies and teaching for generalization. *Analysis of Verbal Behavior, 5,* 15–27.

American Psychological Association. (2005). Policy statement on evidence-based practice in psychology. Retrieved from *www.apa.org/practice/resources/evidence/evidence-basedstatement.pdf.*

Andronis, P. T., Layng, T. J., & Goldiamond, I. (1997). Contingency adduction of "symbolic aggression" by pigeons. *Analysis of Verbal Behavior, 14,* 5–17.

Bambling, M., King, R., Raue, P., Schweitzer, R., & Lambert, W. (2006). Clinical supervision: Its influence on client-rated working alliance and client symptom reduction in the brief treatment of major depression. *Psychotherapy Research, 16*(3), 317–331.

Bordin, E. S. (1983). A working alliance based model of supervision. *Counseling Psychologist, 11*(1), 35–42.

Codd, R. T., III. (2017). Protecting the scientific lexical cannon. *Behavior Therapist, 40*(5), 185–191.

Cooper, Z., Doll, H., Bailey-Straebler, S., Bohn, K., DeVries, D., Murphy, R., et al. (2017). Assessing therapist competence: Development of a performance-based measure and its comparison with a Web-based measure. *JMIR Mental Health, 4*(4), e51.

Creswell, J. D., Welch, W. T., Taylor, S. E., Sherman, D. K., Gruenewald, T. L., & Mann, T. (2005). Affirmation of personal values buffers neuroendocrine and psychological stress responses. *Psychological Science, 16*(11), 846–851.

Crocker, J., Niiya, Y., & Mischkowski, D. (2008). Why does writing about important values reduce defensiveness?: Self-affirmation and the role of positive other-directed feelings. *Psychological Science, 19*(7), 740–747.

Dahl, J., Lundgren, T., Plumb, J., & Stewart, I. (2009). *The art and science of valuing in psychotherapy: Helping clients discover, explore, and commit to valued action using acceptance and commitment therapy.* Oakland, CA: New Harbinger.

Deacon, B. J., Farrell, N. R., Kemp, J. J., Dixon, L. J., Sy, J. T., Zhang, A. R., et al. (2013). Assessing therapist reservations about exposure therapy for anxiety disorders: The Therapist Beliefs about Exposure Scale. *Journal of Anxiety Disorders, 27*(8), 772–780.

Dorsey, S., Kerns, S. E., Lucid, L., Pullmann, M. D., Harrison, J. P., Berliner, L., et al. (2018). Objective coding of content and techniques in workplace-based supervision of an EBT in public mental health. *Implementation Science, 13*(1), 19.

Epstein, R. (1991). Skinner, creativity, and the problem of spontaneous behavior. *Psychological Science, 2*(6), 362–370.

Epstein, R., Kirshnit, C. E., Lanza, R. P., & Rubin, L. C. (1984). "Insight" in the pigeon: Antecedents and determinants of an intelligent performance. *Nature, 308,* 61–62.

Farrell, N. R., Deacon, B. J., Dixon, L. J., & Lickel, J. J. (2013). Theory-based training strategies for modifying practitioner concerns about exposure therapy. *Journal of Anxiety Disorders, 27*(8), 781–787.

Farrell, N. R., Deacon, B. J., Kemp, J. J., Dixon, L. J., & Sy, J. T. (2013). Do negative beliefs about exposure therapy cause its suboptimal delivery?: An experimental investigation. *Journal of Anxiety Disorders, 27*(8), 763–771.

Farrell, N. R., Kemp, J. J., Blakey, S. M., Meyer, J. M., & Deacon, B. J. (2016). Targeting clinician concerns about exposure therapy: A pilot study comparing standard vs. enhanced training. *Behaviour Research and Therapy, 85,* 53–59.

Gambrill, E. (2005). *Critical thinking in clinical practice: Improving the quality of judgments and decisions* (2nd ed.). Hoboken, NJ: Wiley.

Gilovich, T. (2008). *How we know what isn't so.* New York: Simon & Schuster.

Goldberg, S. B., Rousmaniere, T., Miller, S. D., Whipple, J., Nielsen, S. L., Hoyt, W. T., et al. (2016). Do psychotherapists improve with time and experience?: A longitudinal analysis of outcomes in a clinical setting. *Journal of Counseling Psychology, 63*(1), 1–11.

Hannan, C., Lambert, M. J., Harmon, C., Nielsen, S. L., Smart, D. W., Shimokawa, K., et al. (2005). A lab test and algorithms for identifying clients at risk for treatment failure. *Journal of Clinical Psychology, 61*(2), 155–163.

Improving Access to Psychological Therapies. (2008). Adult Improving Access to Psychological Therapies Programme. Retrieved from *www.england.nhs.uk/mental-health/adults/iapt.*

Johnson, K., & Street, E. M. (2004). *The Morningside model of generative instruction: What it means to leave no child behind.* Concord, MA: Cambridge Center for Behavioral Studies.

Johnson, K. R., & Layng, T. J. (1992). Breaking the structuralist barrier. *American Psychologist, 47*(11), 1475–1490.

Kahneman, D. (2011). *Thinking, fast and slow*. New York: Macmillan.

Karlin, B. E., Brown, G. K., Trockel, M., Cunning, D., Zeiss, A. M., & Taylor, C. B. (2012). National dissemination of cognitive behavioral therapy for depression in the Department of Veterans Affairs health care system: Therapist and patient-level outcomes. *Journal of Consulting and Clinical Psychology, 80*(5), 707–718.

Kavanaugh, D. J. (1994). Issues in multidisciplinary training of cognitive-behavioural interventions. *Behaviour Change: Journal of the Australian Behaviour Modification Association, 11,* 38–44.

Kendall, P. C., Kipnis, D., & Otto-Salaj, L. (1992). When clients don't progress: Influences on and explanations for lack of therapeutic progress. *Cognitive Therapy and Research, 16*(3), 269–281.

Kohn, R., Saxena, S., Levav, I., & Saraceno, B. (2004). The treatment gap in mental health care. *Bulletin of the World Health Organization, 82*(11), 858–866.

Kubina, R. M., & Yurich, K. K. (2012). *Precision teaching book*. Lemont, PA: Greatness Achieved.

Ladany, N., Hill, C. E., Corbett, M. M., & Nutt, E. A. (1996). Nature, extent, and importance of what psychotherapy trainees do not disclose to their supervisors. *Journal of Counseling Psychology, 43*(1), 10–24.

Lambert, M. J., Harmon, D., Slade, K., Whipple, J. L., & Hawkins, E. J. (2005). Providing feedback to psychotherapists on their patients' progress: Clinical results and practice suggestions. *Journal of Clinical Psychology, 61,* 165–174.

Liese, B. S., & Beck, J. S. (1997). Cognitive therapy supervision. In C. E. Watkins (Ed.), *Handbook of psychotherapy supervision* (pp. 114–133). Chichester, UK: Wiley.

Lindsley, O. R. (1971). From Skinner to precision teaching: The child knows best. In J. B. Jordan & C. S. Robbins (Eds.), *Let's try doing something else kind of thing* (pp. 1–11). Arlington, VA: Council for Exceptional Children.

Lynch, T. R. (2018). *The skills training manual for radically open dialectical behavior therapy: A clinician's guide for treating disorders of overcontrol*. Oakland, CA: New Harbinger.

McQueen, A., & Klein, W. M. (2006). Experimental manipulations of self-affirmation: A systematic review. *Self and Identity, 5*(4), 289–354.

Milne, D. L., & Reiser, R. P. (2017). *A manual for evidence-based CBT supervision*. Chichester, UK: Wiley-Blackwell.

Mojtabai, R., Olfson, M., Sampson, N. A., Jin, R., Druss, B., Wang, P. S., et al. (2011). Barriers to mental health treatment: Results from the National Comorbidity Survey Replication. *Psychological Medicine, 41*(8), 1751–1761.

Olfson, M., Blanco, C., & Marcus, S. C. (2016). Treatment of adult depression in the United States. *JAMA Internal Medicine, 176*(10), 1482–1491.

Olfson, M., & Marcus, S. C. (2010). National trends in outpatient psychotherapy. *American Journal of Psychiatry, 167*(12), 1456–1463.

Padesky, C. A. (1996). Developing cognitive therapist competency: Teaching and supervision models. In P. M. Salkovskis (Ed.), *Frontiers of cognitive therapy* (pp. 266–292). New York: Guilford Press.

Ruscio, J. (2006). *Critical thinking in psychology: Separating sense from nonsense* (2nd ed.). Belmont, CA: Wadsworth.

Scherr, S. R., Herbert, J. D., & Forman, E. M. (2015). The role of therapist experiential avoidance in predicting therapist preference for exposure treatment for OCD. *Journal of Contextual Behavioral Science, 4*(1), 21–29.

Sherman, D. A. K., & Cohen, G. L. (2006). The psychology of self-defense: Self-affirmation theory. In M. P. Zanna (Ed.), *Advances in experimental social psychology* (Vol. 38, pp. 183–242). New York: Guilford Press.

Sherman, D. A. K., Nelson, L. D., & Steele, C. M. (2000). Do messages about health risks threaten the self?: Increasing the acceptance of threatening health messages via self-affirmation. *Personality and Social Psychology Bulletin, 26*(9), 1046–1058.

Sholomskas, D. E., Syracuse-Siewart, G., Rusaville, B. J., Ball, S. A., Nuro, K. F., & Carroll, K. M. (2005). We do not train in vain: A dissemination trail of three strategies of training clinicians in cognitive-behavioral therapy. *Journal of Consulting and Clinical Psychology, 73,* 106–115.

Simons, A. D., Rozek, D. C., & Serrano, J. L. (2013). Wanted: Reliable and valid measures for the science of cognitive behavioral therapy dissemination and implementation. *Clinical Psychology: Science and Practice, 20*(2), 181–194.

Simpson-Southward, C., Waller, G., & Hardy, G. E. (2016). Supervision for treatment of depression: An experimental study of the role of therapist gender and anxiety. *Behaviour Research and Therapy, 77,* 17–22.

Sudak, D. M., & Goldberg, D. A. (2012). Trends in psychotherapy training: A national survey of psychiatry residency training. *Academic Psychiatry, 36*(5), 369–373.

Tesser, A., Martin, L. L., & Cornell, D. P. (1996). On the substitutability of self-protective mechanisms. In P. M. Golwitzer & J. A. Bargh (Eds.), *The psychology of action: Linking cognition and motivation to behavior* (pp. 48–68). New York: Guilford Press.

Thyer, B. A. (2004). What is evidence-based practice? *Brief Treatment and Crisis Intervention, 4*(2), 167–176.

Walfish, S., McAlister, B., O'Donnell, P., & Lambert, M. J. (2012). An investigation of self-assessment bias in mental health providers. *Psychological Reports, 110*(2), 639–644.

Waller, G., & Turner, H. (2016). Therapist drift redux: Why well-meaning clinicians fail to deliver evidence-based therapy, and how to get back on track. *Behaviour Research and Therapy, 77,* 129–137.

Weissman, M. M., Verdeli, H., Gameroff, M. J., Bledsoe, S. E., Betts, K., Mufson, L., et al. (2006). National survey of psychotherapy training in psychiatry, psychology, and social work. *Archives of General Psychiatry, 63*(8), 925–934.

Wilson, K. G., & Sandoz, E. K. (2008). Mindfulness, values, and the therapeutic relationship in acceptance and commitment therapy. In S. F. Hick & T. Bein (Eds.), *Mindfulness and the therapeutic relationship* (pp. 89–106). New York: Guilford Press.

Young, J. E., & Beck, A. T. (1980). *Cognitive Therapy Scale rating manual.* Unpublished manuscript, University of Pennsylvania Center for Psychotherapy Research, Philadelphia, PA.

Author Index

Subject Index

Note. *f* or *t* following a page number indicate a figure or a table.